MEDICINAL CHEMISTRY
OF ANTICANCER DRUGS

MEDICINAL CHEMISTRY OF ANTICANCER DRUGS

CARMEN AVENDAÑO AND J. CARLOS MENÉNDEZ

Departamento de Química Orgánica y Farmacéutica
Facultad de Farmacia, Universidad Complutense Madrid, Spain

ELSEVIER

Amsterdam • Boston • Heidelberg • London • New York • Oxford
Paris • San Diego • San Francisco • Singapore • Sydney • Tokyo

Elsevier
Radarweg 29, PO Box 211, 1000 AE Amsterdam, The Netherlands
Linacre House, Jordan Hill, Oxford OX2 8DP, UK

First edition 2008

Library of Congress Cataloging-in-Publication Data
A catalog record for this book is available from the Library of Congress

British Library Cataloguing in Publication Data
A catalogue record for this book is available from the British Library

ISBN: 978-0-444-52824-7

For information on all Elsevier publications
visit our website at books.elsevier.com

Printed and bound in Hungary
08   09   10   11   12   10   9   8   7   6   5   4   3   2   1

D
616.99406'1
AVE

CONTENTS

Preface   ix

Abbreviations   xi

1. Introduction   1

    1. Some General Remarks About Cancer and Cancer Chemotherapy   1

    2. A Brief Account of the Role of Chemistry in Cancer Chemotherapy   3

    3. Natural Products in Cancer Chemotherapy   5

    4. A Brief Comment About Cancer Nanotechnology   6

    5. Conclusion   7

    References   7

2. Antimetabolites   9

    1. Introduction   10

    2. Inhibitors of the Biosynthesis of Uridylic Acid   10

    3. Inhibitors of the Biosynthesis of 2′-Deoxyribonucleotides by

       Ribonucleotide Reductase (RNR)   11

    4. Inhibitors of the Biosynthesis of Thymidilic Acid   18

    5. Inhibitors of Dihydrofolate Reductase (DHFR)   32

    6. Inhibitors of the De Novo Purine Biosynthesis Pathway   36

    7. Inhibitors of Adenosine Deaminase   42

    8. Inhibitors of Late Stages in DNA Synthesis   45

    9. Antimetabolite Enzymes   50

    References   51

3. Anticancer Drugs That Inhibit Hormone Action   53

    1. Introduction   54

    2. Estrogens and Their Involvement in Carcinogenesis   54

    3. Antiestrogens as Antitumor Drugs   58

    4. Aromatase Inhibitors   65

    5. Steroid Sulfatase Inhibitors   73

    6. Androgen-Related Antitumor Agents   75

    7. Regulation of Steroidal Hormone Synthesis as a Target for Antitumor Drugs   79

    8. Miscellaneous Steroid Hormone-Related Anticancer Therapy   85

    9. Compounds Acting on Other Proteins of the Nuclear Receptor Superfamily:

       Retinoids   86

    References   90

4. Anticancer Drugs Acting via Radical Species, Photosensitizers and Photodynamic Therapy of Cancer   **93**

    1. Introduction: Radicals and Other Reactive Oxygen Species   93
    2. Biological Effects of ROS   95
    3. Anthracyclines and Their Analogs   102
    4. Mitoxantrone and Related Quinones   112
    5. Actinomycin D   114
    6. Chartreusin, Elsamicin A, and Related Compounds   116
    7. Bleomycins   116
    8. Enediyne Antibiotics   122
    9. Tirapazamine   126
   10. Penclomedine   128
   11. Radiosensitizers   129
   12. Photodynamic Therapy of Cancer   132
    References   135

5. DNA Alkylating Agents   **139**

    1. Introduction   139
    2. Nitrogen Mustards   141
    3. Aziridines (Ethyleneimines)   154
    4. Epoxides   158
    5. Methanesulfonates   159
    6. Nitrosoureas   160
    7. Triazenes   165
    8. Methylhydrazines   166
    9. 1,3,5-Triazines: Hexamethylmelamine and Trimelamol   168
   10. Platinum Complexes   169
   11. Miscellaneous Alkylating and Acylating Antitumor Agents   173
    References   174

6. Alkylating and Non-Alkylating Compounds Interacting with the DNA Minor Groove   **177**

    1. Introduction   177
    2. Netropsin, Distamycin, and Related Compounds   178
    3. Mitomycins   182
    4. Tetrahydroisoquinoline Alkaloids   189
    5. Cyclopropylindole Alkylating Agents   193
    6. Pyrrolo[1,4]Benzodiazepines   195
    References   196

7. DNA Intercalators and Topoisomerase Inhibitors   **199**

    1. DNA Intercalation and Its Consequences   200
    2. Monofunctional Intercalating Agents   201
    3. Bifunctional Intercalating Agents   206
    4. DNA Topoisomerases   209

5. Topoisomerase II Poisons   213
6. Topoisomerase II Catalytic Inhibitors   218
7. Specific Topoisomerase I Inhibitors   220
   References   225

8. Anticancer Drugs Targeting Tubulin and Microtubules   **229**
1. Introduction   229
2. Drugs That Inhibit Microtubule Polymerization at High Concentrations   231
3. Microtubule-Stabilizing Agents: Compounds Binding at the Taxane Site   237
4. Miscellaneous Anticancer Drugs Acting on Novel Sites on Tubuline   245
5. Antivascular Effects of Microtubule-Targeted Agents   245
6. Mitotic Kinesin Inhibitors   246
   References   247

9. Drugs That Inhibit Signalling Pathways for Tumor Cell
   Growth and Proliferation   **251**
1. Introduction: The Role of Protein Kinases in Cancer   252
2. Signalling Pathways Related to Kinases   254
3. Inhibitors of Tyrosine Kinases (TKs)   254
4. Inhibitors of Serine-Threonine Kinases   275
5. Inhibitors of the RAS–RAF–MEK Signalling Pathway and Farnesyl Transferase   286
6. Inhibitors of Farnesyldiphosphate Synthase and Geranylgeranyldiphosphate
   Synthase   295
7. Anticancer Drugs Acting on Apoptotic Signalling Pathways   296
8. Inhibitors of Heat-Shock Proteins (HSP 90)   299
   References   302

10. Other Approaches to Targeted Therapy   **307**
1. Proteasome Inhibitors   307
2. Antiangiogenic Agents Unrelated to Kinase Signaling   312
3. Epigenetic Therapy of Cancer   323
4. Inhibitors of Other DNA-Associated Enzymes   337
5. Therapy Directed at Other Targets   341
   References   347

11. Drug Targeting in Anticancer Chemotherapy   **351**
1. Introduction   351
2. Prodrug-Based Anticancer Drug Targeting: Small-Molecule Prodrugs   352
3. Polymer-Protein Conjugates   368
4. Macromolecular Small-Drug Carrier Systems   369
5. Polymer-Directed Enzyme Prodrug Therapy (PDEPT)   377
6. Folate Receptor-Targeted Chemotherapy and Immunotherapy of Cancer   378
7. Liposomes and Nanoparticles in Anticancer Drug Targeting   380
   References   383

12. Drugs That Modulate Resistance to Antitumor Agents   **387**

    1. ATP-Binding Cassette Efflux Pumps in Anticancer Drug Resistance   388

    2. Glutathione and Glutathione-S-Transferase in Anticancer Drug Resistance   397

    3. Chemosensitizers Targeting DNA-Repair Systems   401

    4. Antitumor Drug Resistance Related to Extracellular pH: Tumor-Associated
       Carbonic Anhydrase as an Anticancer Target   412

    References   414

13. Cancer Chemoprevention   **417**

    1. Introduction   417

    2. Ligands for Nuclear Receptors in Cancer Chemoprevention   418

    3. Anti-Inflammatory Agents and Antioxidants in Cancer Chemoprevention   421

    4. Chromatin Modifiers in Cancer Chemoprevention   425

    5. Miscellaneous Agents for Chemoprevention   426

    6. Cancer Vaccines   428

    References   428

Index   *431*

Chemistry, and organic chemistry in particular, is a very broad subject that bears a profound relationship with all phases of drug discovery, design, and development. The involvement of many facets of chemistry is needed for the translation of the knowledge of the cellular, molecular, and genetic bases of cancer into effective therapies. In the past decades, the boundaries between biology and chemistry are becoming increasingly diffused because biology is close to becoming a chemical science. Indeed, it can be easily verified that in the past years many Nobel prizes in chemistry have been awarded for discoveries that are biological in nature. As our understanding of the basic chemistry of life increases, we begin to understand the complex phenomena at molecular levels, and this level of understanding allows for the design of molecular entities that are selectively suited to interact with a given biological target, since drug action is always a consequence, more or less immediate, of a chemical interaction.

Cancer is presently responsible for about 25% of deaths in developed countries and for 15% of all deaths worldwide. It can therefore be considered as one of the foremost health problems, with about 1.45 million new cancer cases being expected yearly. Antitumor chemotherapy is nowadays a very active field of research, and a huge amount of information on the topic is generated every year. Although there is a large amount of information available dealing with clinical aspects of cancer chemotherapy, we felt that there was a clear need for an updated treatment from the point of view of medicinal chemistry and drug design. Thus, we have attempted to produce a concise but reasonably comprehensive treatment that fills the gap between the elementary medicinal chemistry textbooks and the primary literature and helps readers to achieve a deeper understanding of the molecular basis of the action of antitumor drugs. Our focus has been on the mechanism of action of antitumor drugs from the atomistic point of view of chemistry and on the relationship between chemical structure and chemical and biochemical reactivity of antitumor agents, aiming at the rationalization of the action of these drugs in order to allow the design of new active molecules. We have purposefully excluded the discussion of antitumor drug synthesis, not because we believe that it is not pertaining to a book devoted to medicinal chemistry, but because it would have required a full volume in itself to do some justice to the impressive achievements made in this field. Because of the huge number of agents that have shown high *in vitro* antitumor activities, in compiling the information presented in this book we have needed to make some difficult decisions on the inclusion of certain topics. With some exceptions, most notably in chapters 11 and 12, we have limited our discussion to agents that have been already approved in chemotherapy or chemoprevention regimes or that have at least entered in clinical trials. The organization of the book is based on targets and mechanisms of action from a molecular point of view because we believe that this is the best possible approach to the study of drug design. In this classification, we have attempted to use the main mechanism of action of each drug as the criterion, although some decisions that we have taken in this regard may be debatable. Whenever possible, we have attempted to present concepts in a pictorial way, and hence the large number of figures in the book.

This book is expected to be useful to undergraduate and postgraduate students of medicinal chemistry and their instructors, in courses related both to chemistry and to the health sciences. It should also have some appeal for students of pharmacology or biochemistry courses where a concise overview of the biochemistry of cancer is of interest. We hope that the inclusion of a large number of references to the review and primary literature will also make the book useful for researchers and practitioners of health professions.

We thank some colleagues that contributed to the clarity of the text by thoroughly reviewing parts of the manuscript, especially Drs. Pilar Iniesta, Pilar López-Alvarado, Rosario Perona, and María Teresa Ramos. We are obviously responsible for any remaining errors, and will welcome constructive criticism from readers in this regard.

Carmen Avendaño
José Carlos Menéndez
Madrid, November 2007

ABC	ATP-binding cassette
ACAT	Acyl coenzymeA: cholesterol acyl transferase
ACNU	1-(4-Amino-2-methyl-5-pyrimidinyl)methyl-3-(2-chloroethyl)-3-nitrosourea (nimustine)
ADCC	Antibody-dependent cell-mediated cytotoxicity
ADEPT	Antibody-directed enzyme prodrug therapy
Adiol	5-Androstene-3β,17β-diol
ADME	Absorption, distribution, metabolism, and excretion
AEBS	Antiestrogen binding site
AF	Activating function
AGT	O^6-Alkylguanine-DNA alkyltransferase (alkylguanine transferase)
AICARFT	Aminoimidazolecarboxamide ribonucleotide formyltransferase
AKT	Active human protein kinase (equivalent to PKB)
ALA	5-Aminolevulinic acid
AM	Aminopterin
APL	Acute promyelocytic leukemia
AR	Androgen receptor
Ara-C	Arabinofuranosylcytosine (cytarabine)
AT gene	Ataxia telangiectasia gene
ATP	Adenosine triphosphate
BCL-2	B-cells limphoma 2
BCNU	1,3-Bis(2-chloroethyl)nitrosourea (carmustine)
BCRP	Breast cancer resistance protein
BER	Base excision repair
BLM	Bleomycin
BPU	Benzoylphenylurea
CaM	Calmodulin
CARD	Caspase-associated recruitment domain
CCNU	1-Cyclohexyl-3-(2-chloroethyl)-3-nitrosourea (lomustine)
CDDP	Cisdiamminedichloroplatinum II (cisplatin)
CDHP	5-Chloro-2,4-dihydroxypyridine (gimestat)
CDK	Cyclin-dependent kinase
CF	Coformycin
CHK	Checkpoint kinase
CKI	CDK inhibitor
CLL	Chronic lymphocytic leukaemia
CNDAC	2′-Cyano-2′-deoxy-1-βD-arabinofuranosylcytosine
COX-2	Cyclooxygenase 2
CPT	Camptothecin

CYP3A	Cytochrome P4503A
dATP	Deoxyadenosine triphosphate
DAUF	Daunoform
dCF	2′-Deoxycoformycin (pentostatin)
dFdC	Difluorodeoxycytidine
dG	Deoxyguanosine
dGTP	Deoxyguanosine triphosphate
dGTP	Deoxyguanosine triphosphate
DHEA	Dehydroepiandrosterone
DHEA-S	Dehydroepiandrosterone sulphate
DHF	Dihydrofolate
DHFR	Dihydrofolate reductase
DHFU	Dihydrofluorouracil
DHT	5α-Dihydrotestosterone
DNA	Deoxyribonucleic acid
DNA-PK	DNA protein kinase
DNMT	DNA methyltransferase
DNR	Daunorubicyn (daunomycin)
DON	6-Diazo-5-oxo-L-norleucine
DOX	Doxorubicin (adriamycin)
DOXF	Doxoform
DPD	Dihydropyrimidine dehydrogenase
dR	Deoxyribose
DSB	Double-strand breaks
DTD	DT-diaphorase
DTIC	5-Dimethyltriazeneimidazole-4-carboxamide (dacarbazine)
dUMP	Deoxyuridine monophosphate
E_2	Estradiol
E_2-2,3-Q	Estradiol-2,3-quinone
E_2-3,4-Q	Estradiol-3,4-quinone
EDTA	Ethylenediaminetetraacetic acid
EGFR	Epidermal growth factor receptor (equivalent to HER1)
EMEA	European Medicines Agency
EPI	Epirubicin
EPR effect	Enhanced permeability and retention effect
ER	Estrogen receptor
ERBB2	V-erb-b2 erythroblastic leukemia viral oncogene homolog 2 (HER2)
ERE	Estrogen response element
ERK	Extracellular signal-regulated kinase (equivalent to MAPK)
ESR	Electron spin resonance
ETS	Endothelial transcription factor
FDA	Food and drug administration
5-FdUTP	5-Fluoro-2′-desoxyuridine-triphosphate
FGAR	Formylglycinamide ribonucleotide
FGF	Fibroblast growth factor
FmdC	Fluoromethylenedeoxycytidine

FPGS	Folylpolyglutamate synthetase
FPP	Farnesyl pyrophosphate
FPP	Farnesyldiphosphate synthase
FSH	Follicle stimulating hormone
FTase	Farnesyltransferase
5-FU	5-Fluorouracil
GAP	GTPase activating protein
GAPDH	Glyceraldehyde-3-phosphate dehydrogenase
GAR	Glycinamide ribonucleotide
GARFT	Ribonucleotide formyltransferase
GCSF	Granulocyte colony-stimulating factor
GDEPT	Gene-directed enzyme prodrug therapy
GGPP	Geranylgeranyldiphosphate synthase
GIST	Gastrointestinal stromal tumor
GMP	Guanosine monophosphate (guanylic acid)
GnRH	Gonadotropin-releasing hormone (equivalent to LHRH)
GSH	Glutathione
GST	Glutathione-S-transferase
GTP	Guanosine triphosphate
HAT	Histone acetylase
HDAC	Histone deacetylase
HGPRT	Hypoxantine guanine phosphoribosyl transferase
HIF-1	Hypoxia-inducible factor-1
HMM	Hexamethylmelamine (altretamine)
HMT	Histone methyltransferases
HMTA	Hexamethylenetetraamine
HOMO	Highest Occupied Molecular Orbital
HPMA	N-(2-Hydroxypropylmethacrylamide)
HS	Heparan sulfate
HSP 90	Heat-shock protein 90
HTS	High-throughput screening
IC	Inhibitory concentration
IDA	Idarubicin
IGF	Insulin-like growth factors
IMP	Inosine monophosphate (inosinic acid)
IPMK	Inositolphosphate multikinase
IRP-1	Iron regulatory protein 1
IudR	5-Iodouridine deoxyribose
JNK	Jun N-terminal kinase
L-BSO	L-Buthioninesulfoximine
LH	Luteinizing hormone
LHRH	Luteinizing hormone releasing hormone (equivalent to GnRH)
mAB	Monoclonal antibody
MAO	Monoaminooxidase
MAPK	Mitogen-activated protein kinase (equivalent to ERK)
MDA	Malondialdehyde

MDR	Multidrug resistance
MDS	Myelodysplastic syndrome
MEK	Mitogen activated protein kinase kinase
MFR	Membrane folate receptor (α-FR)
MGB	Minor groove binder
MMP	Matrix metalloproteinase
8-MOP	8-Methoxypsoralen (methoxsalen)
MP	6-Mercaptopurine
mPEG	MethoxyPEG (O-methylPEG)
MRI	Magnetic resonance imaging
MS	Multiple sclerosis
MTA	Multi-targeted antifolate
MTIC	5-Methyltriazeneimidazole-4-carboxamide
MTOR	Mammalian target of rapamycin
MTX	Methotrexate (amethopterin)
NAD	Nicotinamide adenine dinucleotide
NADP	Nicotinamide adenine dinucleotide phosphate
N-BP	Nitrogen-containing biphosphonates
NCEs	New chemical entities
NCI	National Cancer Institute
NCS	Neocarzinostatin
NDPR	Nucleoside diphosphate reductase (equivalent to RNR)
NER	Nucleotide excision repair
NMHE	N-methyl-9-hydroxyellipticinium
NMR	Nuclear magnetic resonance
NPY	Neuropeptide Y
NSCLC	Non-small lung cell cancer
4-OHE$_2$	4-Hydroxyestradiol
PALA	N-phosphonoacetyl-L-aspartate
PAR	Poly(ADP-ribose)
PARP	Poly(ADP-ribose) polymerase
PDGF	Platelet-derived endothelial cell growth factor
PDK1	Phosphoinositide-dependant protein kinase
PDT	Photodynamic therapy
PEG	Polyethyleneglycol
PGA	Polyglutamic acid
P-gp	Glycoprotein P
PKB	Protein kinase B (equivalent to AKT)
PKC	Protein kinase C
PLP	Pyridoxal phosphate
PML	Promyelocite leukemia protein
PNP	Purine nucleoside phosphorylase
Polβ	DNA polimerase β
PPARγ	Peroxysome proliferator activating receptors γ
PRPP	Phosphoribosyl pyrophosphate
PS	Photosensitizer
PTA	cis-3-(9H-Purin-6-ylthio)acrylic acid

PTK	Protein kinase
QSAR	Quantitative structure-activity relationships
RAR	Retinoic acid receptors
RARE	Retinoic acid response elements
REPSA	Restriction endonuclease protection, selection, and amplification
RFC	Reduced folate carrier
RNA	Ribonucleic acid
RNase	Ribonuclease
RNOS	Nitrogen oxide reactive species
RNR	Ribonucleotide reductase (equivalent to NDPR)
ROS	Reactive oxygen species
RPTK	Receptor protein kinase
RXR	Retinoid X receptors
SAHA	Suberoylanilide hydroxamic acid
SAR	Structure-activity relationships
SARM	Selective androgen receptor modulators
SERM	Selective estrogen receptor modulators
SHMT	Serine hydroxymethyl transferase
SMANCS	Styrene maleic acid and neocarzinostatin copolymer
SOD	Superoxide dismutase
SPARC	Secreted protein acidic and rich in cysteine
STI	Signal transduction inhibitor
STS	Steroid sulfatase
TEM	Triethylenemelamine
TEPA	Triethylenephosphoramide
TERT	Telomerase reverse transcriptase
TG	6-Thioguanine
TGFα	Transforming growth factor α
THF	Tetrahydrofolate
TK	Tyrosine kinase
TLM	Tallysomycin
TMP	Thymidine monophosphate (thymidylate)
TP	Thymidine phosphorylase
TPMT	Thiopurine methyltransferase
TPZ	Tirapazamine
TR	Telomerase RNA (TERC)
TRAIL	Tumor necrosis factor-related apoptosis-inducing ligand
TS	Thymidylate synthase
TSA	Trichostatin
TSP-1	Thrombospondin-1
TUA	6-Thiouric acid
UMP	Uridine monophosphate
UTP	Uridine triphosphate
VDEPT	Virus-directed enzyme prodrug therapy
VEGF	Vascular endothelial growth factor
VTA	Vascular-targeting agent
XMP	Xanthosine monophosphate (xantosinic acid, xanthylic acid)

CHAPTER 1

Introduction

Contents

1. Some General Remarks About Cancer and
   Cancer Chemotherapy 1
2. A Brief Account of the Role of Chemistry in
   Cancer Chemotherapy 3
3. Natural Products in Cancer Chemotherapy 5
4. A Brief Comment About Cancer Nanotechnology 6
5. Conclusion 7
   References 7

1. SOME GENERAL REMARKS ABOUT CANCER AND CANCER CHEMOTHERAPY

Cancer is a collective term used for a group of diseases that are characterized by the loss of control of the growth, division, and spread of a group of cells, leading to a primary tumor that invades and destroys adjacent tissues. It may also spread to other regions of the body through a process known as metastasis, which is the cause of 90% of cancer deaths. Cancer remains one of the most difficult diseases to treat and is responsible for about 13% of all deaths worldwide, and this incidence is increasing due to the ageing of population in most countries, but specially in the developed ones.

Cancer is normally caused by abnormalities of the genetic material of the affected cells. Tumorigenesis is a multistep process that involves the accumulation of successive mutations in oncogenes and suppressor genes that deregulates the cell cycle. Tumorigenic events include small-scale changes in DNA sequences, such as point mutations; larger-scale chromosomal aberrations, such as translocations, deletions, and amplifications; and changes that affect the chromatin structure and are associated with dysfunctional epigenetic control, such as aberrant methylation of DNA or acetylation of histones.[1] About 2,000–3,000 proteins may have a potential role in the regulation of gene transcription and in the complex

---

Medicinal Chemistry of Anticancer Drugs
DOI: 10.1016/B978-0-444-52824-7.00001-9

signal-transduction cascades that regulate the activity of these regulators. Cancer is not only a cell disease, but also a tisular disease in which the normal relationships between epithelial cells and their underlying stromal cells are altered.[2]

Cancer therapy is based on surgery and radiotherapy, which are, when possible, rather successful regional interventions, and on systemic chemotherapy. Approximately half of cancer patients are not cured by these treatments and may obtain only a prolonged survival or no benefit at all. The aim of most cancer chemotherapeutic drugs currently in clinical use is to kill malignant tumor cells by inhibiting some of the mechanisms implied in cellular division. Accordingly, the antitumor compounds developed through this approach are cytostatic or cytotoxic. However, the knowledge of tumor biology has exploded during the past decades and this may pave the way for more active, targeted anticancer drugs.[3] The introduction of the tyrosine kinase inhibitor imatinib as a highly effective drug in chronic myeloid lekemia and gastrointestinal stromal tumors[4] was a proof of the concept of effective drug development based on the knowledge of tumor biology.[5]

Effective targeted therapies may be suitable only for small subgroups of patients.[6] Pharmacogenetics, which focuses on intersubject variation in therapeutic drug effects and toxicity depending of polymorphisms, is particularly interesting in oncology since anticancer drugs usually have a narrow margin of safety. The dose of chemotherapeutic agents is generally adjusted by body surface area, but this parameter is not sufficient to overcome differences in drug disposition.[7] DNA microarray technology permits to study alterations in the transcriptional level of entire genomes, and may become an important tool for predicting the chemosensitivity of tumors before treatment.

It is obvious that cancer chemotherapy is a very difficult task.[8] One of its main associated problems is the nonspecific toxicity of most anticancer drugs due to their biodistribution throughout the body, which requires the administration of a large total dose to achieve high local concentrations in a tumor. Drug targeting aims at preferred drug accumulation in the target cells independently on the method and route of drug administration.[9] One approach that allows to improve the selectivity of cytotoxic compounds is the use of prodrugs that are selectively activated in tumor tissues, taking advantage of some unique aspects of tumor physiology, such as selective enzyme expression, hypoxia, and low extracellular pH. More sophisticated tumor-specific delivery techniques allow the selective activation of prodrugs by exogenous enzymes (gene-directed and antibody-directed enzyme prodrug therapy). Furthermore, the increased permeability of vascular endothelium in tumors (enhanced permeability and retention, EPR effect) permits that nanoparticles loaded with an antitumor drug can extravasate and accumulate inside the interstitial space, where the drug can be released as a result of normal carrier degradation (see also Section 4).[10]

Another problem in cancer chemotherapy is drug resistance. After the development of a resistance mechanism in response to a single drug, cells can display cross-resistance to other structural and mechanistically unrelated drugs, a phenomenon known as multidrug resistance (MDR) in which ATP-dependent transporters have a significant role.[11]

Finally, a major problem in the development of anticancer drugs is the large gap from promising findings in preclinical *in vitro* and *in vivo* models to the results of clinical trials. The problems found in this transition arise because experimental cancer models greatly differ from patients, who very often suffer from a much more complex therapeutic situation. Although a large number of clinical trials are in progress and new results are continuously being published, the real clinical efficacy of most of these treatments is usually disappointing and a statistically significant benefit is observed for very few of them.[12] It has been claimed that development and utilization of more clinically relevant cancer models would represent a major advance for anticancer drug research.

2. A BRIEF ACCOUNT OF THE ROLE OF CHEMISTRY IN CANCER CHEMOTHERAPY

Chemistry has had varying roles in the discovery and development of anticancer drugs since the beginning of cancer therapies.[13] In its early history, chemical modification of sulfur mustard gas led to the serendipitous discovery of the still clinically useful nitrogen mustards. Since those years, synthetic chemistry has been extensively used to modify drug leads, especially those of natural origin, and to solve the problem of the often scarce supply of natural products by developing semisynthetic or synthetic strategies (see Section 3).

Since the 1950s, chemistry has also generated many antitumor drug leads through *in vitro* screening programs promoted by the National Cancer Institute (NCI) in the United States by using a range of cancer cell lines. In this early period, transplantable rodent tumors models characterized by a high growth rate were used for *in vivo* screening. Later on, human tumor xenografts, based on transplantation of human tumor tissue into immune-tolerant animals, became also important tools for selecting antitumor drugs because the xenograft models allowed to simulate a chemotherapeutic effect under conditions closer to man. In the late seventies and early eighties, the role of chemotherapy was extended to preoperative and postoperative adjuvants, radiosensitizers to enhance radiation effects, and supportive therapy to increase the tolerance of the organism toward toxicity.[14]

The rationale for the use of conventional cytotoxic antitumor drugs is based on the theory that rapidly proliferating and dividing cells are more sensitive to these compounds than the normal cells.[15] The interactions of cytotoxic agents with DNA are now better defined, and new compounds that target particular base sequences may inhibit transcription factors in a more specific manner. DNA can be considered as a true molecular receptor that is capable of molecular recognition and of triggering response elements which transmit signals through protein interactions.[16] The binding properties of DNA ligands can be rationalized on the basis of their structural and electronic complementarity with the functional groups present in the major and minor grooves of particular DNA sequences which are mainly recognized by specific hydrogen bonds.[17]

Although DNA continues to be an essential target for anticancer chemotherapy, much recent effort has been directed to discover antitumor drugs specifically suited to target molecular aberrations which are specific to tumor cells.[18] This new generation of antitumor agents is based on research in areas such as cell signaling processes, angiogenesis and metastasis, and inhibition of enzymes that, like telomerase, are reactivated in the majority of cancer cells.[19] These goals may use small molecule drugs or other macromolecular structures, such as monoclonal antibodies that bind to antigens present preferentially or exclusively on tumor cells. The aim of other research programs is to develop compounds that interfere with gene expression to suppress the production of damaged proteins involved in carcinogenesis. In the antisense approach, the mRNA translation is interfered thereby inhibiting the translation of the information at the ribosome, while in the antigene therapy, a direct binding to the DNA double strand inhibits transcription.[20]

The knowledge of the three-dimensional structure of these new target macromolecules, which are normally proteins, by using X-ray crystallography, permits the rational design of small molecules that mimic the stereochemical features of the macromolecule functional domains. The principal steps in structure-based drug design using X-ray techniques are summarized in Fig. 1.1. In the absence of a three-dimensional structure of a target protein, homology criteria may be applied using the experimental structure of similar proteins, which is especially useful in the case of individual subfamilies. The knowledge of the three-dimensional structure of a target also permits to design and generate virtual libraries of potential drug molecules to be used for *in silico* screening.

Progress in the development of potential drug molecules is often problematic because it is difficult to convert them into "druggable" compounds, that is, into molecules with adequate pharmaceutical properties. To this end, it is absolutely necessary to know the chemical properties of a lead compound, especially solubility and reactivity, because these properties are relevant for cellular uptake and metabolism in order to transform this lead compound into a real drug. The "druggability" of a drug candidate describes their adequate absorption, distribution, metabolism, and excretion (ADME) properties. In this task, the structural knowledge of important metabolic enzymes, such as cytochrome P450 3A4 (CYP3A4), will permit to improve the effectiveness and patient tolerance for antitumor compounds. A preliminary knowledge of ADME properties may be now gained by using *in silico* techniques, although an experienced chemist can provide

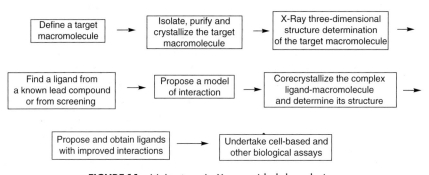

FIGURE 1.1   Main steps in X-ray-guided drug design.

accurate insights into this picture only by simple inspection of a given structure. The chemical properties of a drug candidate also govern its proposed formulation.

In this list of contributions to the development of antitumor agents, it has to be mentioned that chemistry has also made possible important advances in prodrug development and in related targeted approaches, such as antibody-coupled drugs or photoactive agents.

3. NATURAL PRODUCTS IN CANCER CHEMOTHERAPY

Plants, microorganisms, and, more recently, marine organisms of various types have traditionally represented a main source of cytotoxic anticancer agents since the beginning of chemotherapy.[21] Even if the new technologies of combinatorial chemistry and high-throughput screening (HTS) represent an important step in drug discovery, the role of natural sources in providing new cytotoxics should not be disregarded for the future.[22] The number of microbial species studied in this regard is still very low, and the marine ecosystem is largely unexplored.

Around half of the drugs currently in clinical use as anticancer drugs are of natural product origin, and it has been estimated that about 60% of new chemical entities (NCEs) introduced in the 1981–2002 period in this field were natural products or were derived from a natural lead compound.[23] Despite this statistic, pharmaceutical companies have neglected in the recent past the development of potential natural drug candidates in favor of combinatorial chemistry and high-throughput synthesis of large compound libraries. The main reason of this reluctance to use natural products as drug candidates lies primarily in supply problems that make the development of synthetic routes necessary, which are often long and difficult to scale-up owing to their structural complexity. It is becoming increasingly apparent, however, that the unguided production of vast libraries of compounds is unlikely to result in the identification of new drugs.

In general, natural products have several functional groups which are located into a precise three-dimensional position providing specific interactions with target molecules. It is often assumed that secondary metabolites in nature organisms have been optimized through evolution to exert their still not well-defined effects. Consequently, they may be considered as highly advanced lead compounds in which further optimization of activity is difficult.[24] In many cases, some parts of the complex structure of a natural product act only as a framework to position determined atoms, and more simple analogs may be developed without considerable loss of activity. For this reason, structural modification of natural products is often directed to find the simplest portion that maintains most of the biological activity, that is, its pharmacophoric unit. One example of this approach is the development of the antitumor agent E7389 that arose from studies on the total synthesis of the cytotoxic marine compound halichondrin B and is currently in Phase III clinical trials. The development of synthetic strategies to obtain halichondrin B revealed that deletion of a large portion of this compound, as well as the replacement of the unstable lactone by a ketone function, did not affect its antimitotic properties.[25]

Halichondrin B   E7389

The notion that the use of natural product templates combined with chemical modifications leading to more selective analogs will have a better chance of success than combinatorial approaches is gaining acceptance. In other words, it is becoming more and more clear that, at least in the anticancer field, nature has already carried out the combinatorial chemistry and all we have to do is refine the structures.[26] These ideas are leading to a renaissance of natural products as drug candidates.[27]

4. A BRIEF COMMENT ABOUT CANCER NANOTECHNOLOGY

Nanotechnology is a field of applied science that covers a broad range of topics in which matter is controlled on a scale of 1–1,000 nm. Its application to cancer chemotherapy includes the use of nanovectors for the targeted delivery of antitumor compounds and imaging contrast agents, aiming at increasing the efficacy per dose of therapeutic or imaging contrast formulations.[28]

Liposomes, which are the simplest forms of nanovectors, use the EPR effect to increase drug concentration at tumor sites, and were first applied to anthracyclines in order to avoid their cardiotoxicity. The refinement of liposomes and their application in cancer chemotherapy is still an active field of research, although other novel drug delivery modalities have appeared.[29,30] In general, a nanovector has a core constituent material, a therapeutic and/or imaging payload, and biological surface modifiers to enhance biodistribution and tumor targeting. Among several types of nanoparticles directed to enhance the properties of magnetic resonance imaging (MRI) contrast agents,[31] dendrimers, which are self-assembling polymers, have been used in mouse models of breast cancer to study the lymphatic drainage by MRI.[32]

Several nanotechnologies are realistic candidates for the precise patterning of biological molecules, including DNA microarrays and surface-enhanced laser desorption/ionization time-of-flight (SELDI-TOF) mass spectrometry.[33]

DNA microarrays are devices used for molecular diagnostics, genotyping, and biomarking. They are single-stranded DNA probes that are prepared through a sequential procedure that implies selective ultraviolet deprotection of hydroxyl groups. With the ability to control the molecular depositions of polynucleotides in a nanometer range, the information might be packed in nanoarrays directed at nucleic acids[34] or at the detection of proteomic profiles.[35]

5. CONCLUSION

The goal of developing superior therapies that have a meaningful impact on the lives of cancer patients is seen with optimism by considering the huge number of molecules, especially signal transduction signals, that may be targeted. Very high expectations are also being placed on the multiple technologies available to achieve a selective distribution of cytotoxic drugs or to selectively bioactivate prodrugs in a particular tumor. It is also generally accepted that classical anticancer approaches, such as DNA interacting agents, will remain in the antitumor therapeutic arsenal, and that natural products will continue to be an invaluable source of drug prototypes.

REFERENCES

1. Nelson, S. M., Ferguson, L. R., and Denny, W. A. (2004). *Cell Chromosome* **3**, 2.
2. Bissell, M. J., and Radisky, D. (2001). *Nat. Rev. Cancer* **1**, 46.
3. Bradbury, R. H. (ed.) (2007). *Cancer* in "Topics in Medicinal Chemistry," vol. 1. Springer-Verlag, Berlin Heidelberg.
4. Capdeville, R., Buchdunger, E., Zimmermann, J., and Matter, A. (2002). *Nat. Rev. Drug Discov.* **1**, 493.
5. Atkins, J. H., and Gershell, L. J. (2002). *Nat. Rev. Drug Discov.* **1**, 491.
6. Díaz, L. A., and Saurabh, S. (2005). *Nat. Rev. Drug Discov.* **4**, 375.
7. Toffoli, G., Cecchin, E., Corona, G., and Boiocchi, M. (2003). *Curr. Med. Chem. Anti-Cancer Agents* **3**, 225.
8. Nygren, P., and Larsson, R. (2003). *J. Intern. Med.* **253**, 46.
9. Torchilin, V. P. (2000). *Eur. J. Pharm. Sci.* **11**, 81.
10. Jain, R. K. (1987). *Cancer Metastasis Rev.* **6**, 559.
11. Gottesman, M. M., Fojo, T., and Bates, S. E. (2002). *Nat. Rev. Cancer* **2**, 48.
12. Nygren, P., and Larsson, R. (2003). *J. Intern. Med.* **253**, 46.
13. Neidle, S., and Thurston, D. E. (2005). *Nat. Rev. Cancer* **5**, 285.
14. Eckhardt, S. (2002). *Curr. Med. Chem. Anti-Cancer Agents* **2**, 419.
15. Marchini, S., and Broggini, M. (2004). *Curr. Med. Chem. Anti-Cancer Agents* **4**, 247.
16. Hurley, L. H. (2002). *Nat. Rev. Cancer* **2**, 188.
17. Gago, F. (1998). *Methods* **14**, 277.
18. Longley, D. B., Harkin, D. P., and Johnston, P. G. (2003). *Nat. Rev. Cancer* **3**, 330.
19. Nam, N.-H., and Parang, K. (2003). *Curr. Drug Targets* **4**, 159.
20. Segota, E., and Bukowski, R. M. (2004). *Cleve. Clin. J. Med.* **71**, 551.
21. Butler, M. S. (2005). *Nat. Prod. Rep.* **22**, 162.
22. Cozzi, P., Mongelli, N., and Suarato, A. (2004). *Curr. Med. Chem. Anti-Cancer Agents* **4**, 93.
23. Newman, D. J., and Cragg, G. M. (2007). *J. Nat. Prod.* **70**, 461.
24. Cozzi, P., Mongelli, N., and Suarato, A. (2004). *Curr. Med. Chem. Anti-Cancer Agents* **4**, 93.
25. Zheng, W., Seletsky, B. M., Palme, M. H., Lydon, P. J., Singer, L. A., Chase, C. E., Lemelin, C. A., Shen, Y., Davis, H., Tremblay, L., Towle, M. J., *et al.* (2004). *Bioorg. Med. Chem. Lett.* **14**, 5551.
26. Mann, J. (2002). *Nat. Rev. Cancer* **2**, 143.
27. Paterson, I., and Anderson, E. (2005). *Science* **310**, 451.
28. Ferrari, M. (2005). *Nat. Rev. Cancer* **5**, 161.

29. Couvrer, P., and Vauthier, C. (2006). *Pharm. Res.* **23,** 1417.
30. Nishiyama, N., and Kataoka, K. (2006). *Pharmacol. Ther.* **112,** 630.
31. Kircher, M. F., Mahmood, U., King, R. S., Weissleder, R., and Josephson, L. (2003). *Cancer Res.* **63,** 8122.
32. Kobayashi, H., Choyke, P. L., Brechbiel, M. W., and Waldmann, T. A. (2004). *J. Natl. Cancer Inst.* **96,** 703.
33. Vorderwülbecke, S., Cleverley, S., Weinberger, S. R., and Wiesner, A. (2005). *Nat. Methods* **2,** 393.
34. Demers, L. M., Ginger, D. S., Park, S.-J., Li, Z., Chung, S.-W., and Mirkin, C. A. (2002). *Science* **296,** 1836.
35. Brickbauer, A., and Klenerman, D. (2004). *J. Am. Chem. Soc.* **126,** 6508.

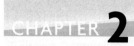

CHAPTER 2

Antimetabolites

Contents
1. Introduction   10
2. Inhibitors of the Biosynthesis of Uridylic Acid   10
3. Inhibitors of the Biosynthesis of 2′-Deoxyribonucleotides by
   Ribonucleotide Reductase (RNR)   11
   3.1. Structure and catalytic cycle of RNR   12
   3.2. Radical scavengers as inhibitors of RNR   13
   3.3. Substrate analogs as RNR inhibitors   15
   3.4. Allosteric inhibition of RNR   18
4. Inhibitors of the Biosynthesis of Thymidilic Acid   18
   4.1. Thymidylate synthase   18
   4.2. 5-fluorouracil (5-FU) and floxuridine   21
   4.3. 5-FU prodrugs   24
   4.4. Modulation of 5-FU activity   27
   4.5. Folate-Based TS inhibitors   29
5. Inhibitors of Dihydrofolate Reductase (DHFR)   32
   5.1. Classical DHFR inhibitors   33
   5.2. Nonclassical (lipophilic) DHFR inhibitors   36
6. Inhibitors of the De Novo Purine Biosynthesis Pathway   36
   6.1. Inhibitors of phosphoribosylpyrophosphate (PRPP)
        amidotransferase   36
   6.2. Inhibitors of glycinamide ribonucleotide formyltransferase
        (GARFT)   37
   6.3. Inhibitors of phosphoribosylformylglycinamidine
        synthetase   39
   6.4. Inhibitors of 5-aminoimidazole-4-carboxamide
        ribonucleotide formyltransferase   41
   6.5. Thiopurines and related compounds   41
7. Inhibitors of Adenosine Deaminase   42
8. Inhibitors of Late Stages in DNA Synthesis   45
   8.1. Pyrimidine nucleosides   47
   8.2. Purine nucleosides   49
9. Antimetabolite Enzymes   50
References   51

Medicinal Chemistry of Anticancer Drugs
DOI: 10.1016/B978-0-444-52824-7.00002-0

1. INTRODUCTION

Antimetabolites can be defined as analogs of naturally occurring compounds that interfere with their formation or utilization, thus inhibiting essential metabolic routes. Although the enzymes inhibited by antimetabolites are also present in normal cells, some selectivity toward cancer cells is possible due to their faster division rates.

Most antimetabolites interfere with nucleic acid synthesis and for this reason we will study in this chapter the antitumor compounds that hamper the production of DNA or RNA by a variety of mechanisms including:

a. Competition for binding sites of enzymes that participate in essential biosynthetic processes.
b. Incorporation into nucleic acids, which inhibits their normal function and triggers the apoptosis process.

Because of this mode of action, most antimetabolites have high cell cycle specificity.

A brief outline of DNA biosynthesis is given in Fig. 2.1, including the main steps where antimetabolite drugs discussed in this chapter exert their action.

Although clinically useful antimetabolites ultimately inhibit DNA (and sometimes RNA) synthesis, their site of action may be many steps removed from these reactions. Specific interference with the *de novo* nucleic acid pathways in cancer cells is probably not possible because tumor and normal cells use the same biosynthetic routes. Nevertheless, some antimetabolites are remarkably effective against some human cancers and are still one of the bases of cancer chemotherapy.

2. INHIBITORS OF THE BIOSYNTHESIS OF URIDYLIC ACID

The biosynthesis of pyrimidine nucleotides starts with the construction of the heterocyclic system by carbamoylation of aspartate followed by cyclization to dihydroorotate. Its dehydrogenation gives orotate, which then reacts with

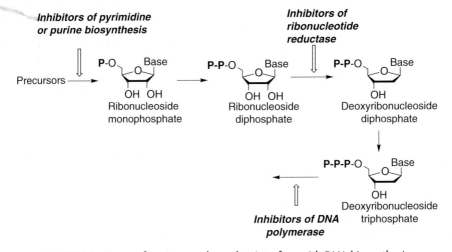

FIGURE 2.1   Types of anticancer drugs that interfere with DNA biosynthesis.

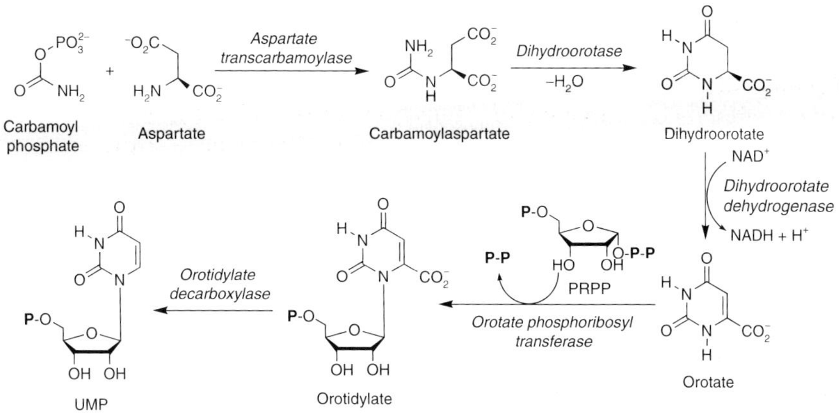

FIGURE 2.2 Biosynthesis of pyrimidine nucleotides.

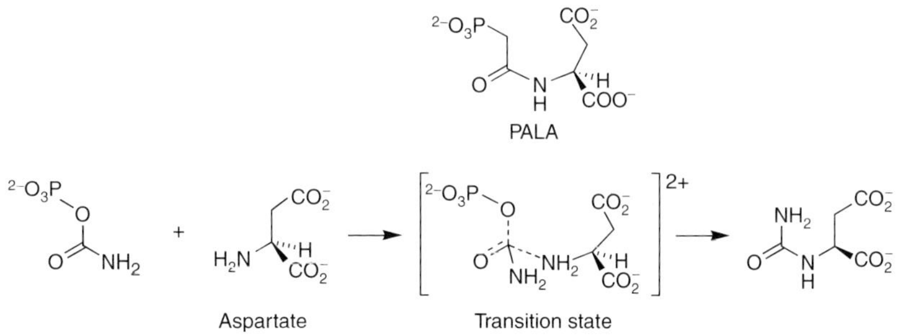

FIGURE 2.3 Inhibition of aspartate transcarbamoylase by PALA.

phosphoribosyl pyrophosphate (PRPP) to give orotidylate. Finally, uridylic acid (uridine monophosphate, UMP) is generated by decarboxylation (Fig. 2.2). UMP is the precursor to other pyrimidine nucleotides, after its conversion to the corresponding nucleoside triphosphate (UTP).

Among the many compounds known to inhibit reactions of this pathway, we will only mention N-phosphonoacetyl-L-aspartate (PALA), an inhibitor of aspartate transcarbamoylase that acts as a transition state analog (Fig. 2.3). This compound has undergone some clinical trials, normally in combination with 5-fluorouracil (5-FU), another pyrimidine antimetabolite.[1]

3. INHIBITORS OF THE BIOSYNTHESIS OF 2′-DEOXYRIBONUCLEOTIDES BY RIBONUCLEOTIDE REDUCTASE (RNR)

The biosynthesis of 2′-deoxyribonucleotides, which are the immediate precursors of DNA, involves the replacement of the 2′-OH group by a hydrogen atom (Fig. 2.4). This reaction takes place on ribonucleoside-5′-diphosphates and is catalyzed by the

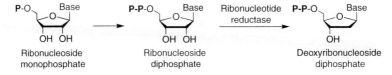

FIGURE 2.4   Biosynthesis of 2-deoxyribonucleotides.

enzyme ribonucleotide reductase (RNR), also known as nucleoside diphosphate reductase (NDPR).

3.1. Structure and catalytic cycle of RNR

RNR plays a central role in cell growth and proliferation by ensuring a balanced supply of nucleotide precursors for DNA synthesis. The most extensively studied RNR is that from *Escherichia coli*, which is considered as a suitable prototype for the mammalian enzyme. In eukaryotes, RNR has two subunits containing each a tyrosine that generates and stabilizes a tyrosyl radical through a redox process that transforms the initial Fe (II) complex into a binuclear oxo-bridged Fe (III) complex. A high-resolution X-ray diffraction study has shown that the first iron atom is pentacoordinate, although it maintains an octahedral structure, while the second one is hexacoordinate[2] (Fig. 2.5).

Although the Tyr-122 radical triggers the reductive process, it is too far away from the catalytic site. Therefore, it must generate a second radical in the vicinity of the substrate, probably a thiyl radical from Cys-439. The cysteine radical then abstracts the $C_{3'}$–H atom of the nucleoside diphosphate substrate and generates the anion-radical **2.1**, with prior or simultaneous deprotonation of the $C_{3'}$–OH group by the Glu-441 residue of the enzyme. Two cysteine residues, probably Cys-225 and Cys-462, form the redox-active sulfhydryl pair responsible for the reduction of this radical. Thus, protonation of the $C_{2'}$–OH and subsequent elimination of a molecule of water yields a cation that is stabilized by migration of the unpaired electron from C-3' to C-2' to give **2.2**. The Cys-462 mercapto group transfers a proton and one electron to this radical to give **2.3**, with concomitant formation of a disulfide anion radical, which then transfers one electron to the carbonyl group in **2.3**, leading to **2.4**. Radical **2.4** is transformed into **2.5** by a mechanism reverse to the one that produced **2.1**, and the active center of the enzyme is finally regenerated by reduction of the newly formed disulfide unit by thioredoxin, a ubiquitous protein that has a pair of proximal cysteine residues, which reacts with the oxidized form of RNR via disulfide exchange (Fig. 2.6).[3]

It is interesting to note that the enzymatic reaction of RNR is initiated by the formation of free radical **2.2**, even though the reactions leading to reductive elimination of the $C_{2'}$–OH group are ionic. The reason for this type of mechanism may be the enhanced stability of **2.2** through the stabilizing effect of the radical at C-3 on the intermediate carbocation formed at C-2, as shown by the resonance structures in Fig. 2.7.

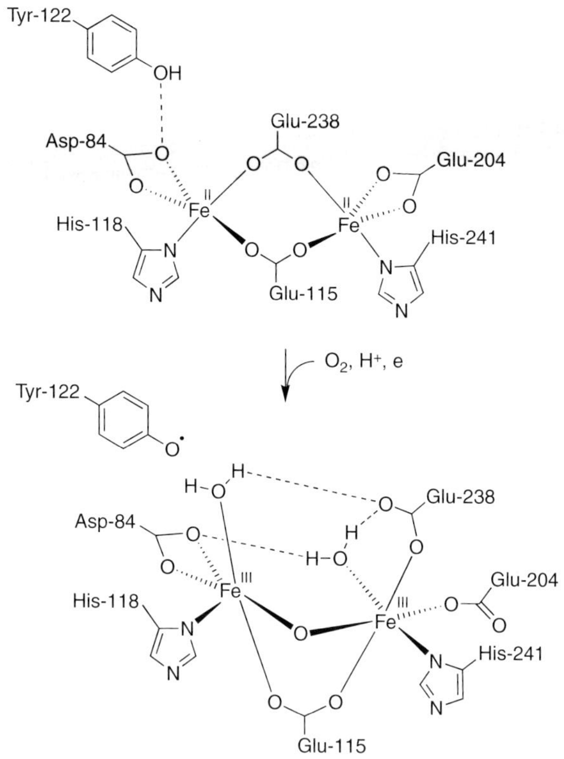

FIGURE 2.5   Generation of a tyrosyl radical in the active site of ribonucleotide reductase.

3.2. Radical scavengers as inhibitors of RNR

The best-known inhibitor of RNR is hydroxyurea, a cell cycle phase-specific (S-phase) inhibitor that is also known to behave as a radiosensitizer. After oral administration, this compound is well absorbed and transported into cells, where it quenches the tyrosyl radical at the active site of RNR, inactivating the enzyme (Fig. 2.8).[4] Hydroxyurea is primarily used in the management of myeloproliferative disorders, such as chronic granulocytic leukemia, polycythemia vera, and essential thrombocytosis, and is sometimes combined with other antitumor drugs such as the tyrosine kinase inhibitor imatinib.[5] Hydroxyurea is also useful in the treatment of sickle cell anemia because it eases the pain of the patients, which has been attributed to its ability to generate nitric oxide, a potent vasodilator.[6] Nitric oxide may also contribute to the antitumor effect of hydroxyurea, since it is known to inhibit RNR probably because it contains an unpaired electron and therefore it is able to quench the tyrosine radical.[7]

Thiosemicarbazones, represented by triapine, are another important class of inhibitors of RNR that are being the subject of Phase I studies.[8] Besides quenching the tyrosyl radical similarly to hydroxyurea, triapine is an iron chelator, which

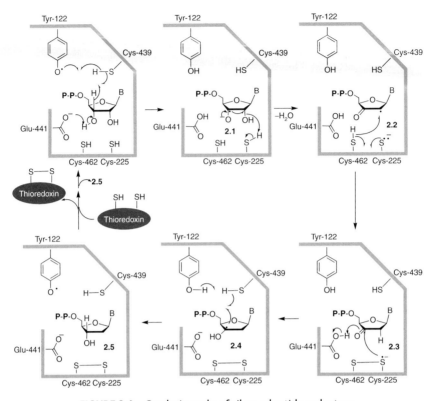

FIGURE 2.6   Catalytic cycle of ribonucleotide reductase.

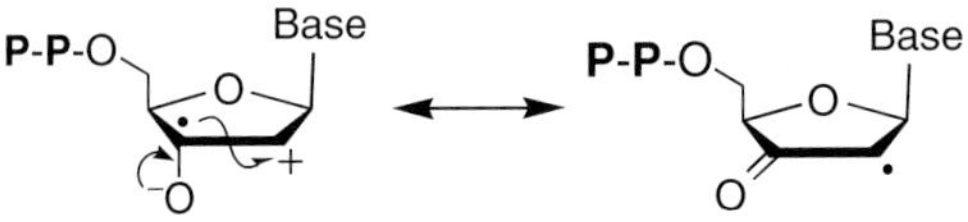

2.2

FIGURE 2.7   Resonance stabilization of radical **2.2**.

enhances its potency because of the key role of iron in RNR. Other promising related inhibitors are hydroxamic acid derivatives such as didox and trimidox.

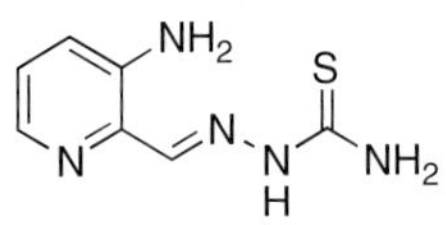

Triapine

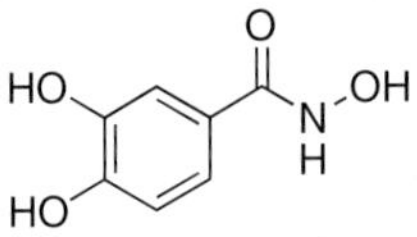

Didox

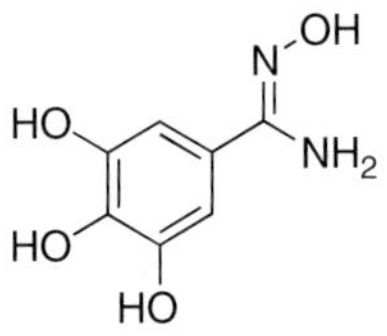

Trimidox

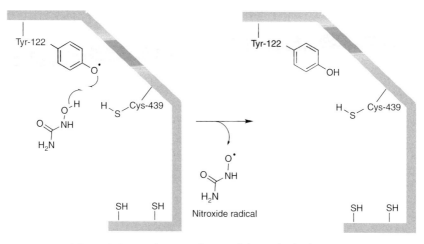

FIGURE 2.8   Mechanism of RNR inhibition by hydroxyurea.

3.3. Substrate analogs as RNR inhibitors

RNR substrate analogs are normally modified at C-2′, which is the position that undergoes reduction in the natural substrate. Many of these compounds bind covalently to the enzyme.

Tezacitabine (fluoromethylenedeoxycytidine, FMdC) is a nucleoside prodrug that shows a dual mechanism of action. Following intracellular phosphorylation, the tezacitabine diphosphate irreversibly inhibits RNR, while the tezacitabine triphosphate can be incorporated into DNA during replication or repair, resulting in DNA chain termination.[9] After initially promising clinical data, analysis of the data from a Phase II trial in patients with gastroesophageal cancer prompted the decision to discontinue further development of tezacitabine.

Tezacitabine (FMdC)

The mechanism of RNR irreversible inhibition by tezacitabine starts by its conversion into tezacitabine diphosphate **2.6**, which, similarly to the natural substrate of the reaction, undergoes H-3′ abstraction by Cys-439, leading to a radical that is stabilized by delocalization onto the adjacent C=C double bond (structure **2.7**). The subsequent evolution of this radical has been studied through theoretical calculations, and the mechanistic pathway that has been proposed to be the major one is summarized in Fig. 2.9.[10] The main steps involved are

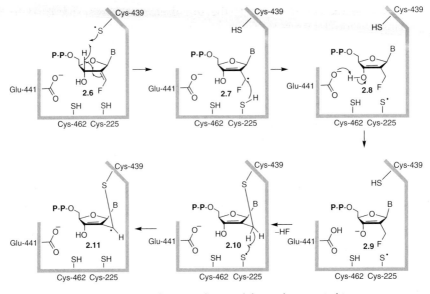

FIGURE 2.9 Mechanism of RNR inhibition by tezacitabine.

abstraction of the Cys-225 mercapto hydrogen by **2.7** to generate **2.8** in which the 3'-OH is deprotonated by Glu-441. The resulting enolate **2.9** evolves through partial protonation of the fluorine atom by Cys-439, which facilitates displacement of HF to give **2.10**. Final abstraction of a hydrogen atom by the Cys-225 radical leads to the proposed final reaction product, the stable radical **2.11**.

Gemcitabine (difluorodeoxycytidine, dFdC) is another nucleoside prodrug that has DNA polymerase inhibition as its primary mechanism of action (see Section 8.1), but it also has some activity as a RNR inhibitor.

NH$_2$

Gemcitabine
(dFdC)

The mechanism of the interaction of gemcitabine diphosphate (**2.12**) with the active site of RNR is very similar to that of the natural substrate, and it only deviates from the natural course after the formation of the bisulfide bridge, as shown by theoretical calculations.[11] The first steps are the abstraction of the 3'-OH proton by the Glu-441 residue and the abstraction of the 3'-H atom by the radical sulfur of Cys-439, leading to anion radical **2.13**. Protonation of the α-fluorine atom by the Cys-225 thiol group facilitates the elimination of a molecule of HF and the formation of radical **2.14**, where the unpaired electron is stabilized by the neighboring carbonyl group and fluorine atom. Transfer of one electron from the Cys-225 anion gives enolate **2.15**, which is protonated by Cys-462 to generate the neutral species **2.16**. The formation of a bisulfide bond and simultaneous transfer of a proton from Glu-441 back to the 3'-O atom leads to radical **2.17**, which on elimination of HF generates the C-2 radical **2.18**. Abstraction of a hydrogen atom from the mercapto group of Cys-439 gives the sulfur radical **2.19**. Although in the natural substrate Cys-439 does not reach the α face of the ribose ring, the conditions in this case are different because **2.19** cannot be stabilized by hydrogen bonds with the active site residues Glu-441 (which are charged) nor with Cys-225 and Cys-462, which are oxidized to a disulfide. This fact, together with possible interactions with the eliminated HF molecules, allows some degree of deviation of the position of the inhibitor, making possible for Cys-439 to reach the 4'-H atom and allowing the generation of the stable radical **2.20** (Fig. 2.10). This prevents the reaction of Cys-439 with Tyr-122 and hence the regeneration of the essential tyrosine radical (see the transformation of **2.4** into **2.5** in Fig. 2.6).

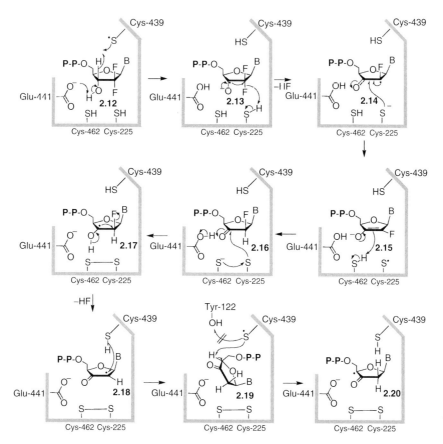

FIGURE 2.10   Mechanism of RNR inhibition by gemcitabine.

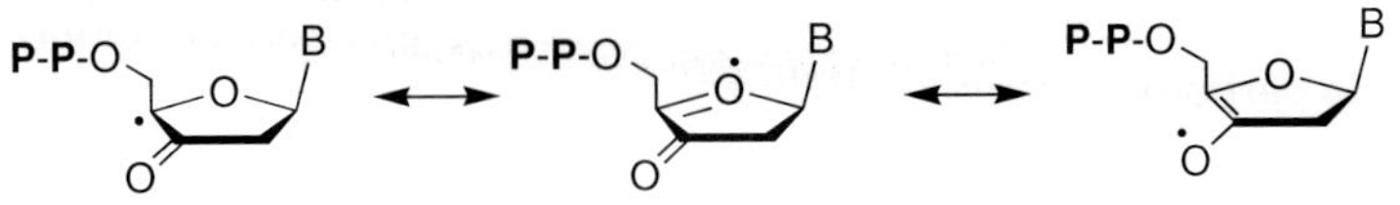

2.20

FIGURE 2.11   Captodative stabilization of radical **2.20**.

The stability of **2.20** is due to the captodative effect of the tetrahydrofuranone oxygen atoms (page 103), since the unpaired electron is adjacent to both an electron-withdrawing and an electron-releasing group (Fig. 2.11).

3.4. Allosteric inhibition of RNR

Therapeutically significant inhibition of RNR can also be achieved through a feedback mechanism by accumulation of deoxyguanosine triphosphate (dGTP) as a consequence of the inhibition of purine nucleoside phosphorylase (PNP), the enzyme that catalyzes the phosphorolysis of the N-ribosidic bonds of purine nucleosides and deoxynucleosides to form purine and α-D-phosphorylated ribosyl products. This inhibition leads to increased blood levels of one of its substrates, deoxyguanosine (dG), which is specifically transported and phosphorylated by T-cell deoxynucleoside kinases. This process leads to pathologically elevated levels of dGTP in these cells, which result in allosteric RNR inhibition (Fig. 2.12). PNP is thus a suitable target for inhibitor development aiming at T-cell immune response modulation, and more specifically in the treatment of relapsed or refractory T-cell lymphoblastic lymphoma, acute leukemia, and T-cell prolymphocytic leukemia.[12]

Immucillin H (forodesine) is a 9-deazanucleoside with a pyrrolidine ring replacing the ribose tetrahydrofuran. It behaves as a very potent inhibitor of PNP because of the analogy of its protonated form with the structure of the transition state, which has oxacarbenium ion character with partial positive charge near C-1'. Immucillin-H has an NH group at N-7 and its charge distribution resembles that of the transition state when N-4' is protonated to the corresponding cation (Fig. 2.13).[13,14]

We will finally mention that some clinically relevant deoxyadenosine derivatives acting primarily as inhibitors of DNA polymerases are also allosteric inhibitors of RNR after their conversion into the corresponding 5'-triphosphates, as will be discussed in Section 8. Therefore, these compounds have a dual action that has been described as "self-potentiation."

4. INHIBITORS OF THE BIOSYNTHESIS OF THYMIDILIC ACID

4.1. Thymidylate synthase

Thymidylate synthase (TS) catalyzes the conversion of deoxyuridine monophosphate (dUMP) to thymidylate (TMP), in a reductive methylation that involves the transfer of a carbon atom from the cofactor 5,10-methylenetetrahydrofolate to the

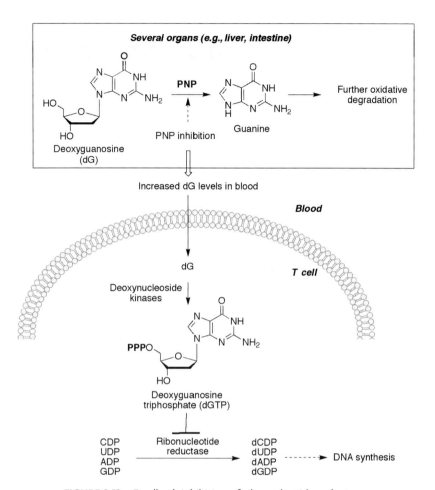

FIGURE 2.12   Feedback inhibition of ribonucleotide reductase.

5 position of the pyrimidine ring. This transformation, that is the only *de novo* source of thymidylate, is part of the so-called thymidylate cycle (Fig. 2.14), where two other enzymes take part, namely serine hydroxymethyl transferase (SHMT) and dihydrofolate reductase (DHFR). SHMT catalyzes the formation of 5,10-methylenetetrahydrofolate from tetrahydrofolate (THF), coupled with the conversion of serine into glycine, with pyridoxal phosphate (PLP) as a cofactor. In the reaction catalyzed by TS, the 5,10-methylene-THF thus formed donates its methylene group to dUMP, being transformed into dihydrofolate (DHF) by a mechanism that will be discussed below (see Fig. 2.15). DHFR finally closes the cycle by reducing DHF to THF. Although methylation of uracil is apparently a small structural change, the extra lipophilicity and bulk associated with the methyl group is essential for the proper discrimination of thymine from the other three bases present in DNA chains by transcription factors, repressors, enhancers, and other DNA-binding proteins.

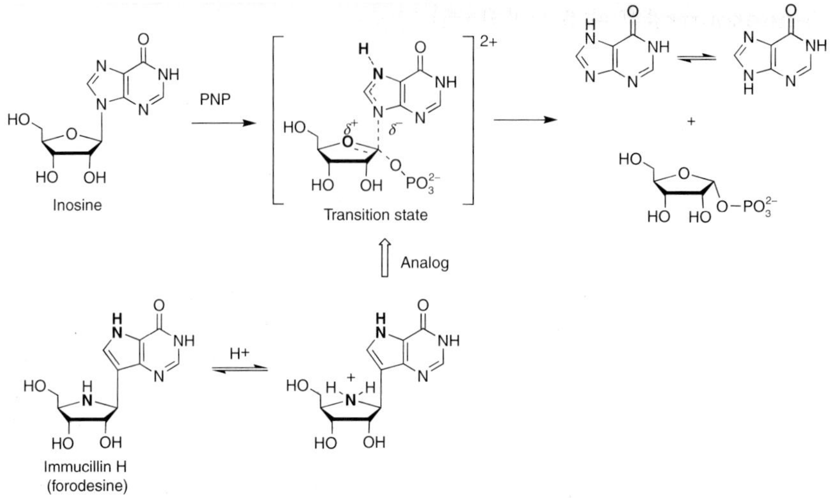

FIGURE 2.13   Mechanism of PNP inhibition by immunocillin H (forodesine).

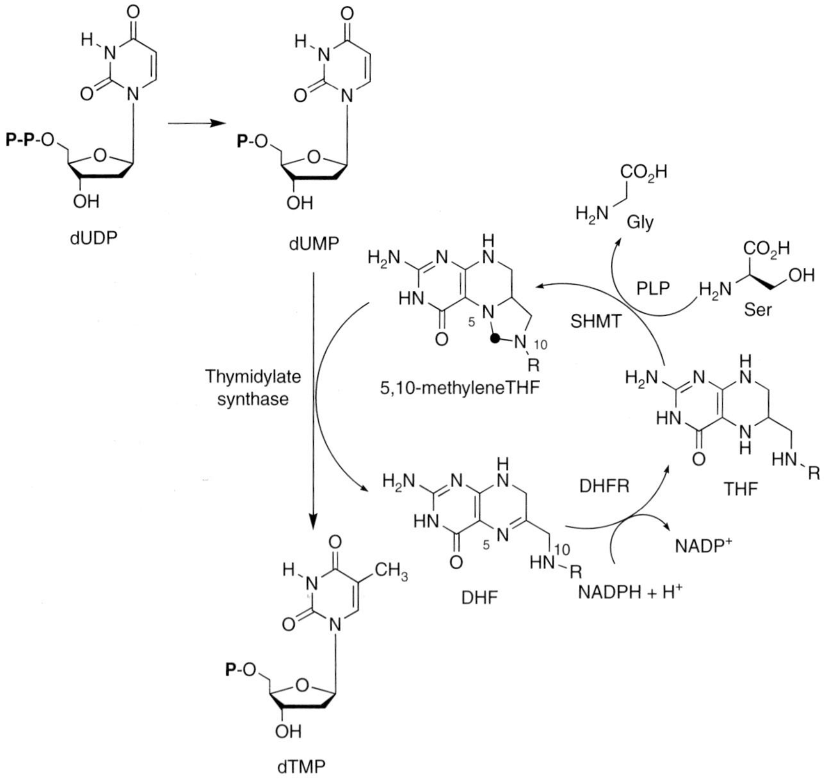

FIGURE 2.14   The thymidylate cycle.

4.2. 5-fluorouracil (5-FU) and floxuridine

The main inhibitors of TS are 5-FU and its deoxynucleoside floxuridine (5-FUdR), and these fluoropyrimidines represent the most widely prescribed class of anti-cancer drugs worldwide.[15] In particular, 5-FU is widely used in the treatment of cancers of the aerodigestive tract, breast, head, and neck, and especially in colo-rectal cancers in combination therapies with oxaliplatin and irinotecan.[16,17] Admi-nistered as a cream, it is also useful for the treatment of some skin cancers. 5-FU was developed in the 1950s following the observation that rat hepatomas utilized uracil at a higher rate than normal tissues, which suggested that uracil metabolism could be a relevant antitumor target. Floxuridine is employed in the treatment of colorectal cancer metastatic to the liver. Because of its nucleoside structure it has a very poor oral bioavailability and is administered in intra-arterial injection.

5-FU is a prodrug that enters the cell using the same facilitated transport mechanism as uracil and is activated to 5-fluoro-2'-deoxyuridine-monophosphate (5-FdUMP) through the complex pathway summarized in Fig. 2.15. Floxuridine

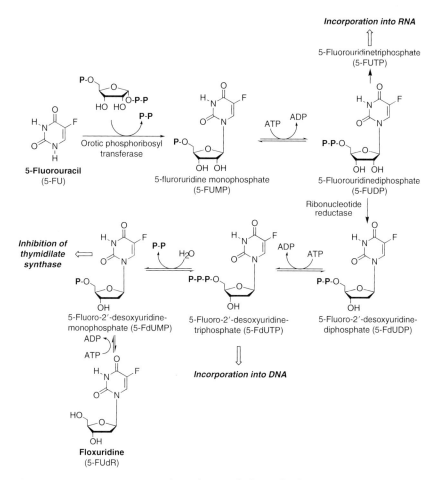

FIGURE 2.15 Antitumor species from the metabolism of 5-fluorouracil and floxuridine.

requires a much simpler bioactivation, consisting of its monophosphorylation. Besides TS inhibition, an additional mechanism that explains the cytotoxic effect of these drugs is based on the misincorporation of their nucleotide and deoxynucleotide triphosphates to RNA and DNA, respectively.

The catalytic cycle of TS involves a two-stage process. Initially, dUMP binds to its recognition site and induces a conformational change that opens an adjacent binding site for the cofactor (5,10-CH$_2$-THF). A cysteine residue in the active site undergoes a Michael addition with the unsaturated carbonyl system in dUMP to give intermediate enolate **2.22**. The nucleophilic attack of this enolate onto the methyleneiminium cation **2.21**, generated from the cofactor, yields the covalent ternary complex **2.23**. An enzyme-catalyzed abstraction of the acidic H-5 proton promotes a β-elimination reaction of a molecule of THF (**2.24**) and generates the methylene intermediate **2.25**. The last step of the sequence involves reduction of **2.25** by hydride transfer from **2.24**, leading to thymidine monophosphate (TMP) and DHF (Fig. 2.16). The overall reaction involves the oxidation of 5,10-methylene-THF to DHF, which must then be recycled by reduction by DHFR and subsequent methylenation, as will be discussed in Section 5.

Fluorine (1.47 Å) and hydrogen (1.20 Å) have very similar van der Waals radii, and this allows 5-FdUMP to bind to TS in the same site and with the same affinity

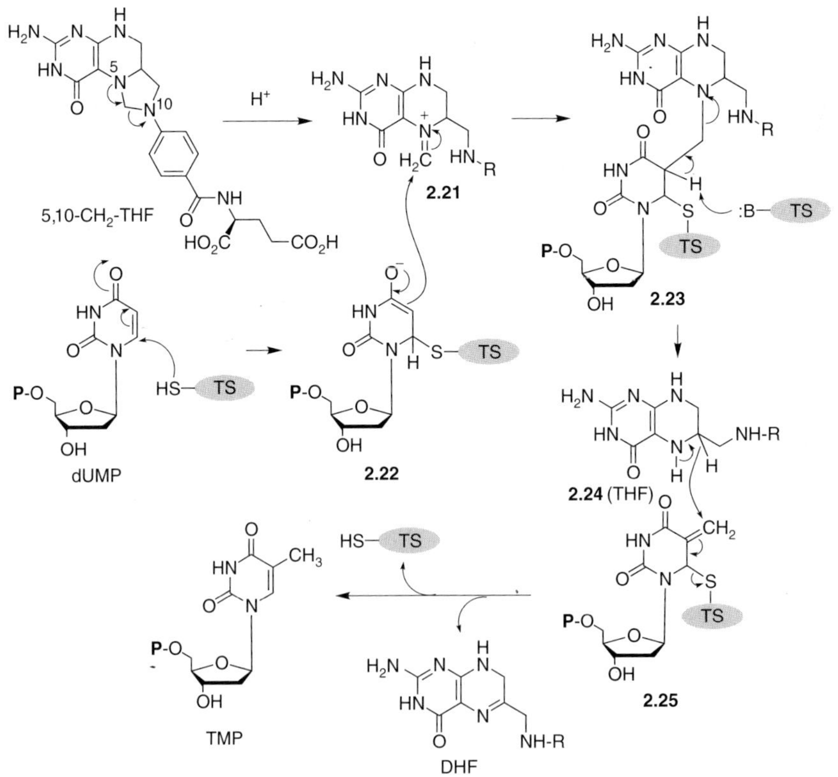

FIGURE 2.16   Catalytic cycle of thymidylate synthase.

as dUMP. The strong electron-withdrawing effect of the fluorine atom increases the electrophilicity of the unsaturated carbonyl system and facilitates the formation of **2.26**, but the final β-elimination reaction is not possible due to the presence of the fluorine atom at C-5 and therefore the ternary complex **2.27** is stable (Fig. 2.17). Because of the need for an activation step by nucleophilic attack of a cysteine residue of TS prior to enzyme inhibition, 5-FdUMP can be considered as a suicide inhibitor.

TS inhibition leads to depletion of TMP and subsequent depletion of dTTP, which induces alterations in the levels of other deoxynucleotides through various feedback mechanisms. These imbalances result in an alteration of the dATP/TTP ratio, among others, which disrupts DNA synthesis and repair and leads to the so-called thymineless death.[18] A cytotoxicity mechanism alternative to TS inhibition is based on the generation of 5-fluoro-2′-deoxyuridine-triphosphate (5-FdUTP), which acts as a false substrate of DNA polymerase and is misincorporated into DNA. As a consequence of the accumulation of dUMP after TS inhibition, dUTP can also be generated and incorporated into DNA. Ultimately this change halts DNA synthesis and promotes DNA fragmentation by repair enzymes. Similarly, transformation of 5-FUDP, a metabolite of 5-FU, into the corresponding triphosphate allows the misincorporation of fluoronucleotides into RNA, leading to profound effects on cell metabolism and viability. Both TS inhibition and misincorporation of 5-FU metabolites in DNA result in the stabilization of p53, a tumor suppressor that maintains DNA integrity by activating genes that arrest cell cycle in response to DNA damage or trigger apoptosis (Fig. 2.18). *In vitro* studies have proved that loss of p53 function is associated to a reduced sensitivity to 5-FU.[19]

The clinical efficacy of 5-FU may be decreased by several mechanisms, the first of which is diminished incorporation of 5-FUTP into RNA as a consequence of competition from high intracellular levels of UTP. On the contrary, the formation

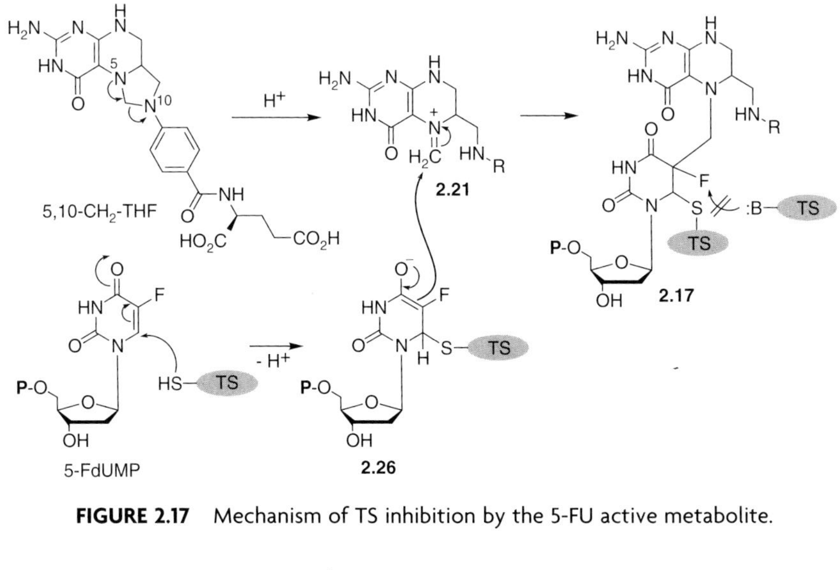

FIGURE 2.17 Mechanism of TS inhibition by the 5-FU active metabolite.

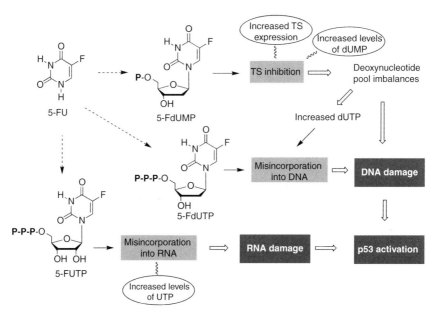

FIGURE 2.18 Mechanisms of the antitumor action of 5-FU.

of the ternary TS-FdUMP-CH_2-THF complex induces TS expression due to the inhibition of a negative feedback mechanism whereby TS binds to its own mRNA and inhibits the translation process. The ternary complex is not able to bind to this mRNA, leading to increased expression of TS and constituting a possible resistance mechanism. Finally, TS inhibition leads to an increase in intracellular dUMP pools, which eventually compete with 5-FdUMP for binding with TS.

4.3. 5-FU prodrugs

5-FU requires intravenous administration, and a number of oral prodrugs have been designed to circumvent this limitation. One of them is ftorafur (tegafur), which is completely absorbed in the gastrointestinal tract and metabolized to 5-FU through two major pathways. The first of them involves microsomal hydroxylation of the C-5′ position of the tetrahydrofuran moiety by cytochrome P450, followed by spontaneous decomposition to 5-FU and succinic aldehyde. An hydrolytic pathway due to cytosolic hydrolases (pyrimidine nucleoside phosphorylase) is also possible, giving 5-FU and 2-tetrahydrofuryl phosphate (Fig. 2.19). Ftorafur was introduced in the clinic in 1967 and showed a significant antitumor response. However, due to severe digestive and cardiac toxicities, it was soon replaced by its combinations with several other enzyme inhibitors, especially UFT and S-1 (see Sections 4.4.1 and 4.4.3).

The levels of the hydrolytic enzyme thymidine phosphorylase (TP) are significantly higher in several solid tumors, such as colorectal, breast, and kidney cancers, compared with normal tissues. This led to assay doxifluridine

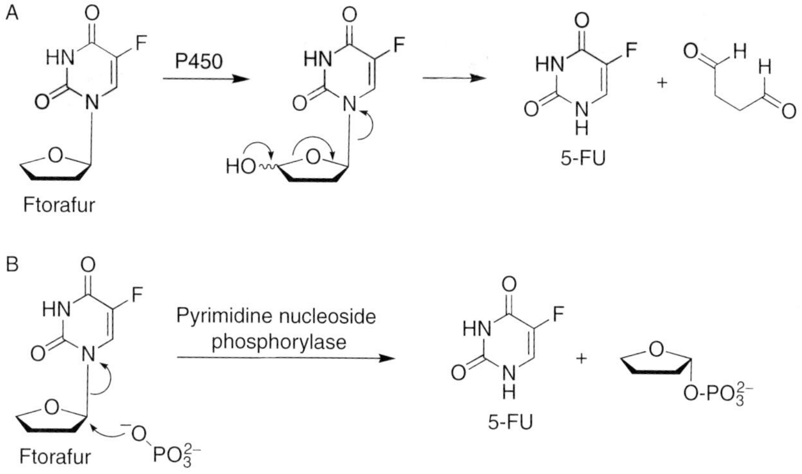

FIGURE 2.19   Bioactivation of ftorafur.

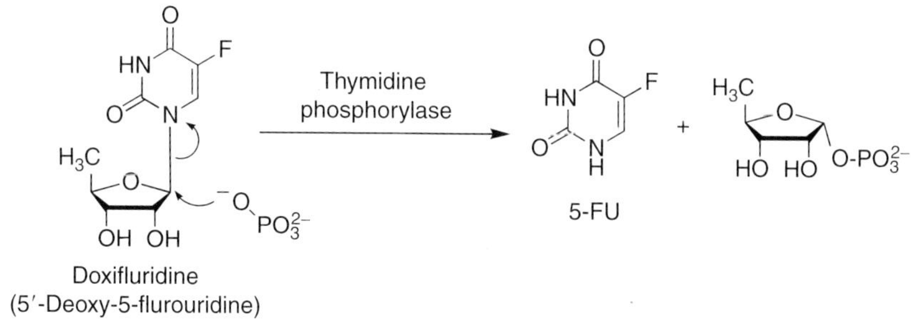

FIGURE 2.20   Bioactivation of doxifluridine.

(5′-deoxy-5-fluorouridine) as a 5-FU prodrug, but this compound showed gastro-intestinal toxicity (diarrhea) after oral administration due to release of 5-FU by intestinal pyrimidine nucleoside phosphorylase (Fig. 2.20). It is worth mentioning that because TP is identical to PDGF (platelet-derived endothelial cell growth factor) and is believed to have angiogenic properties, it is currently being considered as a new cancer target.[20]

Efforts to circumvent the problem of gastric toxicity led to the development of capecitabine as a multiple prodrug, designed to be activated specifically in tumor cells by a three-enzyme cascade process. Because of the increased lipophilicity associated to the presence of the pentyloxycarbonyl chain, this prodrug is rapidly absorbed unaltered after oral administration and metabolyzed by carboxylesterase in the liver to 5′-deoxy-5-fluorocytidine. Subsequent activation steps include deamination by cytidine deaminase and finally transformation into 5-FU by TP (Fig. 2.21). The last step takes place up to 10 times more efficiently in cancer cells than in normal cells, leading to selective delivery of 5-FU into the tumors. In fact, pharmacokinetic data indicate a low systemic exposure to 5-FU and

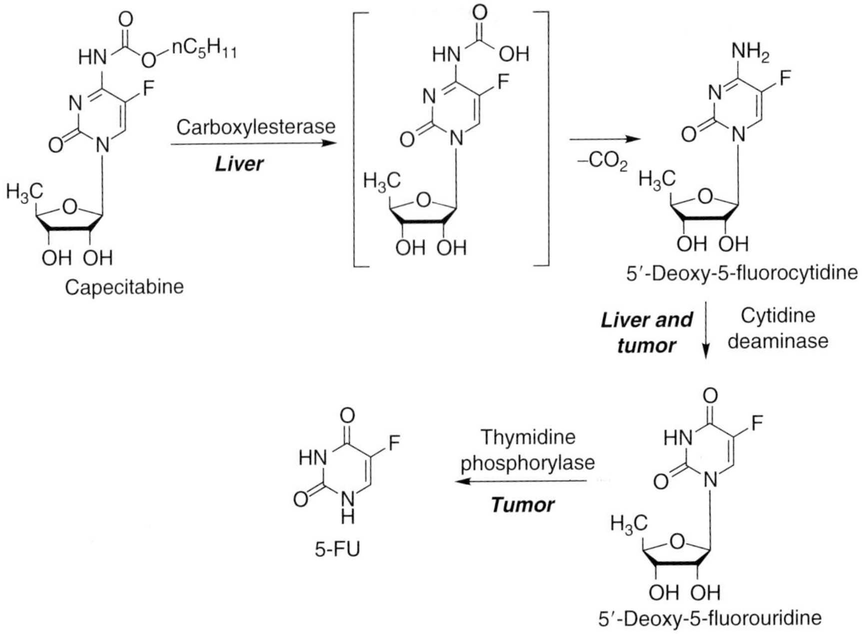

FIGURE 2.21 Bioactivation of capecitabine.

intratumor concentrations of this compound higher than those achieved by administration of equitoxic doses of 5-FU. Capecitabine is indicated as first-line treatment of patients with metastatic colorectal carcinoma when treatment with fluoropyrimidine therapy alone is preferred, and also in combination chemotherapy. Several anticancer drugs such as paclitaxel, docetaxel, and cyclophosphamide enhance the level of TP, facilitating the generation of 5-FU from capecitabine. The combination of capecitabine and some of these drugs (e.g., docetaxel) is under clinical trials for the treatment of patients with metastatic breast cancer after failure of prior anthracycline-containing chemotherapy.[21]

Emitefur is another orally active 5-FU prodrug that avoids high-peak 5-FU levels and decreases the accumulation of toxic metabolites. It is in clinical trials for colorectal cancer.[22]

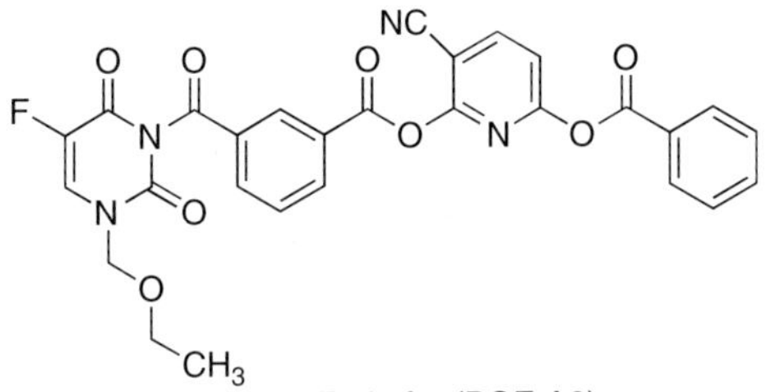

Emitefur (BOF-A2)

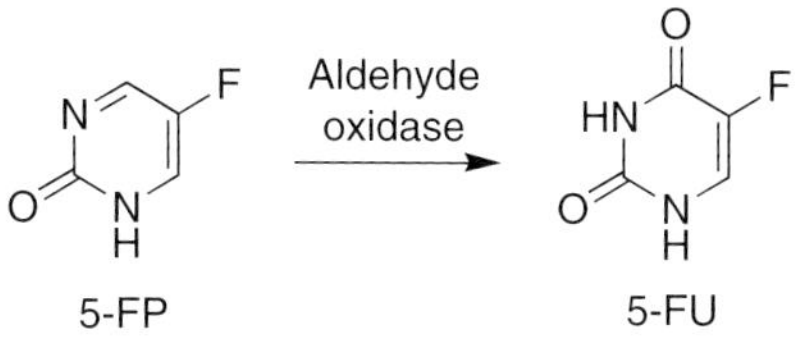

FIGURE 2.22   Bioactivation of 5-FP.

Another prodrug of 5-FU is 5-fluoro-2-pyrimidinone (5-FP), which is activated by hepatic aldehyde oxidase after oral or intravenous administration (Fig. 2.22).

4.4. Modulation of 5-FU activity

Great efforts have been made to modulate the activity of 5-FU, which have focused on (1) decreasing its degradation, (2) enhancing its potency as a TS inhibitor, and (3) increasing 5-FU activation.

4.4.1. Decreased degradation of 5-FU

More than 80% of administered drug is degraded in the liver by dihydropyrimidine dehydrogenase (DPD), which reduces the pyrimidine double bond of 5-FU to give dihydrofluorouracil (DHFU).[23] This metabolite is inactive because it cannot give the initial Michael addition with the nucleophilic site of the active center in TS (Fig. 2.23).

Two different approaches have been developed to improve the biostability of 5-FU. The first of them consists in the coadministration of a large amount of uracil, which saturates the DPD enzyme because uracil is its natural substrate; for instance, the formulation known as UFT uses a 4:1 combination of uracil and the

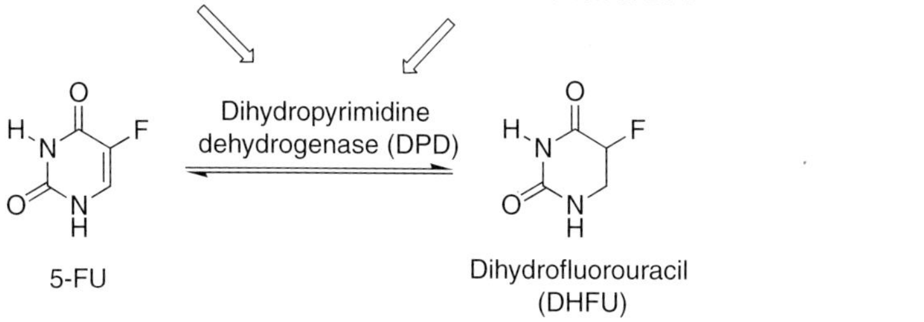

Saturation of DPD by coadministration of uracil

Eniluracil

5-Chloro-2,4-dihydroxy-pyridine (CDHP, gimestat)

Inhibition of DPD

Dihydropyrimidine dehydrogenase (DPD)

5-FU

Dihydrofluorouracil (DHFU)

FIGURE 2.23   Approaches to a decreased degradation of 5-FU.

5-FU prodrug ftorafur.[24] Alternatively, the coadministration of 5-FU with DPD inhibitors, such as 5-chloro-2,4-dihydroxypyridine (CDHP, gimestat) and eniluracil (5-ethynyluracil),[25] is being investigated, as well as the use of the UFT combination plus DPD inhibitors.[26] Eniluracil has received FDA orphan drug designation for its use in combination with fluoropyrimidines in the treatment of hepatocellular cancer.

4.4.2. Enhancement of the inhibition of TS by 5-FU

The action of TS requires the presence of 5,10-methylene-THF, and for this reason the coadministration of precursors of this cofactor increases the cytotoxicity of 5-FU in many cancer cell lines. For instance, the combination of 5-FU or ftorafur with leucovorin (LV, 5-formyl-THF) gave superior response rates than the single agents, and particularly the use of leucovorin to modulate UFT leads to a three-component combination called orzel that has been proposed as first-line chemotherapy of colorectal cancer.[27] Leucovorin enters the cell via the reduced folate carrier (RFC) and is metabolized to 5,10-methylene-THF, without requiring the participation of DHFR, by cyclization to 5,10-methynyl-THF followed by NADP-mediated reduction of the iminium function (Fig. 2.24).

4.4.3. Enhancement of 5-FU activation

It has been proposed that pretreatment with methotrexate (MTX), an antifolate agent, enhances the activity of 5-FU[28] because MTX inhibits the biosynthesis of tetrahydrofolic acid (THF), which is necessary for some steps of purine biosynthesis (see Section 6). This leads to accumulation of PRPP, essential for the activation of 5-FU, even though the levels of the TS cofactor should also be

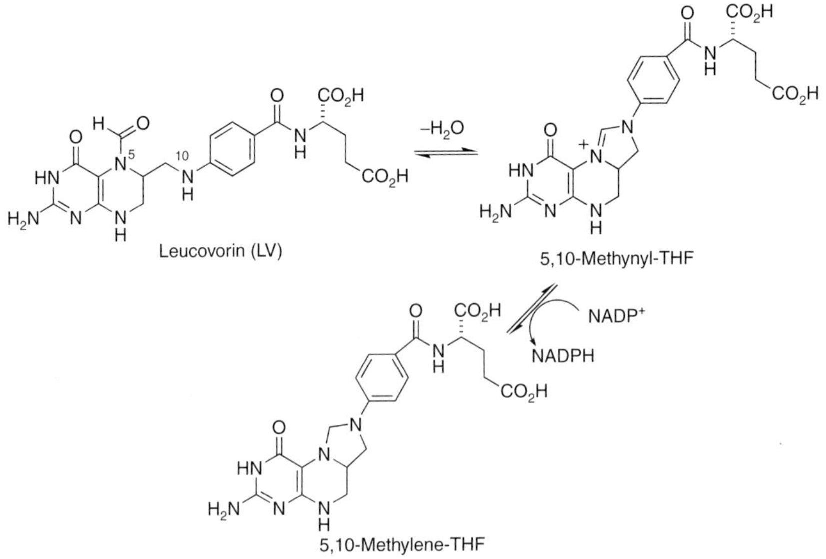

FIGURE 2.24   Biotransformation of leucovorin into 5,10-methylene-THF.

diminished (see Section 4.4.2). Clinically, this combination has not always shown increased antitumor activity.[29] On the contrary, several Phase II studies have shown a modest clinical benefit of 5-FU modulation utilizing MTX and leucovorin in patients with metastatic colorectal cancer.[30]

Diarrhea is the most common dose-limiting toxicity associated to prolonged infusion of 5-FU. In order to prevent this gastrointestinal toxicity, some oral formulations have been proposed that contain oxonic acid, a potent inhibitor of the phosphoriboxylation of 5-FU in the gastrointestinal mucosa. One of these formulations is S-1, which contains ftorafur, oxonic acid, and the previously mentioned gimestat (CDHP), an inhibitor of DPD (see Section 4.4.1).[31] The basis for some of these combinations is summarized in Fig. 2.25.

4.5. Folate-Based TS inhibitors

As previously mentioned, TS inhibition by the fluoropyrimidines is not specific because of the effect of fluorinated nucleotides on other pathways, especially related to RNA (Figs. 2.15 and 2.18). Also, the accumulated dUMP may compete with the antitumor drug for TS. For this reason, there has been much interest in the design of inhibitors that recognize the folate-binding site of TS, which should not have these shortcomings and thus behave as specific TS inhibitors. Four of them (raltitrexed, pemetrexed, ZD-9331, and nolatrexed) have reached therapeutic use

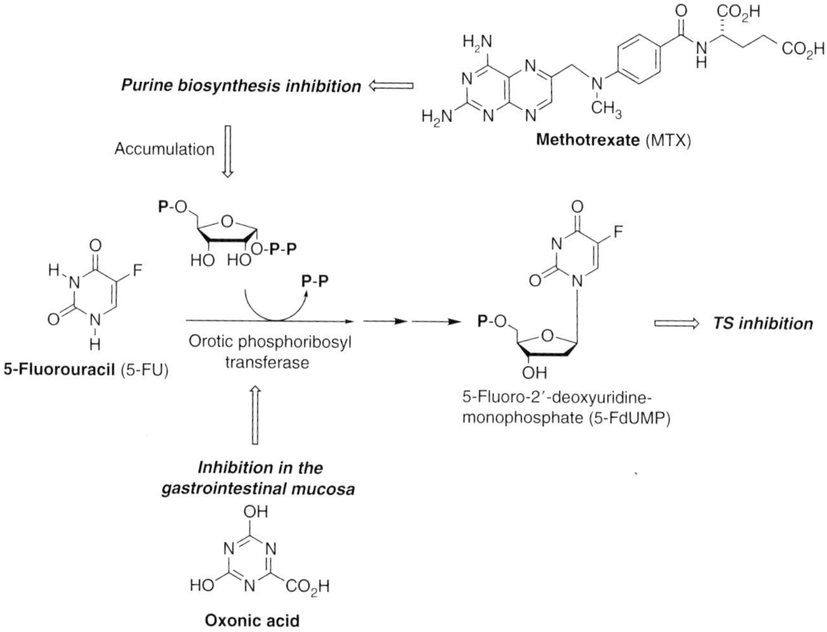

FIGURE 2.25   Strategies to enhance 5-FU activation.

or are under advanced clinical evaluation. These compounds have been designed by manipulation of the folic acid structure.

Folic acid

Raltitrexed

Pemetrexed

ZD 9331

Nolatrexed

Raltitrexed (TOM) was the first specific TS inhibitor to be approved for clinical use, and it is employed for advanced colorectal cancer. Its structure contains two classical bioisosteric modifications, namely replacement of the pteridine ring of folate by a quinazoline unit and replacement of the benzene ring of folate by a thiophene. This drug is transported into the cells by the reduced folate carrier (RFC), and its terminal glutamate residue is converted into a polyglutamate by folylpolyglutamate synthetase (FPGS). The polyglutamate form is more potent as an enzyme inhibitor and it is retained intracellularly, leading to a prolonged action (Fig. 2.26). A related TS inhibitor is pemetrexed (alimta, LY-231514), which also inhibits several other folate-related enzymes and will be discussed in Section 6.2.

ZD-9331 is also a potent inhibitor of TS that is under advanced clinical evaluation[32] and differs from the previously mentioned compounds in several respects. One of them is the presence of a methyl group at C-7, which was designed from X-ray diffraction studies of TS that suggested that a 7-alkyl group would contribute to binding. Another difference is the 2'-fluorine substituent that also increased activity. One final interesting feature of ZD-9331 is the isosteric γ-carboxyl-tetrazole replacement at the glutamic portion which prevents polyglutamation. Because this drug is active against TS in a non-polyglutamated form, it has the advantage over previously mentioned folate-based TS inhibitors of not being subject to resistance by FPGS downregulation.

Nolatrexed (thymitaq, AG-337) is the inhibitor structurally least related to folate. It crosses the cell membrane by passive diffusion rather than using the RFC and, since it is not retained inside the cells because it cannot be polygluta-mated, it requires a prolonged infusion (see Section 5.2). Phase II clinical trials

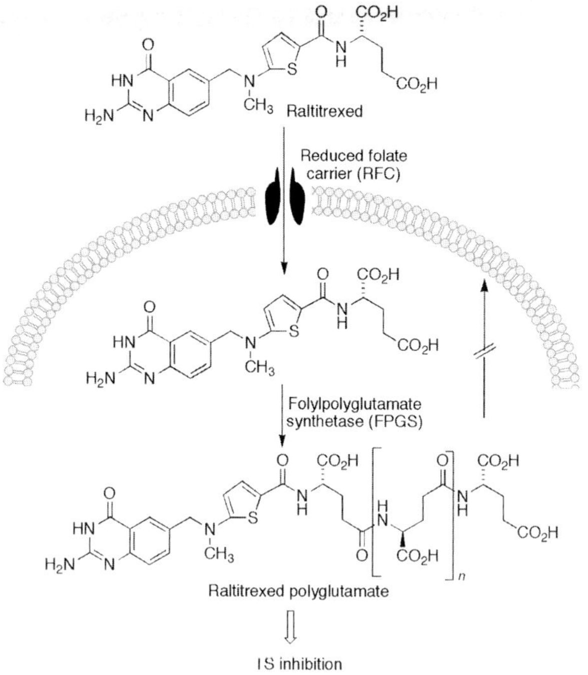

FIGURE 2.26   Active transport and polyglutamation of raltitrexed.

showed activity in patients with hepatocellular carcinoma, head and neck cancer,[33] and adenocarcinoma of the pancreas.

The RFC is ubiquitous and is expressed in normal tissues, leading to increased toxicity of antifolate drugs. Another related membrane transporter is the α-isoform of the membrane folate receptor (MFR, α-FR), which has the advantage of being overexpressed in some tumors. For this reason, it is expected that TS inhibitors with MFR/RFC selectivity will be better tolerated.[34] One of these compounds is CB-300638, which was designed on the basis of the crystal structures of inhibitors bound to TS[35] and has shown promising preclinical data. This compound contains two glutamate units and cannot be further glutamated because of the unnatural *R* configuration at the α carbon of the second residue.[36]

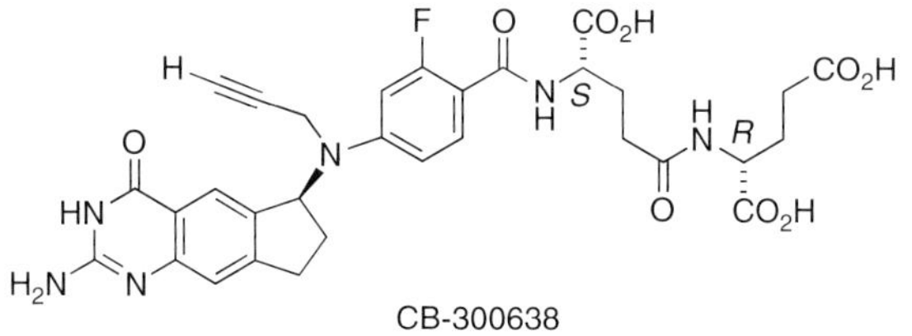

CB-300638

5. INHIBITORS OF DIHYDROFOLATE REDUCTASE (DHFR)

Folic acid and its metabolites (collectively known as folates) are coenzymes of many essential biochemical transformations. Most importantly, they are involved in the previously mentioned transfer of one carbon unit in the *de novo* synthesis of thymidylic acid and purine nucleotides. Folate-dependent enzymes are obvious targets for cancer chemotherapy, but until 1980 only DHFR was exploited in this regard and in fact it was the first enzyme to be targeted for cancer chemotherapy.

In mammals, folic acid is taken with the diet and reduced to THF by dihydro-folic reductase in two stages, using NADPH as a cofactor. Further transformations of THF lead to 5,10-methylene-THF, 5,10-methenyl-THF, 5-formyl-THF, and 10-formyl-THF (Fig. 2.27), which are known as folinic acids and are involved in the transfer of one carbon units. DHFR inhibition leads to cell death due to the essential role of folinic acids in the synthesis of thymidylate and purine bases.

DHFR is a relatively small protein with a large active site in which DHF binds adjacent to the cofactor, NADPH, in a pocket buried deep within the enzyme.

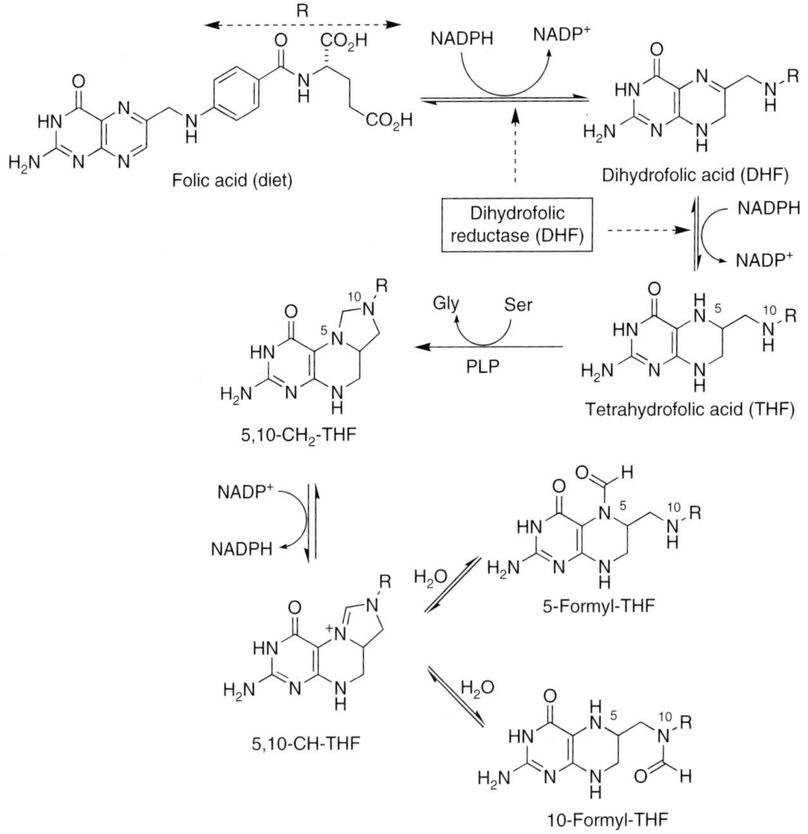

FIGURE 2.27   Biotransformation of folic acid into folinic acids.

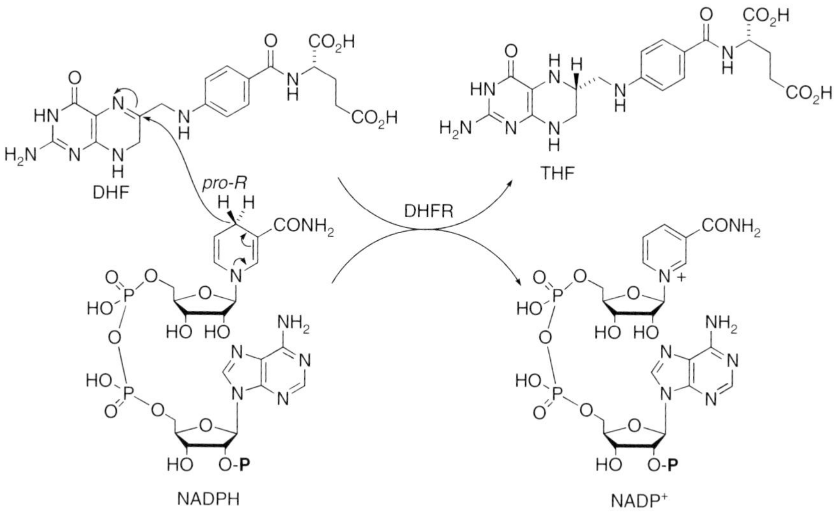

FIGURE 2.28 Reaction catalyzed by DHFR.

It catalyzes the transfer of the *pro-R* hydrogen of the C-4 position of the dihydropyridine ring in the cofactor onto the C=N double bonds of folic acid and dihydrofolic acid (Fig. 2.28).

The most potent inhibitors of DHFR are folic acid analogs that differ from the natural ligand in that they bear a 2,4-diaminopyrimidine unit, as exemplified by aminopterin (AM) and methotrexate (MTX, amethopterin). The inhibitors in which the side chain ends in a glutamic acid residue, as in folic acid, are known as classical antifolates. Other inhibitors with lipophilic substituents are known as nonclassical antifolates.

R = H   Aminopterin (AM)
R = CH$_3$ Methotrexate (MTX)

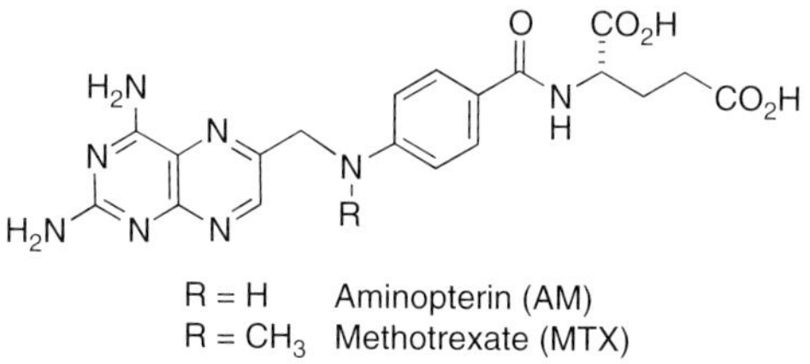

5.1. Classical DHFR inhibitors

MTX and AM were designed by replacing an OH group at C-4 of the natural substrate (DHF) by an amino group. The implicit assumption was that the two ligands would bind similarly and that the 4-amino group of MTX would go to the position in the binding site normally occupied by the DHF oxygen. However, when X-ray diffraction structures of DHFR with DHF and MTX were obtained, different binding modes were observed, with the aminopteridine ring of MTX flipped 180° about the C$_6$–CH$_2$NHR bond in regard to that of DHF (Fig. 2.29).

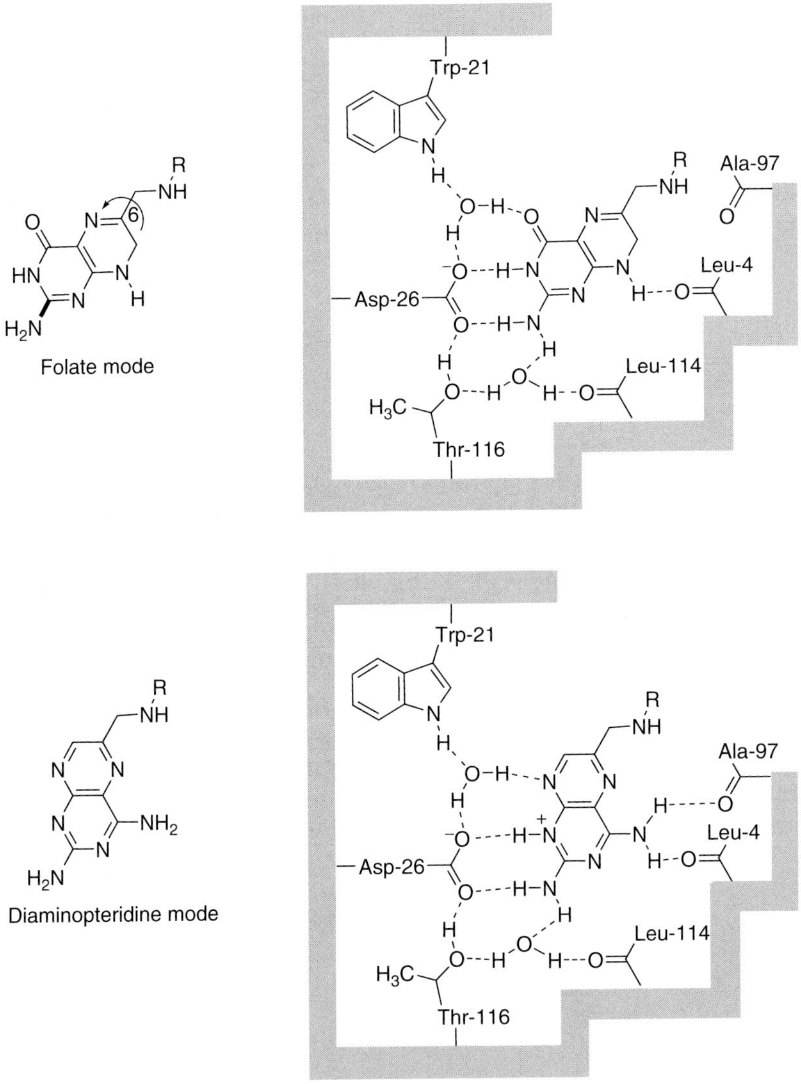

FIGURE 2.29 Binding modes of dihydrofolate and aminopterine to DHFR.

Both ligands bind to the DHFR active site by hydrogen bonds and by additional interactions with bridging water molecules. MTX is about 3 pK_a units more basic than folic acid because it contains an electron-releasing amino group conjugated with the basic guanidine fragment instead of an electron-withdrawing carbonyl, and therefore binds in a protonated state. The electrostatic interaction and an additional hydrogen bond involving the 4-amino group lead to a binding about 10^3 times stronger than that of folate.[37] The binding of MTX to DHFR is dependent on the presence of the NADPH cofactor, and is an example of a type of enzyme inhibition known as slow, tight-binding inhibition.[38] The selective toxicity of MTX in malignant cells with regard to normal ones seems to be partly due to differences in the ratio of NADPH to NADP and NADH in both types of cells.[39]

AM was the first antifolate to be introduced in cancer therapeutics, but it was soon shown that MTX is less toxic and has superior pharmacokinetic properties, and this compound is now the only classical antifolate in clinical use for the treatment of choriocarcinoma, non-Hodgkin's lymphoma and acute lymphocytic leukemia, and also in many combination regimens. Its main side effects are myelosuppression and damage to the gastrointestinal tract, kidneys, and liver. In order to partly alleviate its bone marrow toxicity, MTX is often associated with the calcium salt of leucovorin (N^5-formyltetrahydrofolic acid), one of the folinic acids. As previously mentioned (see Fig. 2.24), leucovorin enters the cell via the RFC and is metabolized to 5,10-methylene-THF without requiring the participation of DHFR thus bypassing its blockade (Fig. 2.30).

Other uses of MTX include the treatment of severe psoriasis and adult rheumatoid arthritis, being the most widely prescribed disease-modifying anti-rheumatic drug. Recently, MTX has been shown to be effective in inducing abortion due to its ability to kill the rapidly growing cells of the placenta.

MTX enters the cells via the RFC and is polyglutamated by FPGS, thereby increasing intracellular retention. Decreased polyglutamation is observed in normal versus malignant cells, which can partly explain the selectivity of MTX for malignant tissue. MTX polyglutamates also inhibit other folate-related enzymes, including TS and also GARFT and AICARFT, two transformylases that participate in the purine *de novo* biosynthesis (Section 6).

Besides MTX and AM, 10-alkyl-10-deaza folate analogs are also classical DHFR inhibitors. These compounds were developed on the basis of the observation that the transport mechanism for normal proliferative tissue such as intestinal epithelium distinguishes AM from its N-alkyl derivative MTX, leading to higher levels of AM in the normal proliferative tissue and hence to increased toxicity. The main compounds

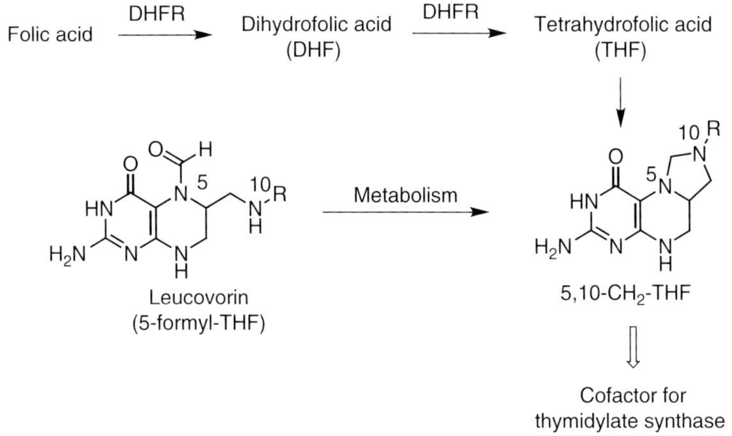

FIGURE 2.30 Bypass of DHFR inhibition by leucovorin.

are 10-ethyl-10-deazaaminopterin (edatrexate) and 10-propargyl-10-deazaaminop-terin (PDX), which are under clinical investigation.[40,41]

R = CH$_2$CH$_3$ Edatrexate
R = CH$_2$-C≡CH   PDX

5.2. Nonclassical (lipophilic) DHFR inhibitors

Suppression of the glutamic chain leads to compounds that are not substrates for the folate active transport systems, and enter the cells by passive diffusion. They have the advantage of being active in cancer cells resistant to MTX because of transport defects. On the contrary, the lack of the glutamic acid side chain prevents polyglutamation and therefore these compounds are not retained within the cells and require more prolonged treatments. Among these compounds, trimetrexate is mainly used to treat pneumonias by *Pneumocystis carinii* and *Toxoplasma gondii*, although it is also used in the treatment of certain cancers, including colon cancer.[42] Piritrexim is being assayed for similar applications, including the treatment of psoriasis, pneumonia, and several cancers.[43]

Trimetrexate   Piretrexim

6. INHIBITORS OF THE *DE NOVO* PURINE BIOSYNTHESIS PATHWAY

In contrast to pyrimidine nucleotide biosynthesis, where a preformed heterocyclic moiety is attached to PRPP, in the case of purine nucleotides the purine ring is constructed gradually. The complete route comprises 10 steps, and is summarized in Fig. 2.31. This *de novo* pathway leads to the formation of inosine monopho-sphate (IMP), the precursor of ATP, GTP, dATP, and dGTP necessary for RNA and DNA formation. Only the steps most relevant to antitumor drug action will be treated in the discussion below.

6.1. Inhibitors of phosphoribosylpyrophosphate (PRPP) amidotransferase

The first irreversible step in the *de novo* purine biosynthesis involves the nucleo-philic displacement of the pyrophosphate group of phosphoribosylpyropho-sphate (PRPP) by a molecule of ammonia, generated by hydrolysis of glutamine to glutamic acid. Both reactions are catalyzed by PRPP amidotransferase, whose

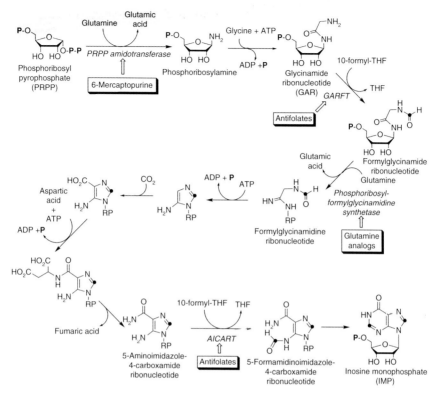

FIGURE 2.31 Biosynthesis of purine nucleotides.

main inhibitors are thiopurines (e.g., 6-mercaptopurine, MP), acting through feedback mechanisms. These antitumor drugs have a complex mechanism of action, involving the inhibition of several enzymes related to purine biosynthesis and misincorporation into nucleic acids, and will be studied in Section 6.5.

6.2. Inhibitors of glycinamide ribonucleotide formyltransferase (GARFT)

The third reaction in the *de novo* purine biosynthesis is the transformation of glycinamide ribonucleotide (GAR) into its formylderivative (FGAR) using 10-formyl-THF as the formyl donor (Fig. 2.32). The enzyme that catalyzes this step is known as glycinamide ribonucleotide formyltransferase (GARFT). In mammals, this enzyme is multifunctional and it also catalyzes the second and fifth steps of the pathway.

The first selective and sufficiently potent GARFT inhibitor was lometrexol, designed as a folate analog lacking the 5 and 10 nitrogen atoms and therefore unable to participate in the transfer of single carbon units.[44] On the contrary, lometrexol has a 2-aminopyrimidin-4-one subunit identical to that found in the THF cofactor, and therefore different from the 2,4-diaminopyrimidine pattern

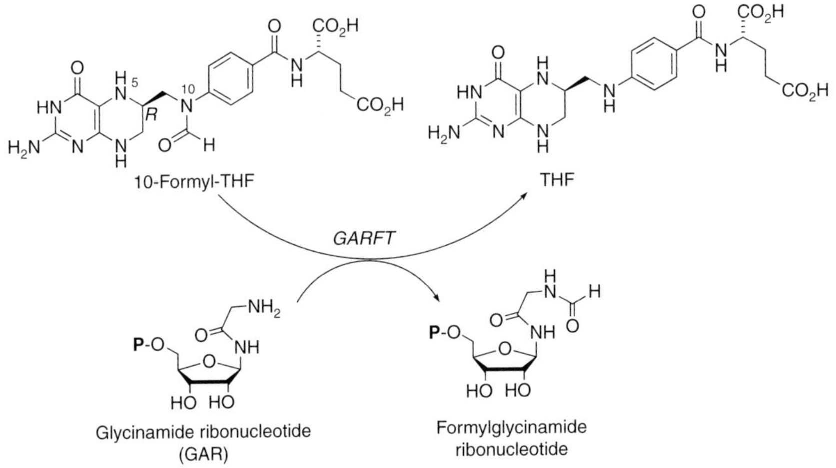

FIGURE 2.32   Reaction catalyzed by GARFT.

commonly present in DHFR inhibitors. Its glutamate side chain allows its ready transport into cells by means of the RFC and MFR as transport systems, and also its polyglutamation by folylpolyglutamate synthase (FPGS). Lometrexol was investigated clinically, but unexpected observations of delayed cumulative toxicity[45] prompted a search for second-generation antimetabolites with a more favorable profile (Fig. 2.33). Some of these compounds are LY-309887, an analog of lometrexol designed by benzene-thiophene bioisosteric replacement with a nine-fold greater potency as a GARFT inhibitor, and AG-2037, an analog with the opposite configuration at C-6. Besides being well tolerated, the latter compound shows an interesting synergism with 5-FU and is being studied in Phase II in patients with metastatic adenocarcinoma of the colon or rectum that failed prior fluorouracil and leucovorin calcium therapies.[46]

Pemetrexed (alimta, MTA, LY-231514) was discovered during structure–activity studies of lometrexol by removal of the C-5 carbon atom and concomitant replacement of the ring fused to the quinazolinone unit by an indole, leading to loss of stereochemical information at C-6. It employs the RFC for entering the cells, and its polyglutamation product inhibits multiple targets in the folate pathway, including TS, DHFR, and two enzymes from the *de novo* synthesis of purines, namely GARFT and aminoimidazolecarboxamide ribonucleotide formyltransferase (AICARFT). This complex mechanism of action has led to its designation as MTA (multitargeted antifolate). Pemetrexed has been approved for the treatment of malignant pleural mesothelioma in association with cisplatin, and as second-line treatment of non-small cell lung cancer.[47] The interaction of pemetrexed with DHFR has been studied based on molecular modeling and NMR studies that suggest that it can bind to the enzyme in a "2,4-diaminopteridine mode," where the pyrrole nitrogen mimics the 4-amino group of MTX. Replacement of the 4-oxo group by a methyl (AAG 113–161) led to a further increase in activity, explained by a hydrophobic interaction of the 4-methyl with Phe-31 and Leu-22.[48]

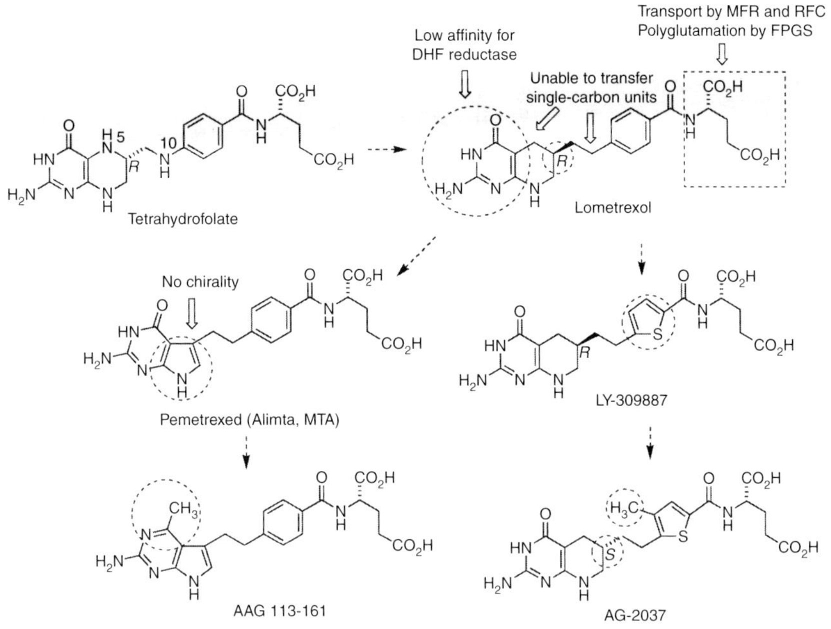

FIGURE 2.33   Representative GARFT inhibitors.

A summary of the main targets for antifolate drugs and their relationships with nucleic acid biosynthesis is given in Fig. 2.34.

6.3. Inhibitors of phosphoribosylformylglycinamidine synthetase

This enzyme catalyzes the reaction of formylglycinamide ribonucleotide with ammonia to give formylglycinamidine ribonucleotide, with glutamine as a cofactor. The enzyme activates the amide group adjacent to the ribose ring to nucleophilic attack by its transformation into iminoether **2.28**. In addition, another catalytic site of the enzyme hydrolyzes glutamine to glutamic acid and ammonia, which is then channeled to the first site and reacts with **2.28** by an addition–elimination mechanism, affording the amidine **2.29** (formylglycinamidine ribonucleotide) (Fig. 2.35).

Some analogs of glutamine bearing a diazomethyl moiety have antitumor activity because of their ability to inhibit several reactions in which glutamine is involved as a cofactor, specially the one catalyzed by formylglycinamidine ribonucleotide synthetase. Azaserine (*O*-diazoacetyl-L-serine) and 6-diazo-5-oxo-L-norleucine (DON) are two antitumor natural products, isolated from *Streptomyces* broths that act as covalent inhibitors of the enzyme. Reversible attachment using the binding points normally employed by the cofactor glutamine positions the diazomethyl group close to a cysteine sulfhydryl group in the active site. After protonation, this unit is transformed into a diazonium group, which covalently links to the cysteine thiol group (Fig. 2.36). Clinical trials have shown good

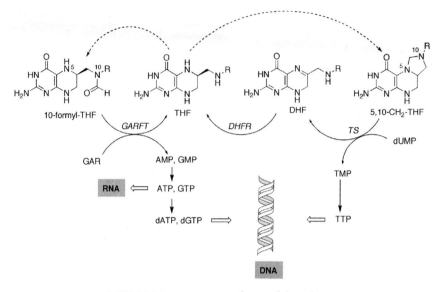

FIGURE 2.34   Main targets for antifolate drugs.

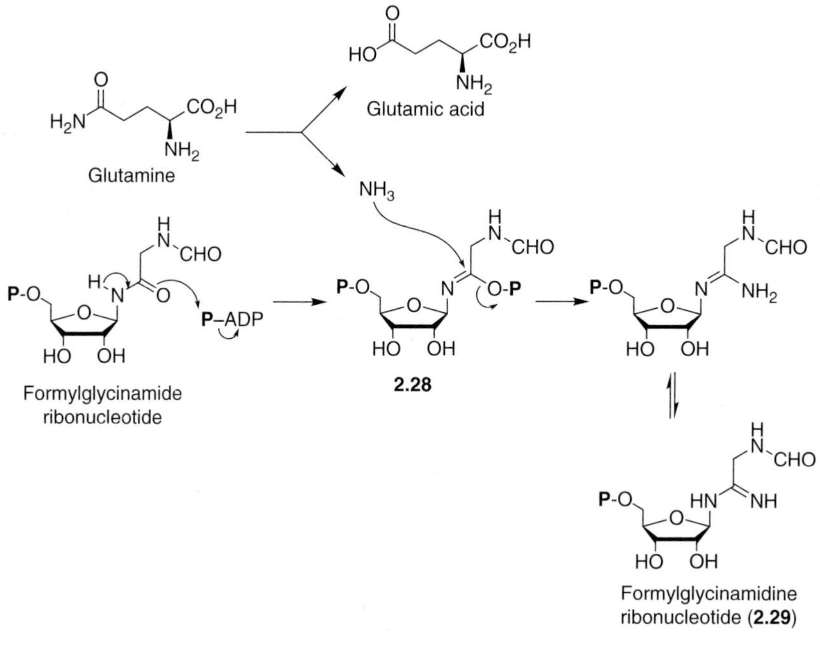

FIGURE 2.35   Biosynthesis of formylglycinamidine ribonucleotide.

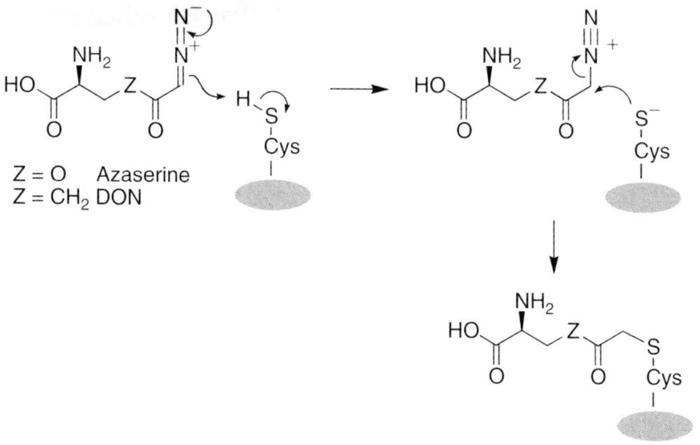

FIGURE 2.36 Covalent inactivation of phosphoribosylformylglycinamidine synthase by azaserine and DON.

response of choriocarcinoma to DON, although in general these compounds are too toxic.

6.4. Inhibitors of 5-aminoimidazole-4-carboxamide ribonucleotide formyltransferase

Some antifolate drugs (e.g., MTX, permetrexed) inhibit this enzyme, although it is not their primary target.

6.5. Thiopurines and related compounds

Among nonnatural purine derivatives assayed as antitumor agents, 6-mercapto-purine (MP) and 6-thioguanine (TG) are the most active. These compounds are among the oldest cancer chemotherapeutic drugs in clinical use; MP is used for lymphoblastic and myeloblastic leukemias, and the more toxic TG is employed for the treatment of acute non-lymphocytic leukemia.

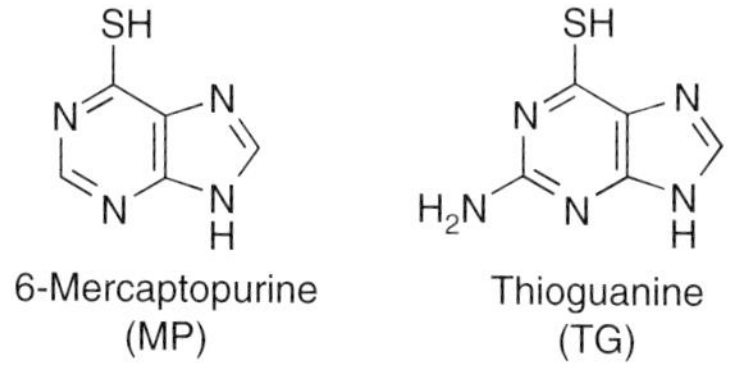

6-Mercaptopurine
(MP)

Thioguanine
(TG)

6-Mercaptopurine requires intracellular metabolism by hypoxanthine guanine phosphoribosyl transferase (HGPRT) to be transformed into the thioinosinic acid, which shows cell cycle S-phase-specific cytotoxicity. Intracellular activation results in the inhibition of several enzymes belonging to the *de novo* purine synthesis pathway and misincorporation into DNA and RNA. Thus, thioinosinic acid, formed by incorporation of a ribose phosphate unit to MP catalyzed by HGPRT, inhibits PRPP amidotransferase, the first enzyme in the *de novo* synthesis of purines, through a retroinhibition mechanism. Several other enzymes which are also inhibited resulting in lower levels of AMP and GMP are the following:

a. HGPRT itself because of competition between MP and its natural substrate, hypoxanthine.
b. Inosinic dehydrogenase, which transforms inosinic acid (IMP) into xanthylic acid (xantosinic acid, XMP), a precursor of guanylic acid (GMP).
c. Adenylosuccinate synthetase, which catalyzes the first step of the transformation of inosinic acid into adenylic acid (AMP).

Finally, thioinosinic acid is transformed into thioguanylic acid, which is mis-incorporated into DNA and RNA. This leads to single strand DNA breaks and DNA–protein cross-links by alteration of DNA repair mechanisms (Fig. 2.37). Thioguanine acts by a very similar mechanism, after its transformation into thioguanylic acid by HGPRT.

The main degradative pathways of MP are its S-methylation by thiopurine methyltransferase (TPMT) and its oxidation by xanthine oxidase to an 8-oxo deriv-ative and further to 6-thiouric acid (TUA) (Fig. 2.38). Allopurinol is a structural analog of hypoxanthine that is a competitive inhibitor of xanthine oxidase. It is also a substrate for xanthine oxidase and is converted slowly to alloxanthine, which also inhibits the enzyme. Since allopurinol interferes with the metabolism of MP, increasing its levels and leading to an interaction between both drugs, patients taking allopurinol should have their MP dose reduced by up to 75%. However, the clinical benefit of this association in cancer patients taking MP is only slight and renal damage may occur. S-Methylation is another catabolic route of MP, since the S-methyl derivative is not a substrate for the purine phosphoribosyl transferases.

Some heterocyclic derivatives of thiopurines have been designed to afford protection from the degradation processes described above, two examples being the nitroimidazole derivatives azathioprine (imuran) and thiamiprine (guaneran). These compounds act as prodrugs and are presumably activated by an S_NAr mechanism involving nucleophilic attack from thiols onto the 5 position the 4-nitroimidazole ring, followed by elimination of the thiopurine as a leaving group (Fig. 2.39). None of these prodrugs are more effective as anticancer agents than the parent compounds although azathioprine is an important immunosuppressant agent, widely used in autoimmune diseases.[49]

Another prodrug that is activated by a related mechanism is cis-3-(9H-purin-6-ylthio)acrylic acid (PTA), which is activated by glutathione through a Michael addition to the acrylic acid moiety followed by elimination (Fig. 2.40).[50]

Considerable efforts are in progress to prepare other novel mercaptopurine and thioguanine analogs and their nucleosides to improve their antitumor efficacy.[51]

7. INHIBITORS OF ADENOSINE DEAMINASE

Coformycin (CF) and pentostatin (2′-deoxycoformycin, dCF) are two natural products isolated from Streptomyces species that are analogs of inosine and 2′-deoxyinosine, respectively, in which the purine ring is modified and contains

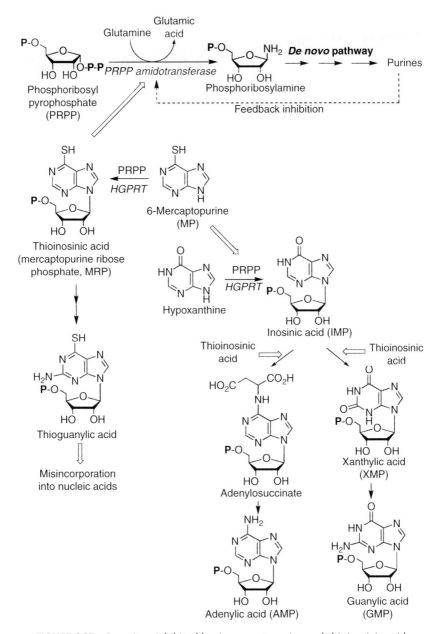

FIGURE 2.37   Reactions inhibited by 6-mercaptopurine and thioinosinic acid.

a seven-membered ring. These compounds behave as very potent inhibitors of adenosine deaminase, the enzyme that degrades deoxyadenosine by its transformation into 2′-deoxyinosine, by analogy with the transition state of this reaction (Fig. 2.41).

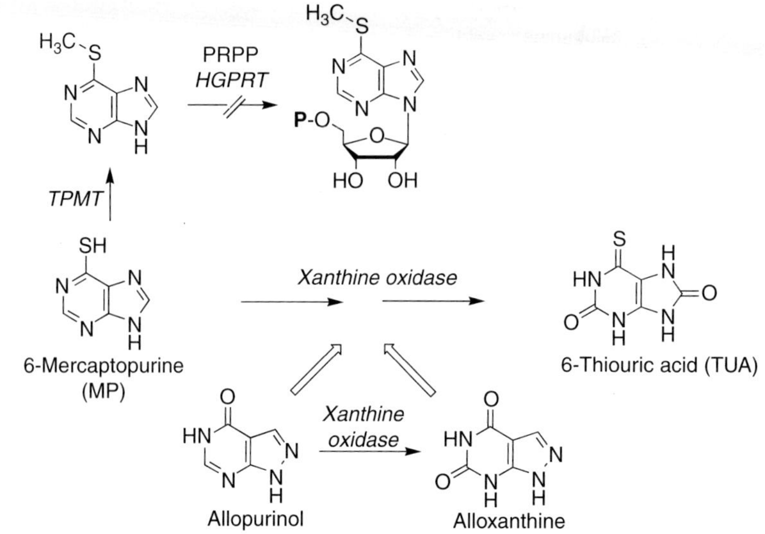

FIGURE 2.38   Main degradative pathways of 6-mercaptopurine.

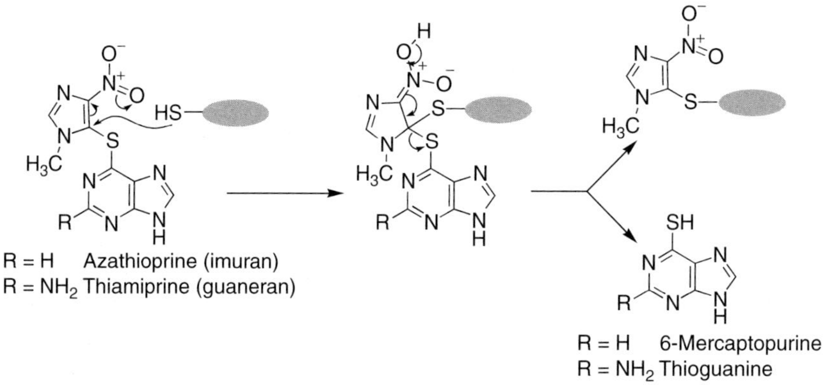

R = H   Azathioprine (imuran)
R = NH$_2$ Thiamiprine (guaneran)

R = H   6-Mercaptopurine
R = NH$_2$ Thioguanine

FIGURE 2.39   Bioactivation of azathioprine and thiamiprine.

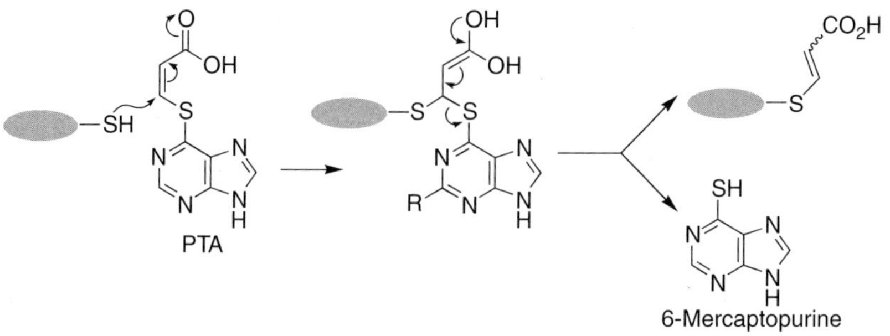

PTA

6-Mercaptopurine

FIGURE 2.40   Bioactivation of the 6-mercaptopurine prodrug PTA.

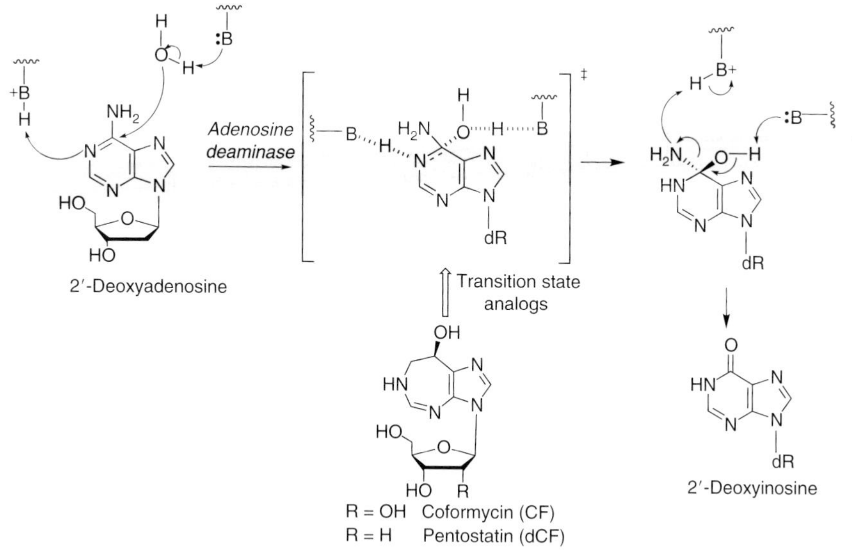

FIGURE 2.41 Inhibitors of adenosine deaminase.

Pentostatin is combined with adenosine-derived antitumor drugs in order to increase their half-life. On its own, pentostatin is also an antitumor agent that is useful in the treatment of some types of leukemias, like hairy cell leukemia. The mechanism of its antitumor activity is unclear and complex, and includes the following events (Fig. 2.42):

a. Pentostatin is triphosphorylated and misincorporated into DNA.
b. Inhibition of adenosine deaminase leads to accumulation of adenosine, and hence to retroinhibition of the enzyme S-adenosylhomocysteine hydrolase. The subsequently accumulated S-adenosylhomocysteine acts as a competitive inhibitor of most of the methyltransferases that use S-adenosylmethionine as a cofactor, and therefore perturbs the processes related to the methylation of nucleic acids (see Section 3.1 of Chapter 10).
c. Accumulation of deoxyadenosine also leads to high levels of deoxyadenosine triphosphate, which is an inhibitor of RNR, the enzyme that removes the 2'-hydroxy group of the ribose ring during the biosynthesis of DNA.

8. INHIBITORS OF LATE STAGES IN DNA SYNTHESIS

Several ribonucleoside and deoxyribonucleoside analogs are anticancer prodrugs that are activated to their triphosphates by phosphorylation catalyzed by kinases.[52] After bioactivation, the triphosphates act by misincorporation into DNA, resulting slower chain elongation and alterations in DNA repair. Another mechanism of antitumor action of these compounds is the inhibition of DNA

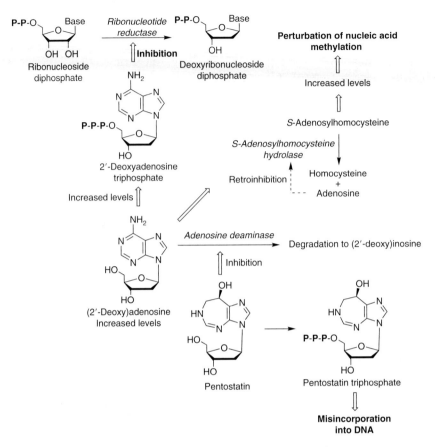

FIGURE 2.42   Events involved in the antitumor activity of pentostatin.

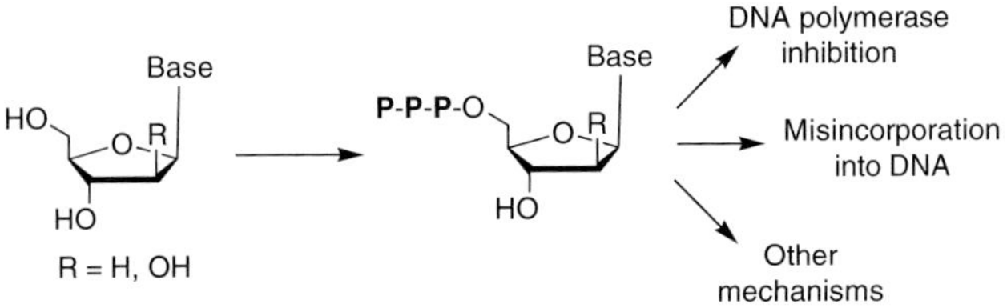

FIGURE 2.43   Antitumor mechanisms of ribonucleoside triphosphates.

polymerase, and other mechanisms (e.g., inhibition of RNR or PNP) are known for particular compounds (Fig. 2.43). A general problem associated with these drugs is due to their cytotoxicity to lymphoid cells, resulting in significant and long-lasting immunosuppression.

8.1. Pyrimidine nucleosides

The main anticancer compounds belonging to this group are cytosine or azacytosine nucleosides with a modified ribose ring, including cytarabine (Ara-C), fazarabine, gemcitabine (dFdC), and azacitidine.

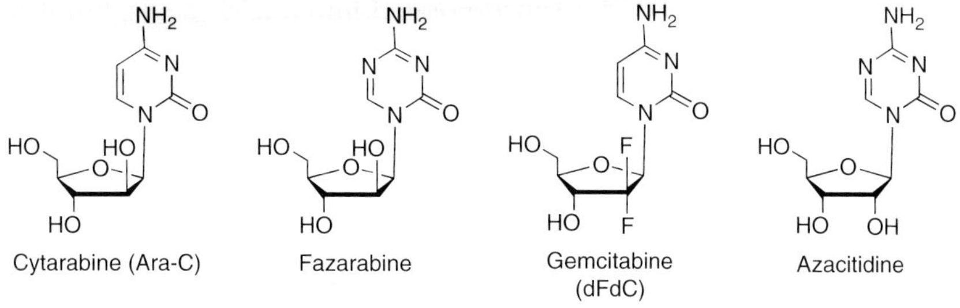

Cytarabine (Ara-C)   Fazarabine   Gemcitabine (dFdC)   Azacitidine

Among the arabinose-derived nucleosides, cytarabine (Ara-C), the 2′-epimer of cytidine, is useful in several leukemias, including acute myelogenous leukemia and non-Hodgkin lymphoma. Cytarabine is employed either as a single agent or in combination with others, specially the anthracyclines, and is the prime example of an antitumor drug specifically acting in the S-phase of the cell cycle because its incorporation into DNA after being activated to the corresponding triphosphate leads to inhibition of strand elongation (Fig. 2.44). Because of this S-phase-specificity, prolonged exposure of cells to cytotoxic concentrations is critical to achieve maximum cytotoxic activity. However, the activity of cytarabine is decreased by its rapid deamination by cytosine deaminase to the biologically inactive metabolite uracil arabinoside.[53] For this reason, the search for effective formulations and derivatives of cytarabine that cannot be deaminated and exhibit better pharmacokinetic parameters is an active field of research.[54]

Fazarabine is an aza analog with a very potent activity in animal models, including solid tumors, and has been submitted to several clinical trials.[55] Gemcitabine blocks the cell cycle at the S-phase similarly to cytarabine and it is also an inhibitor of RNR in its diphosphate form (see Section 3.3). Gemcitabine can be considered as the leading marketed nucleoside analog and is most commonly used to treat

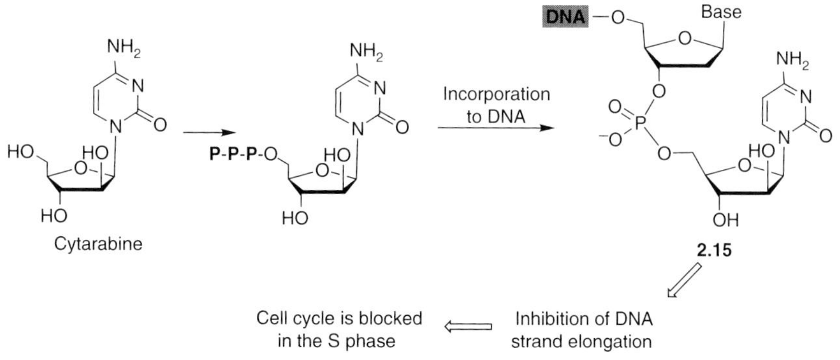

FIGURE 2.44 Antitumor mechanisms of cytarabine.

non-small cell lung cancer, pancreatic, bladder, and breast cancer. It has also been shown to be synergistic in combination with pemetrexed in Phase III studies for pancreatic and non-small cell lung cancer because pemetrexed depletes the intracellular stores of purine and pyrimidine nucleotides, while gemcitabine is incorporated in nascent DNA strands.[56] Finally, azacitidine and its 2′-deoxy analog are also triphosphorylated and misincorporated into nucleic acids, but it will be studied in Chapter 10 in connection with the inhibition of DNA methylation.

One of the main drawbacks of cytarabine is its short half-life in plasma due to rapid deamination to its uracil analog by cytidine deaminase. During the search for cytarabine analogs that could overcome this problem, and also in an effort to achieve activity against solid tumors, the arabinose 2-hydroxy group was replaced with other substituents.[57] The 2-cyano derivative (2′-cyano-2′-deoxy-1-β-D-arabinofuranosylcytosine, CNDAC) is particularly interesting because it acts by a novel mechanism among nucleoside analogs, involving DNA single strand breaking by a β-elimination reaction. CNDAC is less efficient than cytarabine and gemcitabine at inhibiting DNA strand elongation, and the cells can progress through the S-phase, leading to incorporation of its nucleotides at internal positions of DNA (**2.30** and **2.31**). The electron-withdrawing effect of the cyano group at the arabinose 2′-β position increases the acidity of the 2′-α proton and facilitates a β-elimination reaction in **2.31** involving an oxygen of the phosphate group at the 3′-β position that leads to single strand break that affords a DNA molecule lacking a 3′-hydroxyl. This prevents its repair by ligation and leads to inhibition of the cell cycle at the G2 phase (Fig. 2.45).[58]

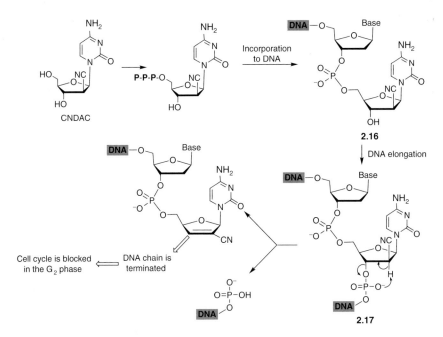

FIGURE 2.45   Antitumor mechanisms of CNDAC.

The N^4-palmitoyl derivative of CNDAC is an oral prodrug known as CYC-682 (CS-682), which is activated by intestinal and plasma amidases.[59] This compound has entered Phase I clinical assays.[60]

Another way to avoid the action of cytidine deaminase is the use of L-nucleosides. For instance, troxacitabine is a dioxolane analog of β-L-deoxycytidine which is a poor substrate for this enzyme. After activation as a triphosphate, troxacitabine inhibits DNA polymerase activity and leads to a complete chain termination. This compound has shown positive responses in clinical trials in patients with metastatic renal cancer.[61]

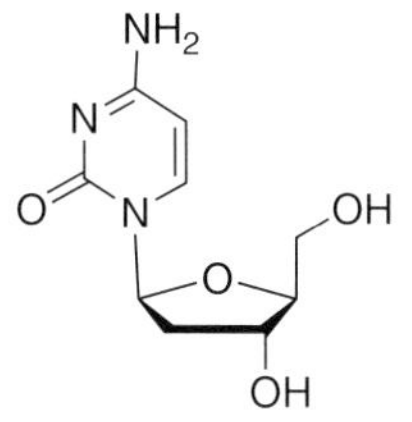

β–L-Deoxycytidine

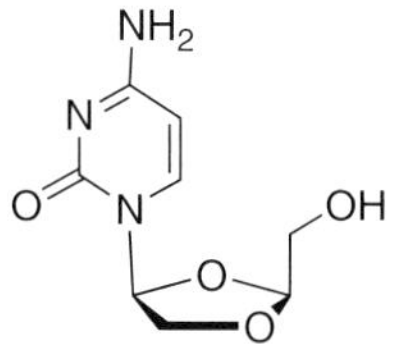

Troxacitabine
(β–L-dioxolanecytidine, L-OddC)

8.2. Purine nucleosides

Fludarabine and cladribine are used in cancer therapy, especially as second-line treatment for patients with B-cell chronic lymphocytic leukemia (CLL) that do not respond to alkylating agents. Other purine nucleosides (clofarabine, nelarabine, and immucillin H) have been recently introduced into clinical trials.[62] These compounds use nucleoside-specific membrane transporters to enter the cells and must then be converted into their active triphosphate forms.

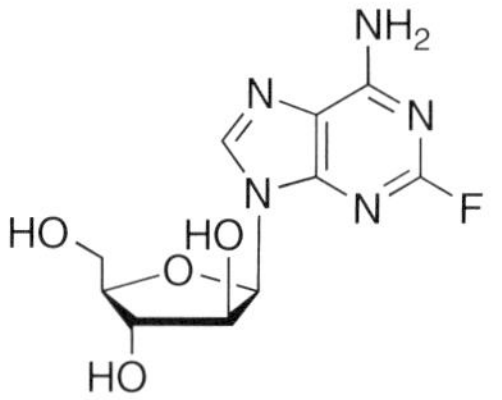

Fludarabine

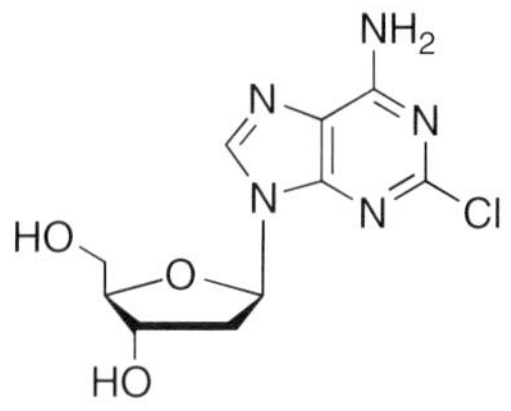

Cladribine

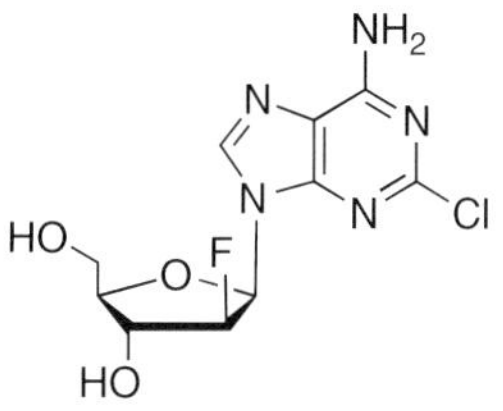

Clofarabine

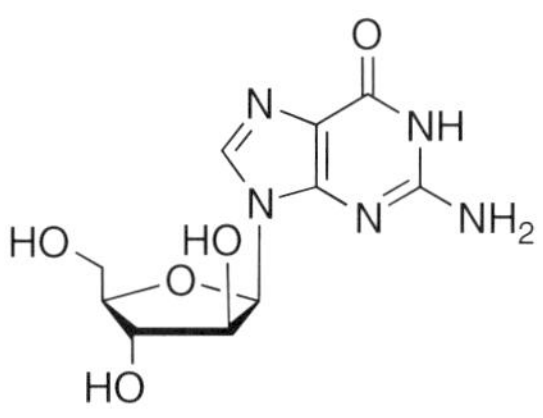

Ara-G

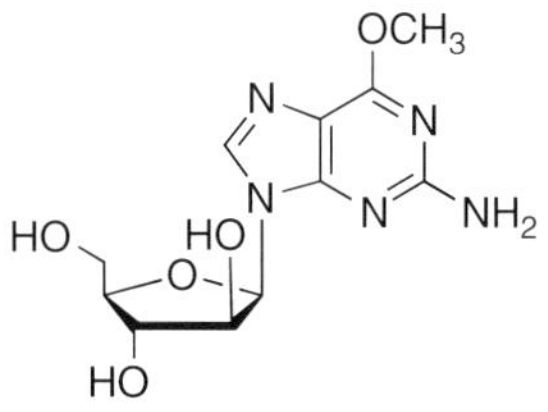

Nelarabine

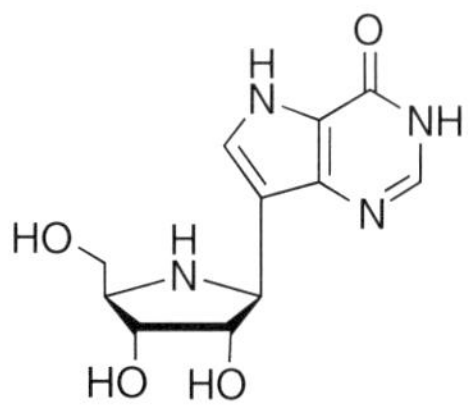

Immucillin H (forodesine)

Fludarabine is very insoluble and is administered as a phosphate prodrug that must be cleaved back to the nucleoside prior to entering the cell. Besides the mechanisms common to this group of drugs, it is an inhibitor of RNR and is active against several lymphoid malignancies. Cladribine is also employed in hairy cell leukemia and has the advantage over other adenine derivatives of being resistant to adenosine deaminase, a property that shares with all 2-halogenated adenine derivatives. The 2'-fluoro derivative of cladribine, called clofarabine, is more acid stable, leading to increased oral bioavailability, and has recently entered clinical trials. Ara-G has a very poor water solubility, and this has led to the development of its prodrug nelarabine, which is 10 times more soluble and has entered clinical trials. Another purine nucleoside that has entered clinical trials is immucillin H, which was studied in Section 3.

9. ANTIMETABOLITE ENZYMES

L-Asparaginase is an enzyme that behaves as an antimetabolite. Its physiological role is the hydrolysis of the amino acid L-asparagine to aspartic acid and ammonia (Fig. 2.46). Normal tissues can synthesize L-asparagine in amounts sufficient for protein synthesis, but some types of lymphoid malignancies take it from plasma. Treatment of these patients with L-asparaginase leads to the hydrolysis of circulating L-asparagine and prevents its uptake into the tumor cells, leading to interruption of protein synthesis and cell death. L-Asparaginase is normally used for the treatment of acute lymphocytic leukemia in combination with other agents, such as MTX, doxorubicin, cytarabine, and vincristine.

L-Asparaginase has been modified by covalent attachment of polyethyleneglycol (PEG) compounds such as monomethoxypolyethyleneglycolsuccinimidyl units. This PEG-modified enzyme is known as pegaspargase (see Section 3 of Chapter 11), and it is employed for the treatment of acute lymphocytic leukemia in patients that have developed hypersensitivity to the native form of L-asparaginase.[63]

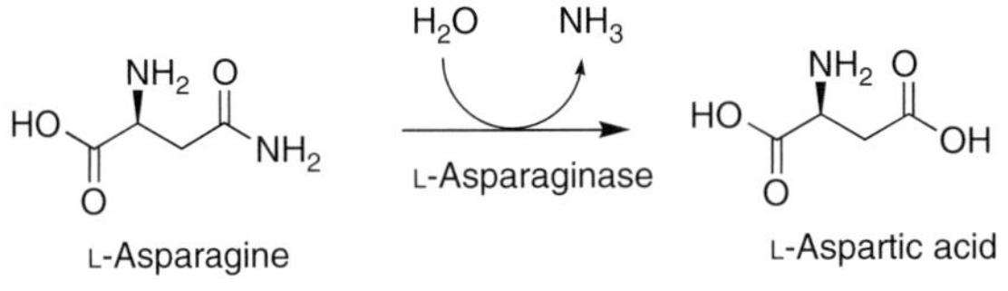

FIGURE 2.46 Reaction catalyzed by L-Asparaginase.

REFERENCES

1. Redei, I., Green, F., Hoffman, J. P., Weiner, L. M., Scher, R., and O'Dwyer, P. J. (1994). *Invest. New Drugs* **12**, 319.
2. Hogbom, M., Galander, M., Andersson, M., Kolberg, M., Hofbauer, W., Lassmann, G., Nordlund, P., and Lendzian, F. (2003). *Proc. Natl. Acad. Sci. USA* **100**, 3209.
3. Pereira, S., Cerqueira, N., Fernandes, P. A., and Ramos, M. J. (2006). *Eur. Biophys. J.* **35**, 125.
4. Yarbro, J. W. (1992). *Semin. Oncol.* **19**(3 Suppl. 9), 1.
5. Reardon, D. A., Egorin, M. J., Quinn, J. A., Rich, J. N., Gururangan, I., Vredenburgh, J. J., Desjardins, A., Sathornsumetee, S., Provenzale, J. M., Herndon, J. E., Dowell, J. M., Badruddoja, M. A., *et al.* (2005). *J. Clin. Oncol.* **23**, 9359.
6. Halsey, C., and Roberts, I. A. G. (2003). *Br. J. Haematol.* **120**, 177.
7. Jiang, J., Jordan, S. J., Barr, D. P., Gunther, M. R., Maeda, H., and Mason, R. P. (1997). *Mol. Pharmacol.* **52**, 1081.
8. Wadler, S., Makower, D., Clairmont, C., Lambert, P., Fehn, K., and Sznol, M. (2004). *J. Clin. Oncol.* **22**, 1553.
9. Taverna, P., Rendahl, K., Jekic-McMullen, D., Shao, Y., Aardalen, K., Salangsang, F., Doyle, L., Moler, E., and Hibner, B. (2007). *Biochem. Pharmacol.* **73**, 44.
10. Fernandes, P. A., and Ramos, M. J. (2003). *J. Am. Chem. Soc.* **125**, 6311.
11. Pereira, S., Fernandes, P. A., and Ramos, M. J. (2004). *J. Comput. Chem.* **25**, 1288.
12. Gandhi, V., Kilpatrick, J. M., Plunkett, W., Ayres, M., Harman, L., Du, M., Banthia, S., Davisson, J., Wierd, W. G., Faderl, S., Kantarjian, H., and Thomas, D. (2005). *Blood* **106**, 4253.
13. Kicska, G. A., Long, L., Hörig, H., Fairchild, C., Tyler, P. C., Furneaux, R. H., Schramm, V. L., and Kaufman, H. L. (2001). *Proc. Natl. Acad. Sci. USA* **98**, 4593.
14. Lee, J. L., Singhy, V., Evans, G. B., Tyler, P. C., Furneaux, R. H., Cornell, K. A., Riscoe, M. K., Schrammy, V. L., and Howell, P. L. (2005). *J. Biol. Chem.* **280**, 18274.
15. Longley, D. B., Harkin, D. P., and Johnston, P. G. (2003). *Nat. Rev. Cancer* **3**, 330.
16. Adjei, A. A. (1999). *J. Clin. Pharmacol.* **48**, 265.
17. Papamichael, D. (2000). *Stem Cells* **18**, 166.
18. Houghton, J. A., Tilman, D. M., and Harwood, F. G. (1995). *Clin. Cancer Res.* **1**, 723.
19. Longley, D. B., Boyer, J., Allen, W. L., Latif, T., Ferguson, P. R., Maxwell, P. J., McDermott, U., Lynch, M., Harkin, D. P., and Johnston, P. G. (2002). *Cancer Res.* **62**, 2644.
20. Ciccolini, J., Evrad, A., and Cuq, P. (2004). *Curr. Med. Chem. Anti-Cancer Agents* **4**, 71.
21. O'Shaughnessy, J., Miles, D., Vukelja, S., Moiseyenko, V., Ayoub, J. P., Cervantes, G., Fumoleau, P., Jones, S., Lui, W. Y., Mauriac, L., Twelves, C., Van Hazel, G., Verma, S., and Leonard, R. (2002). *J. Clin. Oncol.* **20**, 2812.
22. Nemunaitis, J., Eager, R., Twaddell, T., Corey, A., Sekar, K., Tkaczuk, K., Thompson, J., Hoff, P. M., and Pazdur, R. (2000). *J. Clin. Oncol.* **18**, 3423.
23. Diasio, R. B., and Harris, B. E. (1989). *Clin. Pharmacokinet.* **16**, 215.
24. Peters, G. J., van Groeningen, C. J., and Giaccone, G. (2001). *J. Clin. Oncol.* **19**, 4267.
25. Smith, I. E., Johnston, S. R. D., O'Brien, M. E. R., Hickish, T. F., Boer, R. H., Norton, A., Cirkel, D. T., and Barton, C. M. (2000). *J. Clin. Oncol.* **18**, 2378.
26. Hoff, P. M., and Pazdur, R. (1998). *Oncologist* **3**, 155.
27. Eng, C., Kindler, H. L., and Schilsky, R. L. (2001). *Clin. Colorectal Cancer* **1**, 95.
28. Leyland-Jones, B., and O'Dwyer, P. J. (1986). *Cancer Treat. Rep.* **70**, 219.
29. Browman, G. P., Levine, M. N., Goodyear, M. D., Russell, R., Archibald, S. D., Jackson, B. S., Young, J. E., Basrur, V., and Johanson, C. (1988). *J. Clin. Oncol.* **6**, 963.
30. Tomlinson, S. K., Melin, S. A., Higgs, V., White, D. R., Savage, P., Case, D., and Blackstock, A. W. (2002). *BMC Cancer* **2**, 9.
31. Peters, G. J., Noordhuis, P., Van Kuilenburg, A. B., Schornagel, J. H., Gall, H., Turner, S. L., Swart, M. S., Voorn, D., Van Gennip, A. H., Wanders, J., Holwerda, U., Smid, K., *et al.* (2003). *Cancer Chemother. Pharmacol.* **52**, 1.
32. Smith, D., and Gallagher, N. (2003). *Eur. J. Cancer* **39**, 1377.
33. Pivot, X., Wadler, S., Kelly, C., Ruxer, R., Tortochaux, J., Stern, J., Belpomme, D., Humblet, Y., Domenge, C., Clendeninn, N., Johnston, A., Penning, C., *et al.* (2001). *Ann. Oncol.* **12**, 1595.

34. Jackmann, A. L., Theti, D. S., and Gibbs, D. D. (2004). *Adv. Drug Deliv. Rev.* **56**, 1111.
35. Theti, D. S., Bavetsias, V., Gibbs, D. D., Skelton, L. A., and Jackman, A. L. (2001). *Proc. Am. Soc. Cancer Res.* **42**, 291.
36. Bavetsias, V., Marriott, J. H., Melin, C., Kimbell, R., Matusiak, Z. S., Boyle, T., and Jackman, A. L. (2000). *J. Med. Chem.* **43**, 1910.
37. Goodsell, D. S. (1999). *Oncologyst* **4**, 340.
38. Blakley, R. L., and Cocco, L. (1985). *Biochemistry* **24**, 4772.
39. Kamen, B. A., Whyte-Bauer, S., and Bertino, J. R. (1983). *Biochem. Pharmacol.* **32**, 1837.
40. Schornagel, J. H., Verweij, J., de Mulder, P. H., Cognetti, F., Vermorken, J. B., Cappelaere, P., Armand, J. P., Wildiers, J., de Graeff, A., and Clavel, M. (1995). *J. Clin. Oncol.* **3**, 1649.
41. Meyers, F. J., Lew, D., Lara, P. N., Williamson, S., Marshall, E., Balcerzak, S. P., Rivkin, S. E., Samlowski, W., and Crawford, E. D. (1999). *Invest. New Drugs* **16**, 347.
42. Blanke, C. D., Kasimis, B., Schein, P., Capizzi, R., and Kurman, M. (1997). *J. Clin. Oncol.* **15**, 915.
43. Takimoto, C. H. (1996). *Oncologist* **1**, 68.
44. Kisliuk, R. L. (2003). *Curr. Pharm. Des.* **9**, 2615.
45. Sessa, C., de Jong, J., D'Incalci, M., Hatty, S., Pagani, O., and Cavalli, F. (1996). *Clin. J. Cancer Res.* **2**, 1123.
46. http://www.cancer.gov/clinicaltrials/MSKCC-04032
47. Kut, V., Patel, J. D., and Argiris, A. (2004). *Exp. Rev. Anticancer Ther.* **4**, 511.
48. Gangjee, A., Yu, J., Mcguire, J. J., Cody, V., Galitsky, N., Kisliuk, R. L., and Queener, S. F. (2000). *J. Med. Chem.* **43**, 3837.
49. Aberra, F. N., and Lichtenstein, G. R. (2005). *Aliment. Pharmacol. Ther.* **21**, 307.
50. Gunnasdottir, S., and Elfarra, A. A. (1999). *J. Pharmacol. Exp. Ther.* **290**, 950.
51. Elgemeie, G. H. (2003). *Curr. Pharm. Des.* **9**, 2627.
52. Johnson, S. A. (2000). *Clin. Pharmacokinet.* **39**, 5.
53. Ohta, T., Hori, H., Ogawa, M., Miyahara, M., Kawasaki, H., Taniguchi, N., and Komada, Y. (2004). *Oncol. Rep.* **12**, 1115.
54. Hamada, A., Kawaguchi, T., and Nakano, M. (2002). *Clin. Pharmacokinet.* **41**, 705.
55. Ben-Baruch, N., Denicoff, A. M., Goldspiel, B. R., O'Shaughnessy, J. A., and Cowan, K. W. (1993). *Invest. New Drugs* **11**, 71.
56. Henry, J. R., and Mader, M. M. (2004). *Annu. Rep. Med. Chem.* **39**, 161.
57. Matsuda, A., Nakajima, Y., Azuma, A., Tanaka, M., and Sasaki, T. (1991). *J. Med. Chem.* **34**, 2919.
58. Azuma, A., Huang, P., Matsuda, A., and Plunkett, W. (2001). *Mol. Pharmacol.* **59**, 725.
59. Hanaoka, K., Suzuki, M., Kobayashi, T., Tanzawa, F., Tanaka, K., Shibayama, T., Miura, S., Ikeda, T., Iwabuchi, H., Nakagawa, A., Mitsuhashi, Y., Hisaoka, M., *et al.* (1999). *Int. J. Cancer* **82**, 226.
60. Tolcher, A., Cohen, R. B., Benettaib, B., Frenz, L., Gianella-Borradori, A., and Calvo, E. (2005). *J. Clin. Oncol.* **23**, 2026.
61. Townsley, C. A., Chi, K., Ernst, D. S., Belanger, K., Tannock, I., Bjarnason, G. A., Stewart, D., Goel, R., Ruether, J. D., Siu, L. L., Jolivet, J., McIntosh, L., *et al.* (2003). *J. Clin. Oncol.* **21**, 1524.
62. Robak, T., Lech-Maranda, E., Korycka, A., and Robak, E. (2006). *Curr. Med. Chem.* **13**, 3165.
63. Asselin, B. L., Whitin, J. C., Coppola, D. J., Rupp, I. P., Sallan, S. E., and Cohen, H. J. (1993). *J. Clin. Oncol.* **11**, 1780.

CHAPTER 3

Anticancer Drugs That Inhibit Hormone Action

Contents

1. Introduction   54
2. Estrogens and Their Involvement in Carcinogenesis   54
3. Antiestrogens as Antitumor Drugs   58
    3.1. Nonsteroidal antiestrogens (SERMs)   58
    3.2. Steroidal antiestrogens   62
4. Aromatase Inhibitors   65
    4.1. Aromatase mechanism of action   67
    4.2. Steroidal aromatase inhibitors (type I inhibitors)   68
    4.3. Nonsteroidal aromatase inhibitors (type II)   72
5. Steroid Sulfatase Inhibitors   73
6. Androgen-Related Antitumor Agents   75
    6.1. Antiandrogens   76
    6.2. Inhibitors of 14α-demethylase and 17α-hydroxylase   77
    6.3. Inhibitors of 5α-reductase   77
7. Regulation of Steroidal Hormone Synthesis as a Target for Antitumor Drugs   79
    7.1. Introduction   79
    7.2. GnRH (LHRH) agonists   81
    7.3. GnRH (LHRH) antagonists   82
8. Miscellaneous Steroid Hormone-Related Anticancer Therapy   85
    8.1. Gestagens as antitumor agents   85
    8.2. Glucocorticoids and inhibitors of their biosynthesis as antitumor agents   85
9. Compounds Acting on Other Proteins of the Nuclear Receptor Superfamily: Retinoids   86
References   90

Medicinal Chemistry of Anticancer Drugs
DOI: 10.1016/B978-0-444-52824-7.00003-2

1. INTRODUCTION

Hormones, and in particular steroid hormones, are the main determinants in the induction and growth of several types of tumors and for this reason the search for antihormones has been one of the mainstays of cancer chemotherapy. Thus, compounds acting on estrogen and androgen receptors (ARs) are involved in the treatment of breast and prostatic cancers, among others, while corticosteroids are employed in myelomas and lymphomas because of their role in the function of lymphoid tissues.

Steroid hormone receptors are cytoplasmic or nuclear proteins that have a binding site for a particular steroid molecule. Their response elements are DNA sequences that bind to the complex formed by the steroid and its receptor and are part of a gene promoter. This binding activates or represses the gene controlled by that promoter. The steroid hormone receptors consist of at least three domains, namely, a domain needed for the receptor to activate the promoters of the genes being controlled, the zinc-finger domain needed for DNA binding to the response element (a zinc finger can be defined as a configuration of a DNA-binding protein that resembles a finger with an amino acid, usually cysteine or histidine, binding a zinc ion), and finally the domain responsible for binding the particular hormone as well as the second unit of the dimer.

The sequence of events leading to the start of gene transcription by an steroid hormone is as follows (Fig. 3.1): (1) binding of the hormone to the receptor; (2) formation of a homodimer from two molecules of receptor (not shown in Fig. 3.1); (3) transport to the nucleus, if necessary (e.g., in the case of estrogen hormones); (4) binding to the response element; (5) recruitment of coactivators; and (6) final activation of transcription factors to start transcription. The ultimate consequence is the synthesis of an mRNA molecule and the corresponding protein, which triggers the observed biological response.

2. ESTROGENS AND THEIR INVOLVEMENT IN CARCINOGENESIS

Estrogens are a family of related steroidal molecules that stimulate the development and maintenance of female characteristics and sexual reproduction, including regulation of the menstrual cycle, and have several other physiological functions. The most prevalent forms of human estrogens are estradiol and estrone, which are produced and secreted by the ovaries, although estrone is also synthesized in the adrenal glands and other organs.

Estradiol   Estrone

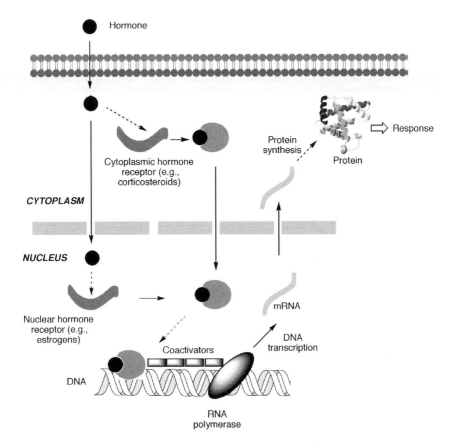

FIGURE 3.1   Sequence of events related to steroid hormone activity.

The estrogen receptor (ER) is a ligand-dependent transcription factor, that is, a DNA-binding protein that regulates the transcription of its target genes. Although early models proposed that the ERs were cytoplasmic and were translocated to the nucleus after binding to the estrogen molecules, subsequent studies with monoclonal antibodies revealed that the ERs were located in the nucleus.

Regulation of gene transcription by estrogens is highly complex. It involves regions of DNA called estrogen response elements (EREs) and also the binding of several nuclear proteins (coactivators) that form a multisubunit transcriptional complex. Occupation of the steroid binding domain in the receptor by the hormone is followed by receptor dimerization, which is essential for DNA binding. On estrogen recognition, a conformational change takes place in the receptor protein that allows the recognition of coactivators and the start of the transcription process.

The natural estrogens induce tumors in a variety of organs in laboratory animals, and high estrogen levels increase the risk of breast and uterine cancer.[1] Several mechanisms have been proposed that explain the development of estrogen-dependent tumors. In the first place, the transcription process initiated by the binding of estrogens to their receptors ultimately induces cell proliferation in some target tissues. Examples are breast tissue, where estrogens trigger the proliferation of cells lining the milk glands, thereby preparing the breast to produce milk in case of pregnancy, and the endometrium of the uterus, where they stimulate cell proliferation in order to prepare the uterus for implantation. This proliferative action is one of the physiological roles of estrogens, but it can also lead to the development of breast or uterine cancer because if cells from these tissues already possess a DNA mutation that increases the risk of developing cancer, they will proliferate (along with normal cells) in response to estrogen stimulation.

An alternative mechanism that explains the carcinogenesis by estrogens is the generation of mutagenic species in their metabolism.[2] Strong evidence supports that tumors may be initiated by metabolic conversion of estradiol (E_2) to the catechol metabolite 4-hydroxyestradiol (4-OHE_2), which is further oxidized to estradiol-3,4-quinone (E_2-3,4-Q) (Fig. 3.2).

Estradiol-3,4-quinone reacts with DNA as a Michael substrate forming a bond between its C-1 atom and the N-7 atom of guanine, affording hydroquinone **3.1**. The positive charge generated at the guanine N-7 position facilitates the hydrolysis of the glycosidic bond of **3.1**, leading to the purine derivative **3.2** and depurinized DNA (**3.3**) (Fig. 3.3).

Alternatively, the nucleophilic attack to the estradiol-3,4-quinone may involve the N-3 atom of adenine residues, leading to hydroquinone **3.4**. Similarly to **3.1**, these covalent adducts are unstable under hydrolytic conditions and evolve to give purine derivatives **3.5** and depurinized DNA **3.3** (Fig. 3.4).

As shown in Fig. 3.5, the alternative catechol metabolite 2-hydroxyestradiol (2-OHE_2) produces the estradiol-2,3-quinone (E_2-2,3-Q), which also gives DNA adducts by forming a covalent bond with a nitrogen atom of a purine base, but these adducts are much less reactive than those derived from E_2-3,4-Q and have less relevance in the carcinogenesis due to estradiol.[3]

The link between ovarian function and breast cancer has been known for more than a century, and endocrine therapy can be considered as the oldest, safest, and best-established systemic treatment for breast cancer. Many breast and endometrial tumors are estrogen-dependent, and for this reason their treatment is based on the modulation of these hormones. This can be achieved directly by

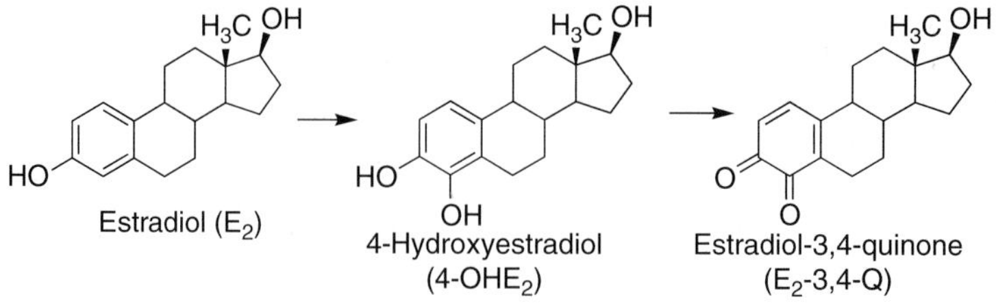

FIGURE 3.2   Metabolism of estradiol.

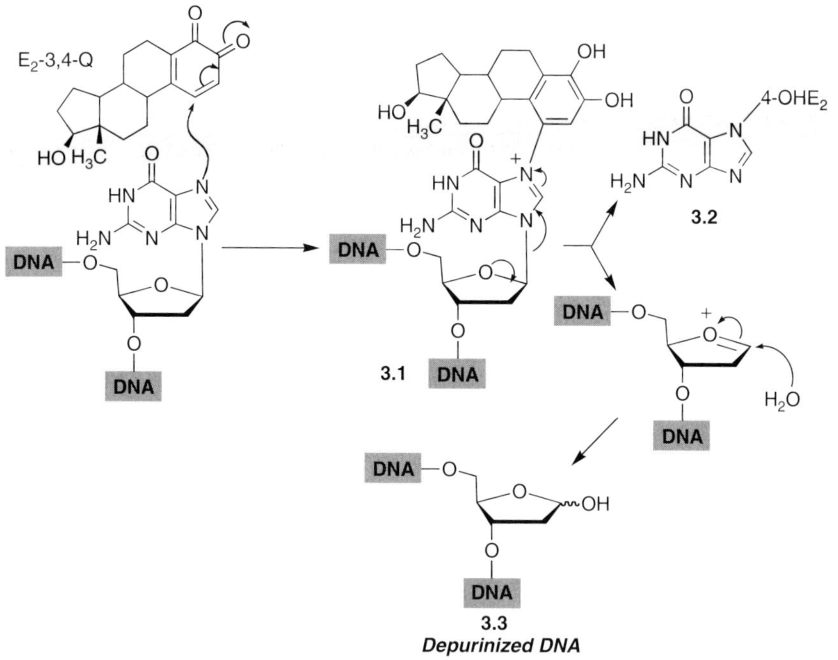

FIGURE 3.3   DNA depurinization by estradiol-3,4-quinone.

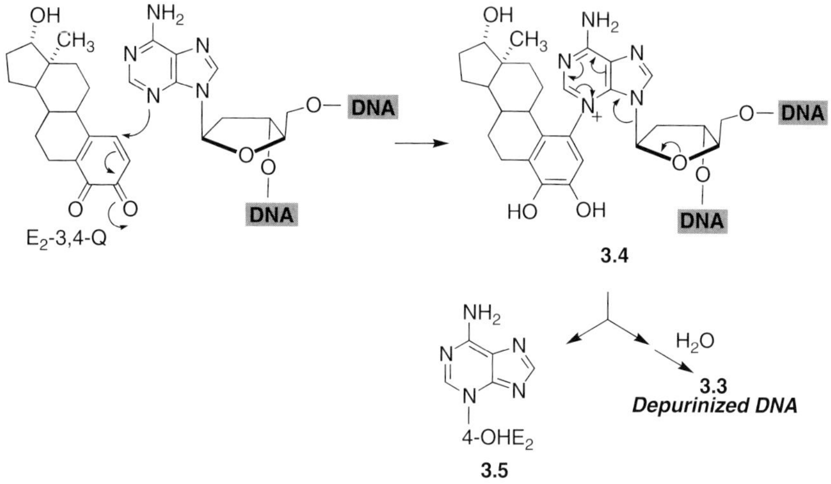

FIGURE 3.4   Alternative mechanism for DNA depurinization by estradiol-3,4-quinone.

administration of antiestrogens or indirectly by inhibition of aromatase, the enzyme responsible for the biosynthesis of estrogens. Finally, estrogen production can also be controlled by inhibition of the release of luteinizing hormone (LH) (see Section 7).

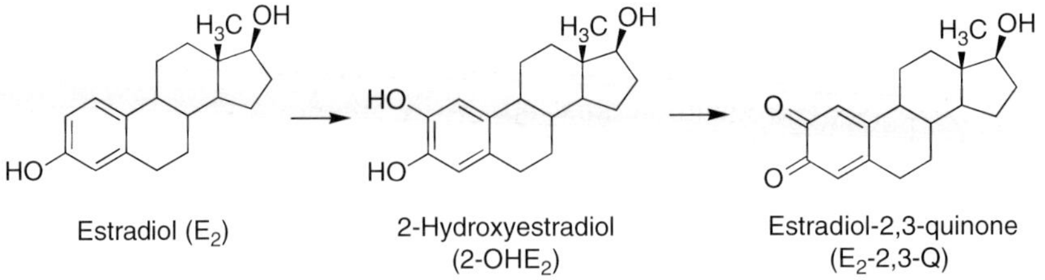

FIGURE 3.5   Metabolic conversion of estradiol into estradiol-2,3-quinone.

3. ANTIESTROGENS AS ANTITUMOR DRUGS

Antiestrogens can be defined as compounds that prevent the stimulation of transcription by the ER. Two main types of antiestrogens are known:

a. Nonsteroidal antiestrogens, which interfere with the transcription process by binding to the hormone recognition site in the ER and preventing the induction of the conformational change necessary for recognition of the coactivators. Since ERs of different target tissues vary in chemical structure, these compounds may show mixed biological responses because they can behave as antagonists in one estrogen target tissue and as agonists in another. In spite of not being completely selective, compounds of this group are often designed as selective estrogen receptor modulators (SERMs).

b. Pure antiestrogens are analogs of the natural hormones that bear long, flexible side chains at C-7. These compounds bind to the ER and prevent receptor binding to DNA, probably because the side chains bind to the receptor outside the steroid-binding region.

3.1. Nonsteroidal antiestrogens (SERMs)

The discovery of this group of compounds is a good example of serendipity. They are derivatives of the triphenylethylene system, developed by molecular manipulation of diethylstilbestrol, the prototype nonsteroidal estrogen agonist. The key structural features of this group of compounds, which are essential for activity, are the presence of a triphenylethylene core and a basic aminoether side chain at the 4-position of one of the phenyl rings.[4]

The first discovered antiestrogen was clomiphene, but its development for the treatment for advanced breast cancer was discontinued because of concerns about potential side effects. In 1974, tamoxifen was the first antiestrogen to be approved for the treatment of advanced breast cancer (Great Britain) and in 1977 a similar approval was given by the FDA. Since then, tamoxifen has become the standard therapy for all types of ER-positive breast cancer. In the 1990s, it was also the first cancer chemopreventive agent approved by the FDA for the reduction of breast cancer in pre- and postmenopausal women with high risk.[5] Tamoxifen also binds with high affinity to other targets, such as the microsomal antiestrogen binding site (AEBS), protein kinase C, calmodulin (CaM)-dependent enzymes, and acyl coenzyme A:cholesterol acyl transferase (ACAT).[6]

Tamoxifen has estrogenic agonist effects in other tissues such as bone and endometrium due to the nonspecific activation of their ERs. For this reason, several antiestrogen compounds, known as SERMs, have been developed which have a reduced agonist profile on breast and gynecological tissues.[7] Some of these compounds belonging to the triphenylethylene family include toremifene,[8] droloxifene,[9] and idoxifene.[10]

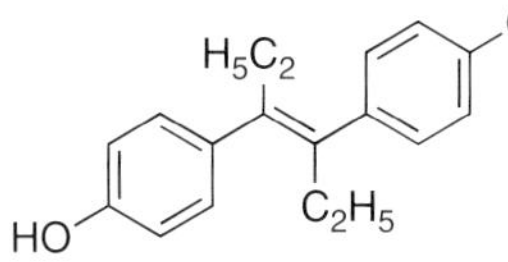

Diethylstilbestrol

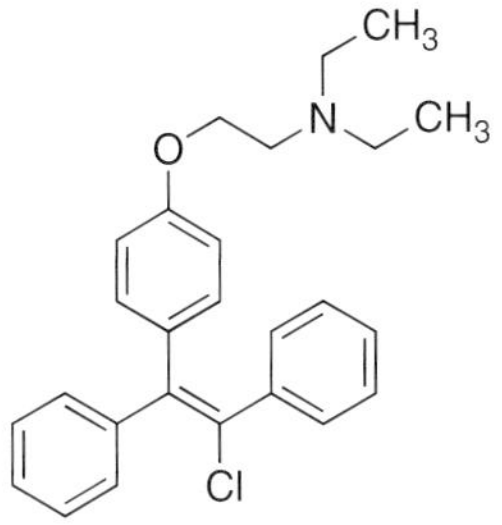

Clomiphene

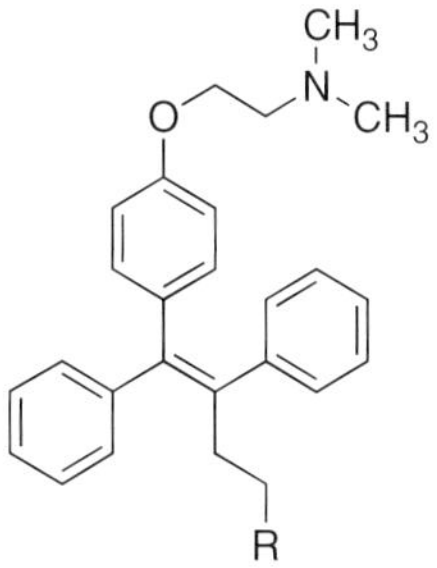

R = H   Tamoxifen
R = Cl   Toremifene

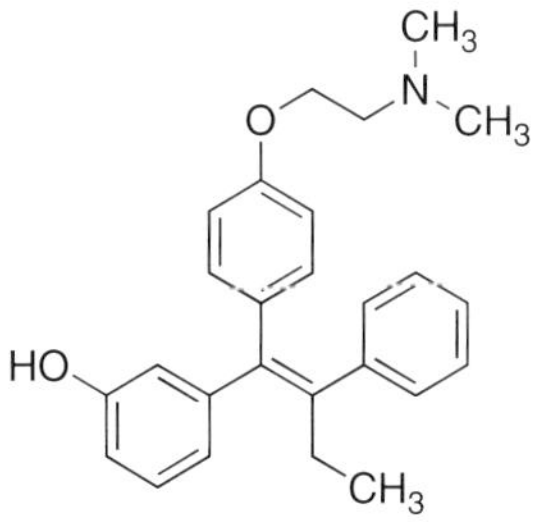

Droloxifene

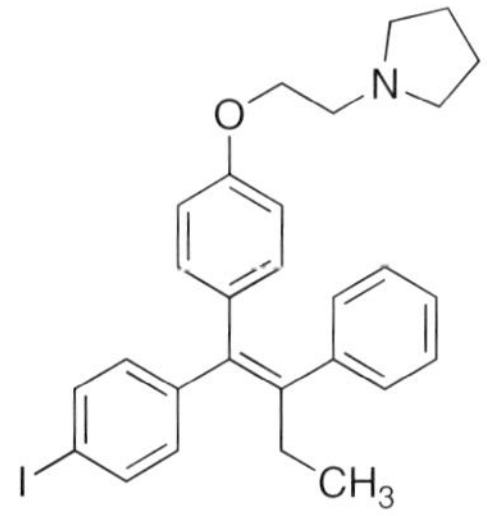

Idoxifene

Most of these compounds may lead to long-term toxic effects. For instance, tamoxifen induces liver cancer in rats after prolonged administration, which has been attributed to the generation of DNA-alkylating species from the metabolism of the stilbene framework. It has been proposed that cytochrome P450 hydroxylates tamoxifen at the allylic position of the ethyl side chain, leading to an alcohol, which can generate a highly delocalized allylic cation **3.6** and therefore alkylate DNA to give product **3.7** through an S_N1 mechanism (Fig. 3.6).

This proposal also explains the lack of carcinogenicity of toremifene, which can be attributed to destabilization of the positive charge in **3.8** by the inductive effect of the chlorine substituent at the position adjacent to the allylic carbon (Fig. 3.7).

Because of the toxic effects associated to the central double bond in triphenylethylene derivatives, a new family of antiestrogens has been developed where the incorporation of this double bond into a cyclic system increases its chemical and metabolic stability. Another structural difference of these compounds with the traditional triphenylethylene derivatives is the presence of a ketone bridging

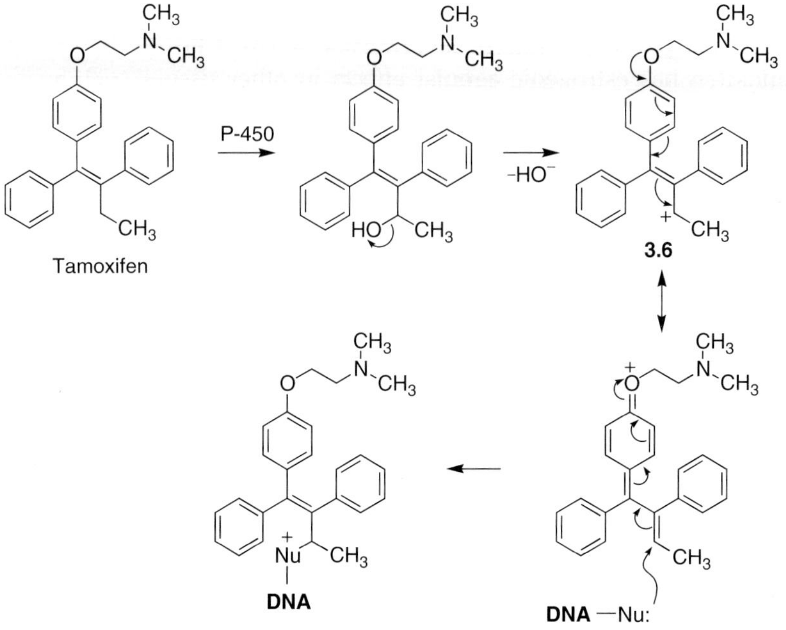

FIGURE 3.6   Mechanism proposed to explain tamoxifen long-term toxicity.

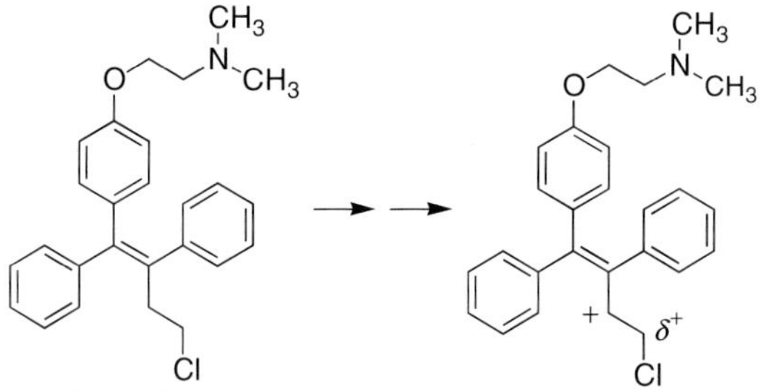

FIGURE 3.7   Destabilization of the electrophilic species derived from toremifene.

group linking the phenyl ring that contains the basic side chain. The main representative of this family is raloxifene, which was identified as an antiestrogen but it was approved by the FDA only for the prevention of osteoporosis, while studies as a treatment for breast cancer were discontinued. However, there is a recent renewal of the interest on raloxifene as a means for breast cancer prevention, with a very large clinical study in progress involving more than 19,000 postmenopausal women at increased risk of breast cancer, aimed at comparing the efficacy of tamoxifen and raloxifene in chemoprevention.[11]

Raloxifene

The inhibition of the ER by the triphenylethylene derivatives and by their cyclic analogs has been rationalized using the structures of their complexes with the receptor, as determined by X-ray diffraction data.[12] The agonists and antagonists bind at the same site, but with different binding modes, as shown in Fig. 3.8. Recognition of estradiol by the ligand-binding domain of the receptor involves a combination of polar and nonpolar interactions. Thus, the A ring and the A/B interface interact with the side chains of Ala-350, Leu-387, and Phe-404, while the D ring contacts with Ile-424, Gly-521, and Leu-525. The hydroxyl at the phenolic ring of ring A establishes hydrogen bonds with the carboxylate of Glu-353, the guanidinium group of Arg-394 and a water molecule. The hydroxyl group at the C-17 position of the D ring establishes a hydrogen bond with the His-524 residue. The antagonists, exemplified by raloxifene, occupy the same binding sites but the interaction is different. The imidazole ring in the His-524 rotates in order to accommodate the difference in position of the hydroxyl group in raloxifen that corresponds to the hydroxyl at C-17 in estradiol. The rest of the interactions are similar in both cases, but the antagonists have additional hydrophobic interactions due to the side chain, and also a hydrogen bond between the basic group present in the side chain and the carboxylate group of Asp-351.

After binding of an agonist to the ligand-binding domain of the ER, a conformational change takes place on which the helix H12 is placed against the

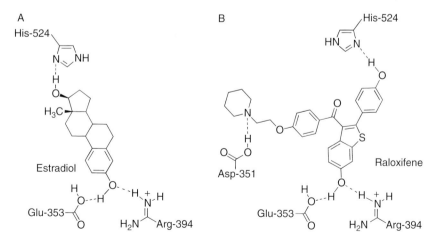

FIGURE 3.8 Binding modes of ER agonists (A) and antagonists (B).

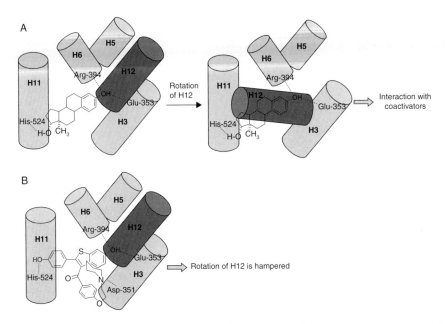

FIGURE 3.9 Conformational changes following the activation of the estrogen receptor and their inhibition by raloxifene.

ligand-binding cavity, projecting its inner, hydrophobic surface toward the ligand. The outer, charged surface, which is essential for the interaction of the receptor with coactivators, is left outside (Fig. 3.9A).[13] The alignment of H12 over the cavity is prevented by the binding of antagonists, exemplified by raloxifene, because their side chain is too long to fit the binding cavity and protrudes from the pocket between H3 and H11, preventing the holding of the helix H12 and hence the transcriptional activation function of ER (Fig. 3.9B). This helix displacement seems to be a common feature of steroidal and nonsteroidal antiestrogens with a bulky side chain.

Some ER-positive breast tumors that also overexpress the peptide growth factor receptor ERBB2 (also known as HER2) and/or epidermal growth factor receptor EGFR (also known as HER1) are relatively resistant to hormonal therapy, especially when tamoxifen is employed.[14]

3.2. Steroidal antiestrogens

The SERMs, especially tamoxifen and toremifene, have been the preferred first-line hormonal therapy in estrogen-responsive postmenopausal breast cancer, but they have several disadvantages that are related to their partial estrogenic agonistic activity. These include tumor stimulation in some patients at the initial stages of the treatment (tumor flare) and increased hot flashes, endometrial cancer, and thromboembolism. These limitations stimulated the search for pure ER antagonists.

Structurally, the main family of selective estrogen antagonists are steroids bearing a long lipophilic chain at C-6, represented by fulvestrant (ICI-182780), which has been approved for the treatment of postmenopausal women with hormone-sensitive advanced breast cancer following prior endocrine therapy.[15]

Fulvestrant

Fulvestrant has a unique mechanism of action,[16] comprising several different aspects (Fig. 3.10). In the first place, fulvestrant is a competitive inhibitor of estradiol binding at the ER, with an affinity of 89% that of estradiol. Another consequence of fulvestrant binding is the impairment of the dimerization of ER, an event that takes place after estrogen binding and is essential for the nuclear localization of the receptor. Because of the inhibition of dimerization, fulvestrant binding leads to accelerated receptor degradation due to the lower stability of the monomer.

On the contrary, the side chain of fulvestrant obstructs the folding of the H12 helix of the receptor and therefore prevents its interaction with coactivators, as mentioned in Section 2.1 (Fig. 3.11).

Figure 3.12 gives a summarized picture of the events associated to fully activated transcription by ER agonists, partially inactivated transcription by SERMs, and full inactivation by antiestrogens. In the first case (Fig. 3.12A), estradiol (E)

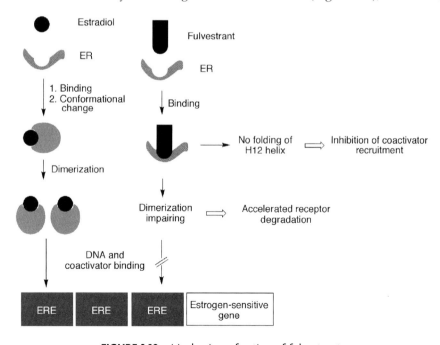

FIGURE 3.10   Mechanism of action of fulvestrant.

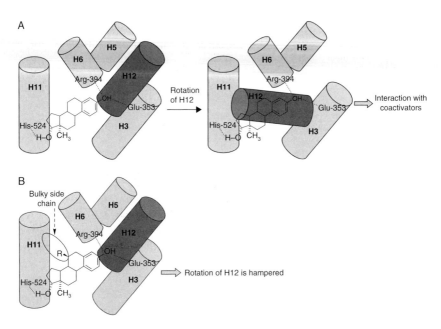

FIGURE 3.11   Binding of fulvestrant to the estrogen receptor. Comparison with estradiol binding.

binds to the ER which in the resting state has a single domain, called activating function (AF1), available for binding with coactivators and/or corepressors. After binding of estradiol, a second activating function (AF2) is exposed. The complex dimerizes and migrates to the cell nucleus, where it binds to the ERE of DNA, leading to recruitment of coactivators by both activation functions, subsequent stimulation of RNA polymerase activity and fully activated transcription. After the binding of SERMs, exemplified by tamoxifene (T) (Fig. 3.12B), activation of AF2 does not take place and therefore coactivator recruitment and transcription activation are only partial. The pure steroidal antagonists, like fulvestrant (Fig. 3.12C), bind to the ER with high affinity. This binding leads to a conformational change in the receptor resulting in the formation of a complex in which neither of the AF1 and AF2 activation functions is active. This complex does not dimerize, which facilitates its degradation. Also, migration to the cell nucleus is markedly reduced, preventing coactivator recruitment and transcription activation.

Trilostane is another steroidal compound that has been occasionally employed in the treatment of breast cancer and is now under reevaluation. It is an inhibitor of 3β-hydroxysteroid dehydrogenase, the enzyme that transforms pregnenolone into progesterone, a gestagen and also a biosynthetic precursor to all other types of steroidal hormones. Because of this property, it has been employed in disorders due to high levels of these hormones, such as Cushing's disease, which is characterized by high levels of cortisol. Further studies have shown that the antitumor effects of trilostane are partially due to the inhibition of steroidogenesis and also to allosteric inhibition of the estrogen, probably binding directly to the DNA-binding domain.[17] Because it modulates ERs differently to tamoxifen and is able to influence internal cell signals and gene expression, it is undergoing clinical trials in

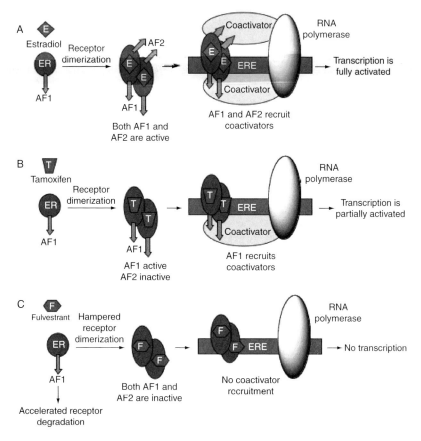

FIGURE 3.12 Events following the interaction of the estrogen receptors with agonists (A), modulators (B) and antagonists (C).

premenopausal women and in a postmenopausal group where both tamoxifen and aromatase inhibitors have failed.

Trilostane

4. AROMATASE INHIBITORS

An alternative strategy for achieving antiestrogenic effects is the inhibition of aromatase, the enzyme responsible for the biosynthesis of estradiol and estrone from androgens.[18] In principle, this strategy has the advantage over the use of antiestrogens of blocking the two pathways involved in the generation of tumors by the estrogenic hormones, which were discussed in Section 2, namely ER activation and the generation of carcinogenic metabolites (Fig. 3.13).

Aromatase catalyzes the loss of the C-19 methyl group as a formic acid molecule, allowing the creation of the aromatic A ring that is characteristic of estrogens (Fig. 3.14). Aromatase inhibitors are employed for the therapy of breast cancer in postmenopausal women, for whom the primary estrogen source is aromatase activity in adipose tissues in the breast, bone, vascular endothelium, and central nervous system and aromatase levels are not under gonadotropin regulation. In premenopausal women, the use of aromatase inhibitors leads to incomplete estrogen suppression and increased gonadal stimulation due to the feedback regulatory mechanism that increases luteinizing hormone and follicle-stimulating hormone after aromatase inhibition (see also Section 3.9). This complication is not observed in postmenopausal women.

Aromatase inhibition, specially by third-generation drugs, results in near-complete estrogen deprivation and for this reason some of the drugs discussed below have improved clinical outcomes over tamoxifen in breast cancer treatment. This difference is probably related to the previously mentioned estrogenic agonistic effects of tamoxifen and to the genotoxicity of the estradiol metabolites, specially its quinones, since aromatase inhibitors prevent the generation of estradiol while antiestrogens do not (Fig. 3.13).[20] The combination of aromatase inhibitors

```
Aromatase          Antiestrogens
inhibitors
    ⇓                   ⇓      ER activation ⟶  Proliferation of
                                                mutated cells
              Aromatase                                          ↘
Androstenedione ⟶  Estrone                                        CANCER
Testosterone       Estradiol                                    ↗
                              ↖ Generation of ⟶ DNA alkylation
                                E₂-3,4-quinone   and depurination
```

FIGURE 3.13   Pathways involved in tumorogenesis by estrogens.

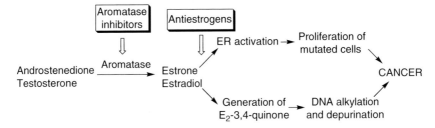

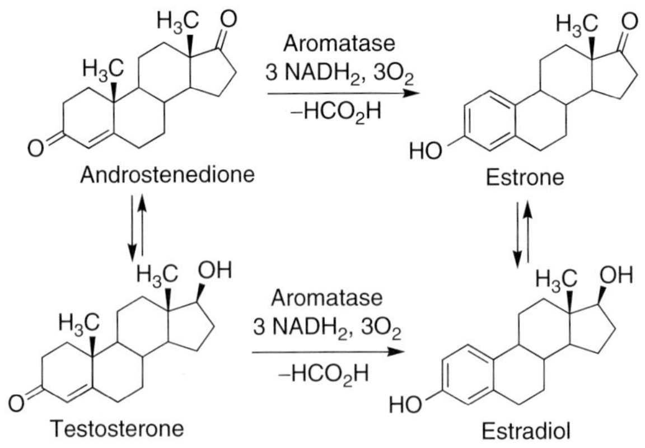

Androstenedione → Estrone

Aromatase, 3 NADH₂, 3O₂, −HCO₂H

Testosterone → Estradiol

Aromatase, 3 NADH₂, 3O₂, −HCO₂H

FIGURE 3.14   Biotransformations catalyzed by aromatase.

with bisphosphonates to compensate for their pro-osteoporotic effects has still not been fully evaluated, and other possible long-term effects remain unknown.[21]

4.1. Aromatase mechanism of action

Aromatase belongs to the group of microsomal cytochrome P450 enzymes responsible for hydroxylation metabolic processes. The overall process catalyzed by aromatase comprises a series of three oxidative steps. The first two are the insertion of two hydroxyl groups at the C-19 methyl group of its substrates leading to **3.9** and then to *gem*-diol **3.10**, which is dehydrated to aldehyde **3.11**. The third reaction is only partly understood, and involves loss of the C-19 carbon atom as a molecule of formic acid, with concomitant aromatization of ring A. One mechanistic possibility is that a third hydroxylation takes place at C-2β, yielding intermediate **3.12**, which can be postulated to rearrange to **3.14** through the intermediacy of the cyclic hemiacetal **3.13**. Loss of a molecule of formic acid, driven by the generation of the aromatic A ring, would finally culminate the process, yielding the estrogens estradiol and estrone (Fig. 3.15). However, experiments with [2β-^{18}O-,19-^{3}H]-2β-hydroxy-10β-formylandrost-4-ene-3,17-dione failed to show incorporation of the β-hydroxyl to formic acid under enzymatic and nonenzymatic conditions.[22]

Similar to other cytochrome P450 enzymes, the catalytic site of aromatase contains a Fe (III) heme group which, after reduction to Fe (II) affording species **3.15**, binds to an oxygen molecule, which becomes activated, giving **3.16**. A further

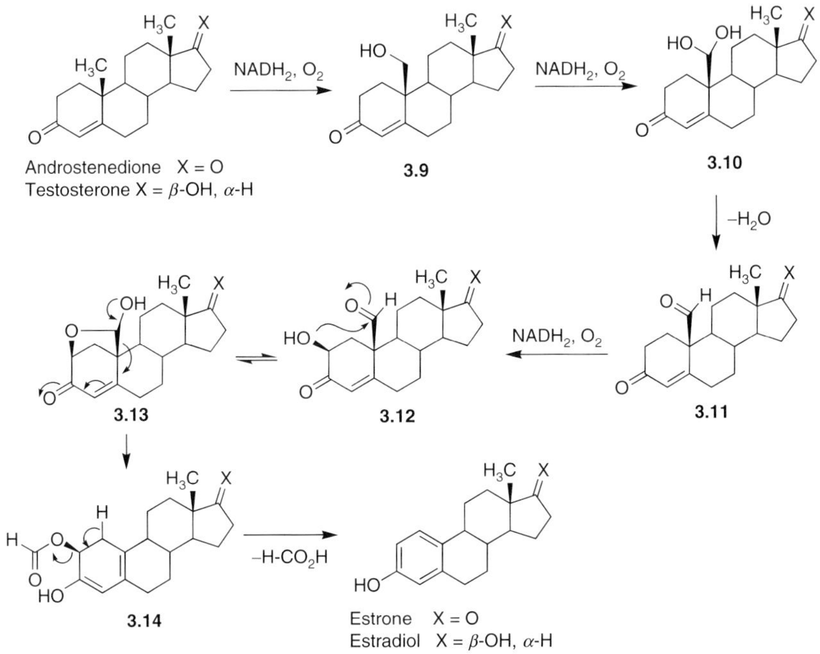

FIGURE 3.15   One possible mechanism to explain aromatase activity.

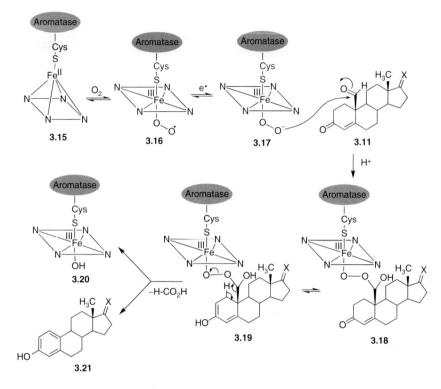

FIGURE 3.16   Alternative mechanism for aromatase activity.

one-electron reduction leads to peroxide anion **3.17**, which can undergo a nucleo-philic attack onto the formyl group of aldehyde **3.11**. The adduct **3.18** thus generated, probably as its enol tautomer **3.19**, evolves by loss of a molecule of formic acid via the ionic mechanism shown in Fig. 3.16, or perhaps through a radical pathway, yielding the estrogen hormones. This mechanism is consistent with all experimental data and is considered more likely than the one via 2-hydroxylation previously discussed and other alternatives that have been proposed.[23]

4.2. Steroidal aromatase inhibitors (type I inhibitors)

Aromatase inhibitors are normally classified as steroidal (type I) or nonsteroidal (type II). Numerous steroidal agents have been developed that exhibit either competitive inhibition, irreversible inhibition, or mechanism-based inhibition of aromatase.[24] Mechanism-based inhibitors are bound to the catalytic site of the enzyme, which transforms them into electrophilic intermediates that become irreversibly attached to the enzyme, blocking its activity, and they are known as "aromatase inactivators." This type of inhibitors have distinct advantages in drug design, since they are highly enzyme specific, produce prolonged inhibition, and exhibit minimal toxicities, and for this reason the steroidal aromatase inhibitors in clinical use behave as mechanism-based irreversible inhibitors.[25]

Although the precise chemical details are sometimes not known, many types of compounds containing latent electrophilic groups intended to be activated by aromatase are known. The most relevant are summarized below.

4.2.1. C-19-modified substrate analogs

The first group steroidal aromatase inhibitors are C-19-modified substrate analogs. One example is the propargyl derivative plomestane, for which two main types of mechanisms have been proposed. The first one postulates its oxidation by aromatase to give the C-19 carbonyl derivative, leading to the Michael acceptor **3.22**, a substrate for nucleophilic attack by nucleophiles at the enzyme active site. The second mechanism is based on the one proposed for the inactivation of cytochrome P450 enzymes by terminal acetylenic compounds and involves epoxidation of the acetylene chain by aromatase to give the unstable oxirene **3.24** that reacts with aromatase to give **3.27** following rearrangement to ketene **3.26** (Fig. 3.17). The development of plomestane as an antitumor drug was halted because of "technical problems."[26]

4.2.2. 4-Hydroxyandrostenedione derivatives

The main representative of this group is formestane. This compound was first described as a competitive inhibitor, but subsequent evidence proved that its binding to aromatase was irreversible. The presence of the C-19 methyl group is essential, since the 19-nor derivative is not an aromatase inactivator, and this suggests that the 19-oxygenated metabolites are the inactivating species. The 4-hydroxy group is also essential, and the ethers and esters of formestane at O-4 are inactive. One possible mechanism that is consistent with these

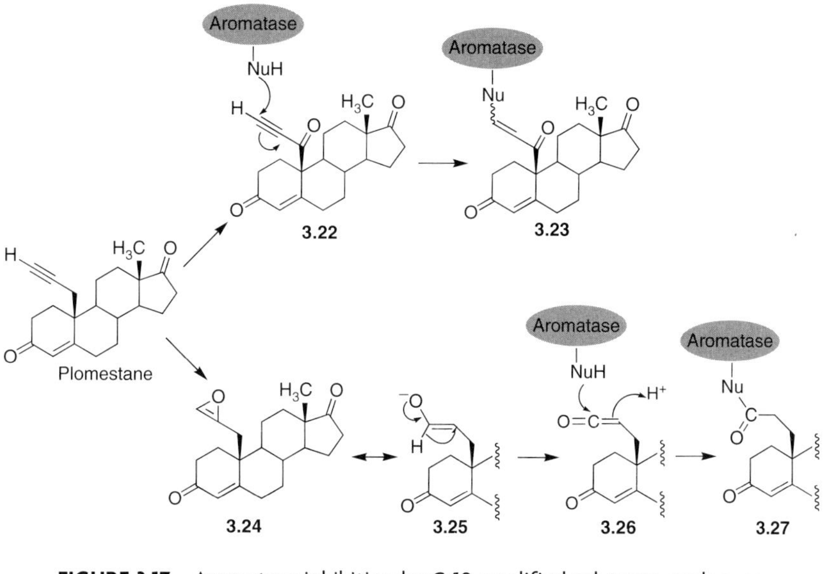

FIGURE 3.17   Aromatase inhibition by C-19-modified substrate analogues.

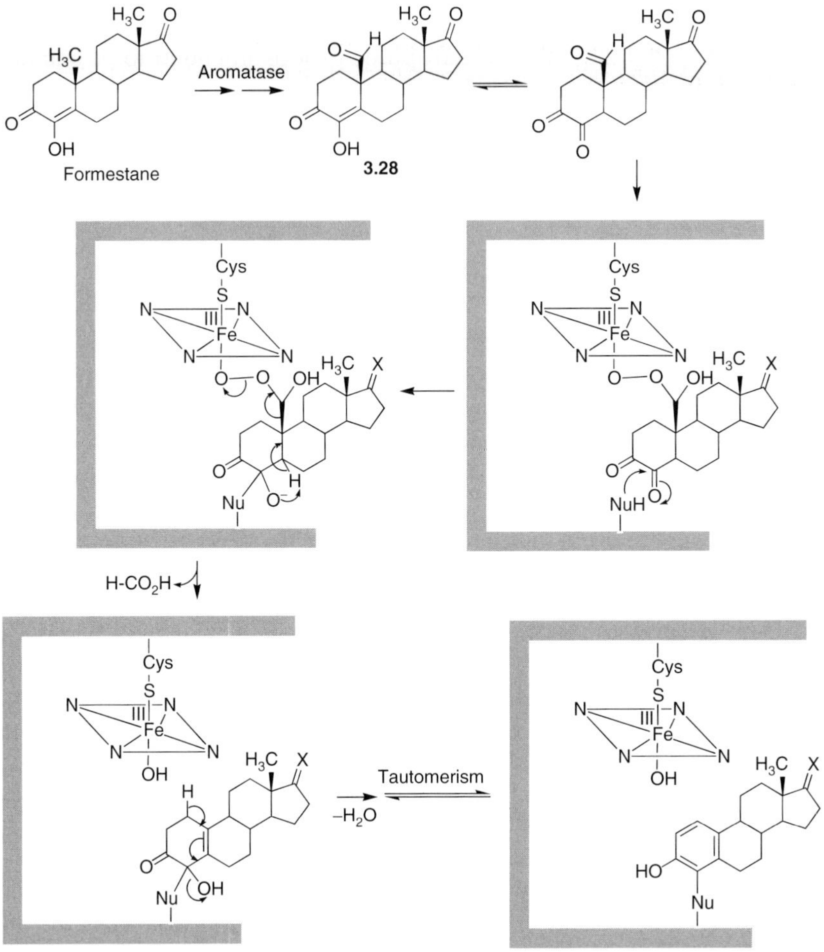

FIGURE 3.18 Aromatase inhibition by 4-hydroxyandrostenedione derivates.

observations is summarized in Fig. 3.18, although the low activity found for the formyl derivative **3.28** proposed as an intermediate would seem to cast doubt on this proposal.

Formestane is a second-generation steroidal aromatase inhibitor, and the first one to reach clinical use during the early 1990s.[27] Its main drawback is that it must be administered intramuscularly in order to avoid its first-pass glucuronidation at the C-4 hydroxyl, a problem that renders it unsuitable for widespread clinical use.

4.2.3. Steroids with additional unsaturations at the A and B rings

The first member of this class of compounds to be recognized as an aromatase inhibitor was testolactone, and subsequently 1,4-androstadiene-3,17-dione. Among other more highly unsaturated compounds, the most relevant is the 6-methylene derivative, known as exemestane.[28] The use of testolactone in the treatment of breast cancer started in 1960, although its ability to inhibit aromatase was not discovered until 1979. It is a weak inhibitor, with a moderate clinical response that has precluded its widespread use. Exemestane was approved more recently for clinical use in some countries and has the advantages over formestane of being more potent and, specially, of allowing oral administration.[29]

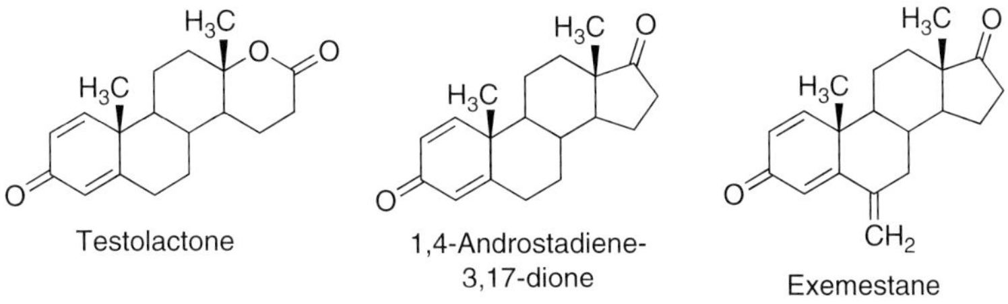

Testolactone   1,4-Androstadiene-   Exemestane
                      3,17-dione

The presence of the double bond at C-1 is essential for activity, and it has been suggested that the mechanism of irreversible inactivation involves its oxidation to a cation radical that would then be intercepted by a nucleophilic group of the active site. The generation of this radical would be facilitated by stabilization of the unpaired electron by delocalization across the adjacent unsaturated carbonyl system (Fig. 3.19).

4.2.4. Structure–activity relationships in steroidal aromatase inhibitors

The spatial requirements for interaction of steroidal compounds with the active site of aromatase are very restrictive, allowing only small structural changes on the A ring and at C-19. Some exceptions to this rule are the incorporation of small polar substituents at the C-4 position, such as a hydroxyl group, or the addition of aryl functionalities at the 7-position of the steroid. Inhibitors with such modifications exhibit enhanced affinity for the enzyme.[24] Several enzyme structure–function studies have revealed two regions that are important parts of the active site and contribute to the binding of the substrate and inhibitors: the I helix, that comprises the portion from Cys-299 to Ser-312, and a hydrophobic pocket that comprises the portion from Ile-474 to His-480. On the contrary, some 3D QSAR studies using steroidal aromatase inhibitors suggested that around the C-6 region of the steroids there are hydrophobic interactions involving the α-face and the β-face with highly hydrophobic aliphatic amino acids, namely Ile-305, Ala-306,

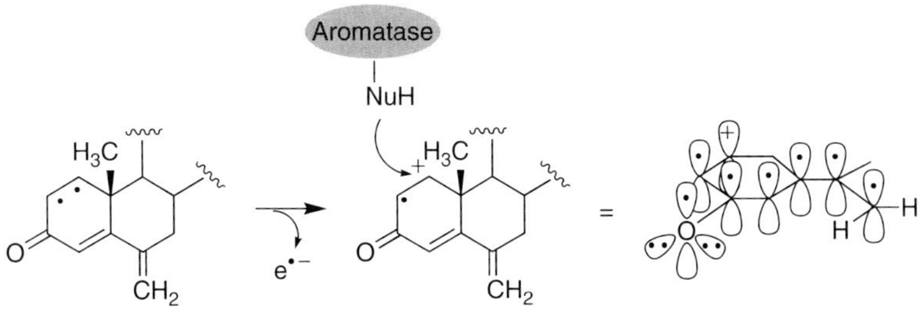

FIGURE 3.19   Inactivation of aromatase by exemestane.

Thr-310, Val-369, and Leu-477. The aromatase selectivity can be attributed to the formation of a hydrogen bond between an acceptor group of the ligand and the hydroxyl group of Ser-478.[30]

4.3. Nonsteroidal aromatase inhibitors (type II)

This group of inhibitors comprises structurally varied compounds that are able to bind to the active site of aromatase through the coordination of an heterocyclic nitrogen atom, usually an imidazole or triazole ring, to the iron atom of the heme group of the enzyme. Because of the similarity of aromatase with other essential enzymes of the cytochrome P450 group, the main problem to be solved is one of selectivity. On the contrary, they have the advantage over steroidal inhibitors of not being subject to metabolism by the cytochrome enzyme system. The structures of the main drugs belonging to this group are given below.

Aminoglutethimide   Dexaminoglutethimide   Fadrozole

Anastrozole   Letrozole   Vorozole

The first nonsteroidal aromatase inhibitor was aminoglutethimide, a derivative of the sedative agent glutethimide that was initially introduced as an anticonvulsant. It was the first aromatase inhibitor approved for use by the FDA for breast cancer treatment but it was withdrawn from use after reports of adrenal insufficiency. Nevertheless, one of its enantiomers, dexaminoglutethimide, is now undergoing clinical trials. The effects of aminoglutethimide are rather nonspecific because it inhibits several cytochrome P450 enzymes thereby affecting a number of hydroxylation steps in the metabolic conversion of cholesterol to active steroid products in adrenal steroid biosynthesis.

The second nonsteroidal aromatase inhibitor to reach the clinic was fadrozole, a fused imidazole derivative, which we will use here as a model compound for describing the interaction of azole derivatives with aromatase. The N-2 atom of fadrozole is involved in a coordinate bond with the heme iron, having also favorable interactions with the side chains of Ile-305, Ala-306, and Thr-310, while the cyano group appears to be hydrogen bonded to the Ser-478 hydroxyl. 3D QSAR data of fadrozole derivatives and other studies support the presence of hydrogen bonding and hydrophobic interactions in the active site of aromatase (Fig. 3.20).[31]

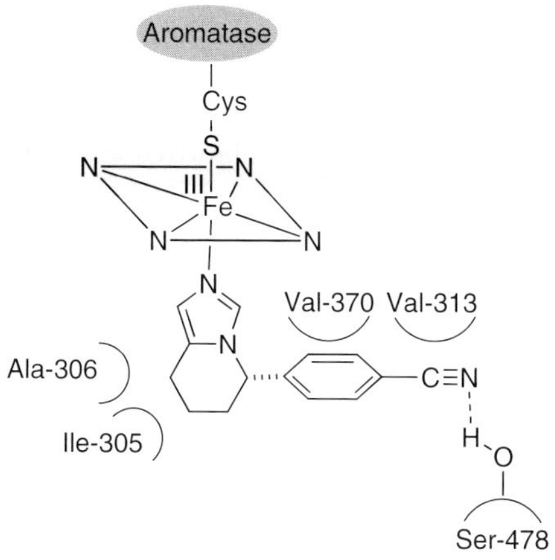

FIGURE 3.20 Interaction of fradozole with the aromatase active site.

The third generation of nonsteroidal aromatase inhibitors includes the triazole derivatives anastrozole, vorozole, and letrozole, which are very potent and specific aromatase inhibitors that allow almost complete estrogen suppression.[32] They have the advantage over aminoglutethimide and fadrozole of not showing affinity for other cytochrome P450-related steroidogenic enzymes because the presence of two electron-withdrawing nitrogen atoms in the triazole ring renders it too electron-deficient for aromatic oxidation. The related triazole derivative finrazole, another selective aromatase inhibitor, is under clinical studies for the treatment of male lower urinary dysfunction, a hitherto intractable disease.

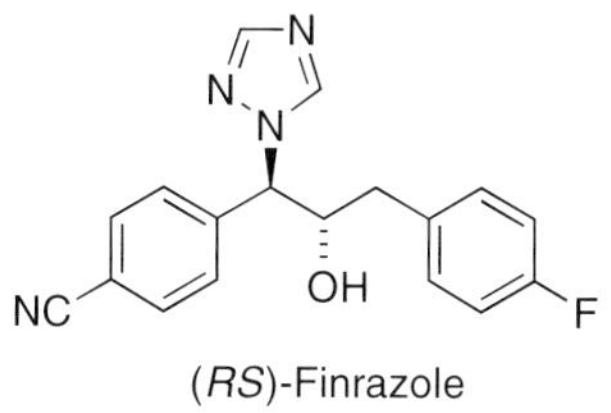

(*RS*)-Finrazole

5. STEROID SULFATASE INHIBITORS

It was previously mentioned that in postmenopausal women, who show the highest incidence of breast cancer, estrogens are produced in adipose tissues and in the breast by the action of aromatase on androstenedione. However, the clinical response to aromatase inhibitors is not as high as expected, and often it is not superior to the one obtained with antiestrogens or with other antihormones. Furthermore, there appears to be no relationship between the clinical response and the degree of suppression of circulating estradiol levels, which suggests that other factors besides the classical estrogens must be involved in tumor growth.[33]

Steroids with estrogenic properties can be biosynthesized by a route involving the steroid sulfatase (STS) enzyme, which regulates the formation of estrone by hydrolysis of estrone sulfate (E_1S) and also controls the hydrolysis of dehydroepiandrosterone sulfate (DHEA-S) to dehydroepiandrosterone (DHEA). The latter compound can be reduced to 5-androstene-3β, 17β-diol (Adiol), a steroid with potent estrogenic properties. On the contrary, there is evidence that in postmenopausal women DHEA is an important source of androstenedione via the peripheral action of 3β-hydroxyesteroid dehydrogenase/isomerase (3-β-HSD/isom), as shown in Fig. 3.21. In consequence, STS inhibitors can be useful for breast cancer therapy, although, in contrast to aromatase inhibitors, they are still in an early stage of development.

Aryl sulfamates have been identified as potent STS inhibitors, and some representative compounds have entered early clinical trials. Although initial research was focused on steroidal compounds, it was realized that many of them were estrogen agonists. For this reason, the first STS inhibitor to enter Phase I clinical trials for treating postmenopausal women with breast cancer was the coumarin derivative 667 coumate (STX-64).[34] Interestingly, this compound

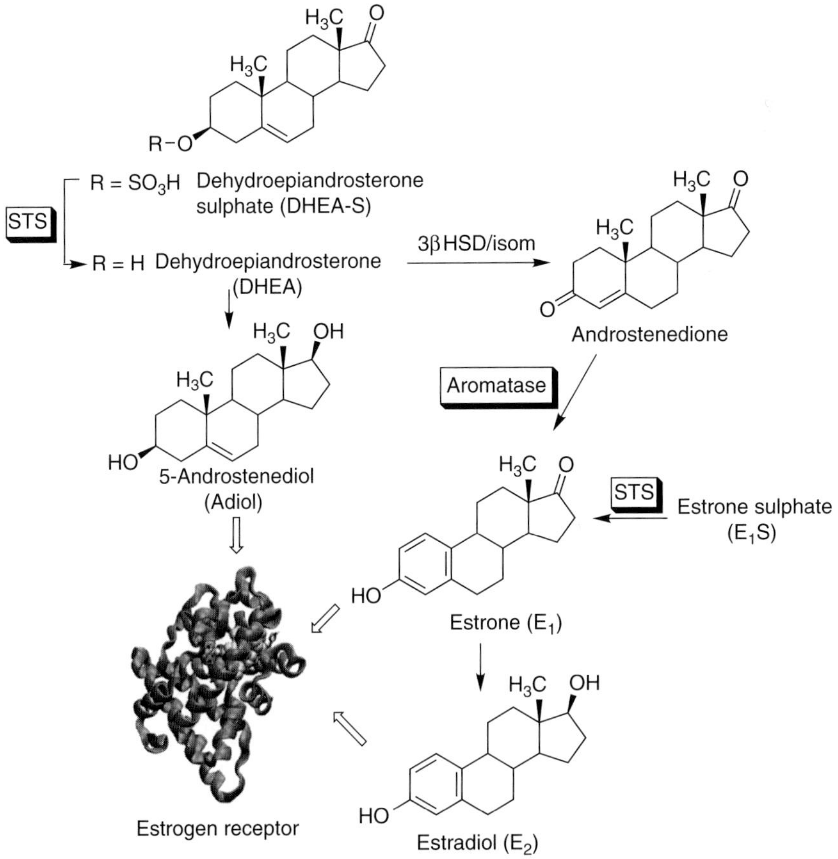

FIGURE 3.21   Role of steriod sulfatase in the biosynthesis of estrogens.

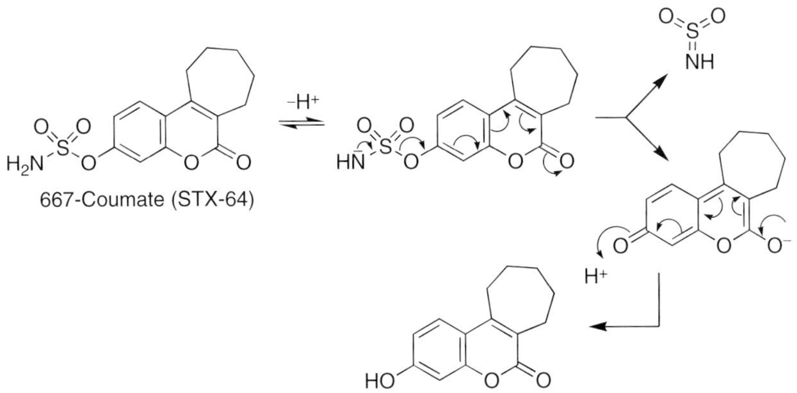

FIGURE 3.22   Metabolism of 667-coumate.

rapidly disappears from plasma because of its low stability, presumably due to the facile E1cB elimination of sulfamate to give the corresponding coumarin (Fig. 3.22), but it shows a long half-life in blood. This increased stability has been ascribed to binding of the drug to carbonic anhydrase II in erythrocytes. The hydrophobic environment in which the coumarin ring system is bound according to modeling studies explains the enhanced stability, since it hampers the generation of charged intermediates through the E1cB mechanism.[35]

Further research in this area is focused toward the development of nonestrogenic steroidal inhibitors of sulfatase by structural manipulation of the A or D rings. Another current goal is the development of dual aromatase-sulfatase inhibitors, which is being pursued by the introduction of the critical sulfamate unit in structures with known aromatase-inhibiting properties. In this connection, it is interesting to note that 667 Coumate shows some activity as an aromatase inhibitor.[33]

6. ANDROGEN-RELATED ANTITUMOR AGENTS

Androgens are steroidal hormones that stimulate and control the masculine primary and secondary characteristics. They exert their action by binding to a nuclear receptor called the androgen receptor (AR)[36] and the complex acts as a transcription factor, in a similar way to estrogens. The main androgens are testosterone and its reduced metabolite 5α-dihydrotestosterone (DHT), which has a higher affinity for the AR and three- to tenfold greater molar potency than testosterone.

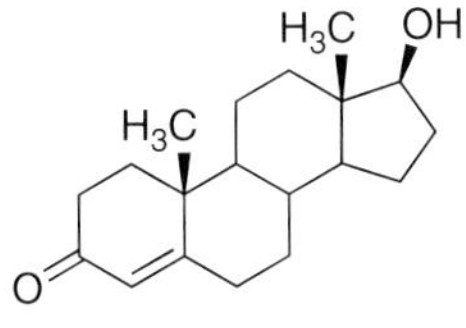

Testosterone 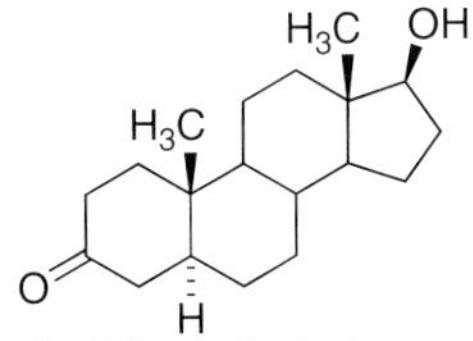   5α-Dihydrotestosterone

Most prostatic tumors are androgen dependent, and for this reason hormone treatment of prostate cancer is based on the modulation of testosterone to achieve medical castration levels. This can be achieved directly by administration of antiandrogens or indirectly by inhibition of 5α-reductase, the enzyme responsible for the reduction of testosterone to its more active metabolite. Androgen production can also be controlled by inhibition of the release of LH (see Section 7).

6.1. Antiandrogens

Androgen antagonists[37] bind to the receptor and prevent binding of the natural steroids, but they do not produce the correct conformational change in the receptor that is essential to elicit normal changes in gene expression. Cyproterone is a steroidal antiandrogen that was initially developed as a synthetic gestagen to be used as a contraceptive, but the observation of feminization of the offspring in gestating rats led to its identification as a competitive inhibitor of the AR. It is used in prostatic carcinoma, but its side effects of gynecomastia and edema, which can be attributed to its analogy with natural gestagens and glucocorticoids, respectively, stimulated the search for nonsteroidal compounds with pure antiandrogenic action (SARM, selective androgen receptor modulators).

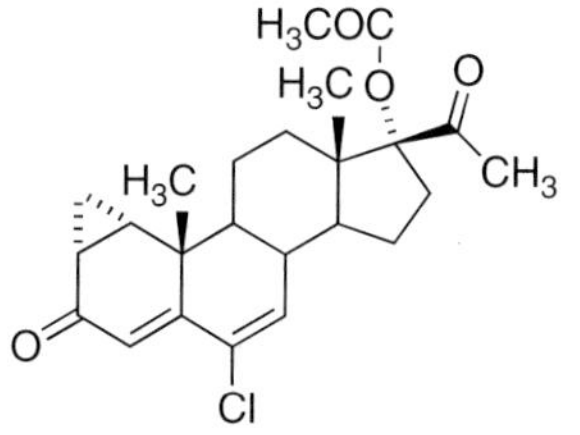

Cyproterone acetate

Flutamide was the first nonsteroidal antiandrogen. In itself it does not act on ARs, but it is metabolized by hydroxylation to the active species. This metabolite inhibits both androgen uptake and binding of androgens to their receptors in target tissues. Other antiandrogens that are in clinical use for the treatment of prostate cancer are bicalutamide and nilutamide, which have the advantage over flutamide of having a higher half-life that allows its administration only once daily.

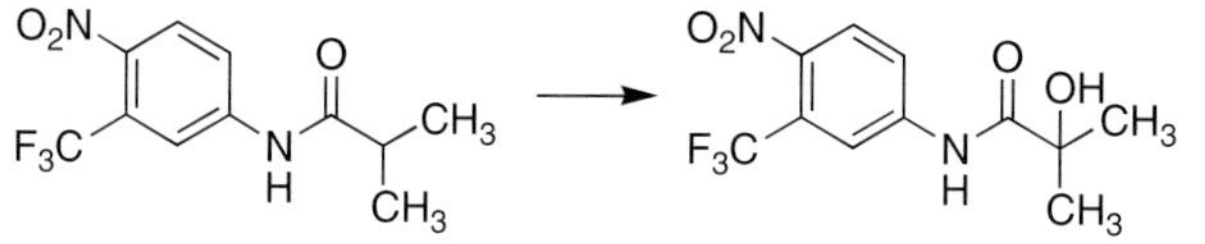

Flutamide

Flutamide active metabolite

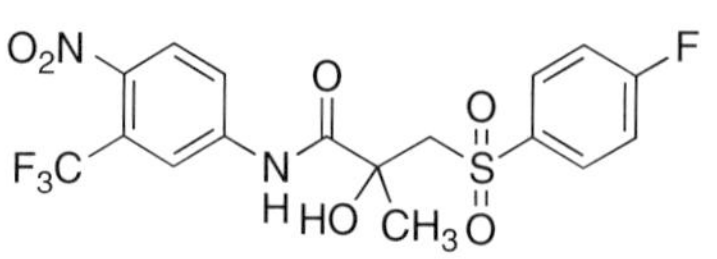

Bicalutamide

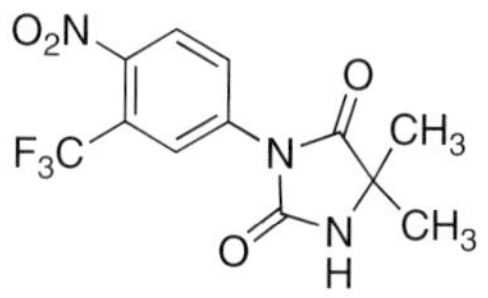

Nilutamide

Antiandrogens are also employed for treatment of benign prostate hyperplasia and as topical antialopecia agents.

6.2. Inhibitors of 14α-demethylase and 17α-hydroxylase

Another way to achieve androgen deprivation consists of the inhibition of the early stages of androgen biosynthesis. Two antitumor compounds that act in this way are ketoconazole and abiraterone acetate.

Ketoconazole   Abiraterone acetate

One procedure for the treatment of metastatic prostate cancers that do not respond to antiandrogens is the administration of ketoconazole, an imidazole derivative that is primarily used as an antifungal agent because it inhibits the biosynthesis of ergosterol, a key component of fungal membranes. Ketoconazole inhibits 14α-demethylase, a cytochrome P450 enzyme necessary for the conversion of lanosterol to ergosterol (in fungal cells) or to cholesterol (in mammalian cells), by coordination of the unsubstituted nitrogen atom to the iron atom in the active site. Since cholesterol is the precursor of all steroidal hormones, in a route that involves the participation of several other cytochrome P450 enzymes (Fig. 3.23), high doses of ketoconazole lead to androgen deprivation.[38] The use of ketoconazole as an antiandrogen normally involves short treatments due to its toxicity, and normally it is associated with corticoids to prevent adrenal insufficiency.

Another compound acting in this pathway is abiraterone acetate (CB7630), an inhibitor of 17α-hydroxylase/C(17,20)-lyase, the enzyme that transforms pregnenolone into 17α-hydroxypregnenolone and the latter into DHEA. A study in humans has shown that repeated treatment of men with intact gonadal function with abiraterone acetate can successfully suppress testosterone levels to the castrate range, although this level of suppression may not be sustained in all patients due to compensatory hypersecretion of LH.[39] Clinical trials are underway to determine the usefulness of abiraterone acetate in patients with prostate cancer.[40]

6.3. Inhibitors of 5α-reductase

The androgenic activity in the prostate is due to 5α-dihydrotestosterone (DHT), since 95% of testosterone entering the prostate is converted to the more potent androgen DHT by the 5α-reductase enzyme of the type 2. Hence, blockade of that enzyme, whose expression is largely restricted to the prostate, facilitates the inhibition of testosterone action on urogenital sinus tissue derivatives, notably

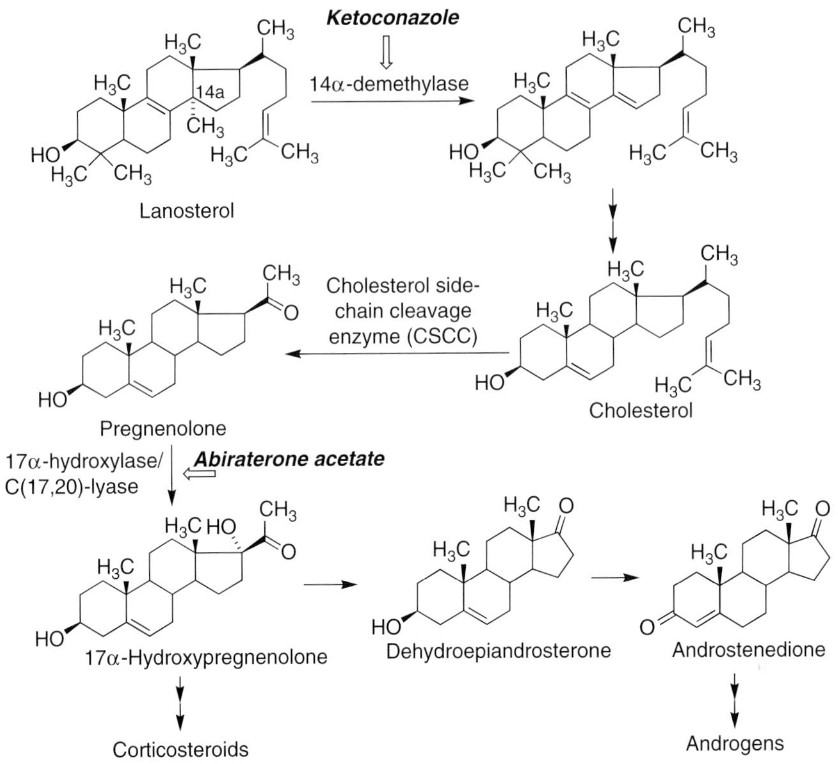

FIGURE 3.23 Antiandrogens that interfere with the conversion of lanosterol into steroidal hormones.

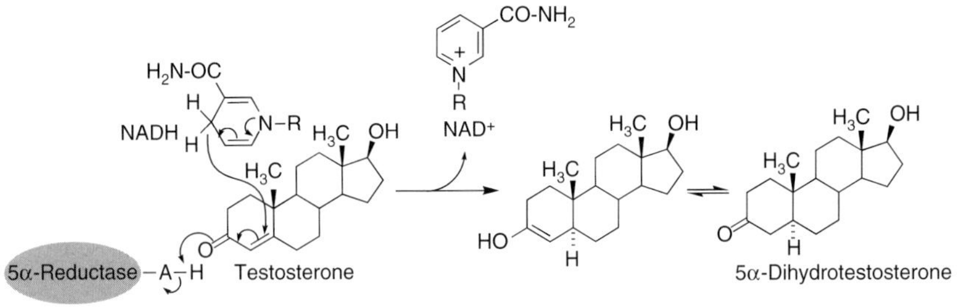

FIGURE 3.24 Reduction of testosterone to 5α-dihydrotestosterone.

the prostate, without blocking peripheral androgenic action due to testosterone. Their main use so far is the treatment of alopecia and benign prostate hyperplasia, and there is interest in their potential use as cancer chemopreventive agents.

5α-Reductase is associated with the nuclear membrane and requires hydride donation from NADH, which acts as a cofactor and is transformed into NAD^+ (Fig. 3.24).

Finasteride, the first inhibitor of this enzyme to reach the market, is believed to be a mechanism-based inhibitor acting through the mechanism shown in Fig. 3.25, which involves the addition of hydride to the unsaturated lactam system in

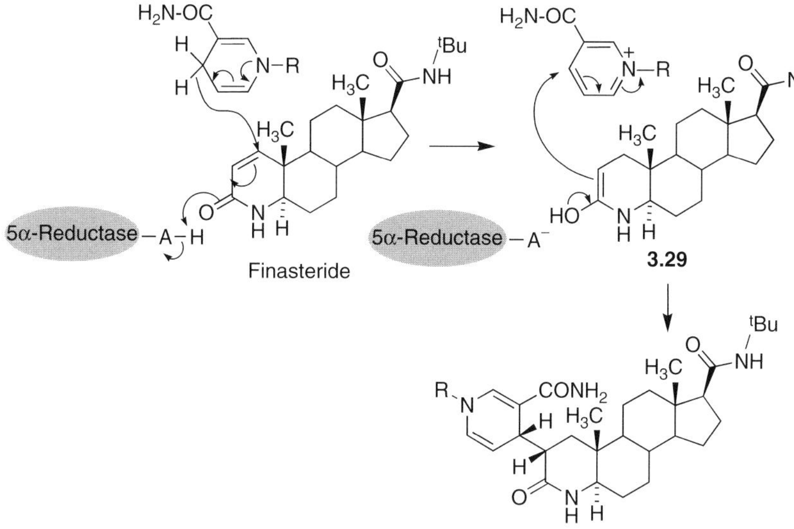

FIGURE 3.25 Inhibition of 5α-reductase by finasteride.

finasteride followed by trapping of the highly electrophilic NAD$^+$ molecule by enol **3.29** generated in the first step.[41]

Dutasteride (GI-198745) is an analog of finasteride that behaves as a dual inhibitor of 5-α-reductase type 1 and 2 isozymes. This compound is approved for benign prostate hyperplasia and has been proposed for the chemoprevention of prostate cancer in men at high risk.[42]

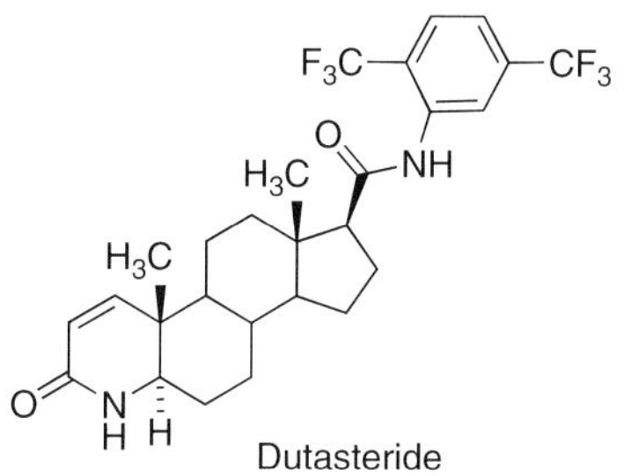

Dutasteride

7. REGULATION OF STEROIDAL HORMONE SYNTHESIS AS A TARGET FOR ANTITUMOR DRUGS

7.1. Introduction

Testosterone production in men is controlled by the hypothalamic–pituitary–gonadal axis. Secretion of gonadotropin-releasing hormone (GnRH, LHRH) from the hypothalamus stimulates the pituitary gland to release luteinizing hormone (LH), which acts on testicular Leydig cells to produce testosterone. The strategies currently employed for achieving a reduction of testosterone levels for the treatment of prostatic cancer,[43] including the ones related to the hormonal control of the process and those studied in Section 8, are summarized in Fig. 3.26.

In women, LH liberation stimulates the onset of ovulation in the first phase of the menstrual cycle and the production of progesterone in the second phase. Another pituitary hormone known as follicle-stimulating hormone (FSH) stimulates the secretion of estrogens in the ovary, although small amounts of LH are also required. A summary of these steps and the drugs used in breast and gynecological cancers discussed so far is presented in Fig. 3.27.

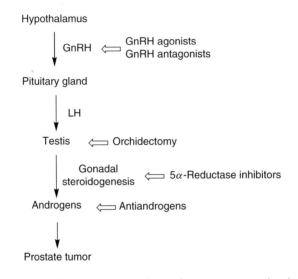

FIGURE 3.26   Strategies used to reduce testosterone levels.

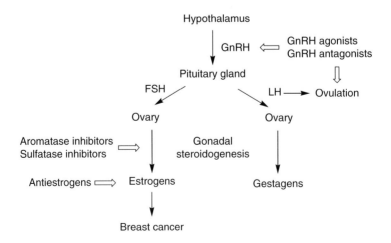

FIGURE 3.27   Regulation of steroidal hormone biosynthesis and interfering drugs.

7.2. GnRH (LHRH) agonists

The main clinical use of these drugs is the treatment of prostatic carcinoma. When a GnRH agonist is given in pulses by injection, it mimics the natural action of GnRH itself and induces the release of LH from the pituitary gland. However, if a GnRH agonist is given continuously, the pituitary is first stimulated, but after some days the response ceases. During the period of initial stimulation, more LH is released and consequently there is a surge in testosterone production, called a flare, and during this time about 1 in 10 men with metastatic cancer may experience a temporary worsening of their symptoms. For this reason, GnRH agonists are associated with an antiandrogen or an inhibitor of androgen synthesis prior and during the first weeks of the treatment. After a few days, the pituitary becomes desensitized by the continuous presence of the hormone, loses its membrane receptors for GnRH and stops releasing LH, leading to a decline of testosterone production and ending in levels similar to those achieved by orchidectomy.

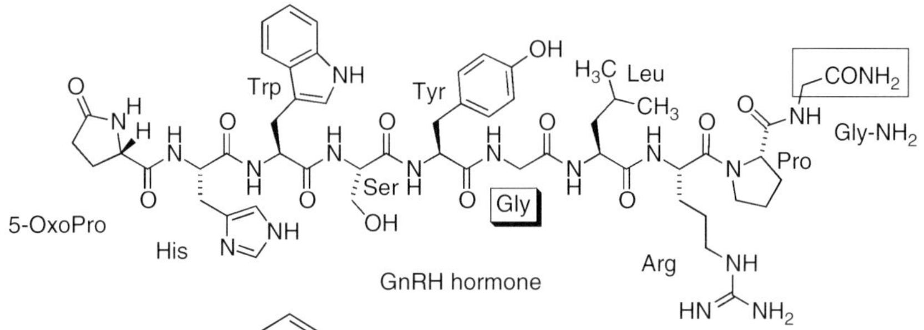

GnRH hormone

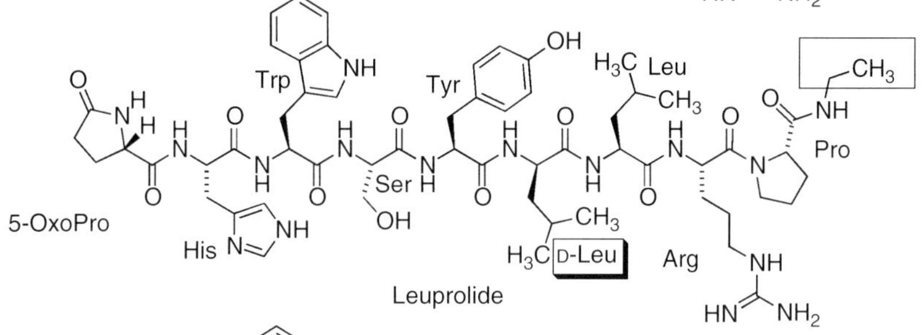

Leuprolide

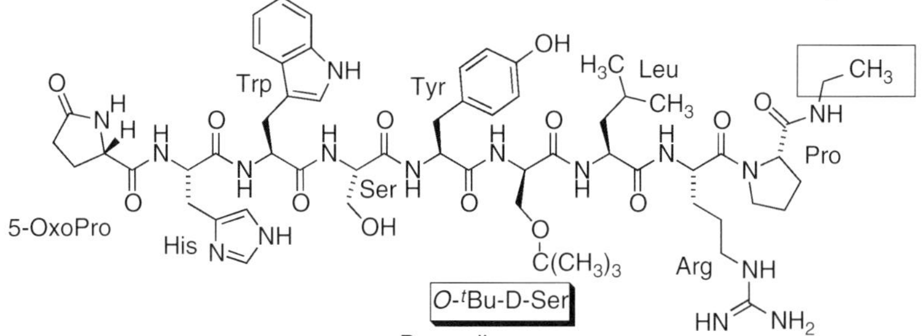

Buserelin

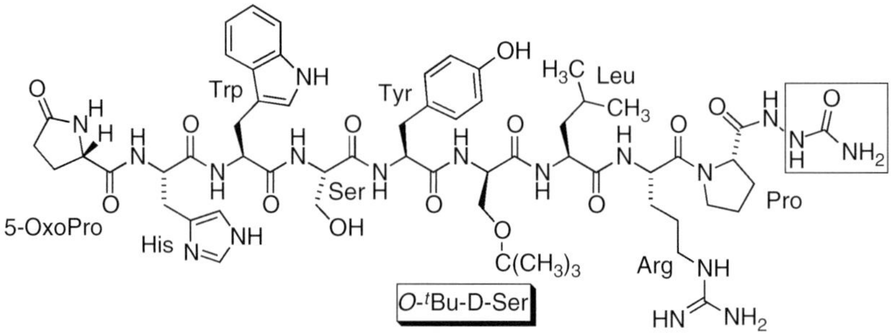

Goserelin

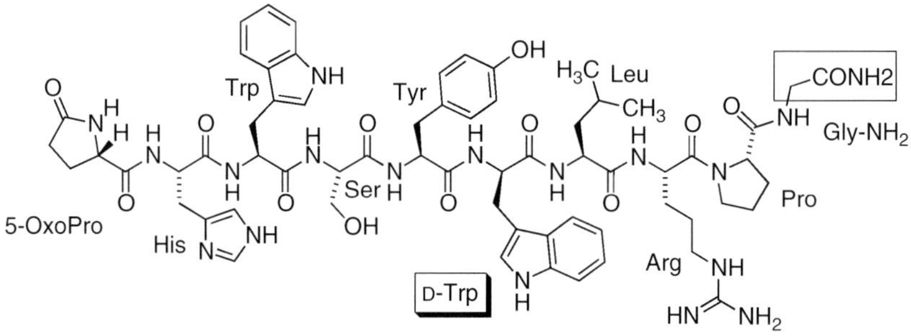

Triptorelin

GnRH is a decapeptide with two isoforms differing in three amino acids, the most important of which is isoform I. Because the *in vivo* half-life of GnRH is very low (4 min) due to fast hydrolysis of the bond between amino acids 6 and 7, a search began for related but more stable molecules. The main strategy employed involved replacement of the sixth amino acid (glycine) by D-amino acids, and the C-terminal glycinamide residue was also replaced by a variety of substituents. The resulting compounds, besides being more stable to enzymatic degradation, are more lipophilic due to the introduction of a side chain at the sixth residue and have higher affinity for their receptor. Among these agonists, leuprorelin (leupro- lide), buserelin, goserelin, and triptorelin are used for prostate cancer. They are administered parenterally or by inhalation to avoid their degradation in the gastrointestinal tract.

Goserelin has also proved useful in premenopausal women with ER-positive early breast cancer, providing an alternative to their chemotherapeutic regimens and avoiding the need for surgical ovariectomy. This means that younger women, when they finish their goserelin treatment, can recover from their bone loss before they reach menopause.

7.3. GnRH (LHRH) antagonists

When administered to patients with prostatic cancer, GnRH antagonists act by direct inhibition of GnRH receptors and therefore LH secretion, leading to a faster onset of the action (hours instead of days) and avoiding the initial rise of testos- terone levels induced by GnRH receptor agonists.

GnRH antagonists currently in clinical use are peptidomimetics obtained by extensive modification of the natural GnRH hormone. The main problems to be overcome were the tendency of the first compounds to induce the release of histamine as well as their low solubility and propension to form gels, which severely limits their formulation.[44] The main modifications that have been explored are the following:

a. Replacement of the first three amino acids by D-amino acids with unnatural side chains. The most widely employed replacements are *N*-acetyl-D-(β-naphthyl)alanine for the first residue, D-(4-chloro)phenylalanine for the second, and D-(2-pyridyl)alanine or D-Trp for the third one.

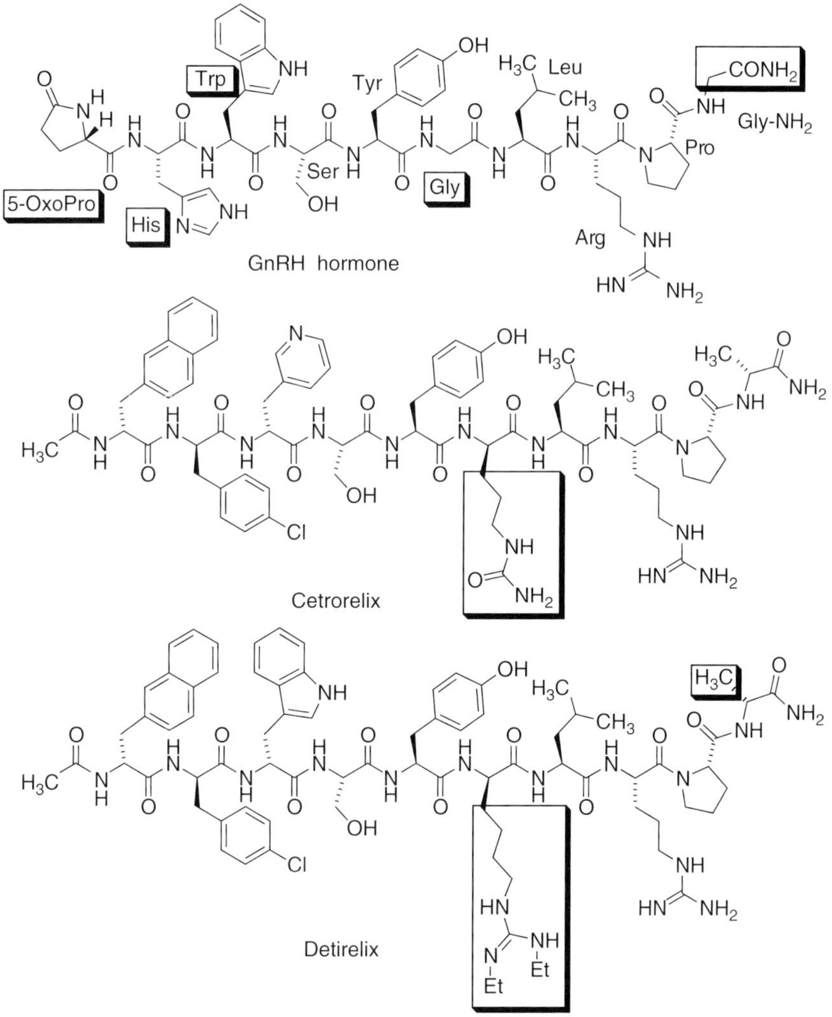

GnRH hormone

Cetrorelix

Detirelix

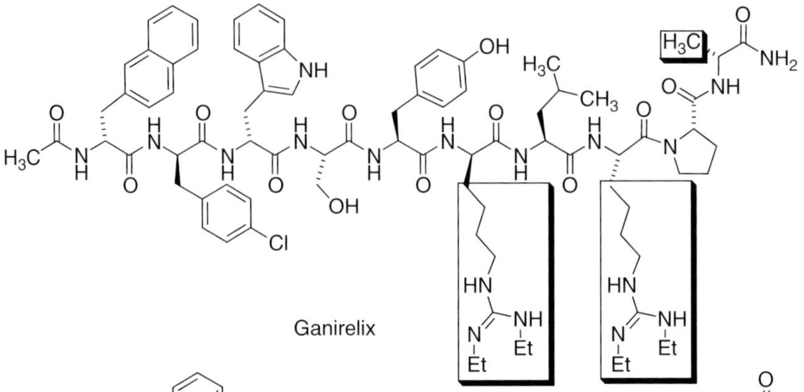

Ganirelix

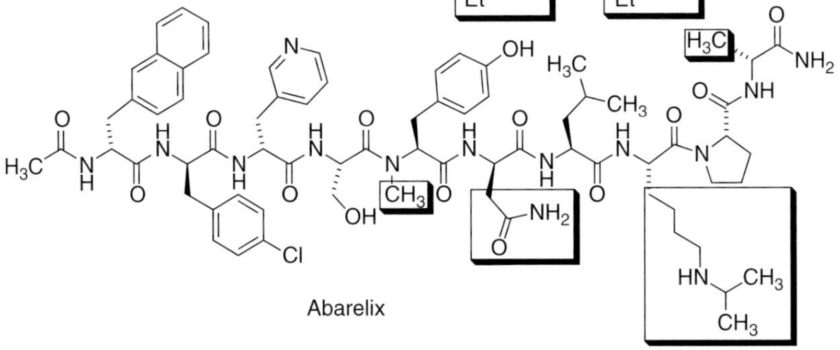

Abarelix

b. Modification of the sixth amino acid, which normally bears chains with amide, urea, or guanidine substituents. The purpose of this substitution is to increase the hydrogen bond-formation capabilities of the molecules and improve their solubilities.

c. Modifications of the side chain in the eighth amino acid.

d. Replacement of the C-terminal glycinamide by D-alaninamide.

The first long-term clinical studies were carried out with cetrorelix and ganirelix. However, the first GnRH antagonist to achieve clinical use as an antitumor agent was abarelix,[45] a short acting antagonist with low histamine-releasing activity that was approved by the FDA in November 2003 and is used as an intramuscular injection for the palliative treatment of advanced symptomatic prostate cancer in patients where LHRH agonist therapy and surgical castration (orchidectomy) are not appropriate. Clinical studies have also shown the usefulness of some of these antagonists, like cetrorelix, in ovarian, endometrial, and breast cancers.[46]

GnRH antagonists have a number of indications other than cancer treatment.[47] For instance, they are employed in assisted reproduction techniques[48] to prevent LH surge in women undergoing controlled ovary stimulation, allowing the follicles to mature for planned oocite collection. The rationale for this treatment is that one of the physiological roles of LH is the initiation of ovulation during the menstrual cycle. When women are undergoing hormone treatment in assisted reproduction techniques sometimes premature ovulation can occur, leading to the release of eggs that are not ready for fertilization.

8. MISCELLANEOUS STEROID HORMONE-RELATED ANTICANCER THERAPY

8.1. Gestagens as antitumor agents

Agonists of the gestagen receptor such as megestrol acetate, medroxyprogesterone acetate, and norethisterone acetate are able to induce apoptosis by binding to progesterone receptors in the cell surface. About 80% of endometrial carcinomas and also some types of breast cancers show a positive response to these drugs.

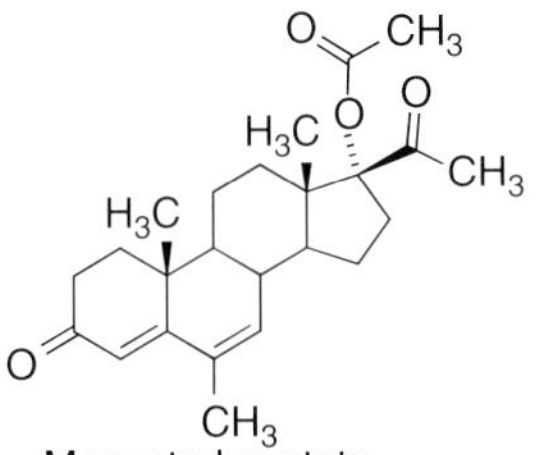

Megestrol acetate 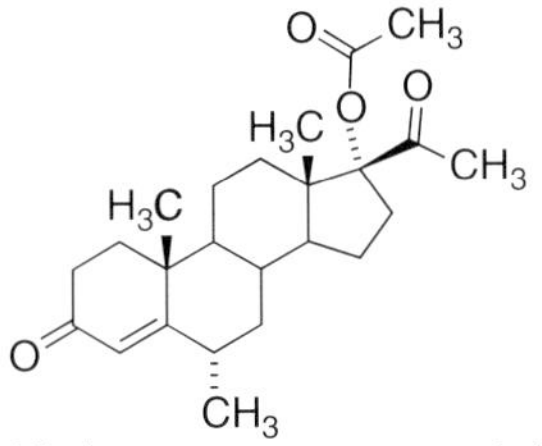   Medroxyprogesterone acetate 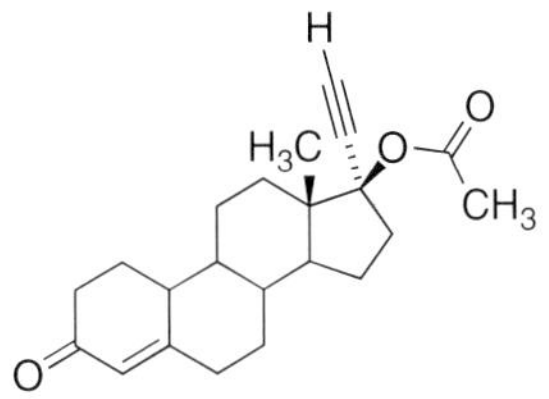   Norethisterone acetate

8.2. Glucocorticoids and inhibitors of their biosynthesis as antitumor agents

The immunosuppressive and anti-inflammatory activities of the glucocorticoids are well known. They exert an influence in human lymphoid tissue (e.g., they can modify the homing of lymphocytes into lymphoid organs), and for this reason they are often useful in the treatment in acute lymphoblastic leukemia and other chronic and acute leukemias. Prednisone is normally employed for this purpose, normally in association with other types of chemotherapy. Because of their anti-inflammatory action, corticosteroids are often included in antitumor regimens to alleviate cancer pain.[49]

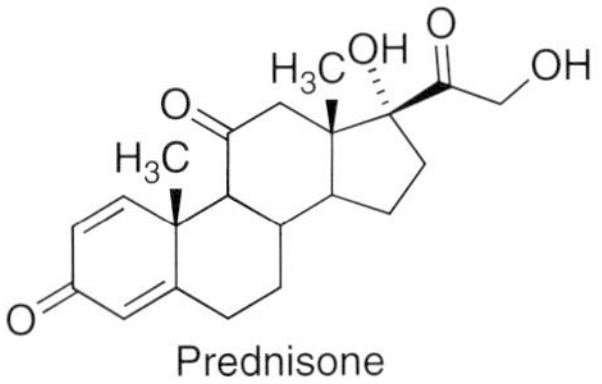

Prednisone

Mitotane (o,p'-DDD) is an analog of the insecticide DDT that has been approved for use in the treatment of human inoperable cancer of the adrenal gland (adrenocortical cancer), and is also being used for treatment of canine Cushing's disease because of its cortex-selective adrenalytic activity. It completely

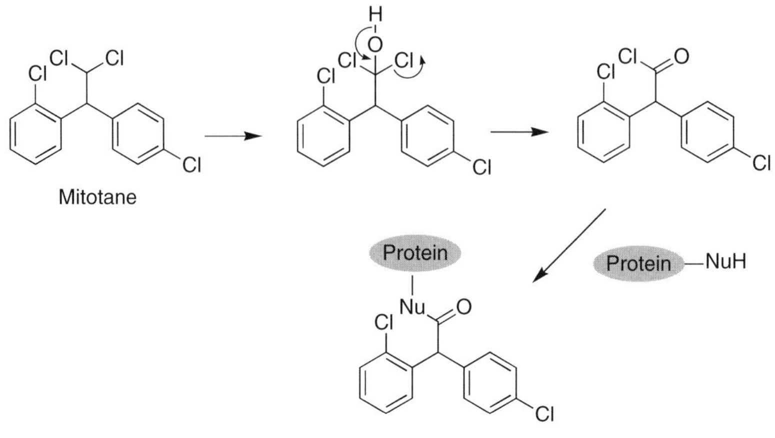

FIGURE 3.28   Biotransformations of mitotane.

obliterates adrenal production of glucocorticoids, mineralocorticoids, and adrenal gland-produced sex hormones.

Adrenal tissue is capable of metabolizing mitotane by action of a novel, non-steroidogenic P450-type enzyme that catalyzes hydroxylation at the position adjacent to the two chlorine atoms. Subsequent dehydrohalogenation of this intermediate leads to a highly electrophilic acyl chloride, which has been shown to react with proteins, leading to direct necrosis and atrophy of the adrenal cortex and hence inhibition of glucocorticoid synthesis (Fig. 3.28). Another possible mechanism is oxidative damage through the production of free radicals.[50]

9. COMPOUNDS ACTING ON OTHER PROTEINS OF THE NUCLEAR RECEPTOR SUPERFAMILY: RETINOIDS

Vitamin A and its analogs, collectively known as retinoids, have profound effects in cell growth and differentiation, and the loss of retinoid function is linked to carcinogenesis in some cancers. The diet-derived all-*trans* retinoic acid is the main retinoid in humans. Several retinoids have shown promising activity as antitumor and cancer chemopreventive agents by inhibiting carcinogenesis at the initiation, promotion, and progression stages.[51]

The anticancer activity of retinoids is mainly due to their binding to nuclear receptors, known as the classical retinoic acid receptors (RARs) and the nonclassical retinoid X receptors (RXRs), each of which has three isoforms (α, β, and γ). They have different ligand-binding domains, and therefore they can be targeted separately. All-*trans* retinoic acid selectively activates the RARs, while 9-*cis*-retinoic acid can activate both RARs and RXRs (Fig. 3.29). Retinoids with selectivity for RXR are known as rexinoids.

RARs can heterodimerize with RXRs, while the latter functions as a master regulator because it can also form heterodimers with other nuclear receptors,

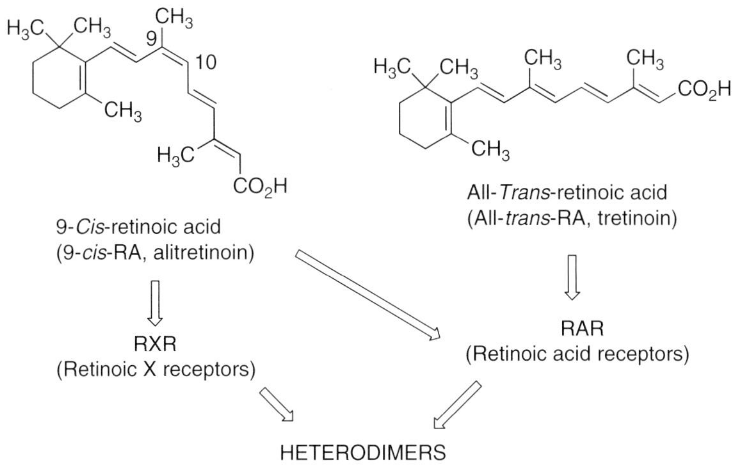

FIGURE 3.29   Retinoids and their receptors.

including the vitamin D receptors, thyroid hormone receptors, and peroxisome proliferator activating receptors (PPARγ). The RAR–RXR heterodimers bind to specific DNA sequences, known as retinoic acid response elements (RARE). In the absence of ligands, the heterodimer–DNA complex is linked to corepressors and histone deacetylases, inducing chromatin compaction and silencing the promoter region of the target genes (gene repression). The binding of ligands to the hetero-dimers induces a conformational change that destabilizes the interaction with core-pressors and allows the union to coactivators, leading to gene transcription (Fig. 3.30).

Some retinoids and their analogs are currently in use or under clinical trials for several types of cancer.[52] The most relevant success of retinoids in this field has been achieved in the therapy of acute promyelocytic leukemia (APL), a previously intractable disease, as well as in the prevention of several other cancers (oral cavity, head and neck, breast, skin, and liver). APL arises from a chromosomal translocation that produces a chimeric protein between RAR-α and promyelocyte leukemia protein (PML). This process interferes with the normal function of both proteins, resulting in the arrest of cell maturation at the stage of promyelocytes. Oral administration of all-*trans* retinoic acid (tretinoin) induces differentiation of these cells to produce mature neutrophils with a high rate of therapeutic success, and a combination of tretinoin with anthracycline and ara-C has become the standard therapy for this disease. The mechanism of action of tretinoin in this tumor is not fully understood, although it has been shown that it induces the cleavage of the PML portion from the chimeric protein and its degradation.[53] 9-*Cis*-retinoic acid (alitretinoin) has been approved for the topical treatment of Kaposi's sarcoma in combination with interferon,[54] and 13-*cis*-retinoic acid (isotretinoin), an RAR ligand, is one of the standard treatments for the prevention of oral cancer.[55] The three mentioned retinoids are also under clinical trials for many other tumors.

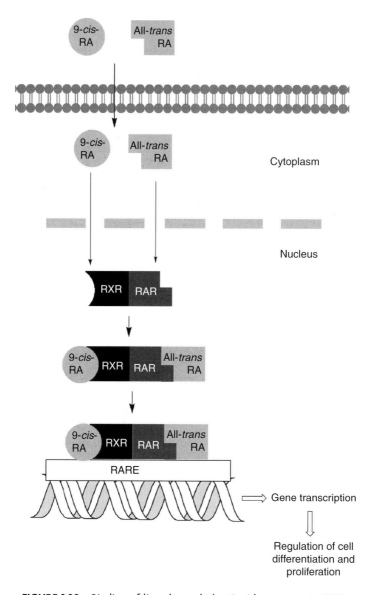

FIGURE 3.30   Binding of ligand-coupled retinoid receptors to DNA.

13-*cis*-retinoic acid
(isotretinoin)

Despite the above-mentioned successes, the full potential of retinoids as anti-cancer agents has not yet been realized because of the problem of intrinsic or acquired resistances. Strategies to overcome this problem include the combination of retinoids with other chemotherapeutic agents acting by related mechanisms and the use of nonclassical retinoids.[56]

Several atypical retinoids have also been assayed for cancer chemoprevention. Fenretinide, an amide of tretinoin that acts as a ligand of RAR-β and RAR-γ receptors, has entered clinical trials showing a beneficial effect in the prevention of premenopausal breast cancer in combination with tamoxifen.[57] Polyprenoic acid, also called acyclic retinoid, has shown RAR, RXR, and PPAR activities and is useful in the prevention of hepatocellular carcinoma.[58] Finally, adapalene prevents cancer in patients with cervical intraepithelial neoplasia.

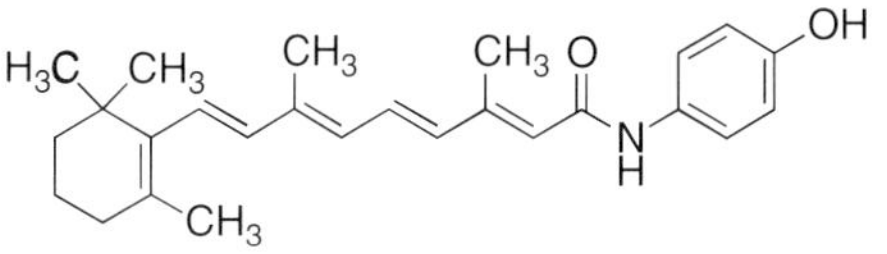

4-Hydroxyphenylretinamide (fenretinide)

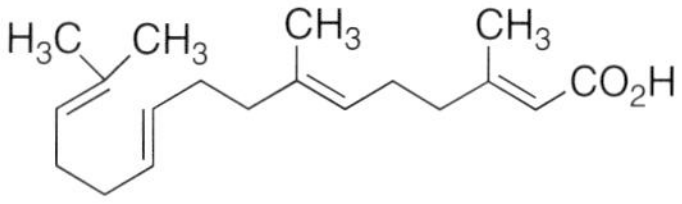

Acyclic retinoid
(polyprenoic acid)

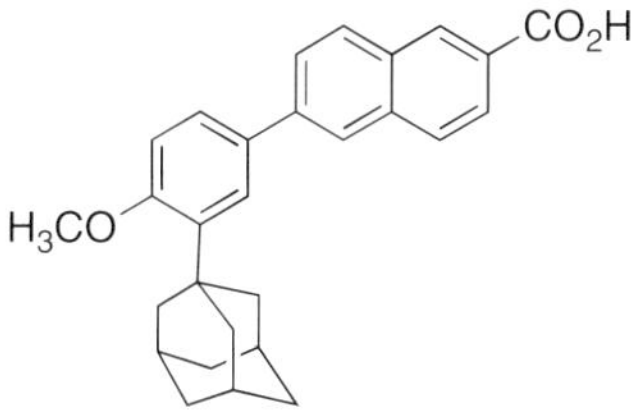

Adapalene

Bexarotene is selective for RXRs (rexinoid) and has been approved by the FDA for cutaneous T-cell lymphoma.[59] In combination with chemotherapeutic agents, such as cisplatin and vinorelbine, bexarotene has demonstrated encouraging results in patients with advanced non-small cell lung cancer, and two Phase III trials are currently under way to fully characterize its role in the treatment of this disease.[60]

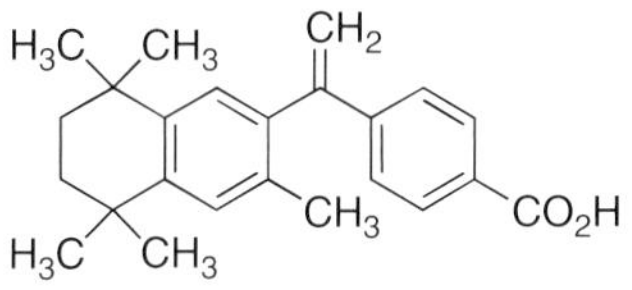

Bexarotene

PPAR ligands have also been studied as antitumor agents. Promising results were obtained in initial clinical trials for liposarcoma and prostate cancers with the PPAR-γ ligand troglitazone, normally employed as an oral antidiabetic. Unfortunately, more recent studies in colorectal and breast cancers have been disappointing.[61]

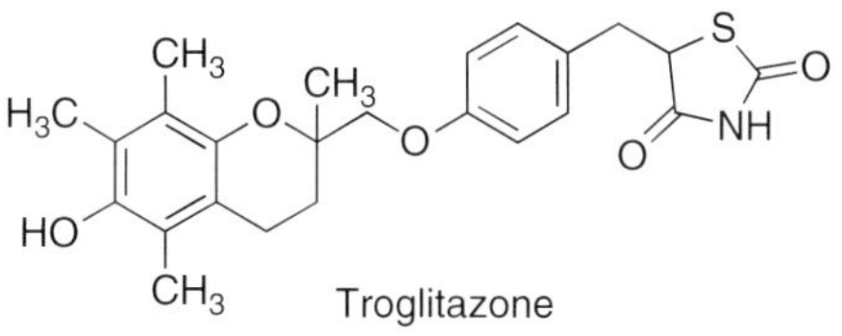

Troglitazone

REFERENCES

1. Liehr, J. G. (2000). *Endocr. Rev.* **21,** 40.
2. Santen, R. J., Yue, W., and Wang, J.-P. (2005). *Breast Cancer Res* **7,** S.08.
3. Zahid, M., Kohli, E., Saeed, M., Rogan, E., and Cavalieri, E. (2006). *Chem. Res. Toxicol.* **19,** 164.
4. Watts, C. K. W., and Sutherland, R. L. (1987). *Mol. Pharmacol.* **31,** 541.
5. Jordan, V. C. (2003). *Nat. Rev. Drug Discov.* **2,** 205.
6. De Médina, P., Favre, G., and Poirot, M. (2004). *Curr. Med. Chem. Anticancer Agents* **4,** 491.
7. Howell, S. J., Johnston, S. R., and Howell, A. (2004). *Best Pract. Res. Clin. Endocrinol. Metab.* **18,** 47.
8. Pagani, O., Gelber, S., Simoncini, E., Castiglione-Gertsch, M., Price, K., Zahrieh, D., Gelber, R., Coates, A., and Goldhirsch, A. (2004). *Ann. Oncol.* **15,** 1749.
9. Buzdar, A., Hayes, D., El-Khoudary, A., Yan, S., Lønning, P., Lichinitser, M., Gopal, R., Falkson, G., Pritchard, K., Lipton, A., Wolter, K., Lee, A., *et al.* (2002). *Breast Cancer Res. Treat.* **73,** 161.
10. Howell, S. J., Johnston, S. R., and Howell, A. (2004). *Best Pract. Res. Clin. Endocrinol. Metab.* **18,** 47.
11. http://www.cancer.gov/star.
12. Brzozowski, A. M., Pike, A. C. W., Dauter, Z., Hubbard, R. E., Bonn, T., Engström, O., Öhman, L., Greene, G. L., Gustaffson, J.-A., and Carlquist, M. (1997). *Nature* **389,** 753.
13. Dardes, R. C., and Jordan, V. C. (2000). *Br. Med. Bull.* **56,** 773.
14. Lake, D. E., and Hudis, C. (2002). *Cancer Control* **9,** 490.
15. Vergote, I., and Robertson, J. F. R. (2004). *Br. J. Cancer* **90**(Suppl. I), S11.
16. Osborne, C. K., Wakeling, A., and Nicholson, R. I. (2004). *Br. J. Cancer* **90**(Suppl. I), S2.
17. Puddefoot, J. R., Barker, S., Glover, H. R., Malouitre, S. D. M., and Vinson, G. P. (2002). *Int. J. Cancer* **101,** 17.
18. Grubjesic, S., Moriarty, R. M., and Pezzuto, J. M. (2002). *Expert Opin. Ther. Pat.* **12,** 1647.
19. Chen, S. (1998). *Front. Biosci.* **3,** 922.
20. Santen, R. J. (2003). *Steroids* **68,** 539.
21. Osborne, C., and Tripathy, D. (2005). *Annu. Rev. Med.* **56,** 103.
22. Brueggemeier, R. W. (1990). *J. Enz. Inh.* **4,** 101.
23. Cole, P. A., and Robinson, C. H. (1990). *J. Med. Chem.* **33,** 2933.
24. Brueggermeier, R. W. (1994). *Breast Cancer Res. Treat.* **30,** 31.
25. Narashimamurty, J., Rao, A. R. R., and Sastry, G. N. (2004). *Curr. Med. Chem. Anticancer Agents* **4,** 523.
26. Reddy, P. (1998). *J. Clin. Pharm. Ther.* **23,** 81.
27. Brodie, A. M., and Njar, V. C. (2000). *Steroids* **65,** 171.
28. Dixon, J. M. (2002). *Expert Rev. Anticancer Ther.* **2,** 267.
29. Zilembo, N., Noberasco, C., and Bajetta, E. (1995). *Br. J. Cancer* **72,** 1007.
30. Opera, T. I., and García, A. E. (1996). *Comput. Aided Mol. Des.* **10,** 186.
31. Cavelli, A., Greco, A. E., Novellino, E., and Recanatini, M. (2000). *Bioorg. Med. Chem.* **8,** 2771.
32. Johnston, S. R. D., and Dowsett, M. (2003). *Nat. Rev. Cancer* **3,** 821.
33. Purohit, A., Woo, L. W. L., Chander, S. K., Newman, S. P., Ireson, C., Ho, Y., Grasso, A., Leese, M. P., Potter, B. V. L., and Reed, M. J. (2003). *J. Steroid Biochem. Mol. Biol.* **86,** 423.
34. Stanway, S. J., Purohit, A., Woo, L. W. L., Sufi, S., Vigushin, D., Ward, R., Wilson, R. H., Stanczyk, F. Z., Dobbs, N., Kulinskaya, E., Elliott, M., Potter, B. V. L., *et al.* (2006). *Clin. Cancer Res.* **12,** 1585.
35. Lloyd, M. D., Pederick, R. L., Natesh, R., Woo, L. W. L., Purohit, A., Reed, M. J., Achayra, K. R., and Potter, B. V. L. (2005). *Biochem. J.* **385,** 715.
36. Sack, J. S., Kish, K. F., Wang, C., Attar, R. M., Kiefer, S. E., An, Y., Wu, G. Y., Scheffler, J. E., Salvati, M. E., Krystek, S. R., Weinmann, R., and Einspahr, H. M. (2001). *Proc. Natl. Acad. Sci. USA* **98,** 4904.
37. Allan, G. F., and Sui, Z. (2003). *Nucl. Rec. Signal.* **1:e009,** doi:10.1621/nrs.01009.
38. Ryan, C. J., and Eisenberger, M. (2005). *J. Clin. Oncol.* **23,** 8242.
39. O'Donnell, A., Judson, I., Dowsett, M., Raynaud, F., Dearnaley, D., Mason, M., Harland, S., Robbins, A., Halbert, G., Nutley, B., and Jarman, M. (2004). *Br. J. Cancer* **90,** 2317.
40. Madan, R. A., and Arlen, P. M. (2006). *IDrugs* **9,** 49.

41. Bull, H. G., García-Calvo, M., Andersson, S., Baginsky, W. F., Chan, H. K., Ellsworth, D. E., Miller, R. R., Stearns, R. A., Bakshi, R. K., Rasmusson, G. H., Tolman, R. L., Myers, R. W., *et al.* (1996). *J. Am. Chem. Soc.* **118,** 2359.
42. Andriole, G., Bostwick, D., Brawley, O., Gomella, L., Marberger, M., Tindall, D., Breed, S., Somerville, M., and Rittmaster, R. (2004). *J. Urol.* **172,** 1314.
43. Denmeade, S. R., and Isaacs, J. T. (2002). *Nat. Rev. Cancer* **2,** 389.
44. Jiang, G., Stalewski, J., Galyean, R., Dykert, J., Schteingart, C., Broqua, P., Aebi, A., Aubert, M. L., Semple, G., Robson, P., Akinsanya, K., Haigh, R., *et al.* (2001). *J. Med. Chem.* **44,** 433.
45. Hedge, S., and Schmidt, M. (2004). *Annu. Rep. Med. Chem.* **40,** 443.
46. Emons, G., Grundker, C., Gunthert, A. R., Westphalen, S., Kavanagh, J., and Verschraegen, C. (2003). *Endocr. Relat. Cancer* **10,** 291.
47. Huirne, J. A. F., and Lambalk, C. B. (2001). *Lancet* **358,** 1793.
48. Hernández, E. R. (2000). *Hum. Reprod.* **15,** 1211.
49. Tannock, I. F., de Wit, R., Berry, W. R., Horti, J., Pluzanska, A., Chi, K. N., Oudard, S., Théodore, C., James, N. D., Turesson, I., Rosenthal, M. A., and Eisenberger, M. A. (2004). *N. Engl. J. Med.* **351,** 1502.
50. Schteingart, D. E. (2000). *Braz. J. Med. Biol. Res.* **33,** 1197.
51. Okuno, M., Kojima, S., Matsushima-Nishigaki, R., Tsurumi, H., Muto, Y., Friedman, S. L., and Moriwaki, H. (2004). *Curr. Cancer Drug Targets* **4,** 285.
52. Altucci, L., and Gronemeyer, H. (2001). *Nat. Rev. Cancer* **1,** 181.
53. Grignani, F., De Matteis, S., Nervi, C., Tomassoni, L., Gelmetti, V., Cioce, M., Fanelli, M., Ruthardt, M., Ferrara, F. F., Zamir, I., Seiser, C., Lazar, M. A., *et al.* (1998). *Nature* **319,** 815.
54. Von Roenn, J. H., and Cianfrocca, M. (2001). *Cancer Treat. Res.* **104,** 127.
55. Lee, J. J., Hong, W. K., Hittelman, W. N., Mao, L., Lotan, R., Shin, D. M., Benner, S. E., Xu, X.-C., Lee, J. S., Papadimitrakopoulou, V. M., Geyer, C., Pérez, C., *et al.* (2000). *Clin Cancer Res.* **6,** 1702.
56. Freemantle, S. J., Spinella, M. J., and Dmitrovsky, E. (2003). *Oncogene* **22,** 7305.
57. Decensi, A., and Costa, A. (2000). *Eur. J. Cancer* **36,** 694.
58. Muto, Y., Moriwaki, H., and Saito, A. (1999). *N. Engl. J. Med.* **340,** 1046.
59. Hurst, R. E. (2001). *Curr. Opin. Invest. Drugs* **1,** 514.
60. Rigas, J. R., and Dragnev, K. (2005). *Oncologist* **10,** 22.
61. Rumi, M. A. K., Ishihara, S., Kazumori, H., Kadowaki, Y., and Kinoshita, Y. (2004). *Curr. Med. Chem. Anticancer Agents* **4,** 465.

CHAPTER 4

Anticancer Drugs Acting via Radical Species, Photosensitizers and Photodynamic Therapy of Cancer

Contents

1. Introduction: Radicals and Other Reactive Oxygen Species   93
2. Biological Effects of ROS   95
   2.1. Membrane phospholipid peroxidation   95
   2.2. Malondialdehyde generation and its consequences   96
   2.3. DNA strand cleavage   98
   2.4. Oxidation of DNA bases   100
   2.5. Formaldehyde generation   102
   2.6. ROS as signaling molecules   102
3. Anthracyclines and Their Analogs   102
4. Mitoxantrone and Related Quinones   112
5. Actinomycin D   114
6. Chartreusin, Elsamicin A, and Related Compounds   116
7. Bleomycins   116
8. Enediyne Antibiotics   122
9. Tirapazamine   126
10. Penclomedine   128
11. Radiosensitizers   129
12. Photodynamic Therapy of Cancer   132
References   135

1. INTRODUCTION: RADICALS AND OTHER REACTIVE OXYGEN SPECIES

A radical (sometimes called *free radical*) is a chemical species capable of independent existence that contains one or more unpaired electrons. Molecular oxygen is the main promoter of the formation of radicals within the cells because ground state oxygen contains two unpaired electrons, each one in a different π^*

Medicinal Chemistry of Anticancer Drugs
DOI: 10.1016/B978-0-444-52824-7.00004-4

antibonding orbital, and hence it can be considered as a biradical. Both electrons have the same spin quantum number and therefore oxygen tends to accept electrons one at a time because a pair of electrons in an atomic or molecular orbital will have opposite spin numbers in accordance with Pauli's principle, and for this reason it will not be able to form two pairs of electrons with antiparallel spins by combination with the oxygen molecule electrons, which have parallel spins. Singlet oxygen species, on the contrary, do not have this restriction because the two electrons of the π^* antibonding orbitals have opposite spins and are more potent oxidants than ground state oxygen. Addition of one electron to oxygen gives the superoxide radical anion, and incorporation of a new electron to the latter leads to the peroxide dianion (Fig. 4.1).

Another oxidizing species found in biological systems is hydrogen peroxide (H_2O_2), arising from diprotonation of peroxide (O_2^{2-}). The main source of peroxide is the enzyme superoxide dismutase (SOD), which catalyzes the one-electron transfer between two superoxides. Because the second electron is added to an antibonding orbital, the O-O bond in peroxide or hydrogen peroxide is weak and can be homolyzed under certain conditions (e.g., exposure to UV radiation), leading to two hydroxyl radicals. Alternatively, electron transfer from superoxide to hydrogen peroxide gives a hydroxide anion and a hydroxyl radical (Haber-Weiss reaction, Fig. 4.2).

The production of hydroxyl radical through the mechanisms in Fig. 4.2 is very slow, but it can be catalyzed by the presence of certain relatively common cations like Fe^{2+} or Cu^+. For instance, Fe^{2+} can decompose hydrogen peroxide to a hydroxyl radical and a hydroxy anion in the so-called Fenton reaction, which is coupled to the regeneration of Fe^{2+} through one-electron reduction of Fe^{3+} by superoxide radical (Fig. 4.3). The extremely reactive hydroxyl radical cannot diffuse from its site of formation and therefore drugs that act through this radical must generate it very close to the target biomolecule.

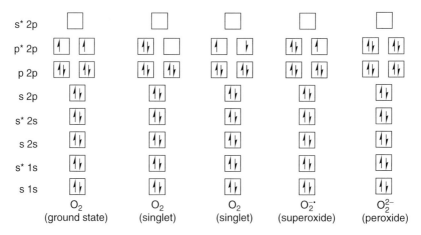

FIGURE 4.1   Different molecular oxygen species.

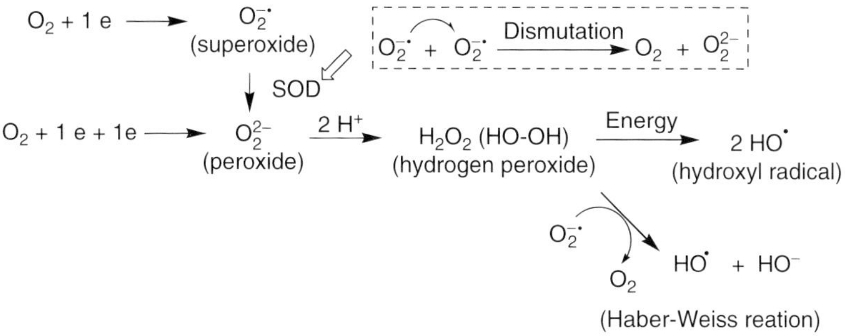

$$O_2 + 1\,e \longrightarrow O_2^{-\bullet} \text{ (superoxide)}$$

$$O_2^{-\bullet} + O_2^{-\bullet} \xrightarrow{\text{Dismutation}} O_2 + O_2^{2-}$$

$$\downarrow \text{SOD}$$

$$O_2 + 1\,e + 1e \longrightarrow O_2^{2-} \text{ (peroxide)} \xrightarrow{2\,H^+} H_2O_2 \text{ (HO-OH)} \xrightarrow{\text{Energy}} 2\,HO^{\bullet} \text{ (hydroxyl radical)}$$
$$\text{(hydrogen peroxide)}$$

$$O_2^{-\bullet} \searrow \quad HO^{\bullet} + HO^-$$
$$O_2$$

(Haber-Weiss reation)

FIGURE 4.2   Redox processes involving molecular oxygen.

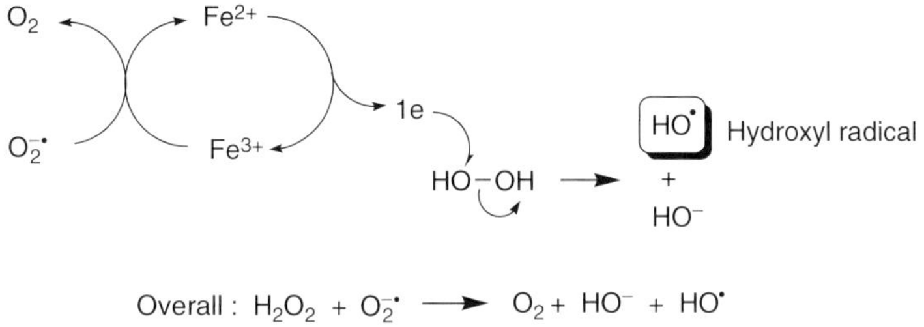

$$O_2 \leftarrow \quad Fe^{2+}$$
$$O_2^{-\bullet} \quad Fe^{3+} \xrightarrow{1e}$$
$$HO-OH \longrightarrow \boxed{HO^{\bullet}} \text{ Hydroxyl radical}$$
$$+ \quad HO^-$$

Overall : $H_2O_2 + O_2^{-\bullet} \longrightarrow O_2 + HO^- + HO^{\bullet}$

FIGURE 4.3   The Fenton reaction.

Oxygen radicals, such as superoxide, and hydroxyl radicals, as well as some nonradical derivatives of oxygen, like hydrogen peroxide, are collectively known as "reactive oxygen species" (ROS).

2. BIOLOGICAL EFFECTS OF ROS

The main biological effect of ROS is the induction of oxidative stress, which can be defined as a situation of imbalance between the production of radical species and antioxidant defense systems. Oxidative stress can cause damage to all kinds of biomolecules, including lipids, proteins, and DNA. For this reason, the mechanism of action of several kinds of antitumor agents is based, at least partly, on the production of hydroxyl radicals and other ROS and the subsequent damages that they cause on biological molecules by a number of mechanisms that will be summarized in this chapter.[1] Most of these mechanisms have been discovered during the course of studies on the anthracyclines.[2]

2.1. Membrane phospholipid peroxidation

Cell membranes are one of the biological structures more sensitive to damage by radicals because of the presence of polyunsaturated fatty acids in them, containing methylene groups that are simultaneously adjacent to two double bonds.

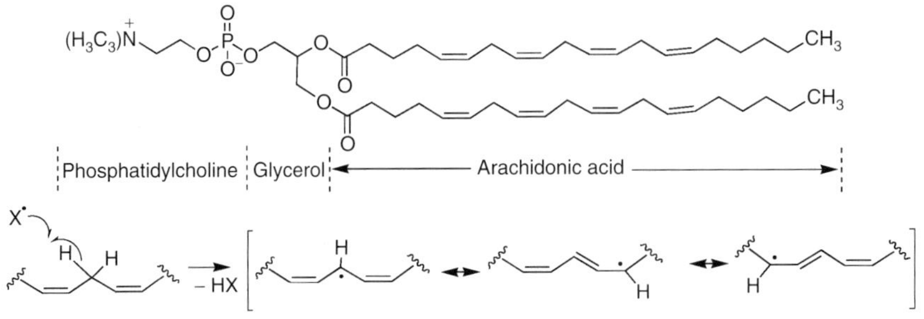

FIGURE 4.4   Radical generation in membrane phospholipids.

The C-H units in these methylenes are particularly suitable points of attack by hydroxyl and other radicals because of the stabilization of the resulting carbon radical by double resonance (Fig. 4.4).

The reaction of these polyunsaturated side chains with oxygen radicals leads to *phospholipid peroxidation* and subsequent membrane injury. This process is initiated by the attack of a hydroxyl radical to one of the previously mentioned bisallylic positions existing in the fatty acid side chains, leading to the generation of an alkyl radical **4.1**. Superoxide radical is not sufficiently reactive to initiate lipid peroxidation, and in any case its negative charge precludes its transport across the highly lipophilic cell membrane. Carbon radical **4.1** reacts rapidly with a molecule of oxygen, which is sufficiently hydrophobic to access the interior of the membranes, generating a peroxyl radical (R-O-O$^\bullet$, **4.2**), which can abstract a new hydrogen atom from a doubly allylic C-H bond in the adjacent fatty acid side chain. This leads to a hydroperoxide **4.3** and a new radical **4.1**, allowing a self-maintained radical process that extends to an expanding area of the membrane, as long as there is sufficient oxygen (propagation phase). If traces of cations, such as Fe^{2+}, are present, they can generate new oxygen radicals (RO$^\bullet$ and HO$^\bullet$) from hydroperoxides **4.3** through Fenton chemistry, contributing to the extension of the peroxidation process (Fig. 4.5).

2.2. Malondialdehyde generation and its consequences

Peroxyl radicals **4.2** can also evolve to cyclic endoperoxides by attack onto a neighboring C=C double bond in the same chain, as shown in Figure 4.6 for the case of a molecule of arachidonic acid, in a process resembling the one catalyzed by cyclooxygenase. Peroxyl radicals **4.2** may lead to lipid peroxidation, as previously mentioned (Fig. 4.5). Alternatively, they can cyclize to radical **4.4**, which then undergoes a new cyclization, coupled with the addition a second oxygen molecule and subsequent reduction of the hydroperoxyl radical thus generated, to give **4.5**. Together with other products, these intermediates generate malondialdehyde (MDA) through a retro Diels-Alder mechanism.

MDA can link covalently to amino groups in proteins, especially at Lys residues, resulting in intra- and intermolecular protein cross-links (Fig. 4.7A).

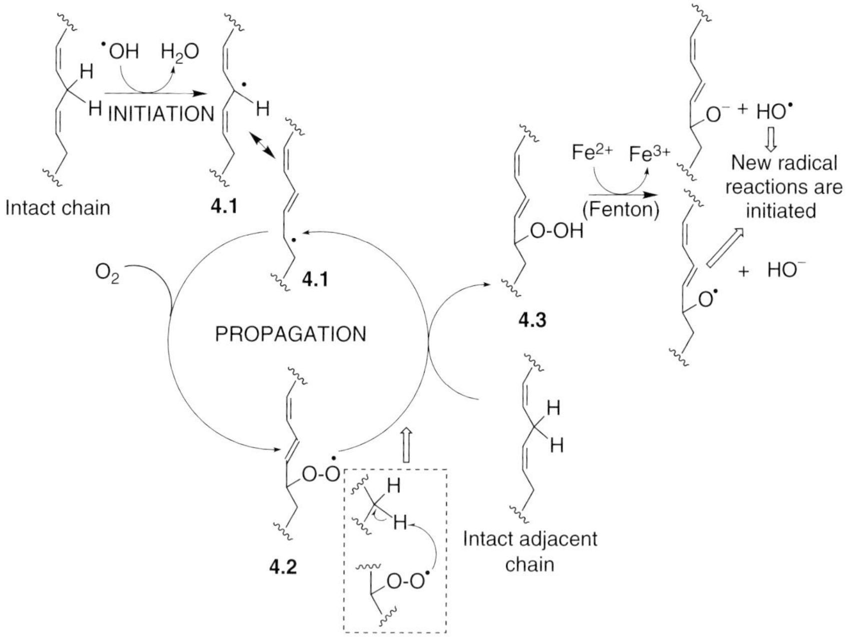

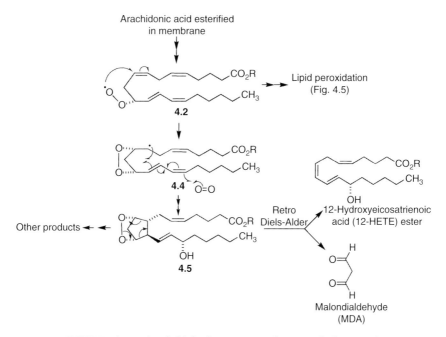

FIGURE 4.5 Phospholipid peroxidation.

FIGURE 4.6 Malondialdehyde generation from arachidonic acid.

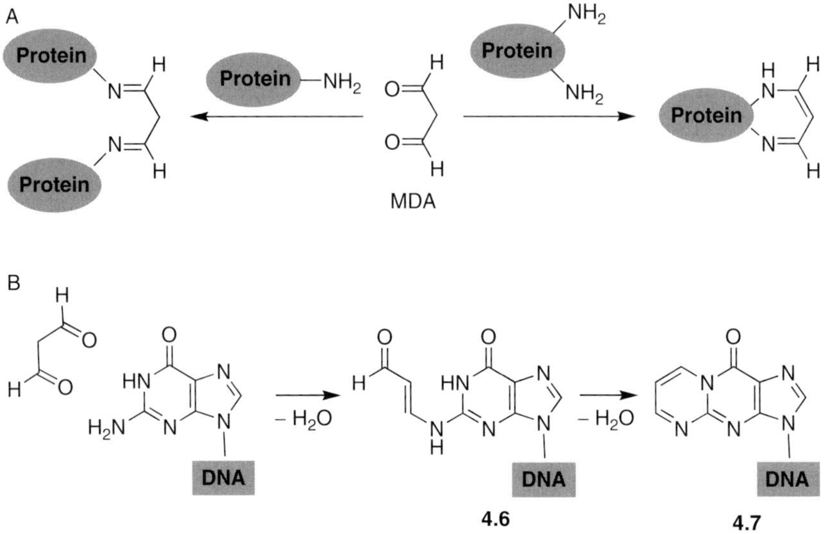

FIGURE 4.7 Covalent derivatives from malondialdehyde and proteins (A) or DNA (B).

It may also react with DNA bases and cause mutagenic lesions, consisting of large insertions and deletions at GC base pairs, by reaction with guanine amino groups to give the oxopropenyl derivatives **4.6** which are finally cyclized to pyrimido-purine derivatives **4.7**, known as M_1dG adducts (Fig. 4.7B).[3] For many years, there has been insufficient evidence for the implication of lipid peroxidation in the antitumor effects of radical-generating drugs like the anthracyclines, but recent studies have shown the involvement of MDA in DNA damage.[4] In proliferating cells, the formation of M_1dG adducts is accompanied by cell cycle arrest and inhibition of cyclin-associated kinase activities. It has been proved that antitumor compounds of the anthracyclin group, at low concentrations, increase MDA-dependent DNA oxopropenylation several fold,[5] establishing a potential link between antitumor drug-dependent generation of ROS, induction of lipid peroxidation, and DNA damage.[6]

2.3. DNA strand cleavage

Oxidative stress by hydroxyl radical also causes direct DNA damage, mainly by strand cleavage and oxidation of pyrimidine and purine bases. DNA, because of the negative charge of its phosphate groups, acts as an anion and is therefore capable of binding many cations, including those required for Fenton chemistry, like Fe^{2+} and Cu^+. Additionally, deoxyribose has also good iron-binding properties. This allows "site-specific" hydroxyl radical generation that cannot be countered by radical scavengers. Perhaps for this reason, antitumor compounds that act by DNA strand cleavage are also normally chelating agents.

The main products of DNA strand scission, which have been studied mainly for the case of the antitumor drug bleomycin, are free DNA bases and N-(3-oxopropenyl) bases, which are accompanied by 5′-phosphate-modified DNA fragments and 3′-phosphoglycolate DNA derivatives (see Fig. 4.9 below). The formation of N-(3-oxopropenyl) bases requires additional oxygen,[7] while that of free bases does not,[8] as shown by isotope studies with $^{18}O_2$ and $H_2^{18}O$.

This process starts by the radical-induced abstraction of a proton from any position of the desoxyribose moiety and can lead to a large number of products. For instance, oxidation at C-4 leads to carbon radical 4.8, stabilized by resonance with the ring oxygen. Addition of an oxygen molecule gives the sugar peroxyl radicals 4.9, which are transformed into hydroperoxide 4.10 by incorporation of one proton and one electron. If their source is the desoxyribose unit of another DNA molecule, the radical process becomes self-maintained, as shown in Fig. 4.8.

One possible degradation pathway that explains some of the products observed in the presence of additional oxygen involves a ring expansion through a modified Criegee rearrangement, where isotope studies with $^{18}O_2$ and $H_2^{18}O$ prove that hydroxide is released from 4.10.[7] The stabilized cation 4.11 resulting from the rearrangement undergoes an elimination reaction to 4.12, which is subsequently decomposed to the observed fragments 4.13, 4.16, and 4.17, which come from 4.14 and 4.15 by the mechanism shown in Fig. 4.9.

The liberation of DNA bases can be explained by the mechanism shown in Fig. 4.10, where the 4′-radical 4.8 evolves to the oxonium cation 4.18 by one-electron oxidation. Nucleophilic attack by a water molecule gives the hydroxy derivative 4.19, which then decomposes to the free base and finally to fragments 4.13 and 4.20. This mechanism predominates in oxygen-limited environments.

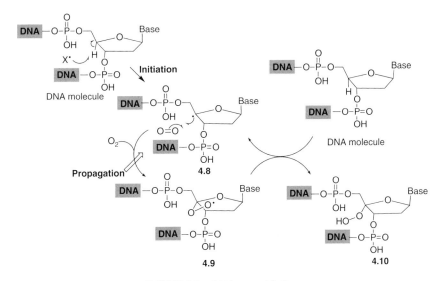

FIGURE 4.8   DNA peroxidation.

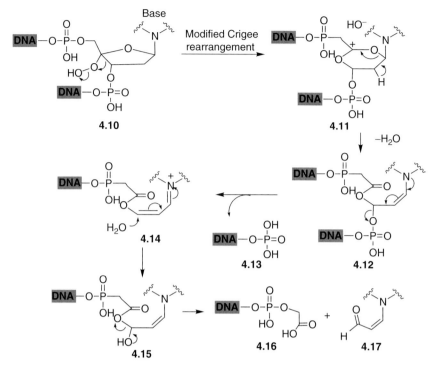

FIGURE 4.9 Degradation of DNA hydroperoxide **4.10**.

2.4. Oxidation of DNA bases

Attack of hydroxyl radicals to purine or pyrimidine bases produces other DNA damages. The structures of the degradation products arising from this reaction have been established mainly from studies with ionizing radiation,[9] but many of them were similarly isolated from patients receiving anthracyclines for the treatment of breast cancer.[10]

The main site for the reaction of hydroxyl radical with pyrimidines is the 5,6-double bond. For instance, thymidine is transformed into the hydroxy hydroperoxides **4.21**, which can be reduced to give thymidine glycols (ThyGly) or be degraded to 5′-hydroxyhydantoin (5′-OH-Hyd) through the intermediacy of open intermediate **4.22**. Thymidine can also suffer hydrogen abstraction from its methyl group, giving the deoxyriboside of 5-(hydroxymethyl)uracil (5-OH-MeUra) after coupling with a hydroxyl radical (Fig. 4.11).

Among other reactions, hydroxyl radicals can add to the guanine C-8 position to give radical **4.23** that can be reduced by addition of one electron and one proton to the unstable aminal intermediate **4.24**, which finally gives the ring-opened product known as FapyGua. Alternatively, **4.23** can undergo one-electron oxidation to 8-hydroxyguanine (8-OHGua). A very similar process transforms adenine into the ring-opened derivative FapyAde (Fig. 4.12).

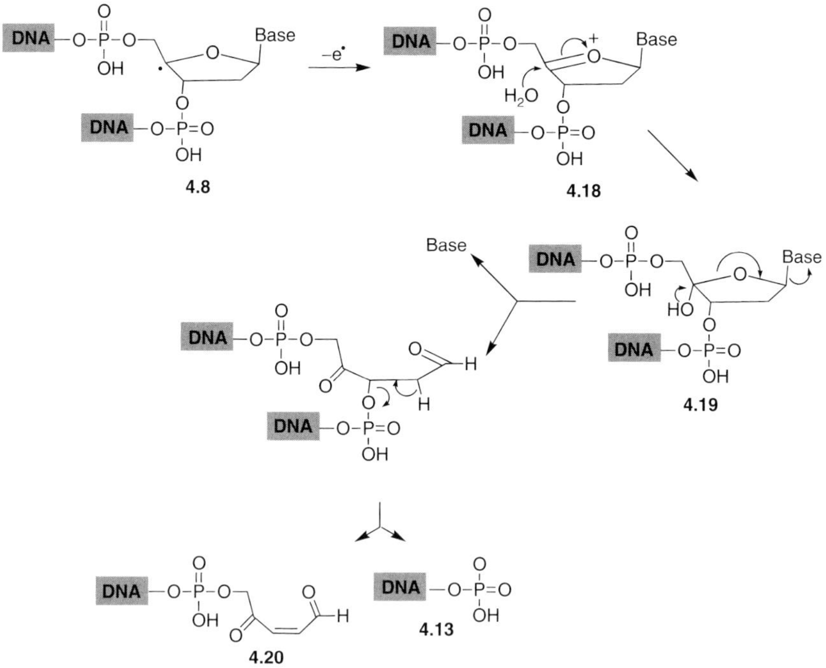

FIGURE 4.10 Liberation of bases from DNA following attack by radicals.

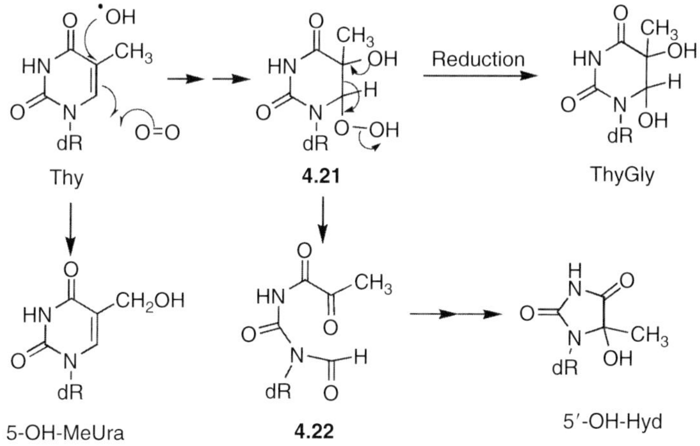

FIGURE 4.11 Oxidation products from thymidine.

The mutagenic potential of some of these degradation products has been clearly established, as in the case of the GC-CG transversions induced by Fapy-Gua. Furthermore, FapyGua and ThyGly block DNA replication or increase reading error frequencies by DNA polymerase, resulting in mutations.[11]

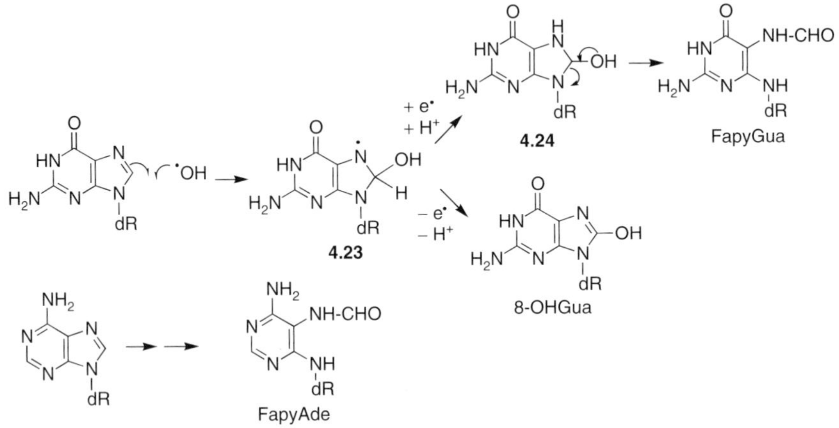

FIGURE 4.12   Oxidation products from purine nucleosides.

This polymerase dysfunction may also be due to oxidation-induced conformational changes in DNA. Nuclear proteins can also be attacked by radicals, especially at Tyr residues, and the resulting protein-derived radicals can cross-link to base-derived radicals that interfere with chromatin unfolding and DNA repair and transcription.[12]

2.5. Formaldehyde generation

Another consequence of the formation of hydroxyl radicals can be the generation of formaldehyde by reaction with certain cell components like spermine and lipids. This mechanism seems to be relevant only in the case of some anthracyclines and will be discussed in Section 3.

2.6. ROS as signaling molecules

Besides their role as mediators of oxidative modifications of cell constituents, ROS can also function as signaling molecules, even at very low concentrations.[13] Some examples of this type of response are ROS activation of neutral sphingomyelinase leading to ceramide formation, and modulation by ROS of several kinases or transcription factors controlling the cell cycle.[14,15] One mechanism by which ROS transmit signals is by oxidation of thiol residues in cysteines of the target proteins to sulfenic acids. This transformation serves as a chemical switch that can either activate or deactivate the protein function.

3. ANTHRACYCLINES AND THEIR ANALOGS

Anthracyclines are a group of antibiotics characterized by the presence of a planar chromophore containing an anthraquinone fragment, attached to an amino sugar. Daunomycin or daunorubicin (DNR) and doxorubicin (DOX), previously called adriamycin, were isolated from a *Streptomyces* species and were the first anthracycline antibiotics introduced in the clinic for cancer treatment. They are widely used for the treatment of human cancers, and, despite its very similar structure, their antitumor spectra of activity differ widely. Thus, daunorubicin is effective in acute lymphocytic and myeloid leukemia, while doxorubicin is an essential component of the chemotherapy of a large number of solid tumors, including breast cancer, childhood solid tumors, soft tissue sarcomas, and aggressive lymphomas. Despite their long-standing clinical utilization, their mechanism of action is still unclear and subject to controversy.[2,16] We will deal here with the mechanisms related to the generation of radical species, while some other mechanisms (intercalation into DNA and consequent inhibition of macromolecular biosynthesis and inhibition of topoisomerase II), will be studied in Sections 5 and 6 of Chapter 7.

R = CH$_2$OH Doxorubicin (DOX)
R = CH$_3$ Daunorubicin (daunomycin, DNR)

The main drawback of anthracyclines is their ability to cause chronic cardiomyopathy, which is related to damages associated to ROS generation and consequent apoptosis induction. These damages are specially important in cardiac tissue because of the low levels of catalase and the easy inhibition of cardiac selenium-dependent glutathion peroxidase by the anthracyclines, both being key enzymes in the detoxification of hydrogen peroxide.[17] Apoptosis induction in cardiac tissue proceeds through activation of NF-κB.[2] This is opposite to what is observed in cancer cells in which NF-κB activation usually inhibits apoptosis induced by anthracyclines, a difference that is still not well understood.

The production of radical species by quinone-containing antibiotics was first demonstrated in 1975, and 2 years later DOX and DNR were shown to generate free radicals through redox cycling.[18] Because of their ability to bind to nucleic acids, these drugs can be considered as site-specific free radical generators.

From a chemical point of view, the generation of radicals from quinones is based on the captodative effect. While cations are stabilized by electron-releasing groups and anions by electron-withdrawing groups, radicals are best stabilized by the simultaneous presence of both types of substituents (captodative effect). In the case of quinones, the ease of formation of the so-called semiquinone radicals by one-electron reduction is due to their stabilization through the captodative effect of the electron-releasing negatively charged oxygen atom and the electron-withdrawing carbonyl groups (Fig. 4.13).

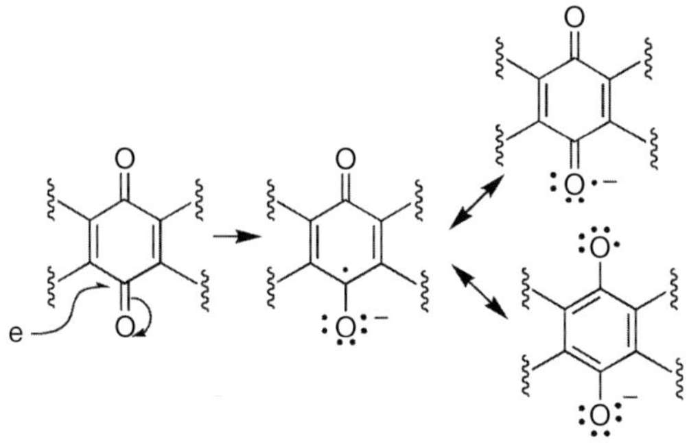

Semiquinone

FIGURE 4.13 Captodative stabilization of semiquinone radicals.

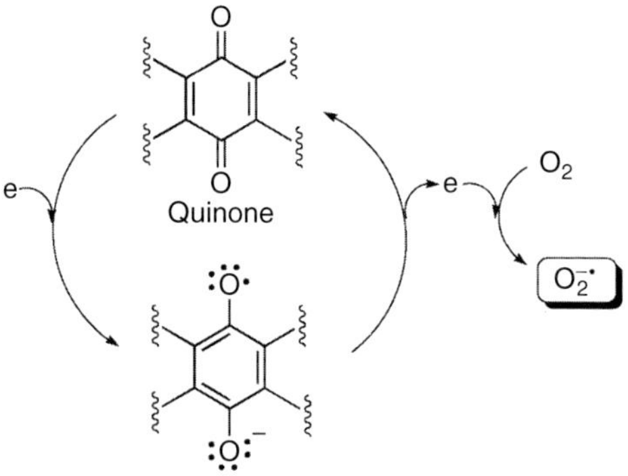

Semiquinone
4.25

FIGURE 4.14 Electron flow from semiquinone radicals to oxygen molecules.

The reversibility of semiquinone formation allows these radicals to induce one-electron reduction of oxygen molecules to superoxide radical anions, leading to an overall increase of the electron flow to oxygen derived from the activity of enzymes such as NADPH dehydrogenase, xanthine dehydrogenase, and the reductase domain of nitric oxide synthase[19] (Fig. 4.14).

A competitive reaction of semiquinone **4.25** can take place, involving loss of daunosamine. Thus, two molecules of **4.25** can disproportionate to give the starting quinone and hydroquinone **4.26**, which is unstable and evolves by elimination of the sugar moiety to give the anthracycline aglycon (Fig. 4.15).[20] Because of their relatively high lipophilicity with regard to the glycosides, these aglycons tend to accumulate in the inner mitochondrial membrane. The oxidative deterioration of mitochondrial functions due to the formation of radicals from these aglycons is one of the factors responsible for the cardiomyopathy associated with the use of anthracyclines.[20]

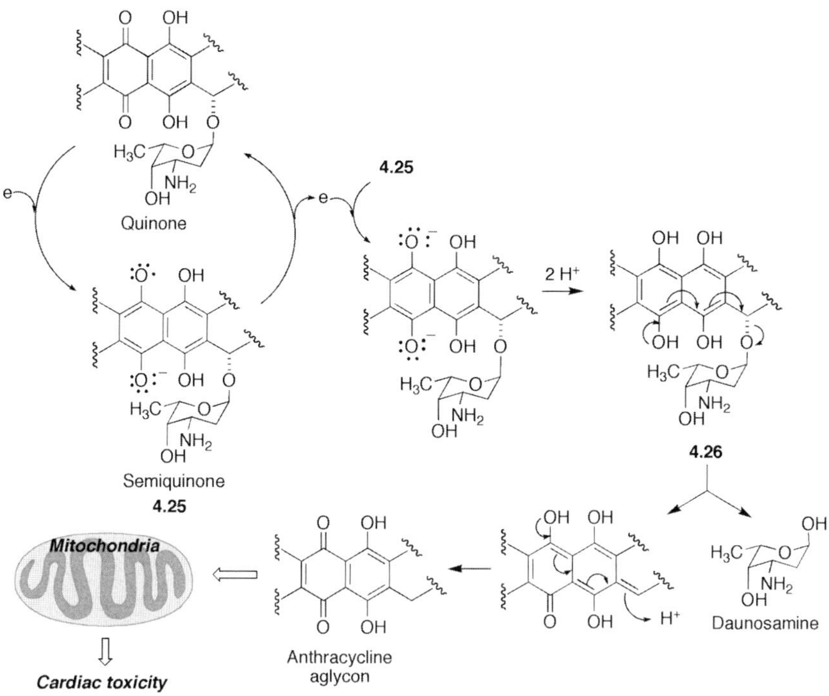

FIGURE 4.15   Elimination of the sugar moiety from anthracyclines.

Another important chemical property of the anthracyclines relevant to their antitumor activity is their chelating ability due to the presence of β-hydroxycarbonyl moieties in their structure, especially at the C-11 and C-12 positions.[21] Probably because of ionic interactions with the phosphate groups, the anthracycline-Fe^{3+} chelate binds to DNA much more tightly than the anthracycline itself and can then generate Fe^{2+} by reaction with superoxide anion. As previously mentioned, Fe^{2+} cations thus generated *in situ* can form hydroxyl radicals through their Fenton reaction with hydrogen peroxide (Fig. 4.16). The high efficiency of DNA fragmentation by these hydroxyl radicals is reflected in the routine use of the Fenton reaction in DNA footprinting, a technique that fragments DNA indiscriminately and allows to determine where DNA-protein interactions take place.[22]

Anthracyclines also induce a severe dysregulation of iron homeostasis, possibly mediated by the release of iron from intracellular stores. This helps to explain why the Fenton reaction takes place in spite of the fact that cells normally have very little or no free iron available,[23] and is also very important in explaining the cumulative cardiotoxicity of the anthracyclines. The main target responsible for this dysregulation of iron homeostasis by the anthracyclines seems to be aconitase, a Krebs cycle enzyme that reversibly isomerizes citrate to isocitrate and is characterized by a catalytic [4Fe-4S] cluster. The anthracycline-mediated release of one of the four Fe atoms from this cluster leads to loss of aconitase activity and converts the enzyme into an iron regulatory protein called (IRP-1). This protein

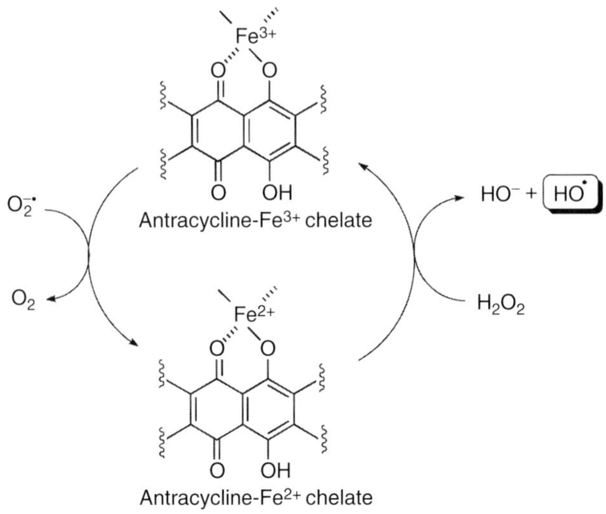

FIGURE 4.16   Anthracycline-mediated Fenton reaction.

has a high affinity for mRNAs corresponding to transferrin receptor and ferritin, an iron storage protein, resulting in an increased synthesis of the former and decreased synthesis of the latter. The overall effect leads to an increase of iron uptake upon iron sequestration, and therefore to an increase in available iron (Fig. 4.17A).

Regarding the mechanism of anthracycline-mediated loss of iron from the aconitase [4Fe-4S] cluster, it has been shown that the secondary alcohols (doxorubicinol, DOXol and daunorubicinol, DNRol, Fig. 4.17B) derived from two-electron reduction of the C-13 carbonyl in anthracyclines by NADPH-dependent cytoplasmic reductases are more reactive than superoxide or hydrogen peroxide toward artificially generated mimics of the cluster.[24] Further research using intact tumor cells has shown, however, that the effects of anthracyclines on IRP-RNA binding activity are not due to DOXol or free generation of free radicals, but due to formation of Fe complexes with DOX itself.[25]

In summary, while the oxidant activity of anthracycline aglycons seems to be responsible for the acute toxicity of anthracyclines, the alterations in iron homeostasis have been proposed to be responsible for the life-threatening chronic toxicity of anthracyclines.[26]

Since ROS-associated toxicity is iron dependent, the association of anthracyclines with chelating agents, such as dexrazoxane (ICRF-159), prevents anthracycline-induced cardiotoxicity without seriously compromising antitumor activity. This compound is a prodrug that can enter the cells easily and is then hydrolyzed in two stages to the iron chelator ADR-925, an EDTA analog (Fig. 4.18).[27] After its approval by the FDA and other regulating agencies for patients receiving anthracyclines and its introduction in the clinic,[28] it has been recently proved that, besides their cardioprotecting activity, dexrazoxane and

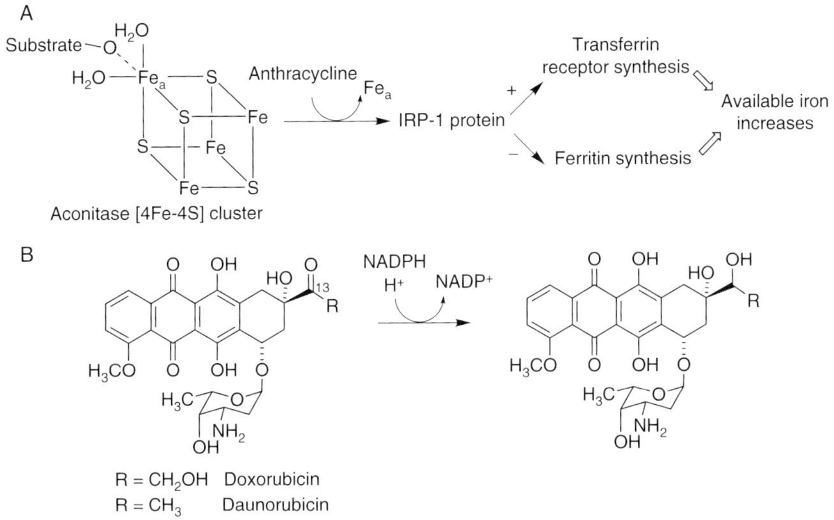

FIGURE 4.17   A. Effects of anthracyclines on iron regulation. B. Biosynthesis of doxorubicinol and daunorubicinol.

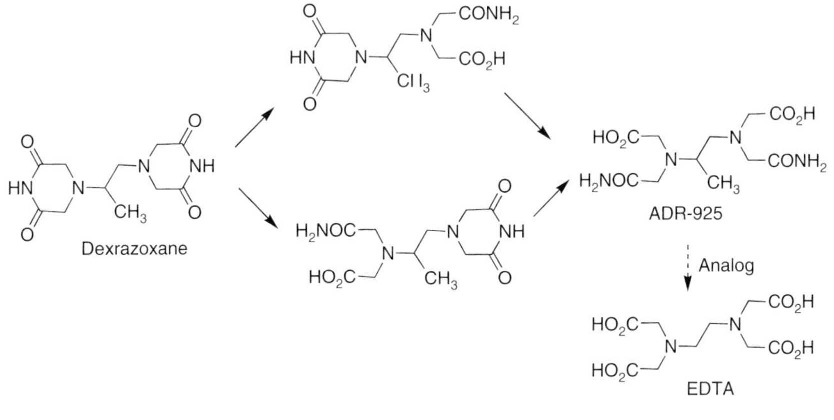

FIGURE 4.18   Bioactivation of dexrazoxane.

other bis(dioxopiperazines) have antitumor activity in themselves due to topoisomerase II inhibition[29] (see Section 6.3 of Chapter 7).

Anthracyclines have been long known to form unstable drug-DNA cross-links at 5′-GC-3′ sequences after redox activation in the presence of iron, leading to transcription blockade.[30] Kinetic studies showed the presence of two bonds with different half-lives, and a model was proposed involving a more labile covalent bond to an isolated G base on one strand of DNA and a less labile one involving cross-linking of both strands by the drug aglycon.[31] However, during studies of the less-labile complex, negative ion electrospray mass spectrometric studies showed the presence of an additional carbon atom for each cross-linked drug molecule, the source of the extra carbon being a molecule of formaldehyde generated from the tris buffer employed in the experiments. These mass spectral data were consistent with the X-ray structure of a complex formed from $(CG)_3$, DNR, and formaldehyde, which in this case was present as an impurity of the crystallization solvent.[32] Further experiments proved that several biomolecules such as spermine and lipids can yield formaldehyde in the presence of anthracycline-induced ROS,[33] which provided a link between these *in vitro* experiments and the mode of action of the anthracyclines *in vivo*. It was shown later that DNR and DOX react with formaldehyde to yield dimeric oxazolidine structures called doxoform (DOXF) and daunoform (DAUF), shown in Figure 4.19, that would liberate by hydrolysis the monomeric structures **4.27** predicted to be the active metabolites of the anthracyclines. Coadministration of DOX and known formaldehyde precursors, like pivaloyloxymethyl butyrate or hexamethylenetetraamine (HMTA), increases the levels of anthracycline-DNA adducts, which can be considered another proof of the role of formaldehyde in this process.[34] Formaldehyde adducts, like DAUF and DOXF, are responsible for the formation of a covalent bond with the 2-amino group of a guanine in the DNA minor groove through the formation of an intermediate Schiff's base **4.28**, as shown in Fig. 4.19.

DAUF and DOXF can be considered as anthracycline prodrugs, and are more active than the parent drugs in some cell lines.

Formation of species **4.29** is accompanied by intercalation and formation of hydrogen bonds with the G-base in the opposite strands (Fig. 4.20). This combination of intercalation, covalent bond, and hydrogen bonding is known as virtual cross-linking. This mechanism has prompted the synthesis of anthracycline formaldehyde conjugates as novel drugs potentially less cardiotoxic and active than the parent compounds against resistant cancer cells.[35]

Among other cardiovascular effects,[36] anthracyclines are thought to be modulators of angiogenesis, a key process in tumor growth and metastasis, inducing a breakdown of tumor vasculature. This is partly due to their effects on nitric oxide (NO) production by inhibition of endothelial NO synthase and inhibition of the expression of inducible NO synthase.[37]

Because anthracyclines are among the most widely employed antitumor drugs, intensive research has been developed in the last two decades trying to find a "better anthracycline," lacking cumulative cardiotoxicity and susceptibility to cell efflux pumps responsible for resistance, such as P-gp (see Chapter 12), but all studies indicate that this goal is yet to be achieved. More than 300 new compounds have been discovered through biosynthetic studies and more than 2000 analogs have been obtained from structural modifications of natural compounds or from total synthesis, but only a few of them have been submitted to clinical studies and even fewer have reached approval.[38,39] Among them, epirubicin (EPI)[40] and idarubicin (IDA)[41] can be mentioned as useful alternatives to DOX or DNR, respectively. EPI is an epimer of DOX at the daunosamine C(4')-position that induces pharmacokinetic and metabolic changes related to the increased 4'-O-glucuronidation and increased elimination. In spite of this

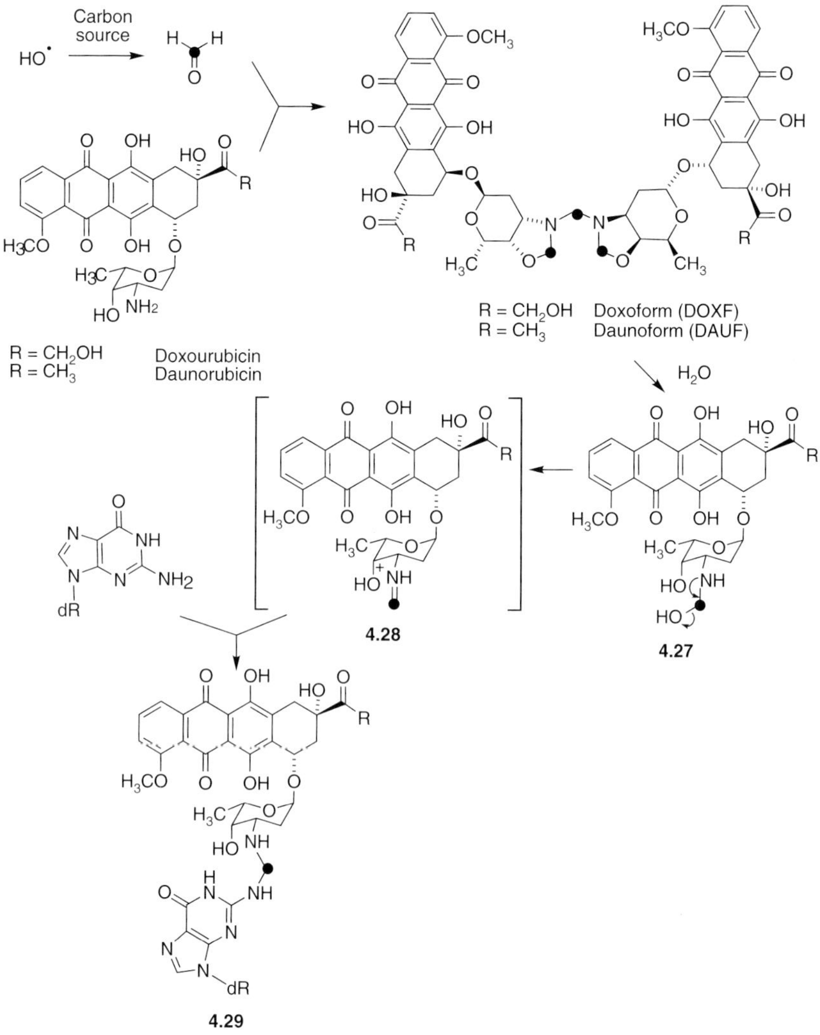

FIGURE 4.19   Generation of formaldehyde adducts of anthracyclines.

finding, clinical studies have shown that replacing DOX with EPI does not eliminate the risk of chronic cardiotoxicity. IDA, an analog of DNR obtained by removal of the methoxy group, has a broader spectrum of activity. This is probably related to its increased lipophilicity, which facilitates the cellular uptake and contributes to stabilize the ternary complex that forms the drug with DNA and topoisomerase II (see Chapter 7). The last effect is important, since a major mechanism of anthracycline activity depends on the formation of this complex. However, the cardiac safety of IDA has not been clearly established.

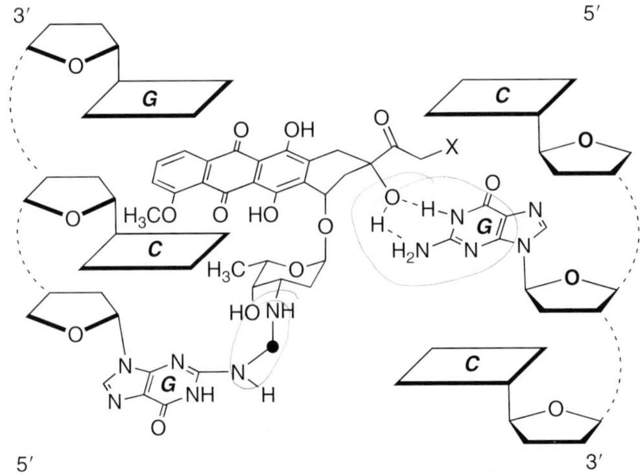

FIGURE 4.20   Interaction of anthracycline-formaldehyde adducts with DNA.

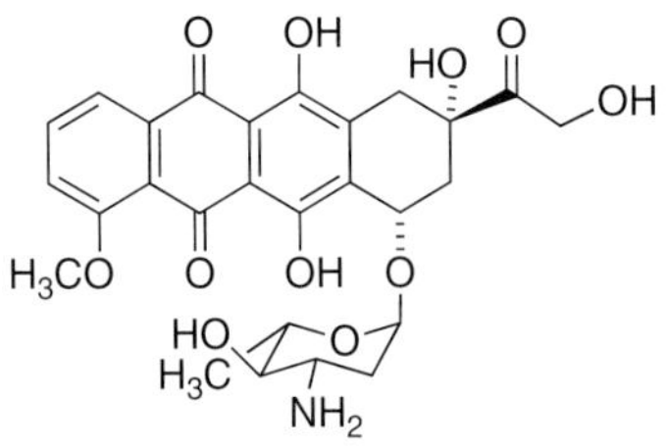

Epirubicin

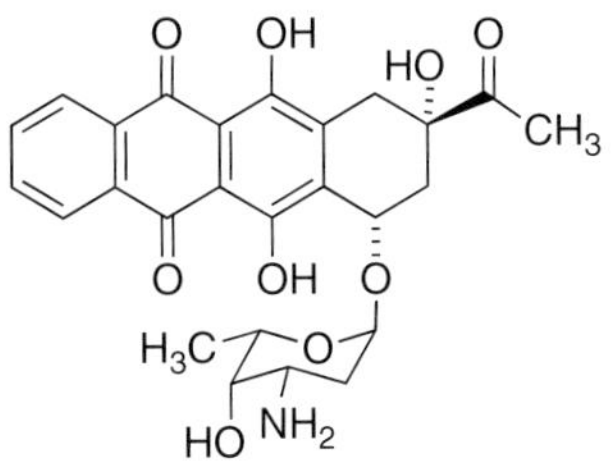

Idarubicin

Pirarubicin, a 4′-tetrahydropyranyl doxorubicin,[42] and aclarubicin (aclacino-mycin A), a trisaccharide anthracycline,[43] showed only modest improvements over DOX and DNR in terms of drug resistance without relevant cardiotoxic safety. Zorubicin, the daunorubicin benzoylhydrazone,[44] and valrubicin,[45] have also been marketed. The latter compound is indicated for *in situ* intravesical therapy[46] of BCG-refractory carcinomas of the urinary bladder.[47]

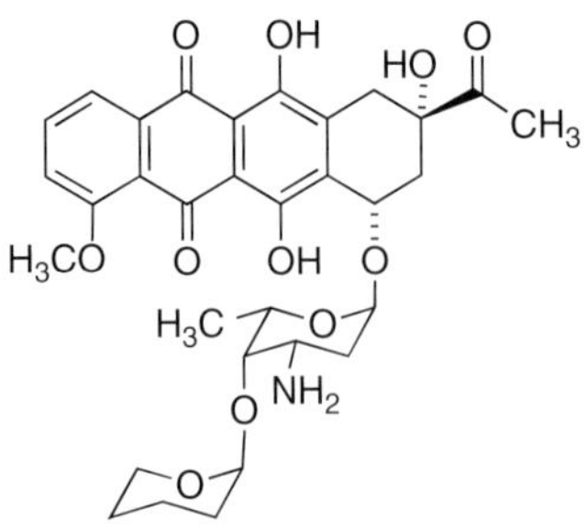

Pirarubicin

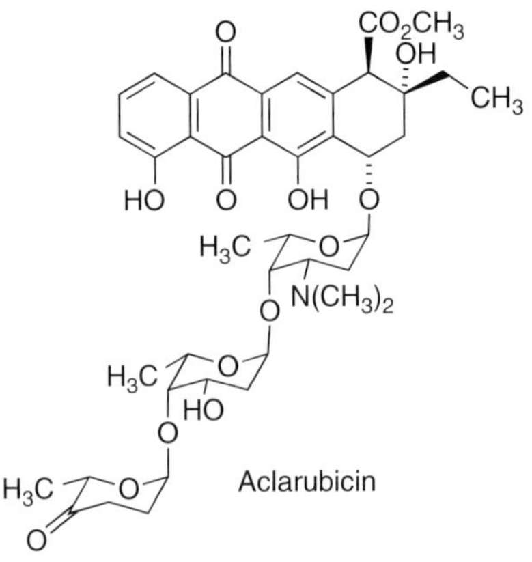

Aclarubicin

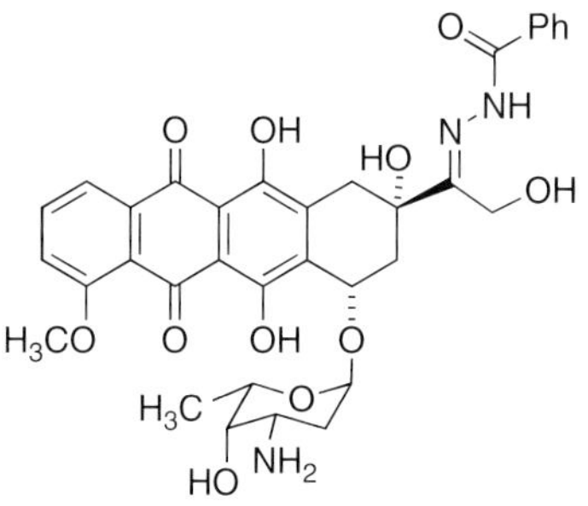

Zorubicin 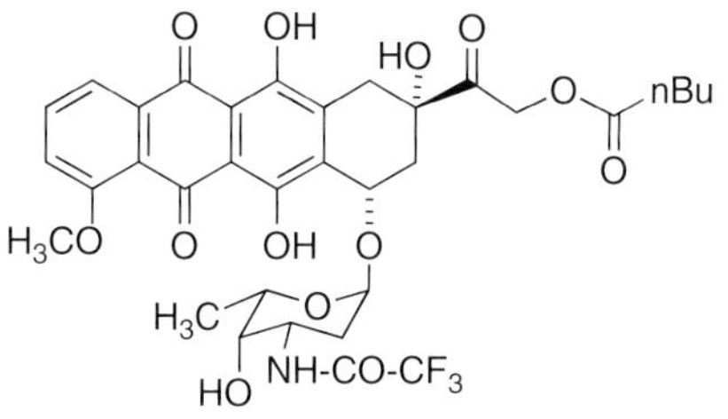   Valrubicin

Among other analogs that have reached clinical trials we can mention nogalamycin that was first isolated in 1968 and lately modified to give menogaril (TUT-7).[48] In this compound, the daunosamine is replaced by a methoxy group and other amino-sugar is attached to the D-ring through a glycosidic linkage and a C-C- bond. Menogaril is active against several human lymphomas and has been advanced to Phase II clinical trials in patients with previously treated multiple myeloma or chronic lymphocytic leukemia.[49]

Another interesting compound is nemorubicin (MMRA), a DOX analog bearing 2(S)-methoxy-4-morpholinyl, for which faster cell extravascular diffusion and cell uptake and lower cardiotoxic effects were claimed,[50] and which is in Phase III clinical studies.

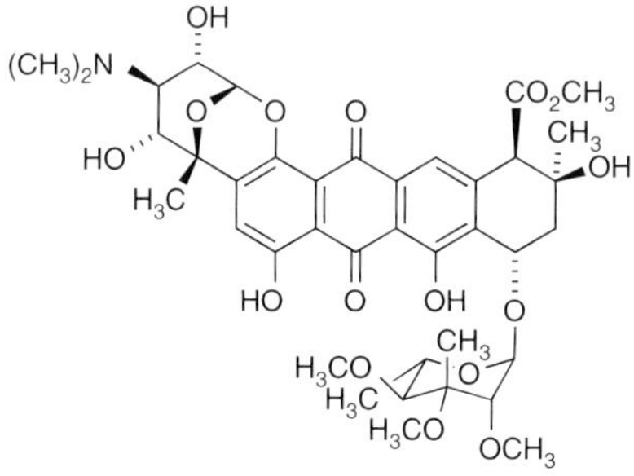

Nogalamycin 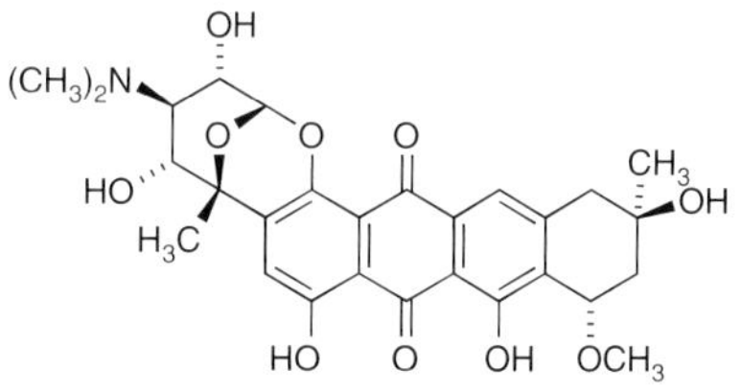   Menogaril

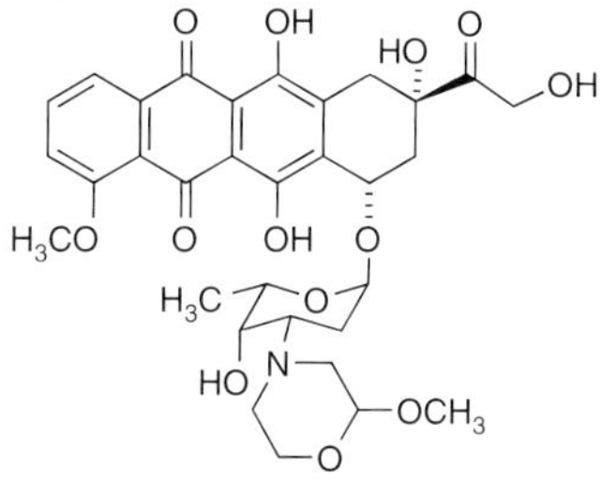

Nemorubicin (MMRA)

Based on the concept of drug hybridization, several molecules with both DNA alkylating and intercalation properties, such as PNU-159548, a 4-demethoxy-3'-deamino-3'-aziridinyl-4'-methylsulfonyl-daunorubicin,[51] have been studied.

Because of its high lipophilicity, it may cross the blood-brain barrier and it is effective against intracranial tumors. Another approach for designing more effective anthracyclines was directed to less basic compounds having a more stable glycosidic bond. One of them is anamycin,[52] which after incorporation into liposomes went into clinical trials. In order to increase the topoisomerase II-mediated DNA cleavage, some groups have prepared 8- and 10-fluoroderivatives.[53]

PNU-159548   Anamycin

We will finally mention that drug carrier technology, either implying specific recognition or simply preferential drug distribution, has been widely employed for targeting anthracyclines to tumors in the last 10 years, as will be discussed in Chapter 11.

4. MITOXANTRONE AND RELATED QUINONES

Mitoxantrone, an anthraquinone derivative bearing polyamine side chains, can be considered as a partial analog of the anthracyclines including the hydroxyquinone function. This compound was obtained as an analog of ametantrone, which was initially prepared as a ballpoint pen ink, but a routine screening by NCI led to recognition of its antitumor activity. The reasoning that led to its design[54] was based on the observation that a large number of antileukemic agents shared a common N-O-O triangular pharmacophore, which was also present in the anthracyclines and involved the daunosamine amino group (Fig. 4.21). The introduction of the two phenolic hydroxy groups in ametantrone allowed to envision two sets of N-O-O triangles, and had the advantage of eliminating the daunosamine amino group, which was considered to have some influence in the cardiotoxicity of the anthracyclines.[55]

Mitoxantrone is active in breast cancer, acute promyelocitic or myelogenous leukemias, and androgen-independent prostate cancer. Although early reports seemed to indicate that its cardiotoxicity was lower than that of the anthracyclines,[56] this claim has been subsequently challenged.[57] Mitoxantrone has been recently approved for treatment of secondary progressive multiple sclerosis (MS).[58] The rationale for this application stems from the fact that MS is considered to be an autoimmune disease where a heightened immune action results in the destruction of the myelin of the central nervous system, causing nerve impulses to be slowed or halted and leading to the symptoms of MS. Since chemotherapeutic

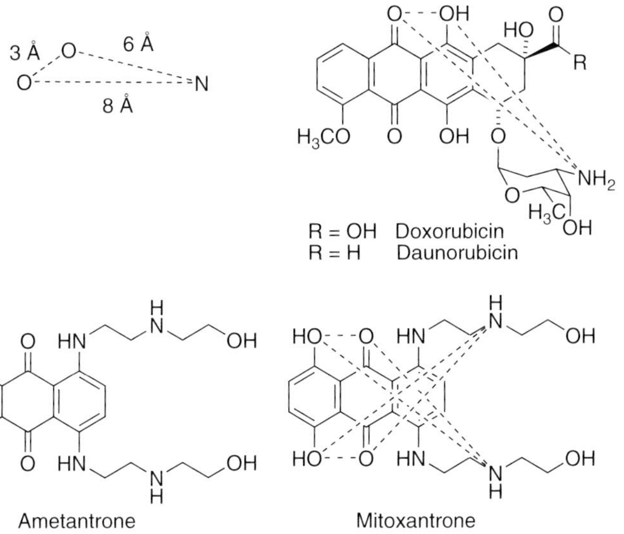

FIGURE 4.21 Similarities between anthracyclines, ametantrone and mitoxantrone.

agents diminish the numbers of white blood cells, it should slow down or halt this autoimmune destruction.

The mechanism of action of mitoxantrone has not yet been fully elucidated. As it will be mentioned in Chapter 7, this drug is a classic intercalating agent that acts as a topoisomerase II poison. Mitoxantrone can also be oxidatively activated to bind DNA; although the mechanism and binding properties have not been resolved, peroxidase-mediated free radical formation suggested that a mitoxantrone reactive intermediate may be involved in the observed DNA strand damage.[59] More recently, it was found that mitoxantrone can be activated by formaldehyde and is able, like adriamycin, to form adducts which stabilize double-stranded DNA, blocking the progression of RNA polymerase during transcription and producing truncated RNA transcripts.[60] This explains why mitoxantrone is particularly active in myeloid tumors, which are known to have increased levels of formaldehyde, formed from spermine and other polyamines by neutrophile-generated ROS.[61] Although mitoxantrone can be reductively activated to a semiquinone free radical, this process has a low efficiency and the compound undergoes less redox cycling *in vitro* than the anthracyclines.[62] The adducts of formaldehyde-activated mitoxantrone occur preferently at CpG and CpA sequences, and their formation is stimulated by cytosine methylation.[63] Thus, the reaction of mitoxantrone with formaldehyde leads to the hydroxymethyl derivative **4.30**, which forms a covalent bond with a guanine amino group to give the covalent adduct **4.32**, presumably through iminium cation **4.31** as an intermediate. The involvement of a single covalent bond has been proved by mass spectrometry, and further stabilization of the complex by hydrogen bonding has been suggested on the basis of molecular modeling studies (Fig. 4.22).[64]

6. CHARTREUSIN, ELSAMICIN A, AND RELATED COMPOUNDS

Chartreusin and elsamicin A are structurally related antibiotics with antitumor activity.

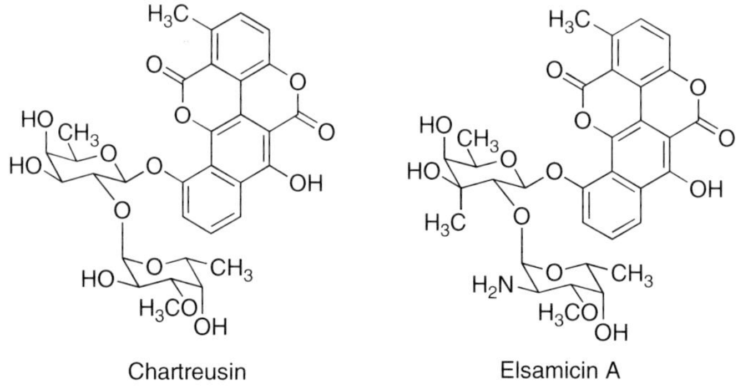

Chartreusin   Elsamicin A

These compounds cause single-strand scission of DNA in the presence of reducing agents via the formation of free radicals. ESR spin-trapping experiments showed that the elsamicin A-iron complex produces hydroxyl radicals in the presence of dithiothreitol as reducing agent.[67] The most probable mechanism involves reduction of either carbonyl group followed by reoxidation by oxygen (Fig. 4.24).

Because elsamicin A is an extremely potent inhibitor of topoisomerase II, these compounds will be further discussed in Chapter 7.

7. BLEOMYCINS

The bleomycins (BLMs) are a family of natural glycopeptidic antibiotics produced by *Streptomyces verticillus* with clinical efficacy against several types of tumors, specially squamous cell carcinoma, testicular carcinoma, and malignant lymphomas.[68] The anticancer drug blenoxane is a mixture of compounds, consisting primarily of the bleomycins A_2 (ca. 60%) and B_2 (ca. 30%). Bleomycins differ from other chemotherapeutic agents in that they produce very little bone marrow depression, and are routinely used in cancer chemotherapy, mostly in

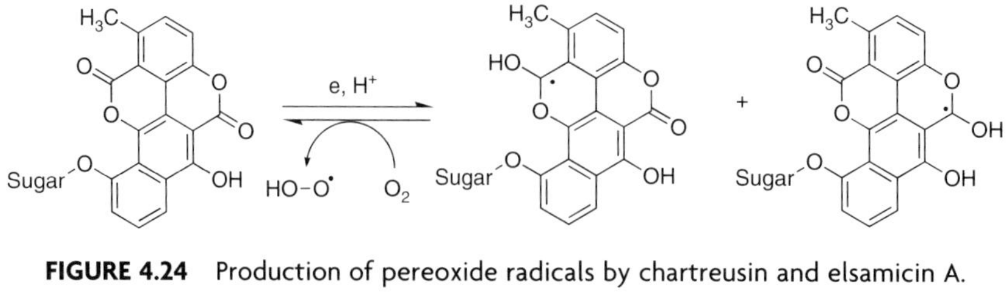

FIGURE 4.24   Production of pereoxide radicals by chartreusin and elsamicin A.

combination with radiotherapy or other chemotherapeutic agents. Their most serious side effect is a dose-dependent induction of interstitial pneumonitis in about 45% of patients, with 3% developing fatal lung fibrosis;[69] this lung toxicity is probably unrelated to their toxicity to tumor cells. Bleomycin A_2 is the most thoroughly studied of the DNA-cleaving reagents.

The structure of the bleomycins is complex and is shown below. A large number of semisynthetic bleomycins, most notably BAPP and liblomycin, have been prepared by addition of alkylamines to the fermentation media.[70]

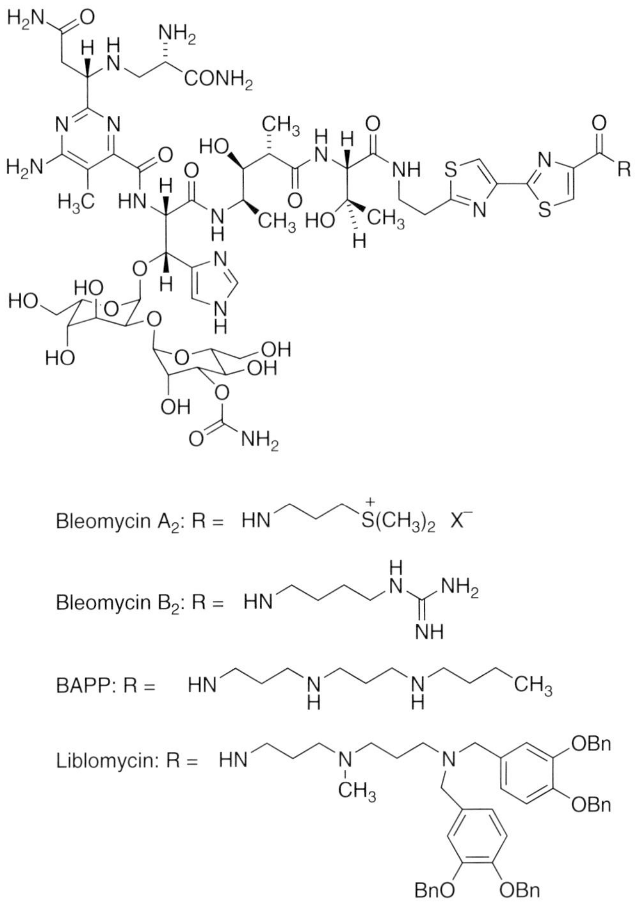

Bleomycin A_2: R =

Bleomycin B_2: R =

BAPP: R =

Liblomycin: R =

Tallysomycin S_{10b} (TLM S_{10b}) is another member of the bleomycin family that has reached clinical trials in patients with advanced head and neck tumors, showing a response similar to that of bleomycin A_2.[71] Its high toxicity prompted the development of immunoconjugates for intracellular targeting (see Section 4.5 of Chapter 11).

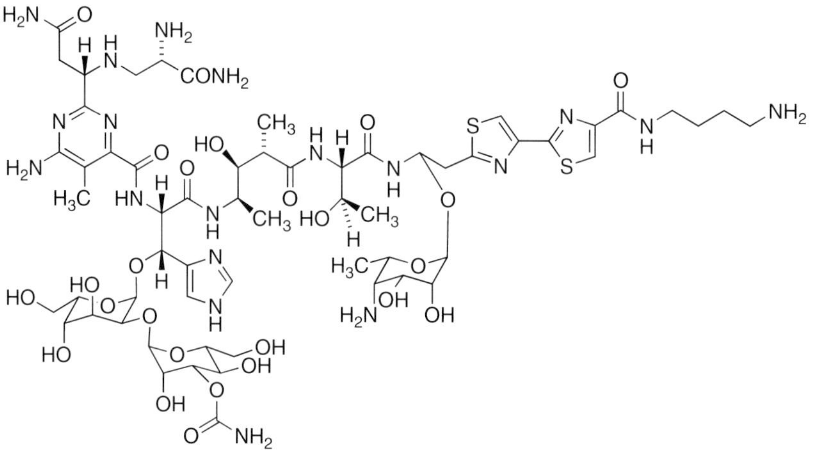

Tallysomycin S_{10b} (TLM S_{10b})

The bleomycins require a reduced transition metal, Fe (II) or perhaps Cu (I), oxygen, and a one-electron reduction to generate an "activated" bleomycin. The primary mechanism of action of the bleomycins is the generation of single- and double-strand DNA breaks and is initiated by the abstraction of a desoxyribose 4'-hydrogen. The species directly responsible for the removal of this hydrogen atom is an "activated" bleomycin complex **4.35**, arising from one-electron reduction of the bleomycin-Fe (II)-oxygen ternary complex. The electron may come from external reductors such as ascorbic acid or thiols, or from another molecule of **4.34**, which would then be transformed into the inactive Fe (III) species **4.36**. Reaction of **4.35** with DNA involves abstraction of the ribose 4'-hydrogen, and proceeds as previously discussed (Figs. 4.8–4.10). Finally, **4.33** can be regenerated from **4.36** by an NADH-dependent enzyme system in the nucleus or by reduction of external thiols, creating a cyclic process. This redox cycling (Fig. 4.25) is important for bleomycin activity because very small amounts of the drug enter the tumor cells.

A mechanism explaining the chemical details of the activation of the bleomycin ternary complex is shown in Fig. 4.26. Addition of one electron and one proton to the bleomycin-Fe (II)-oxygen ternary complex **4.34** gives an Fe (III) hydroperoxy complex **4.37**, which has been detected experimentally by a variety of techniques.[72] One possible mechanism explaining the formation of the activated bleomycin species **4.35**, which is analogous to the one postulated for the case of heme-dependent enzymes like cytochrome P450, involves the heterolytic cleavage of the O-O bond, initiated by a protonation step. This reaction gives a bleomycin-Fe (V)=O species **4.35** or its alternative Fe (IV) resonating form, which can abstract a hydrogen atom from DNA, initiating the series of events that culminate in strand cleavage.

Alternatively, the O-O bond in **4.37** could break homolytically, giving the bleomycin-Fe (IV)=O species **4.39** and a hydroxyl radical, either of which can abstract the DNA 4'-hydrogen (Fig. 4.27). A concerted reaction of **4.37** with DNA with concomitant O-O bond homolysis to give **4.39** is also possible.[73]

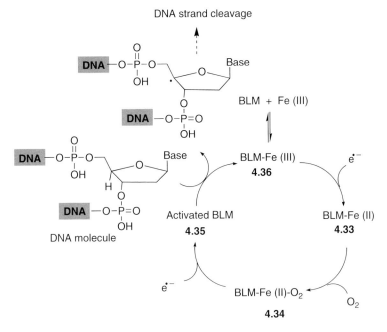

FIGURE 4.25   Redox cycling of bleomycin.

The bleomycin molecule is finely tuned for its function, and its various structural portions act synergistically to affect efficient DNA cleavage, with the roles summarized in Fig. 4.28.[74] The bleomycin-iron complex is formed at the metal-binding domain, comprising the β-aminoalanine-pyrimidine-β-hydroxyhistidine moiety. This portion of the molecule contains five nitrogen atoms at a distance suitable to form a stable chelate with Fe (II), leaving a sixth coordination valence available for a molecule of oxygen. Regarding the mode of interaction of the bleomycins with DNA, it involves two types of interactions, one of them being electrostatic binding of the cationic or protonated amino side chain with DNA phosphate groups, as proved by the observation that nonbasic side chains, although more easily transported into the cells, are much less active. The role of the bisthiazole system in DNA interaction has also been thoroughly studied, and two binding modes seem possible, namely intercalation and binding into the minor groove. Since DNA strand scission starts by abstraction of the deoxyribose 4′-hydrogen, which lies in the minor groove, it seems likely that bleomycin binds there, but intercalation has also been proved by the lengthening of linear DNA or the uncoiling of circular DNA.[75] Bleomycin shows selectivity toward 5′-GC-3′ and 5′-GT-3′ sequences because of hydrogen bonding recognition, either of the bithiazole unit or of the aminopyrimidine function.[76,77] Finally, the sugar moiety may be responsible for the uptake of the drug into cells but it does not seem to be involved in DNA cleavage, although it has been proposed that it has a role in the capability of the bleomycins to accommodate oxygen.[78] The linker region is also essential for

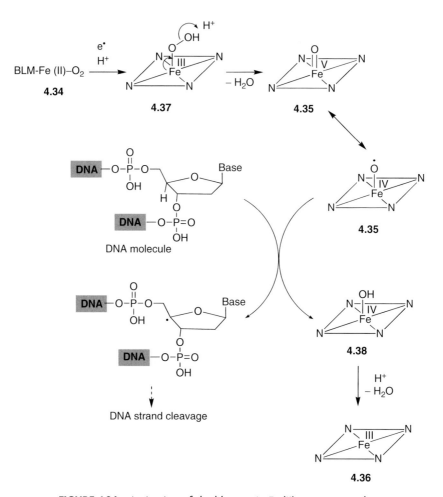

FIGURE 4.26   Activation of the bleomycin-Fe (II)-oxygen complex.

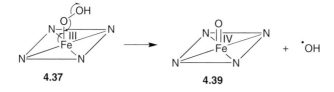

FIGURE 4.27   Homolytic cleavage of the Fe (III) hydroperoxy complex.

activity because it is responsible for the preorganization and stabilization of a compact conformation implicated in DNA cleavage.[74]

Bleomycins are large molecules (ca. 1.5 kDa) and therefore they are probably unable to diffuse through cell membranes. After administration, it has been proposed that they bind rapidly and irreversibly to Cu (II) in plasma. It is believed that

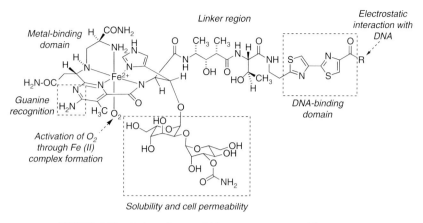

FIGURE 4.28   Roles of several blemoycin structural fragments.

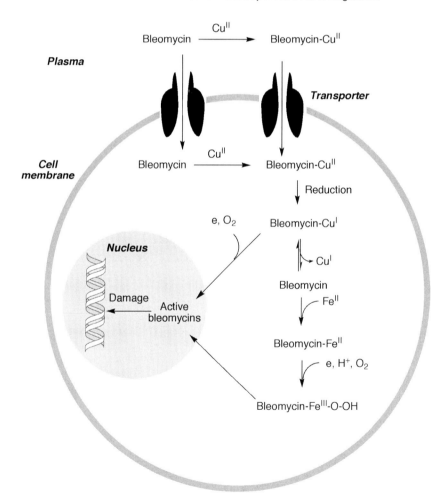

FIGURE 4.29   Bleomycin transport and bioactivation.

both the free bleomycin and the bleomycin-Cu (II) complex are transported into the cells. The Cu (II) complex is intracellularly reduced to bleomycin-Cu (I), which can react with oxygen to initiate a series of reactions leading to DNA strand scission. On the contrary, this complex is less stable than the one from Cu (II) and it can dissociate, allowing the formation of the bleomycin-Fe (II) complex and its trans-formation into the activated bleomycin species (Fig. 4.29).[68] Bleomycin transport is probably critical to the success of chemotherapy, and the use of internalizing antibodies for this purpose is currently being studied[79] (see Chapter 11).

8. ENEDIYNE ANTIBIOTICS

This family of antitumor antibiotics contains as a common structural feature a macrocyclic ring with a conjugated system containing at least one double and two triple bonds. Some members of the group are neocarzinostatin (zinostatin), the oldest of them, isolated from various microorganisms, the esperamicins/calichea-micins, from a *Micromonospora echinospora* spp. *Calichensis*, and dynemicin A, from *Micromonospora chersina*, which combines the structural features of the anthracyclines and the enediynes. In their natural environments, these com-pounds are stabilized by embedding in a protein, which protects the producing microorganism from their cytotoxic action.

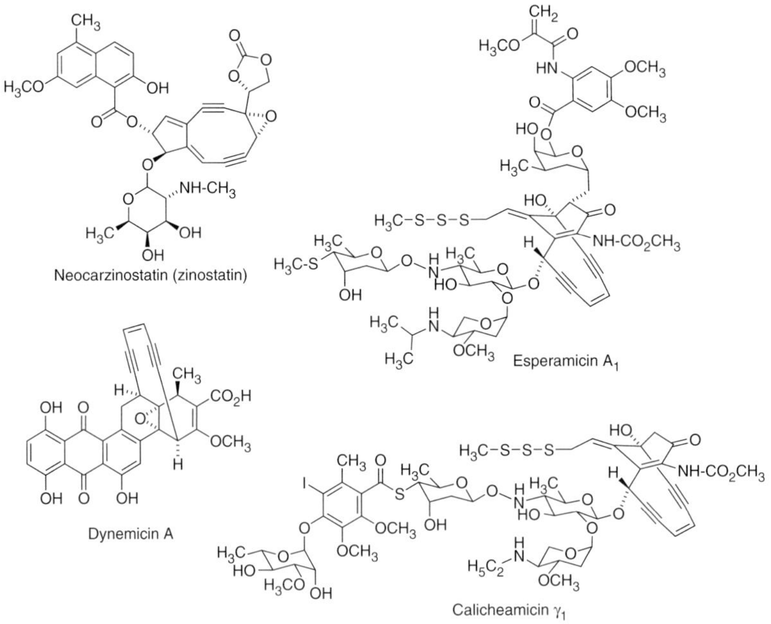

Neocarzinostatin (zinostatin)

Esperamicin A$_1$

Dynemicin A

Calicheamicin γ$_1$

Generally speaking, the enediynes are too toxic for clinical use, and only neocarzinostatin and calicheamicin have found limited application in some countries. For instance, a chemical conjugate of a synthetic copolymer of styrene maleic acid (SMA) and neocarzinostatin (NCS), known as SMANCS, has been proposed for the treatment of hepatocellular carcinoma.[80] More recently, a conjugate of a calicheamicin derivative with an antibody for the CD33 antigen, known as gemtuzumab ozogamicin, has been approved for the treatment of acute myeloid leukemia, which is the most common type of leukemia in adults[81] (see also Section 5.2 of Chapter 10 and Section 4.5 of Chapter 11).

These compounds bind to DNA by interaction of parts of the molecule with the minor groove[82] and activation to DNA-cleaving biradical species, either by reaction with thiols or by reduction.

The chemical basis for enediyne activation is the Bergmann reaction,[83] through which enediyne systems **4.40** undergo cycloaromatization to benzene derivatives, with the intermediacy of the highly reactive 1,4-benzenoid biradical species **4.41** (Fig. 4.30A). In the related Myers reaction, one of the triple bonds can be replaced by an allene unit (**4.42**), leading to biradical **4.43** (Fig. 4.30B). These processes do not take place in the natural products because their spatial arrangement prevents coplanarity of the three bonds involved in Bergmann-type chemistry, and therefore an activation reaction or cascade of reactions that alters the compound geometry is necessary.

In the case of neocarzinostatin, conjugate nucleophilic addition of a thiol results in epoxide opening and formation of a highly strained cumulene **4.45**, which has the correct geometry to undergo a Myers cycloaromatization to biradical **4.46** (Fig. 4.31A).[84] In the absence of thiols, a base-catalyzed intramolecular addition reaction takes place, leading to cumulene **4.47** and subsequently to biradical **4.48** (Fig. 4.31B).[85]

The calicheamicins and esperamicins are also activated by attack of a thiol, in this case to the trisulfide portion, giving the thiolate **4.49**, which undergoes a Michael addition to the bridgehead α,β-unsaturated ketone to give the dihydrothiophene derivative **4.50**. The accompanying change in hybridization of the bridgehead atom triggers a Bergmann cyclization to biradical **4.51** (Fig. 4.32).

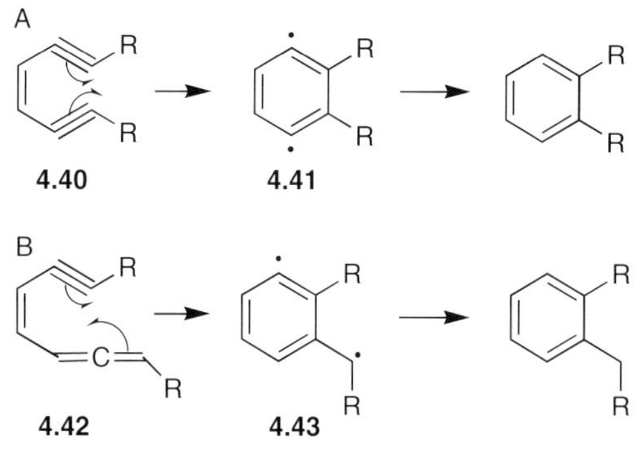

FIGURE 4.30   Radical generation from enediyne antibiotics through the Bergmann (A) and Myers (B) reactions.

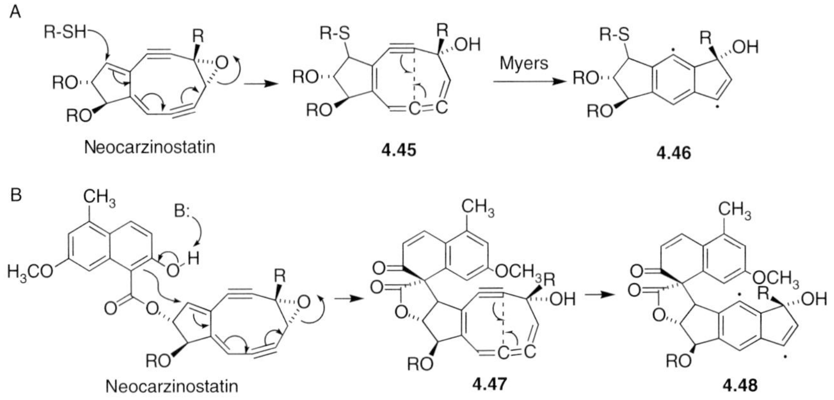

FIGURE 4.31   Activation of enediynes through a thiol addition (A) or an intramolecular addition (B).

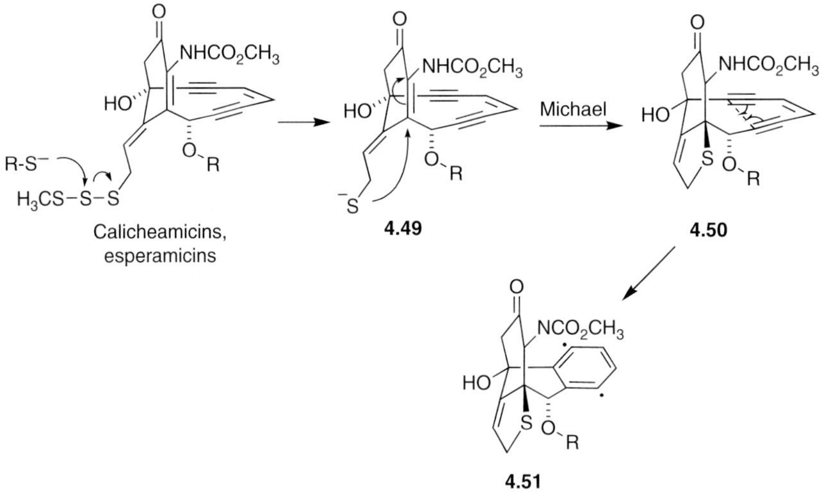

FIGURE 4.32   Generation of radicals from calicheamicins and esperamicins.

In the case of dynemicin A, its rigid structure keeps the alkynes separate, preventing the Bergmann cyclization. The anthraquinone part intercalates into the minor groove, and subsequent activation may involve nucleophilic attack by a thiol or a reductive mechanism mediated by NADPH. In the first case, epoxide opening gives the highly electrophilic quinonimine methide **4.52**. Addition of a thiol gives **4.53**, the precursor of biradical **4.54** through a Bergmann reaction (Fig. 4.33).

In the NAD-mediated mechanism, formation of hydroquinone **4.55** is followed by epoxide ring opening with formation of an extended quinone methide **4.56**. This intermediate can behave both as a nucleophile (Fig. 4.34A) and as an electrophile (Fig. 4.34B).[86] In the first case, protonation leads to **4.57** and in the second

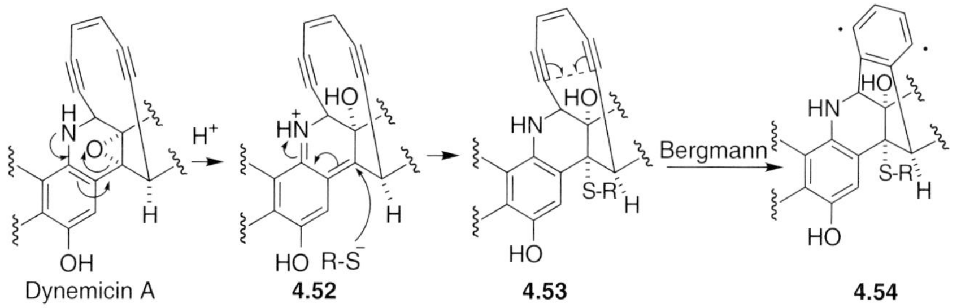

FIGURE 4.33   Generation of a diradical from dynemicin A through a thiol addition.

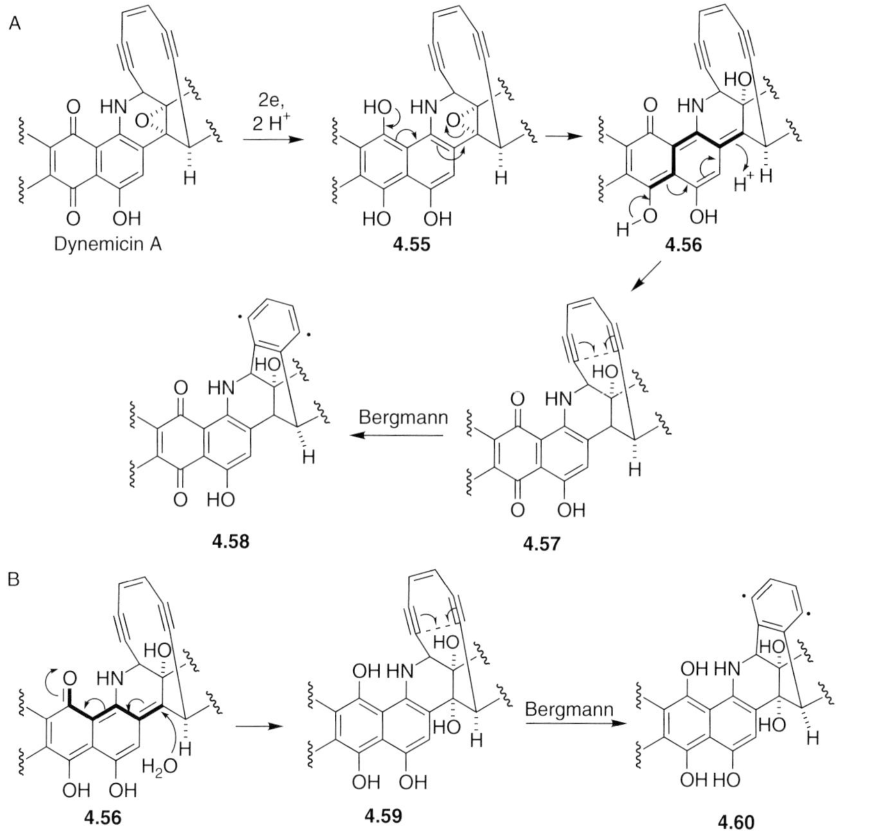

FIGURE 4.34   NAD-mediated generation of a diradical from a dynemicin A extended quinone methide acting as a nucleophile (A) or as an electrophile (B).

case trapping by water gives bishydroquinone **4.59**, both compounds being suitable biradical precursors by Bergmann chemistry.

DNA strand scission by the enediyne biradicals involves hydrogen abstraction from DNA molecules. Both H-4′ and H-5′ of DNA desoxyribose residues in the minor groove are accessible to the biradicals. In the case of H-4′ abstraction, a mechanism similar to that discussed in Figs. 4.8–4.10 operates, but about 80% of DNA lesions correspond to the abstraction of H-5′ from thymidine or deoxyadenosine residues. As shown in Fig. 4.35, radical **4.61** formed in this reaction consumes a molecule of oxygen, one electron, and one proton to give hydroperoxide **4.62**. Fragmentation of **4.62** by nucleophilic attack from a thiol leads to the 3′-phosphate portion **4.63** and the nucleoside-5′-aldehyde **4.64**.

9. TIRAPAZAMINE

Tirapazamine (TPZ) is the lead compound in the benzotriazine-di-N-oxide class of hypoxic cytotoxins that selectively act in hypoxic tumor cells through bioreductive mechanisms (see also Section 2.2.1 of Chapter 11).[87] The mechanism for the selective toxicity toward hypoxic cells is the result of a one-electron reduction of the parent molecule to a free radical species that interacts with DNA to produce single- and double-strand breaks. It has also shown activity when combined with some chemotherapy agents, particularly cisplatin and carboplatin, or radiotherapy, whose efficacy it enhances under hypoxic conditions.[88] Several clinical studies have been undertaken to study the effectiveness of these combinations in non-small cell lung cancer and other refractory solid

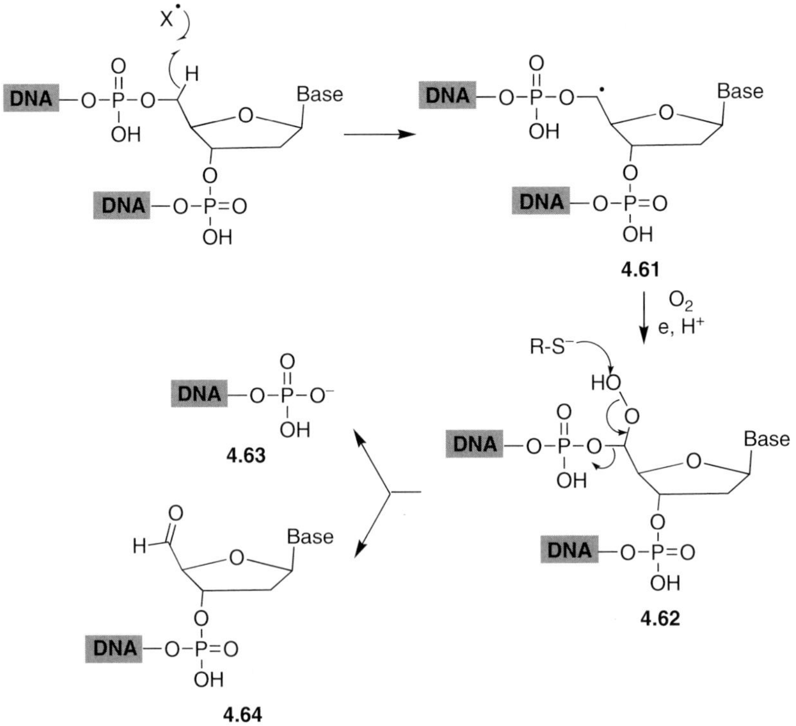

FIGURE 4.35   DNA strand scission induced by enediyne radicals.

tumors.[89,90] It has also been shown that electric pulses combined with TPZ and radiotherapy (electroradiochemotherapy) are more efficient than TPZ and radiation (radiochemotherapy).[91]

One-electron reduction of TPZ by NADPH-dependent cytochrome P450 reductase (P450R) leads to the formation of the TPZ radical, which is rapidly destroyed by oxygen in normal cells, leading to superoxide radical, which is thought to be responsible for the muscle cramps seen in patients given the drug. Under hypoxic conditions, the TPZ radical can undergo homolytic cleavage to the reduced species SR 4317 and a hydroxyl radical. Both radicals can react with DNA, but damage caused by TPZ can be detected both at the DNA backbone and the heterocyclic bases and can therefore be considered as typical of hydroxyl radicals.[92] Another DNA-damaging species generated in the metabolism of TPZ is the benzotriazinyl (BTZ) radical,[93] formed by loss of water (Fig. 4.36). Double-strand breaks are caused, at least partially, by poisoning of topoisomerase II, either by direct damage from the radical species derived from TPZ or from radicals generated on the DNA molecules, which are the topoisomerase II substrates.[94]

Another reactive species that is generated by loss of a molecule of water from the TPZ radical is the BTZ radical, which is also responsible for DNA and topoisomerase damage (Fig. 4.37).

Besides its ability to generate DNA-damaging radicals, TPZ itself can also react with DNA radicals arising from these reactions, playing a role similar to the oxygen molecule. This dual role helps to explain the very high efficiency of TPZ

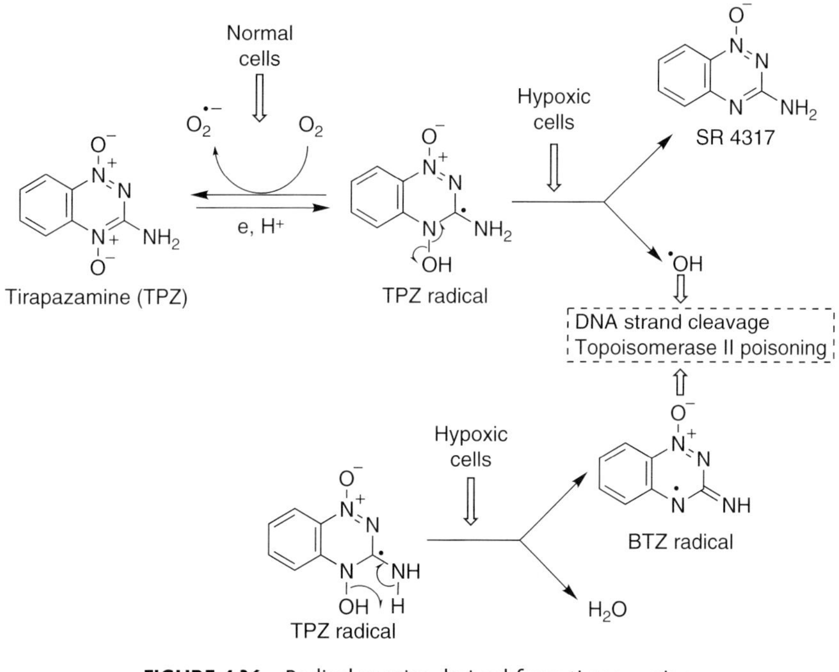

FIGURE 4.36   Radical species derived from tirapazamine.

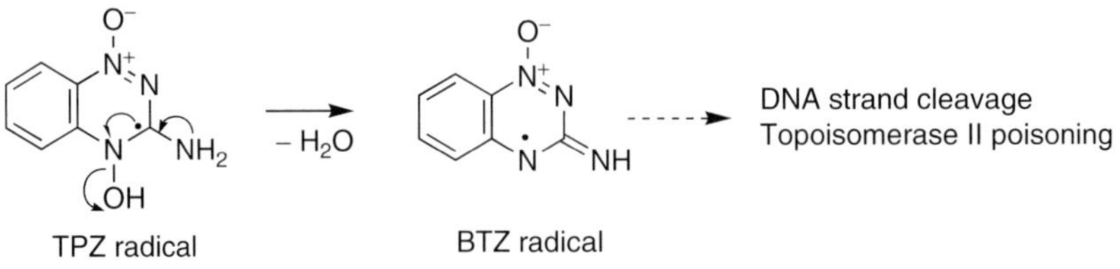

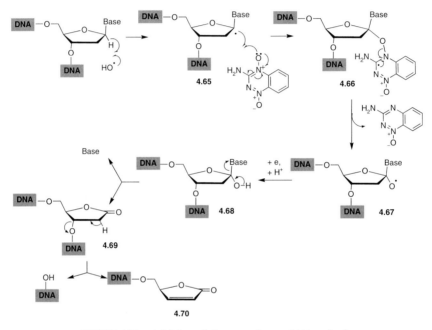

FIGURE 4.37   Formation of the benzotriazinyl radical from tirapazainine.

FIGURE 4.38   Addition of tirapazamine to DNA radicals.

in hypoxic cells. Thus, the reaction of DNA radical **4.65** with a molecule of inactivated TPZ gives intermediates **4.66** and **4.67**, leading to the hydroxylation of the DNA molecule after further reduction and protonation. Evolution of **4.68** leads finally to strand breaks, as shown in Fig. 4.38.

10. PENCLOMEDINE

Penclomedine, a 2-trichloromethylpyridine derivative, entered clinical trials for solid malignancies[95] after initial observations of its strong antitumor properties in animal brain tumor models. It has been shown to be a DNA monoalkylating agent, and it has been proposed that its alkylating properties stem from the

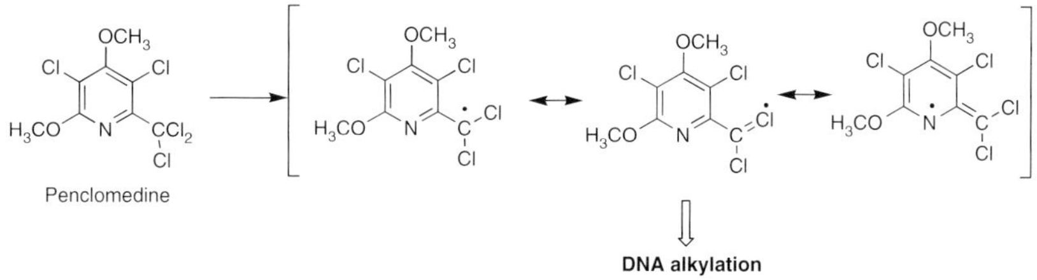

FIGURE 4.39   Generation of radicals from penclomedine.

homolytic cleavage of one of the C-Cl bonds by reductive microsomal metabolism (Fig. 4.39).

11. RADIOSENSITIZERS

Radiotherapy is one of the major approaches to cancer therapy, and can be defined as the medical use of ionizing radiation as part of cancer treatment. It is based on the generation of hydroxyl radicals from homolytic fragmentation of water molecules on local application of ionizing radiation. This fragmentation can be preceded by ionization of water molecules (Fig. 4.40A) or by their excitation (Fig. 4.40B).

As previously mentioned, the main mechanism of cytotoxicity of hydroxyl radicals is based on the generation of radicals from biomolecules (Fig. 4.41A). Cellular defenses against this process are varied, but they are normally based on the reaction of these radicals with an antioxidant molecule such as glutathione, which reacts with the biomolecule radicals, repairing them and leading to a glutathione radical. The latter species is harmless because of its tendency to dimerize to a disulfide (Fig. 4.41B).

Damage by ionizing radiation is enhanced by the presence of oxygen by a factor of 2- to 3.5-fold and therefore oxygen can be considered to act as a radiosensitizer. This so-called "oxygen effect" is due to the property of oxygen of reacting with biomolecule radicals to generate other radicals that cannot be

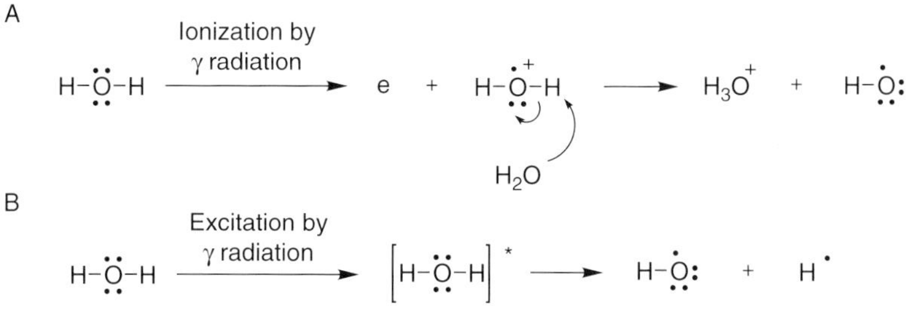

FIGURE 4.40   Generation of hydroxyl radicals from water during radiotherapy.

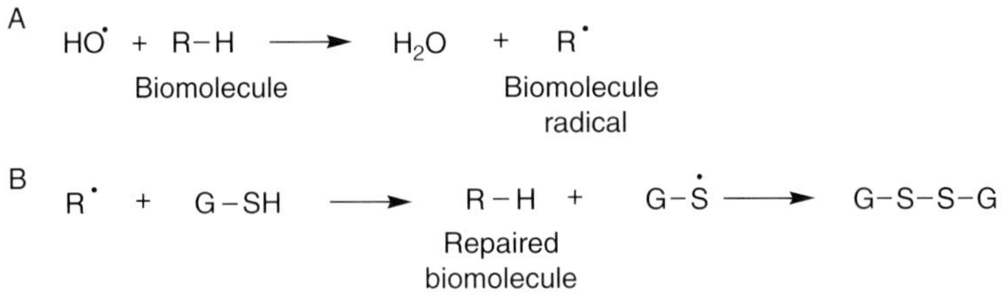

A

HO$^{\bullet}$ + R–H $\longrightarrow$ H$_2$O + R$^{\bullet}$

     Biomolecule   Biomolecule
                                      radical

B

R$^{\bullet}$ + G–SH $\longrightarrow$ R–H + G–S$^{\bullet}$ $\longrightarrow$ G–S–S–G

                          Repaired
                        biomolecule

FIGURE 4.41   Repair of biomolecule radicals by glutathione.

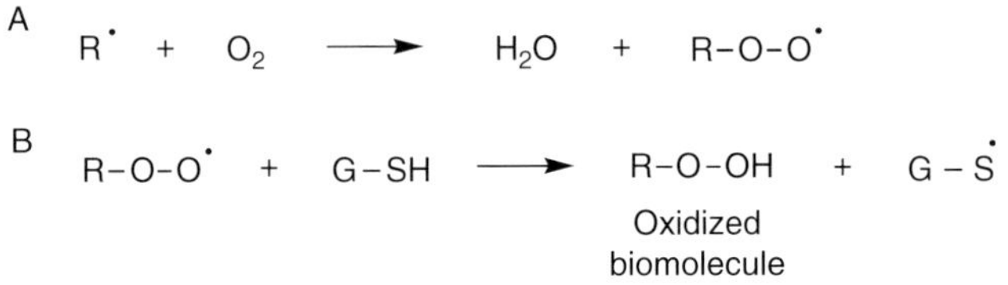

A

R$^{\bullet}$ + O$_2$ $\longrightarrow$ H$_2$O + R–O–O$^{\bullet}$

B

R–O–O$^{\bullet}$ + G–SH $\longrightarrow$ R–O–OH + G–S$^{\bullet}$

                                Oxidized
                                biomolecule

FIGURE 4.42   Enhancement of the effects of ionizing radiation by oxygen.

repaired because the action of glutathione on them does not lead back to the biomolecule, but to an oxidized derivative (Fig. 4.42).

For this reason, tumor hypoxia is associated with resistance to radiotherapy and also to some types of chemotherapy. In these hypoxic tumors, some types of chemical agents can play a similar role to oxygen, and therefore they can be used to increase the sensitivity toward radiotherapy. These compounds are known as radiosensitizers[96] and are being applied to a growing number of human cancers like those of cervix, head and neck, or lung cancer.[97] Another interesting application of some radiosensitizers is their use as hypoxia markers to accurately measure oxygen gradients at the cellular level.[98]

The first compounds that were studied in clinical trials as hypoxic radiosensitizers were nitroimidazoles. The mechanism of hypoxic-cell sensitizing by the nitro derivatives is based on their ability to react with biomolecule radicals giving a radical adduct that cannot be repaired, thereby acting as oxygen surrogates (Fig. 4.43A). Alternatively, addition of the biomolecule radical to the nitro group gives nitro radical anions (Fig. 4.43B).

Nitro radical anions are cytotoxic in themselves in hypoxic environments, although normally only at doses too high to be achieved in clinical situations. However, this cytotoxicity is reinforced by the generation of other radical species, some of which are shown in Fig. 4.44. It is interesting to mention in this context that the antibacterial and antiprotozoal activity of many nitroheterocycles is explained by one-electron reduction of the nitro group to nitro radical anions.

The first nitro compounds to be clinically studied as radiosensitizers, in the early 1970s, were metronidazole and specially misonidazole, which were studied in a large number of clinical assays. Despite initial promise, these clinical studies

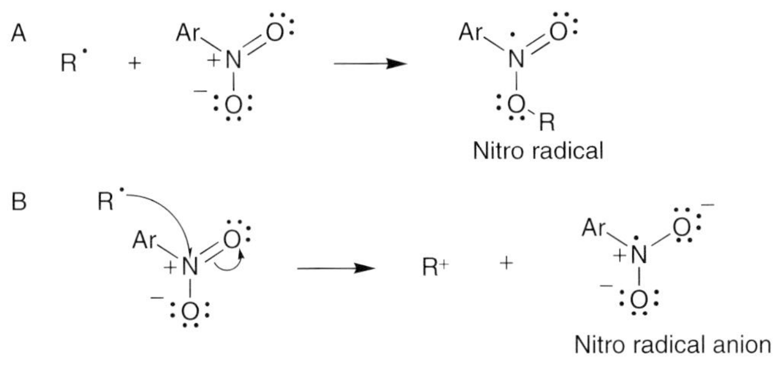

FIGURE 4.43   Generation of nitro radicals (A) and nitro radical anions (B).

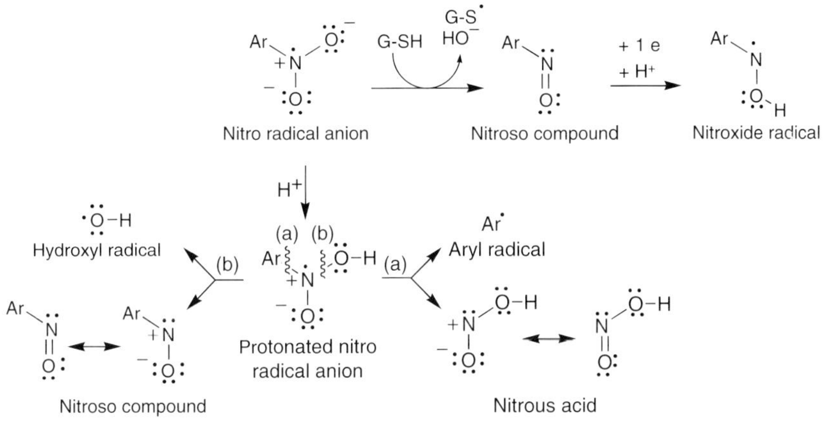

FIGURE 4.44   Cytotoxic radical species generated from nitro radical anions.

were disappointing and the combination of misonidazole with radiotherapy failed to show significant benefits, with some studies reported a significant neurotoxicity. In 1980s, other 2-nitroimidazoles (etanidazole and pimonidazole) were studied as radiosensitizers. Because of their lower lipophilicity as compared with misonidazole, both compounds showed lower penetration in the nervous system and a more rapid excretion, which result in lower neurotoxicity, but their clinical data did not demonstrate any benefit for radiotherapy. Subsequently, some of the newer 5-nitroimidazoles, like nimorazole and ornidazole, entered the clinical trials, with similarly discouraging results.

In the case of RSU-1069, a high efficiency has been observed with certain tumors such as the KHT sarcoma, but this effect seems to be due to cytotoxicity of the compound toward hypoxic cells rather than radiosensitization. Other bioreductive antitumor agents (hypoxic cytotoxins), particularly the previously mentioned porfiromycin and TPZ, have shown a great efficacy in combination with radiotherapy.[99] For a more detailed discussion of the cytotoxicity of these hypoxia-selective nitro compounds, see Section 2.2.3 of Chapter 11.

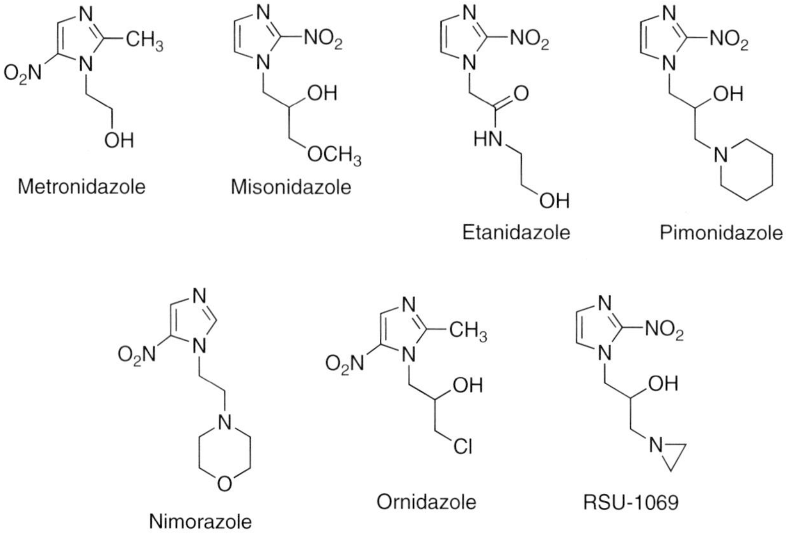

Metronidazole   Misonidazole   Etanidazole   Pimonidazole

Nimorazole   Ornidazole   RSU-1069

12. PHOTODYNAMIC THERAPY OF CANCER

Photodynamic therapy (PDT) of cancer is based on the use of compounds that are able to absorb harmless visible light energy and transfer it efficiently to other molecules in their vicinity or alternatively use it for photochemical reactions with biomolecules.[100] These compounds are normally known as photosensitizers (PS). After irradiation with light of the suitable wavelength, the PS molecules are excited from the ground state ($^1PS^0$) to a singlet excited state ($^1PS^*$) that can reverse to the ground state by nonradiative internal crossing (IC) or by fluorescent emission (F), the latter of which can be used for imaging and detection (photo-diagnosis). Alternatively, it may undergo an electronic rearrangement to the excited triplet state ($^3PS^*$) by intersystem crossing (ISC, Fig. 4.45). Most reactions of relevance to PDT take place in the triplet state, which must be sufficiently long-lived to give intermolecular reactions before its deactivation by emission of phosphorescence (P). In the Type 1 reactions, the PS triplet state reacts with an organic molecule (e.g., a component of the cell membrane) and transfers an electron to form a radical. These radicals may react further with oxygen, giving superoxide and other ROS. In Type 2 reactions, the PS triplet state transfers its energy directly to oxygen, leading to the formation of excited state singlet oxygen, a very potent oxidizer that is believed to be the main damaging agent acting by nonspecific oxidation of intracellular targets. The efficiency of these processes can be improved by increasing the stability of the triplet state, which can be achieved by spin-orbit coupling. In more familiar chemical terms, this involves the inclusion of heavy atoms in the structure of the photosensitizer, for example, by replacement of oxygen by sulfur, sulfur by selenium, or hydrogen by bromine or iodine.

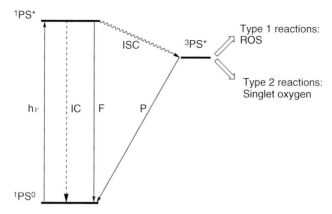

FIGURE 4.45 Events following the irradiation of photosensitizers.

Among the many compounds studied,[101] only two classes have been approved for clinical use, namely porphyrins and psoralens, although most work on PDT has been carried out with porphyrin-based drugs. One major problem of PDT is the lack of selective accumulation of photoactivable molecules within tumor tissues, and for this reason the development of targeted photosensitizers is an active research area.[102]

Initial preparations of hematoporphyrin were complex mixtures of porphyrin oligomers, which were later replaced by photophrin (porfimer sodium oligomer), which has a more regular composition.[103] The semisynthetic derivative talaporphin (mono-L-aspartylchlorin e6) has been approved for early stage lung cancer and, compared with other photosensitizers, it has the advantage of its high aqueous solubility and of being associated with minimum cutaneous photosensitivity. It has a long activation wavelength of 664 nm (in the red part of the visible spectrum), allowing deeper tissue penetration (Fig. 4.46).[104]

An alternative treatment that has also been used in the clinic involves the use of 5-aminolevulinic acid (ALA), a biosynthetic precursor of the natural photosensitizer protoporphirin IX (Fig. 4.47). This compound is normally employed as ester prodrugs, which have an improved absorption when administered as creams.[105] Protoporphyrine thus generated is selectively accumulated in some tumors because of their accelerated metabolism, which includes a faster processing of ALA.

After administration of the photodynamic agent, selective irradiation of the target tissue is achieved by use of a fiber optic diffuser inserted through an endoscope, which leads to local activation. Because of the low stability of the toxic species involved, diffusion to surrounding healthy tissues is not significant and therefore the method is minimally invasive and is well tolerated, although there are obvious limitations in light delivery to the tumor.

Porphyrin-based PDT has been in clinical use for about 20 years, initially for skin cancers. Subsequently it has established itself as a therapeutic strategy for

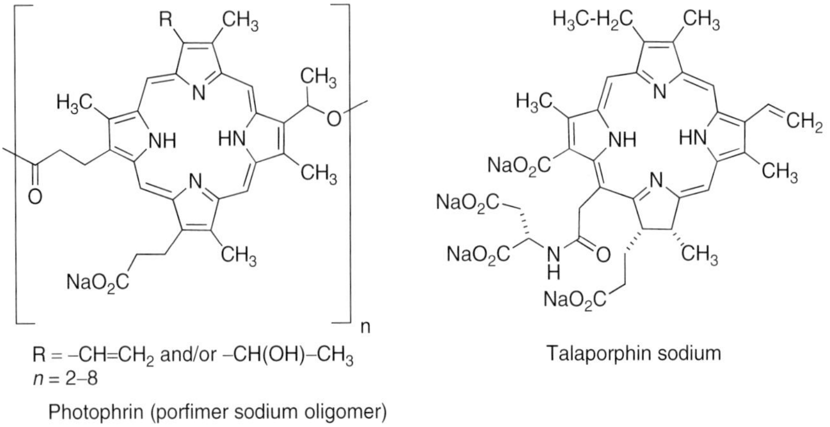

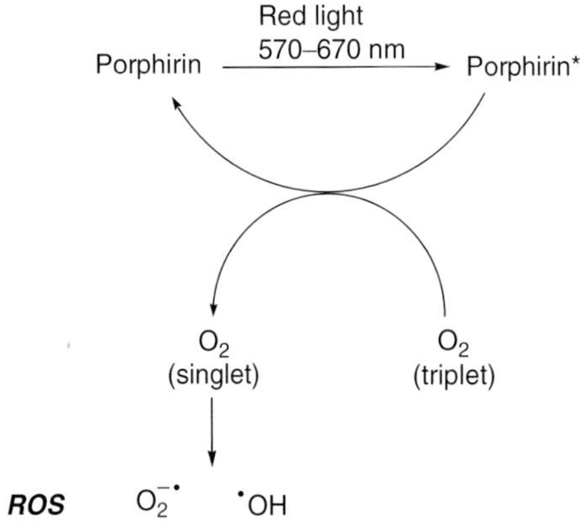

R = –CH=CH₂ and/or –CH(OH)–CH₃
n = 2–8

Photophrin (porfimer sodium oligomer)

Talaporphin sodium

FIGURE 4.46   Photoactivation of porphirins.

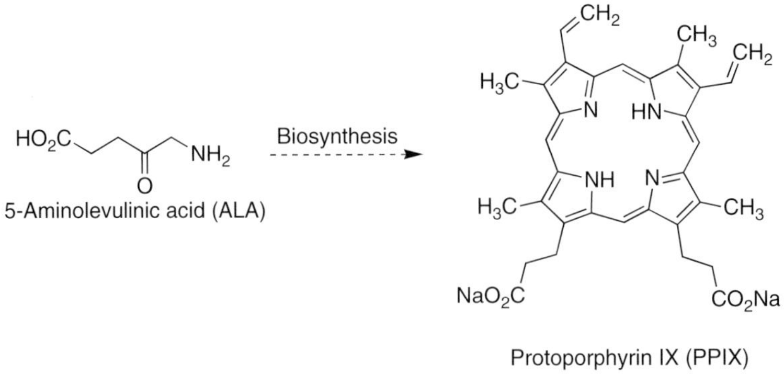

5-Aminolevulinic acid (ALA)

Protoporphyrin IX (PPIX)

FIGURE 4.47   ALA as a precursor of protoporphyrin IX.

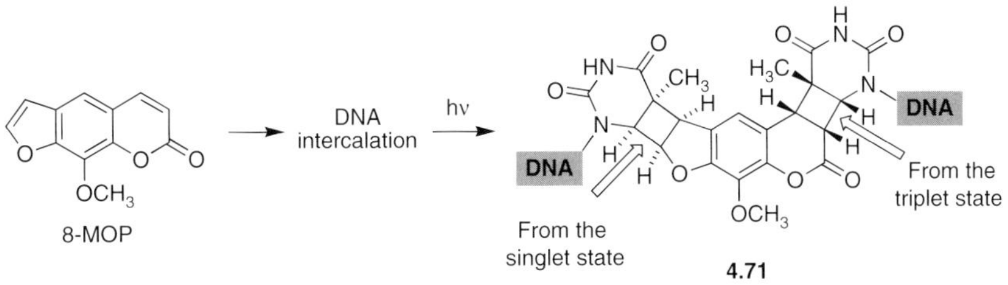

FIGURE 4.48   DNA adducts with 8-methoxypsoralen.

other types of cancer, such as cervical cancer, esophageal, early stage central type lung cancer,[106] and head and neck cancers,[107] among other applications.[108]

Psoralens have been traditionally employed for skin diseases, including psoriasis, but the only member of the group approved for cancer treatment is 8-methoxypsoralen (8-MOP, methoxsalen, Uvadex), which is used in the treatment of cutaneous T cell lymphoma. This compound is administered orally and then some blood is withdrawn, the aberrant white cells are separated and irradiated and then recombined with the other blood constituents and reinjected.[109] In this process, after weakly intercalating into DNA, irradiation of 8-MOP promotes the formation of [2 + 2] cycloadducts between its 3–4 and 5–6 double bonds and the 5–6 double bonds of adjacent thymidine bases of DNA (Fig. 4.48). Both possible monoadducts and bisadducts **4.71** have been isolated, the formation of the latter leading to DNA cross-links.[110]

REFERENCES

1. Halliwell, B., and Gutteridge, J. M. C. (2007). "*Free Radicals in Biology and Medicine.*" 4th ed. Oxford University Press, New York.
2. Minotti, G., Menna, P., Salvatorelli, E., Cairo, G., and Gianni, L. (2004). *Pharmacol. Rev.* **56**, 185.
3. Marnett, L. J., Riggins, J. N., and West, J. D. (2003). *J. Clin. Investig.* **111**, 583.
4. Niedernhofer, L. J., Daniels, J. S., Rouzer, C. A., Greene, R. E., and Marnett, L. J. (2003). *J. Biol. Chem.* **278**, 31426.
5. Plastaras, J. P., Dedon, P. C., and Marnett, L. J. (2002). *Biochemistry* **41**, 5033.
6. Otteneder, M., Scott Daniels, J., Voehler, M., and Marnett, L. J. (2003). *Anal. Biochem.* **315**, 147.
7. McGall, G. H., Rabow, L. E., Ashley, G. W., Wu, S. H., Kozarich, J. W., and Stubbe, J. (1992). *J. Am. Chem. Soc.* **114**, 4958.
8. Rabow, L. E., McGall, G. H., Stubbe, J., and Kozarich, J. W. (1990). *J. Am. Chem. Soc.* **112**, 3203.
9. Gajewski, E., Rao, G., Nackerdien, Z., and Dizdaroglu, M. (1990). *Biochemistry* **29**, 7876.
10. Doroshow, J. H., Synold, T. W., Somlo, G., Akman, S. A., and Gajewski, E. (2001). *Blood* **97**, 2839.
11. Marnett, L. J., Riggins, J. N., and West, J. B. (2003). *J. Clin. Investig.* **111**, 583.
12. Altman, S. A., Zastawny, T. H., Randers-Eichhorn, L., Cacciuttolo, M. A., Akman, S. A., Dizdaroglu, M., and Rao, G. (1995). *Free Radic. Biol. Med.* **19**, 897.
13. Laurent, G., and Jaffrezou, J. P. (2001). *Blood* **98**, 913.
14. Bezombes, C., de Thonel, A., Apostolou, A., Louat, T., Jaffrezou, J. P., Laurent, G., and Quillet-Mary, A. (2002). *Mol. Pharmacol.* **62**, 1446.
15. Martin, D., Salinas, M., Fujita, N., Tsuruo, T., and Cuadrado, A. (2002). *J. Biol. Chem.* **277**, 42943.
16. Gewirtz, D. A. (1999). *Biochem. Pharmacol.* **57**, 727.
17. Siveski-Iliskovic, N., Hill, M., Chow, D. A., and Singal, P. K. (1995). *Circulation* **91**, 10.

18. Goodman, J., and Hochstein, P. (1977). *Biochem. Biophys. Res. Commun.* **77**, 797.
19. Vázquez-Vivar, J., Martasek, P., Hogg, N., Masters, B. S., Pritchard, K. A., and Kalyanaraman, B. (1997). *Biochemistry* **36**, 11293.
20. Gille, L., and Nohl, H. (1997). *Free Radic. Biol. Med.* **23**, 775.
21. Fiallo, M. M. L., Drechsel, H., Garnier-Suillerot, A., Matzanke, B. F., and Kozlowski, H. (1999). *J. Med. Chem.* **42**, 2844.
22. Tullius, T. D., Dombrowski, B. A., Churchill, M. E. A., and Kam, L. (1987). *Methods Enzymol.* **155**, 537.
23. Cairo, G., Recalcati, S., Pietrangelo, A., and Minotti, G. (2002). *Free Radic. Biol. Med.* **32**, 1237.
24. Minotti, G., Ronchi, R., Salvatorelli, E., Menna, P., and Cairo, G. (2001). *Cancer Res.* **61**, 8422.
25. Kwok, J. C., and Richardson, D. R. (2002). *Mol. Pharmacol.* **62**, 888.
26. Licata, S., Saponiero, A., Mordente, A., and Minotti, G. (2000). *Chem. Res. Toxicol.* **13**, 414.
27. Wiseman, L. R., and Spencer, C. M. (1998). *Drugs* **56**, 385.
28. Schuchter, L. M., Hensley, M. L., Meropol, N. J., and Winer, E. P. (2002). *J. Clin. Oncol.* **20**, 2895.
29. Hasinoff, P. B., Abram, M. E., Bernabe, M., Khélifa, T., Allan, W. P., and Yalowich, J. C. (2001). *Mol. Pharmacol.* **59**, 453.
30. Skladanowski, A., and Konopa, J. (1994). *Biochem. Pharmacol.* **47**, 2279.
31. Van Rosmalen, A., Cullinane, C., Cutts, S. M., and Phillips, D. R. (1995). *Nucleic Acids Res.* **23**, 42.
32. Wang, A. H. J., Gao, Y. G., Liaw, Y. C., and Li, Y. K. (1991). *Biochem.* **30**, 3812.
33. Taatjes, D. J., Gaudiano, G., and Koch, T. H. (1997). *Chem. Res. Toxicol.* **10**, 953.
34. Cutts, S. M., Rephaeli, A., Nudelman, A., Hmelnitzky, I., and Phillips, D. R. (2001). *Cancer Res.* **61**, 8194.
35. Taatjes, D. J., and Koch, T. H. (2001). *Curr. Med. Chem.* **8**, 15.
36. Wakabayashi, I., and Groscher, K. (2003). *Curr. Med. Chem.* **10**, 427.
37. Ziche, M., and Morbidelli, L. (2000). *J. Neurooncol.* **50**, 139.
38. Lown, J. W. (ed.) (1988). "Anthracycline and Anthracenedione-Based Anticancer Agents," Elsevier, Amsterdam.
39. Monneret, C. (2001). *Eur. J. Med. Chem.* **36**, 483.
40. Coukell, A. J., and Faukds, D. (1997). *Drugs* **53**, 453.
41. Arcamone, F., Bernardi, L., Giardino, P., Patelli, B., DiMarco, A., and Casazza, A. M. (1976). *Cancer Treat. Rep.* **60**, 829.
42. Umezawa, H., Takahashi, Y., Kinoschita, M., Naganawa, H., Matsuda, T., and Ishizuka, M. (1979). *J. Antibiot.* **32**, 1082.
43. Oki, T., Matsizawa, Y., Yoshimoto, A., Numata, K., Kitamura, I., and Hori, S. (1975). *J. Antibiot.* **28**, 830.
44. Maral, R., Ponsinet, G., and Jolles, G. (1972). *C. R. Acad. Sci. Ser. Ser. D* **275**, 301.
45. Israel, M., Modest, E. J., and Frei, E. (1975). *Cancer Res.* **35**, 1365.
46. Melekos, M. D., and Moutzouris, G. D. (2000). *Curr. Pharm. Design* **6**, 345.
47. Van der Heidjen, A. G., and Witjes, J. A. (2003). *Curr. Opin. Urol.* **13**, 389.
48. Wiley, P. F., Elrod, D. W., Houser, D. J., Johnson, J. L., Pschigoda, L. M., Krueger, W. C., and Moscowitz, A. (1979). *J. Org. Chem.* **44**, 4030.
49. Kukuk, O., Kilton, L., Wade, J. L., Blough, R., and Benson, A. B. (2000). *Am. J. Clin. Oncol.* **23**, 379.
50. Sessa, C., Zucchett, M., Ghielmini, M., Bauer, J., D'Incalci, M., de Jong, J., Naegele, H., Rossi, S., Pacciarini, M. A., Domenigoni, L., and Cavalli, F. (1999). *Cancer Chemother. Pharmacol.* **44**, 403.
51. Marchini, S., González, O., Ripamonti, M., Geroni, C., Bargiotti, A., and Caruso, M. (1995). *Anticancer Drug Des.* **10**, 641.
52. Priebe, W., and Pérez-Soler, R. (1993). *Pharmacol. Ther.* **60**, 215.
53. Arcamone, F. (1998). *Biochimie* **80**, 201.
54. Cheng, C. C. (1983). *Progress Med. Chem.* **20**, 83.
55. Adamson, R. H. (1974). *Cancer Chemother. Rep.* **58**, 293.
56. Estorch, M., Carrio, I., Martínez-Duncker, D., Berna, L., Torres, G., Alonso, C., and Ojeda, B. (1993). *J. Clin. Oncol.* **11**, 1264.
57. Thomas, X., Le, Q. H., and Fiere, D. (2002). *Ann. Hematol.* **81**, 504.
58. Gonsette, R. E. (2003). *J. Neurol. Sci.* **206**, 203.
59. Kapuscinski, J., and Darzynkiewicz, Z. (1986). *Proc. Natl. Acad. Sci. USA* **83**, 6302.

60. Parker, B. S., Cutts, S. M., Cullinane, C., and Phillips, D. R. (2000). *Nucleic Acids Res.* **28,** 982.
61. Edwards, S. W., and Swan, T. F. (1986). *Biochem. J.* **237,** 601.
62. Kharasch, E. D., and Novak, R. F. (1985). *J. Biol. Chem.* **260,** 500.
63. Parker, B. S., Cutts, S. M., and Phillips, D. R. (2001). *J. Biol. Chem.* **276,** 15953.
64. Parker, B. S., Buley, T., Evison, B. J., Cutts, S. M., Neumann, G. M., Iskanders, M. N., and Phillips, D. R. (2004). *J. Biol. Chem.* **279,** 18814.
65. Bachur, N. R., Gee, M. V., and Gordon, S. L. (1978). *Proc. Am. Assoc. Cancer Res.* **19,** 75.
66. Flitter, W. D., and Mason, R. P. (1988). *Arch. Biochem. Biophys.* **267,** 632.
67. Portugal, J. (2003). *Curr. Med. Chem. Anticancer Agents* **3,** 411.
68. Chen, J., and Stubbe, J. A. (2005). *Nature Rev. Cancer* **5,** 102.
69. Sleijfer, S. (2001). *Chest* **120,** 617.
70. Takahashi, K., Ekimoto, H., Minamide, S., Nishikawa, K., Kuramochi, H., Motegi, A., Nakatani, T., Takita, T., Takeuchi, T., and Umezawa, H. (1987). *Cancer Treat. Rev.* **14,** 169.
71. Nicaise, C., Hong, W. K., Dimery, W., Usakewicz, J., Rozencweig, M., and Krakoff, I. (1990). *Invest. New Drugs* **8,** 325.
72. Westre, T. E., Loeb, K. E., Zaleski, J. M., Hedman, B., Hogdson, K. O., and Solomon, E. I. (1995). *J. Am. Chem. Soc.* **117,** 1309.
73. Solomon, E. I., Brunold, T. C., Davis, M. I., Kemsley, J. N., Lee, S. K., Lehnert, N., Neese, F., Skulan, A. J., Yang, Y. S., and Zhou, J. (2000). *Chem. Rev.* **100,** 235.
74. Boger, D. L., and Cai, H. (1999). *Angew. Chem. Int. Ed. Engl.* **38,** 449.
75. Povirk, L. F., Hogan, M., and Dattagupta, N. (1979). *Biochemistry* **18,** 96.
76. Carter, B. J., Murty, V. S., Reddy, K. S., Wang, S. N., and Hecht, S. M. (1990). *J. Biol. Chem.* **265,** 4193.
77. Wu, W., Vanderwall, D. E., Stubbe, J., Kozarick, J. W., and Turner, C. J. (1994). *J. Am. Chem. Soc.* **116,** 10843.
78. Ohno, M. (1989). *Pure Appl. Chem.* **61,** 581.
79. Walker, M. A., Dalton King, H., Dalterio, R. A., Trail, P., Firestone, R., and Dubowchik, G. M. (2004). *Bioorg. Med. Chem. Lett.* **14,** 4323.
80. Abe, S., and Otsuki, M. (2002). *Curr. Med. Chem. Anticancer Agents* **2,** 715.
81. Takeshita, A., Shinjo, K., Naito, K., Matsui, H., Sahara, N., Shigeno, K., Horii, T., Shirai, N., Maekawa, M., Ohnishi, K., Naoe, T., and Ohno, R. (2005). *Leukemia* **19,** 1306.
82. Kumar, R. A., Ikemoto, N., and Patel, D. J. (1997). *J. Mol. Biol.* **265,** 187.
83. Bergmann, R. G. (1973). *Acc. Chem. Res.* **6,** 25.
84. Myers, A. G., and Proteau, P. J. (1989). *J. Am. Chem. Soc.* **111,** 1146.
85. Kappen, L. S., and Goldberg, I. H. (1993). *Science* **261,** 1319.
86. Nicolau, K. C., and Dai, W. M. (1992). *J. Am. Chem. Soc.* **114,** 8908.
87. Brown, J. M. (1999). *Cancer Res.* **59,** 5863.
88. Brown, J., and Wang, L. H. (1998). *Anticancer Drug Des* **13,** 529.
89. Lara, P. N., Frankel, P., Mack, P. C., Gumerlock, P. H., Galvin, I., Martel, C. L., Longmate, J., Doroshow, J. H., Lenz, H. J., Lau, D. H. M., and Gandara, D. R. (2003). *Clin. Cancer Res.* **9,** 4356.
90. Aquino, V. M., Weitman, S. D., Winick, N. J., Blaney, S., Furman, W. L., Kepner, J. L., Bonate, P., Krailo, M., Qu, W., and Bernstein, M. (2004). *J. Clin. Oncol.* **22,** 1413.
91. Maxim, P. G., Carson, J. J. L., Ning, S., Knox, S. J., Boyer, A. L., Hsu, C. P., Benaron, D. A., and Walleczek, J. (2004). *Radiat. Res.* **162,** 185.
92. Kotandeniya, D., Ganley, B., and Gates, K. S. (2002). *Bioorg. Med. Chem. Lett.* **12,** 2325.
93. Anderson, R. F., Shinde, S. S., Hay, M. P., Gamage, S. A., and Denny, W. A. (2003). *J. Am Chem. Soc.* **125,** 748.
94. Peters, K. B., and Brown, J. M. (2002). *Cancer Res.* **62,** 5248.
95. Liu, G., Berlin, J., Tutsch, K. D., Van Ummersen, L., Dresen, A., Marnocha, R., Arzomanian, R., Alberti, D., Feierabend, C., Binger, K., and Wilding, G. (2002). *Clin. Cancer Res.* **8,** 706.
96. Weinmann, M., Welz, S., and Bamberg, M. (2003). *Curr. Med. Chem. Anticancer Agents* **3,** 364.
97. Eschwege, F., Sancho-Garnier, H., Chassagne, D., Brisgand, D., Guerra, M., Malaise, E. P., Bey, P., Busutti, L., Cionini, L., N'Guyen, T., Romanini, A., Chavaudra, J., *et al.* (1997). *Int. J. Radiat. Oncol. Biol. Phys.* **39,** 275.
98. Bennewith, K. L., Raleigh, J. A., and Durand, R. E. (2002). *Cancer Res.* **62,** 6827.

99. Cowen, R. L., Williams, K. J., Chinje, E. C., Jaffar, M., Sheppard, F. C. D., Telfer, B. A., Wind, N. S., and Stratford, I. J. (2004). *Cancer Res.* **64,** 1396.
100. Castano, A., Demidova, T. N., and Hamblin, M. R. (2004). *Photodiagn. Photodyn. Ther.* **1,** 279.
101. Wainwright, M. (2004). *Rev. Prog. Color* **34,** 95.
102. Tacquet, J. P., Frochot, C., Manneville, V., and Barberi-Heyob, M. (2007). *Curr. Med. Chem.* **14,** 1673.
103. Marcus, S. L., and McIntyre, W. R. (2002). *Emerg. Drugs* **7,** 321.
104. Kikuchi, T., Asakura, T., Aihara, H., Shiraki, M., Takagi, S., Kinouchi, Y., Aizawa, K., and Shimosegawa, T. (2003). *Anticancer Res.* **23,** 4897.
105. Brunner, H., Hausmann, F., Krieg, R. C., Endlicher, E., Scholmerich, J., Knuechel, R., and Messmann, H. (2001). *Photochem. Photobiol.* **74,** 721.
106. Kato, H. J. (1998). *Photochem. Photobiol.* **42,** 96.
107. Allison, R. R., Cuenca, R. E., Downie, G. H., Camnitz, P., Brodish, B., and Sibata, C. H. (2005). *Photodiagn. Photodyn. Ther.* **2,** 205.
108. Allison, M. R., Mota, H. C., and Sibata, C. H. (2004). *Photodiagn. Photodyn. Ther.* **1,** 263.
109. Cimino, G. D., Gamper, H. B., Isaacs, S. T., and Hearst, J. E. (1997). *Ann. Photochem. Photobiol.* **66,** 141.
110. Kanne, D., Straub, K., Hearst, J. E., and Rapopport, H. (1982). *J. Am. Chem. Soc.* **104,** 6754.

CHAPTER 5

DNA Alkylating Agents

Contents

1.	Introduction	139
2.	Nitrogen Mustards	141
	2.1. Introduction	141
	2.2. DNA alkylation by nitrogen mustards and cytotoxicity mechanisms	142
	2.3. Structure–activity relationships in nitrogen mustards	144
	2.4. Site-directed nitrogen mustards	147
3.	Aziridines (Ethyleneimines)	154
4.	Epoxides	158
5.	Methanesulfonates	159
6.	Nitrosoureas	160
7.	Triazenes	165
8.	Methylhydrazines	166
9.	1,3,5-Triazines: Hexamethylmelamine and Trimelamol	168
10.	Platinum Complexes	169
11.	Miscellaneous Alkylating and Acylating Antitumor Agents	173
	References	174

1. INTRODUCTION

Anticancer drugs that target DNA have been used in the clinic for more than 60 years.[1] Despite the recent major advances in cancer research, the mechanism by which most clinically relevant anticancer drugs kill cells consists of interference with replication, which can be achieved most simply by DNA alkylation. Alkylating agents can be defined as compounds capable of covalently binding an alkyl group to a biomolecule under physiological conditions (aqueous solution, 37 °C, pH 7.4). DNA alkylating agents interact with resting and proliferating cells in any phase of the cell cycle, but they are more cytotoxic during the late G1 and S phases

Medicinal Chemistry of Anticancer Drugs
DOI: 10.1016/B978-0-444-52824-7.00005-6

because not enough time is available to repair the damage before DNA synthesis takes place.

In principle, covalent bonds can arise from attack of either nucleophilic or electrophilic species to DNA, and indeed some nucleophiles (e.g., hydrazine, hydroxylamine, bisulfite) are known to attack DNA bases under physiological conditions. On the contrary, with the exception of the nitrogen atoms involved in the nucleoside bond (N^9 and N^1 in purines or pyrimidines), all nitrogen and oxygen atoms of purine and pyrimidine bases are nucleophiles and, consequently, therapeutically useful drugs always behave as carbon electrophiles.[2] Attraction between nucleophiles and electrophiles is governed by two related but independent interactions: electrostatic attraction between positive and negative charges (electrostatic control) and orbital overlap between the highest occupied molecular orbital (HOMO) of the nucleophile and the lowest unoccupied molecular orbital (LUMO) of the electrophile (orbital control). These two types of reactivities have been termed as "hard" and "soft," respectively. Thus, the highly electronegative oxygen atoms tend to react under electrostatic control and are considered as "hard" nucleophiles, and accordingly they react with "hard" electrophiles, that is, those with a more pronounced cationic character. Because nitrogen atoms of DNA bases are softer nucleophiles than oxygen atoms and that many therapeutically useful alkylating agents are relatively "soft" electrophiles, they react mainly at nitrogen sites, in the following order: N^7 of guanine $> N^1$ of adenine $> N^3$ of cytosine $> N^3$ of thymine. Diazonium salts, generated from nitrosoureas and other antitumor agents, are examples of therapeutically relevant "hard" electrophiles, which tend to preferentially alkylate oxygen atoms at phosphate residues and carbonyl oxygen atoms in DNA bases, specially O-6 of guanine. DNA alkylation is governed to a great extent by steric effects, and nucleophilic sites placed inside the double helix are less exposed to alkylation, while those in the major and minor groove are more easily attacked.[3]

Structure and dynamics of DNA are greatly affected by base alkylation, which leads to several types of effects. In the first place, alkylation prevents DNA replication and RNA transcription from the affected DNA. It also leads to the fragmentation of DNA by hydrolytic reactions and also by the action of repair enzymes when attempting to remove the alkylated bases. Alkylation also induces the mispairing of the nucleotides by alteration of the normal hydrogen bonding between bases. Finally, compounds capable of bisalkylation can form bridges within a single DNA strand (intrastrand cross-linkage). It can also lead to cross-linking between DNA and associated proteins or between two complementary DNA strands (interstrand cross-linkage), preventing their separation during DNA replication or transcription (Fig. 5.1). It has been proved that bifunctional alkylating compounds are considerably more cytotoxic than their monofunctional counterparts, and also that there is a direct correlation between the degree of interstrand cross-linking and cytotoxicity.

The main types of DNA alkylating drugs that will be covered in this chapter have been classified as follows:

- Nitrogen mustards
- Aziridines (ethyleneimines)

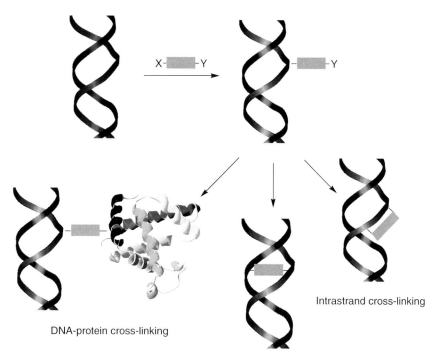

FIGURE 5.1   Different modes of DNA cross-linking.

- Epoxides
- Methanesulfonates
- Nitrosoureas
- Triazenes
- Methylhydrazines
- 1,3,5-Triazines
- Platinum complexes
- Miscellaneous alkylating and acylating antitumor agents

2. NITROGEN MUSTARDS

2.1. Introduction

Sulfur mustard (mustard gas, yperite) was used in World War I for chemical warfare because it is an extremely irritant vesicant agent. After the war, it was realized that it also caused systemic effects such as leukopenia, aplasia of the bone marrow, dissolution of lymphoid tissue, and ulceration of the gastrointestinal tract. This suggested a possible role for this compound in cancer treatment, but after an exploratory study it was considered too toxic for systemic use.[4] A nitrogen analog of sulfur mustard known as mechlorethamine (mustine), the first nitrogen mustard, was also initially conceived as a chemical weapon, but it was applied to a lymphosarcoma patient in 1943 following the observation in autopsies that exposure to mechlorethamine led to profound lymphoid and myeloid suppression after an air attack on a ship carrying a stock of this substance. This study was classified at the time and was not published until 1946, starting the modern era of cancer chemotherapy.[5] Even at this early stage, it was soon apparent that the therapeutic effect was limited by marrow toxicity and the development of resistance, which are still a source of problems in cancer chemotherapy nowadays. These problems notwithstanding, mechlorethamine is still used for the chemotherapy of Hodgkin's lymphoma as part of some antitumor regimes.

Sulfur mustard   Mechlorethamine

2.2. DNA alkylation by nitrogen mustards and cytotoxicity mechanisms

Because of the relative unreactivity of alkyl chlorides as electrophiles, direct attack of DNA nucleophilic centers to nitrogen mustards under physiological conditions is too slow to be of therapeutic relevance. The reason why nitrogen mustards have a high reactivity as alkylating agents under mild conditions is the anchimeric assistance from the nitrogen atom, that is, the formation through an intramolecular nucleophilic substitution of the aziridinium cation **5.1**, which is highly reactive because of the positive charge at the leaving group and the high strain of the three-membered ring, which is relieved in the alkylation process. Since the most nucleophilic atom in DNA is the N-7 nitrogen of guanine, the most common species arising from alkylation is **5.2** (Fig. 5.2).

As mentioned in Section 1 , one consequence of alkylation is the alteration of the normal pairing of DNA bases between adenine-thymine and guanine-cytosine (Watson–Crick base pairs). For instance, the three hydrogen bonds normally linking guanine and cytosine require the existence of a carbonyl group at the purine C-6 position. Because alkylation at N-7 creates a positive charge on this center, which is adjacent to the partial positive charge at C-6 due to the electron deficiency of the carbonyl group, the tautomeric equilibrium in guanine is displaced to the more stable 6-hydroxy form.[6] This change in the normal tautomeric form converts hydrogen bond acceptor groups into donors, and vice versa.

Guanine   Cytosine   Alkylated guanine

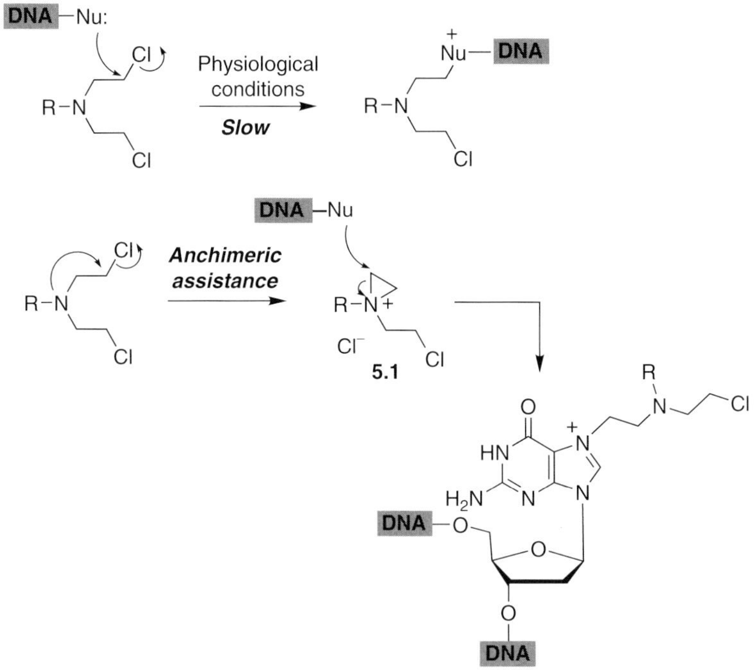

FIGURE 5.2   Mechanism of DNA alkylation by nitrogen mustards.

As a consequence of tautomerism, hydrogen bonding with cytosine is weakened because only two bonds can be established at best. On the contrary, pairing of the 6-hydroxy species with thymine leads to a more stable complex (three hydrogen bonds), and hence the base pairing is altered to guanine-thymine, leading to mutations.

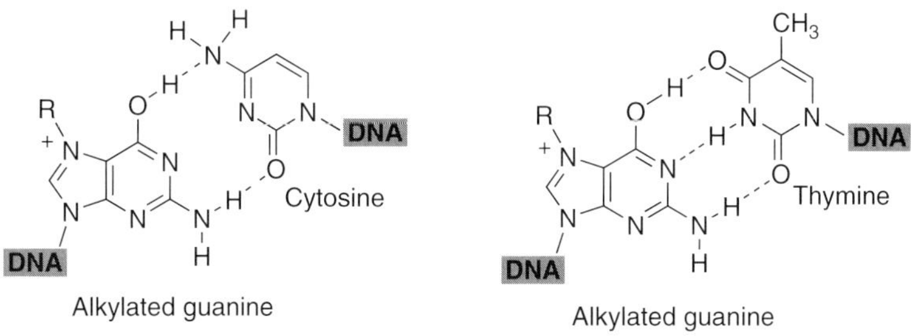

Another consequence of guanine alkylation is an increase in the electrophilicity of positions adjacent or conjugated to the positive charge at N-7, which leads to several hydrolytic reactions that alter the DNA structure. Thus, cleavage of the heteroside bond in structure **5.2**, although slow[7], induces DNA depurination to give **5.3**. This structure is in equilibrium with the open form **5.4**, which has a good

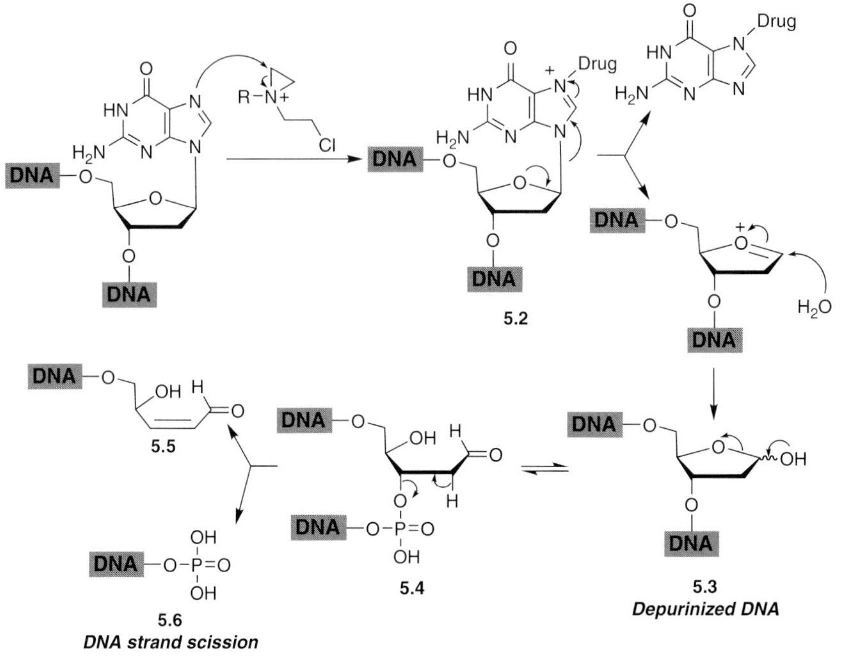

FIGURE 5.3   DNA fragmentation triggered by guanine alkylation.

leaving group (phosphate oxygen) at the β position with respect to the carbonyl group. This arrangement leads to an easy elimination process whereby DNA is fragmented to **5.5** and **5.6** (Fig. 5.3).

Another position of the purine ring with increased electrophilicity is C-8, which is adjacent to the positive charge induced on alkylation. Water addition to C-8 leads to intermediate **5.7**, which then evolves to **5.8**. This compound has an imine structure that allows hydrolysis and gives **5.4** with subsequent DNA strand scission (Fig. 5.4).

Because nitrogen mustards are bifunctional alkylating agents, one of their cytotoxicity mechanisms is related to the ability of DNA-monoalkylated species **5.9** to give covalent DNA interstrand and intrastrand cross-links (**5.10**) or DNA–protein complexes (**5.11**) from the monoalkylated species **5.9**, leading to disruption of replication or transcription (Figs. 5.1 and 5.5).

2.3. Structure–activity relationships in nitrogen mustards

Although mechlorethamine was an improvement over sulfur mustard, it was still highly vesicant and chemically labile because of its very rapid reaction with biological material and water, respectively. Replacement of its methyl group by an aromatic ring lowers its reactivity because the electron-withdrawing effect of this type of substituents hampers anchimeric assistance to alkylation by the nitrogen atom. The increased stability gives enough time for absorption and

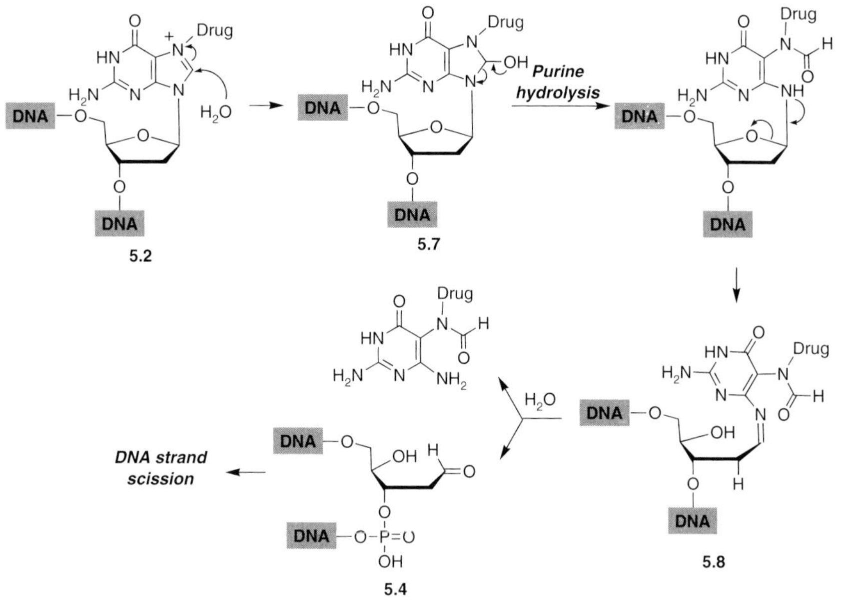

FIGURE 5.4   Other DNA fragmentation processes taking place after guanine alkylation.

distribution before alkylation takes place, and therefore allows oral administration. The simplest aromatic nitrogen mustard is compound **5.12**, which has the disadvantage of not being water soluble. Addition of a carboxyl group led to the soluble analog **5.13**, which was inactive. However, simple separation of the carboxylic group from the aromatic ring by a spacer yielded active compounds such as chlorambucil, which contains a butyric acid side chain. This compound is used to treat chronic lymphocytic leukemia and lymphomas. Bendamustin is a related nitrogen mustard where the benzene ring has been replaced by a benzimidazole.

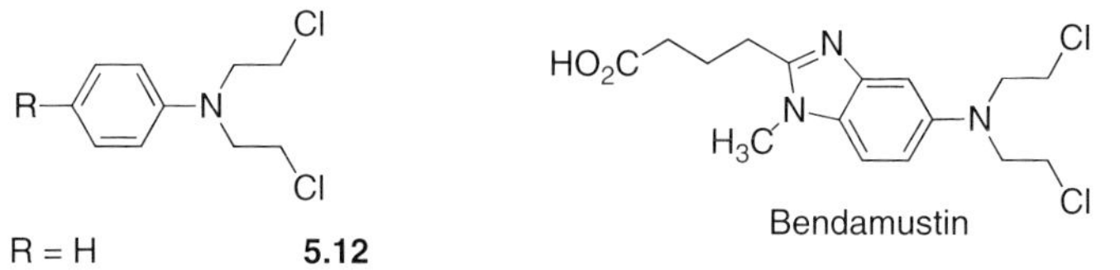

R = H   **5.12**
R= CO$_2$H   **5.13**
R = (CH$_2$)$_3$CO$_2$H   Chlorambucil

Bendamustin

   The butyric acid moiety modulates not only the aqueous solubility and reactivity as alkylating agents of the nitrogen mustards, but also their metabolism. Thus, a significant fraction of chlorambucil is metabolically degraded to an active phenylacetic acid mustard via β-hydroxylation following the biochemical pathway employed for fatty acid degradation. In the case of bendamustin, the active hydroxy metabolite is more stable and is apparently not transformed into the acetic acid analog.[8]

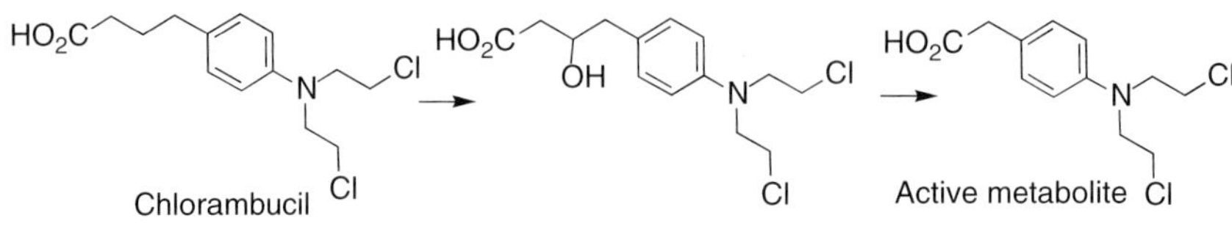

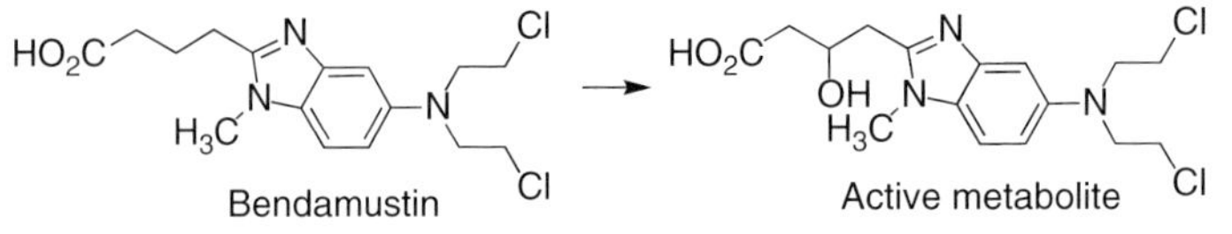

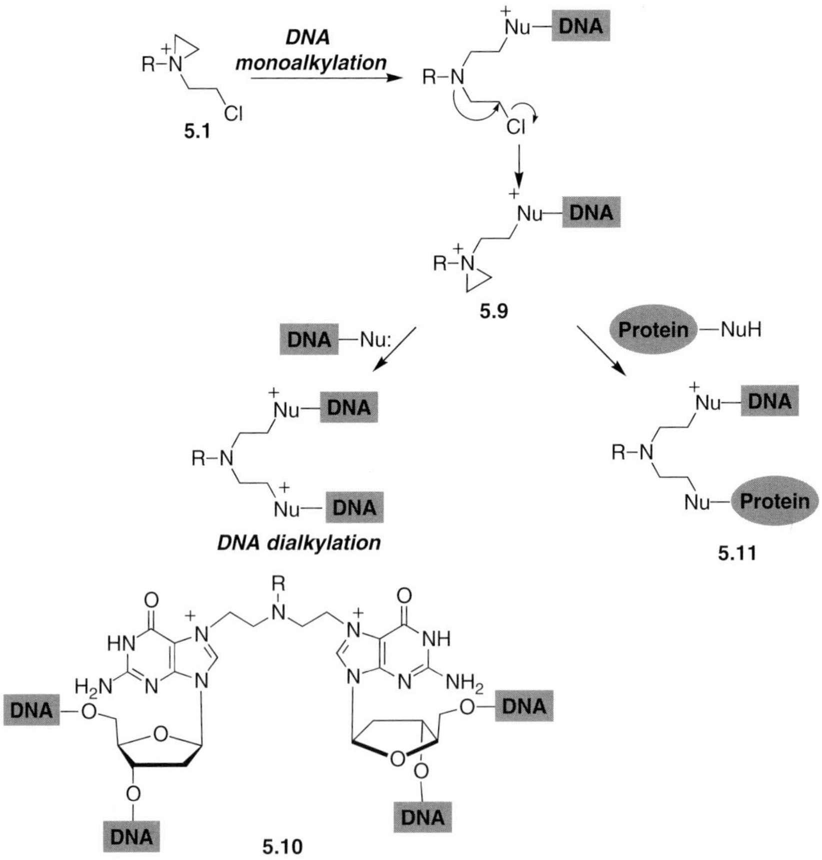

FIGURE 5.5   DNA cross-linking by nitrogen mustards.

2.4. Site-directed nitrogen mustards

Because of their high toxicity, considerable effort has been devoted to the development of site-directed mustards. Initial strategies were based on the incorporation of moieties that were expected to be accumulated preferentially in tumor cells. Thus, melphalan, which contains an L-phenylalanine unit, was postulated to concentrate in melanomas, since melanin is a product of phenylalanine metabolism. Although the original rationale was not correct, melphalan is used in certain types of bone marrow tumors, such as multiple myeloma, and ovarian or breast cancers. The main role of the side chain is to facilitate drug uptake by employing two amino acid transport system to enter tumor cells, that is, the sodium-independent L-amino acid system and the sodium-dependent ASC system for alanine, serine and cysteine. Other compounds designed on similar principles are uracyl mustard and estramustine, which consists of a β-estradiol unit linked to a nitrogen mustard portion via a carbamate bridge.

Melphalan
(L-Phenylalanine mustard)

Uracyl mustard

Estramustine

In contrast to chlorambucil, the bioavailability of orally administered melphalan is very variable, which can be attributed to its very rapid chemical degradation to the mono- and dihydroxy derivatives **5.14** and **5.15**.[9] *In vitro* studies have shown that this hydrolysis is pH dependent and takes place preferentially under neutral or basic conditions,[10] suggesting that the electron-withdrawing effect of the protonated amino group hampers aziridinium ion generation and its subsequent hydrolysis (Fig. 5.6).

The hydrolytic stability of melphalan has been improved by the preparation of analog **5.16**, containing a naphthoate portion that can be found in the antitumor enediyne antibiotic neocarzinostatin. Design of **5.16** was based on the knowledge of the role of this structural fragment in the complexation of neocarzinostatin to a protein called apo-neocarzinostatin, which greatly increases its stability.[11]

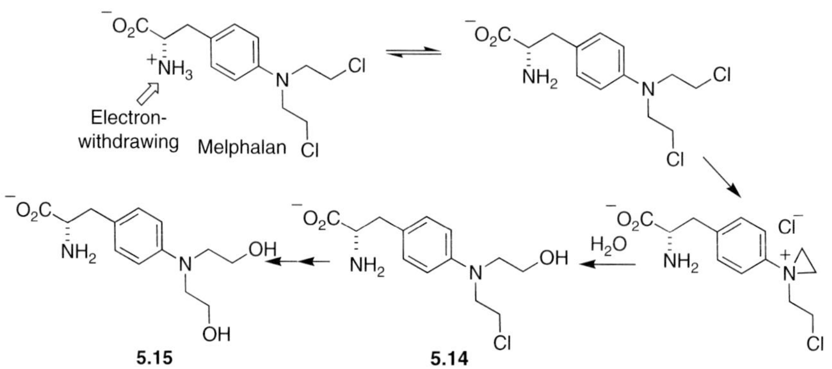

FIGURE 5.6   Chemical degradation of melphalan.

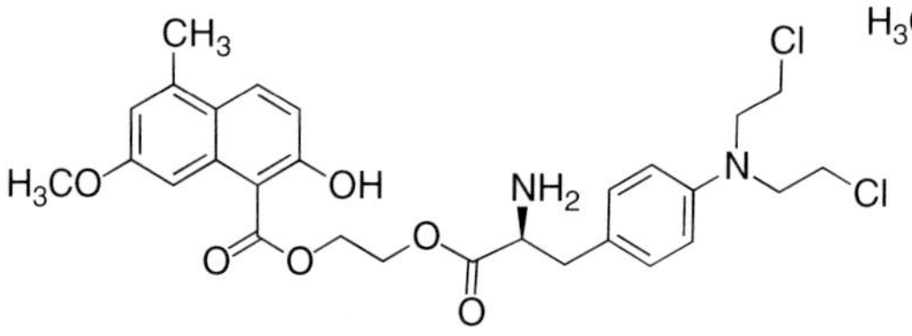

Estramustine was designed as a prodrug, since the electron density of its nitrogen atom is not sufficient to trigger aziridinium formation because of the electron-withdrawing effect of the carbonyl group. Estramustine was thus expected to target estrogenic hormone receptors before release of the active nitrogen mustard group following cleavage of the carbamate ester link. However, this function was stable to enzymatic cleavage, and therefore estramustine did not possess alkylating activity.[12] On the other hand, estramustine is also active in tissues and cell lines which lack estrogen receptors, and therefore its antitumor activity is not hormone related. On exposure to estramustine, cells were arrested in the metaphase and the mitotic spindle was absent, which suggested that estramustine acts by interaction with microtubules to promote microtubule disassembly (see Section 4 of Chapter 8). It has been subsequently proved that estramustine acts via a direct interaction with microtubule-associated proteins and with tubulin.[13] Estramustine has moderate activity against prostate cancers because of the existence in the prostate of the so-called estramustine binding protein (EMBP), which facilitates its uptake.[14]

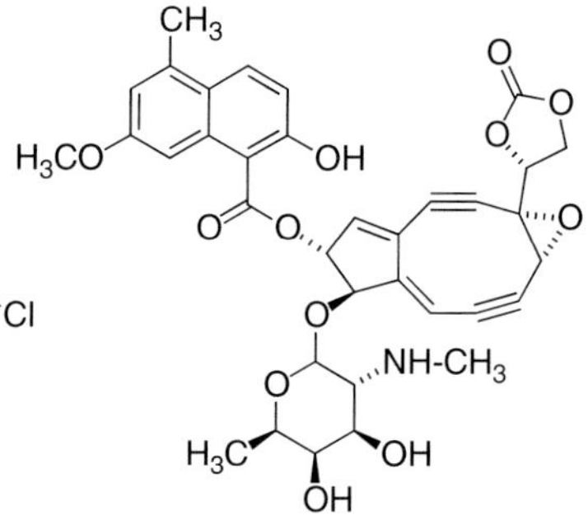

Another strategy for the development of site-directed nitrogen mustards can be selective bioactivation of prodrug forms if biochemical differences can be found between a tumor and normal tissue. Thus, a report stating that some tumors contain high levels of phosphoramidases led to the design of prodrug nitrogen mustards, which were expected to be activated by phosphoramide enzymatic hydrolysis. This assumption led to the preparation of cyclophosphamide, first reported in 1958, which has become the main antitumor drug of the alkylating class, being used to treat Hodgkin's disease, lymphomas, leukemias, and often in combination with other drugs to treat breast cancer, leukemia, and ovarian cancer. Other uses include the treatment of Wegener's granulomatosis, severe rheumatoid arthritis, and lupus erythematosus; the drug also has immunosuppressant action in smaller doses. Ifosfamide, a related compound, is used in testicular cancer. In both compounds, the electron-withdrawing effect of the P=O bond prevents their activation to aziridinium cations.

Cyclophosphamide

Ifosfamide

The initial working assumption soon proved wrong, since several studies showed that the drug is not activated by hydrolysis, but by hepatic P450 oxidation to 4-hydroxycyclophosphamide, which is in equilibrium with its acyclic form aldophosphamide. Hepatic alcohol dehydrogenase transforms these compounds into the inactive metabolites 4-ketocyclophosphamide and carboxyphosphamide, respectively, which explains the low hepatic toxicity of this drug. Some of the hydroxycyclophosphamide is carried throughout the body by the bloodstream and is further activated by a spontaneous elimination reaction that yields acrolein and phosphoramide mustard, the main cytotoxic species. The negative charge on the phosphoramidate oxygen atom balances the electron-withdrawing effect of the P=O group, and allows its activation to an aziridinium cation. Phosphoramide mustard can be hydrolyzed to nornitrogen mustard, which is also active (Fig. 5.7).

In spite of their structural similarity, ifosfamide metabolism is different from that of cyclophosphamide. Thus, although the active metabolite, isofosforamide mustard, is generated from the 4-hydroxy derivative by the same mechanism described for cyclophosphamide, this hydroxylation is slower than that of the chloroethyl side chains attached to the exocyclic nitrogen, probably because of steric hindrance on the C-4 position, which allows formation of inactive metabolites by competing N-dealkylation. These differences explain the need for higher doses to achieve the same effect, when compared to cyclophosphamide (Fig. 5.8).

Acrolein, the second product from the elimination reaction, is less active as an antitumor agent but appears to be responsible for a major side effect of cyclophosphamide, that is, hemorrhagic cystitis.[15] This problem can be reduced by coadministration of a thiol acrolein scavenger, like N-acetylcystein or mesna (sodium 2-mercaptoethanesulfonate). These thiol compounds do not react with the alkylating species responsible for the cytotoxic activity. They are found as disulfides in

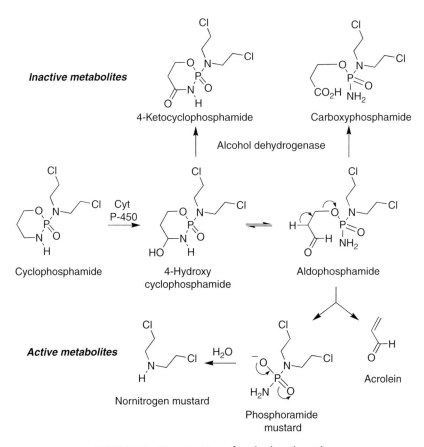

FIGURE 5.7   Bioactivation of cyclophosphamide.

plasma, but the disulfide is reduced by glutathione transferase in the kidney, liberating the thiol that inactivates acrolein through a conjugate addition, giving compounds such as **5.17** for the case of mesna (Fig. 5.9).

Another biochemical difference between some tumors and normal tissues is based on their different reducing capacities. The inner regions of solid tumors have little vascularization and therefore their oxygen content is low (for a more detailed treatment of hypoxia-based strategies for tumor-specific prodrug activation, see Section 2.2 of Chapter 11). Because molecular oxygen reverts some of the reactions of reductive metabolism, the latter is enhanced in hypoxic tissues. Some of these reactions are nitro and azo reduction, which are multistep processes where oxygen reverts the first equilibrium (Fig. 5.10).

On this basis, some aromatic nitrogen mustard prodrugs bearing nitro or azo groups have been designed to be activated in these hypoxic environments. In the simplest of them, the presence of these electron-withdrawing groups in the *p*-position with respect to the nitrogen atom prevents cyclization to an

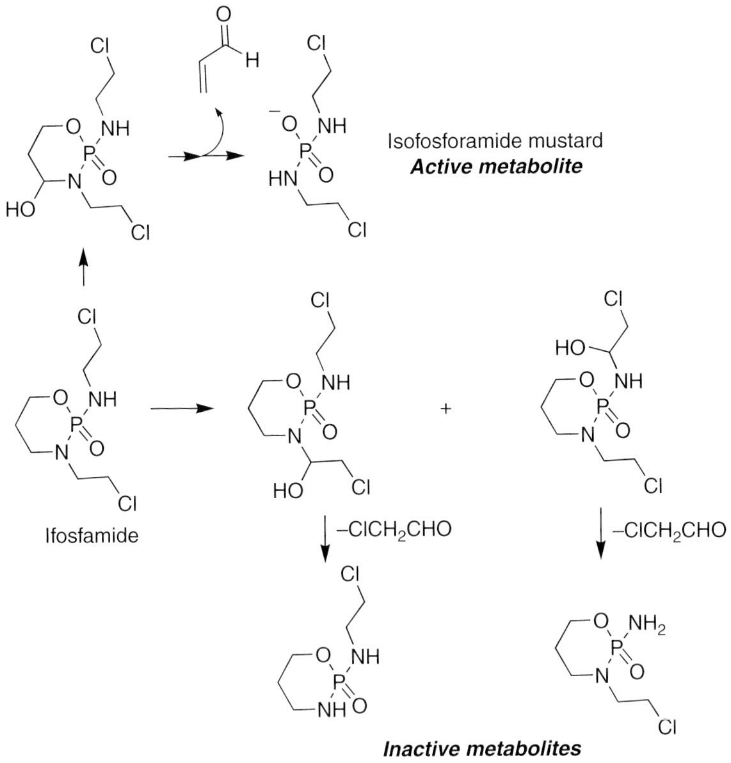

FIGURE 5.8   Metabolism of ifosfamide.

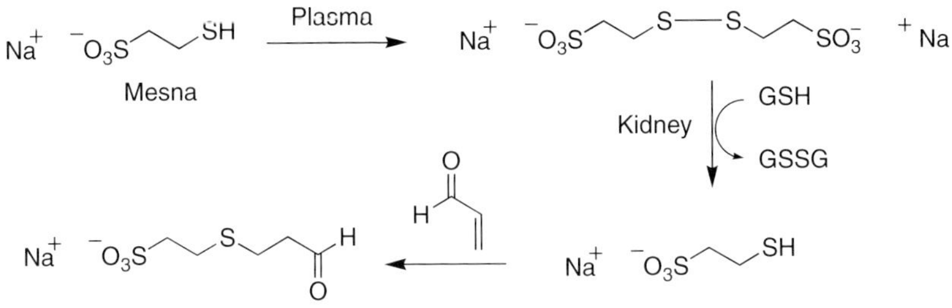

FIGURE 5.9   Detoxification of acrolein by mesna.

aziridinium cation, but after metabolic reduction they are transformed into an electron-releasing group[16] (Fig. 5.11).

Similarly, some nitrogen mustard Co (III) complexes such as SN 24771 are activated by reduction in hypoxic tumor microenvironments because one-electron reduction of Co (III) to Co (II) greatly labilizes the Co–N bonds, causing the release of the active nitrogen mustard (Fig. 5.12).[17] See Section 2.2.4 of Chapter 11 for

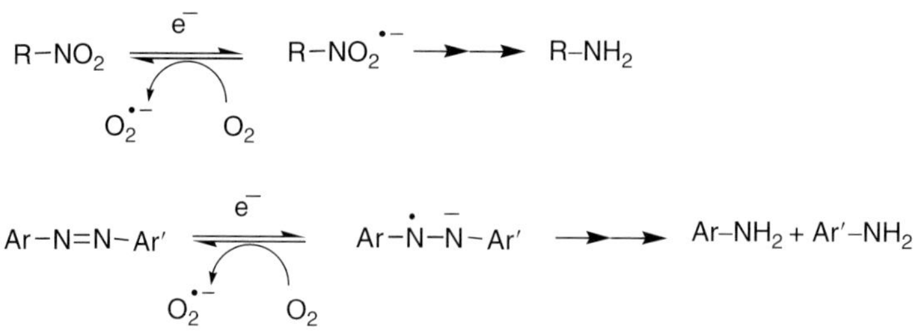

FIGURE 5.10   Reduction of nitro and azo compounds.

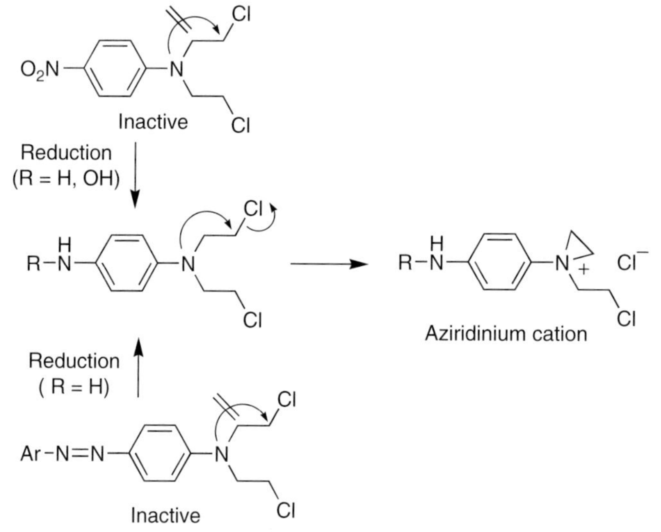

FIGURE 5.11   Aromatic nitrogen mustard prodrugs for selective activation in hypoxic tissues.

further details on the use of Co (III) complexes in hypoxia-based strategies for tumor-specific prodrug activation.

More complex approaches are based on the distal activation concept, where the reductive process uncovers a nucleophilic or basic center that then triggers the liberation of the alkylating agent by reaction with a distant part of the molecule. Thus, the phosphoramide mustard prodrug **5.18** is activated by reduction of its nitro group to amino, which increases the basicity of the quinoline nitrogen sufficiently to allow the elimination reaction depicted in Fig. 5.13.

A related example is based on the reduction of a quinone system, which uncovers two nucleophilic hydroxyl groups, as shown in Fig. 5.14 for the case of the melphalan prodrug **5.19**.[18] The conformation needed for the reaction that liberates the active drug is favored by the presence of the methyl groups because it is less sterically compressed than alternative conformations (Thorpe-Ingold effect).

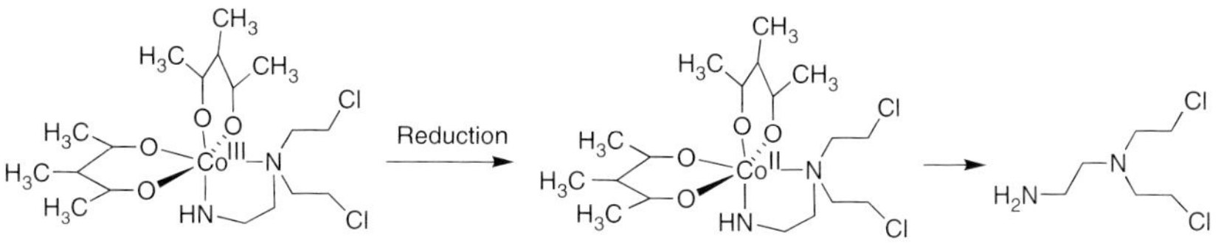

FIGURE 5.12 Nitrogen mustard Co (III) complexes and their activation in hypoxic tissues.

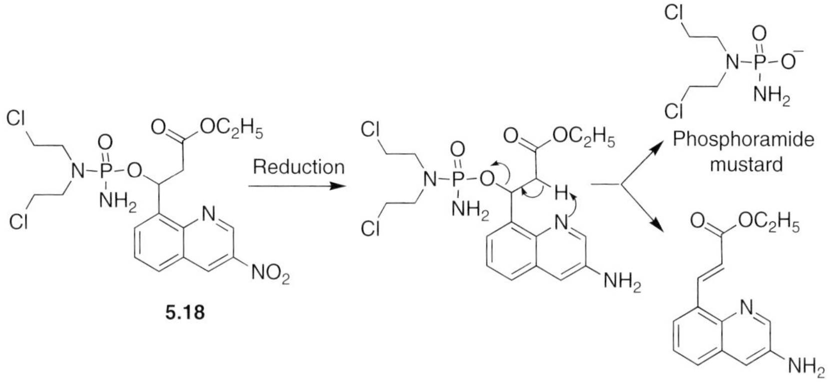

FIGURE 5.13 Distal activation of a nitrogen mustard prodrug mediated by reductive processes.

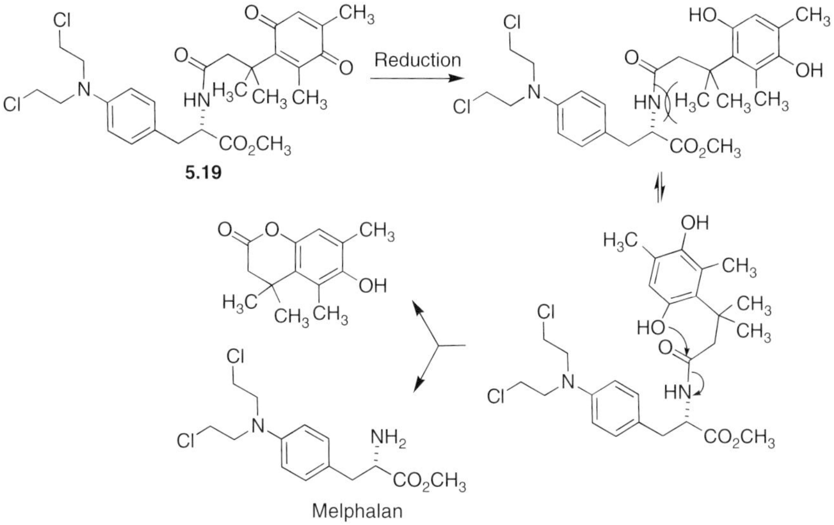

FIGURE 5.14 Bioreductive activation of a melphalan prodrug.

3. AZIRIDINES (ETHYLENEIMINES)

Since the active species involved in DNA alkylation by nitrogen mustards is an aziridinium cation, several aziridine derivatives were also tested as antitumor agents.

Electron-releasing substituents raise the aziridine nitrogen pK_a and lead to a high concentration of aziridinium cations **5.20**, which renders these compounds too reactive to be of therapeutic value. For this reason, the aziridine units are attached to electron-withdrawing groups, which reduce their reactivity as bases but still allow formation of DNA-alkylation products such as **5.22**, which then are protonated to **5.21**. The driving forces of this reaction are the stabilization of the nitrogen negative charge by the electron-withdrawing group and the liberation of ring strain on opening of the aziridium (Fig. 5.15).

Early studies showed that at least two aziridine units were necessary for good activity, which did not improve by addition of a third or fourth aziridine, suggesting that cytotoxicity is mainly due to a cross-linking mechanism, as in the case of nitrogen mustards. The first compounds of this family to be introduced in therapeutics were triethylenemelamine (TEM) and thiotepa, so called because it is a sulfur analog of triethylenephosphoramide (TEPA). Thiotepa is still used in bladder carcinoma by intracavitary administration because of its low stability in the acid conditions prevalent in the stomach. The previously discussed acid-assisted activation process is probably the main mechanism of DNA alkylation by these compounds.[19]

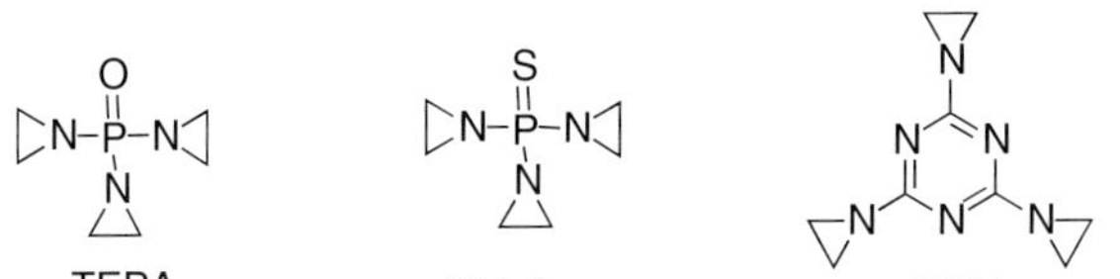

TEPA
(Triethylenephosphoramide)

Thiotepa

TEM
Triethylenemelamine

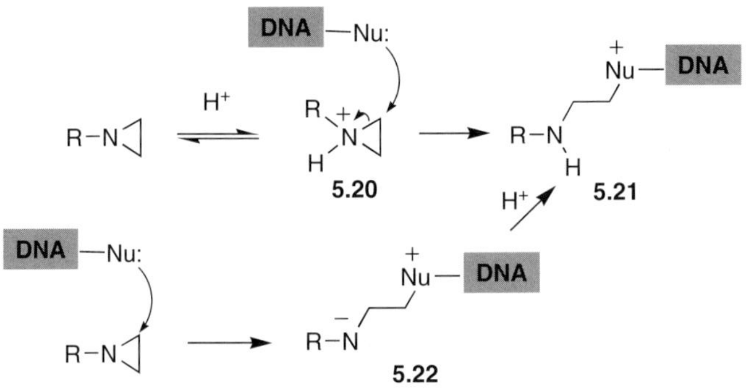

FIGURE 5.15   DNA alkylation by aziridines.

Other antitumor compounds contain two or three aziridine rings linked to a benzoquinone system and can act as DNA bisalkylators and cross-linking agents. They were designed to cross the blood–brain barrier because of their high lipophilicity and low ionization. Some of them have been used in the clinic, as in the case of carboquone (carbazilquinone), diaziquone (AZQ), triaziquone, and BZQ.[20] AZQ, one of the most active compounds, has been studied in a number of clinical trials up to Phase II[21] and was the first "orphan drug" selected by the FDA in the early 1980s, but it showed no clear advantage over preexisting drugs. BZQ and triaziquone[22] also underwent clinical trials, but they were withdrawn because of their toxicity. EO9 contains only one aziridine moiety and has shown very good activity *in vitro* but disappointing results in clinical trials that were attributed to its short half-life.

Carboquone   Diaziquone (AZQ)   Triaziquone

BZQ   RH1   EO9

Generally speaking, the mechanism of DNA alkylation[19] by aziridinylbenzoquinones involves bioreductive processes[23] that are activated by the action of one-electron or two-electron reductases. The oxidation state of the quinone function modulates the alkylating activity, and it also bears a relationship with the generation of cytotoxic reactive oxygen species. Indeed, the quinone group is a structural motif commonly found in reductively activated antitumor agents due to the fact that quinones exhibit reduction potentials similar to substrates of endogenous reductases.[24] Reduction of the quinone to a hydroquinone increases the pK_a of the aziridine nitrogen because of the replacement of the electron-withdrawing carbonyls by two electron-releasing hydroxy groups and therefore allows its protonation to a more reactive aziridinium cation. Furthermore, intramolecular hydrogen bonding of these groups with the aziridine nitrogen may assist this protonation (Fig. 5.16). In some cases (e.g., BZQ) alkylation is possible in the absence of reduction.[25] Indeed, it has been proved that simple aziridinylbenzoquinones can cross-link DNA in the absence of reduction, in a pH-dependent process presumably related to the protonation mechanism shown in Fig. 5.15.[26]

DT-diaphorase (DTD), an obligate two-electron reductase, is a particularly interesting target for antitumor compounds[27] because it is present in the cell nucleus and its levels are increased in a number of tumors,[28] although they are varying in clinical tumors. Since the recognition of the importance of DTD in the

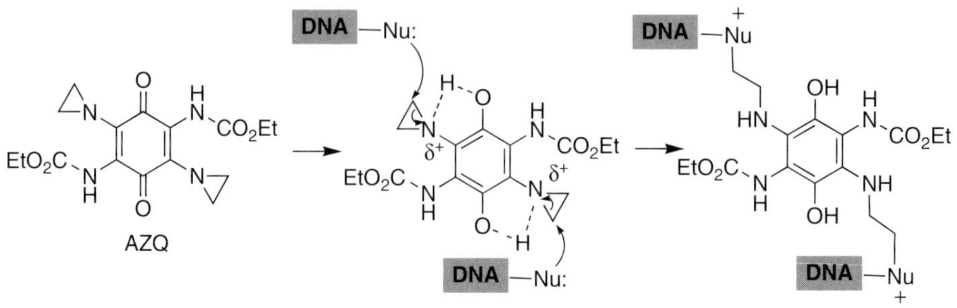

FIGURE 5.16   Bioreductive activation of aziridinylbenzoquinones.

activation of aziridinylbenzoquinones,[29] there has been much effort to produce novel agents that efficiently target this enzyme.[30] Electron-donating groups on the benzoquinone ring increased DNA damage, whereas electron-withdrawing groups and sterically bulky groups at the C-6 position led to inactive compounds or decreased their ability to produce DNA damage.[31] Some of them, like Me-DZQ, are limited by their poor solubility, which has been overcome by introduction of hydrophilic hydroxyl groups in the side chains. For instance, RH1[32] is an excellent substrate for DTD that has a good solubility and antitumor potency *in vitro* and *in vivo*,[33] and is currently undergoing Phase I clinical studies in patients with solid tumors under the auspices of Cancer Research UK.

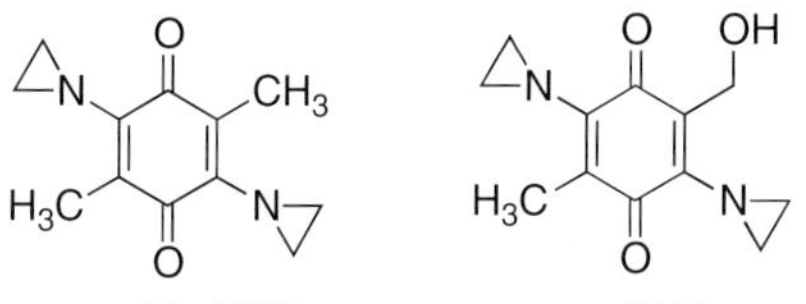

Me-DZQ   RH1

Besides alkylation, other reactions are possible on the hydroquinone form of aziridinylquinones such as **5.23** that lead to its inactivation. One of them is a 1,5-sigmatropic shift of hydrogen to give **5.24**,[34] which is then transformed into ethylaminoquinone **5.25** by tautomerism or into aminoquinone **5.26** through a second 1,5-sigmatropic shift followed by hydrolysis (Fig. 5.17).

An additional transformation that inactivates **5.23** takes place by loss of the aziridine ring on its tautomer **5.27**, leading to quinone **5.28** (Fig. 5.18).

One-electron metabolic reduction of aziridinylquinones is also possible, leading to semiquinones. Their protonated derivatives **5.29** also undergo a 1,5-sigmatropic shift, leading to inactive compounds **5.25** and **5.26**, the same as in the two-electron reduction process (Fig. 5.19). As expected, semiquinone intermediates can also generate oxygen radical species on reaction with O_2.[35]

These degradation pathways have therapeutic implications, since the lower pharmacokinetic stability of indoloquinone aziridines such as EO9 with regard to their benzoquinone analogs is due to higher concentrations of the corresponding protonated semiquinone **5.29** due to the fact that the electron-releasing effect of

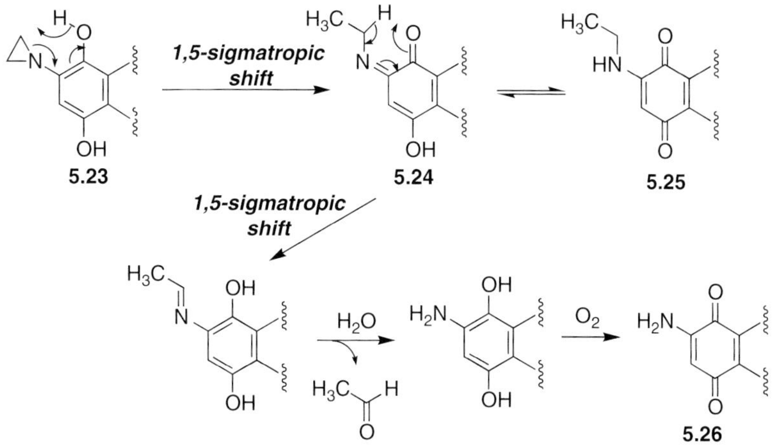

FIGURE 5.17   Inactivation of aziridinylbenzoquinones through a 1,5-sigmatropic shift.

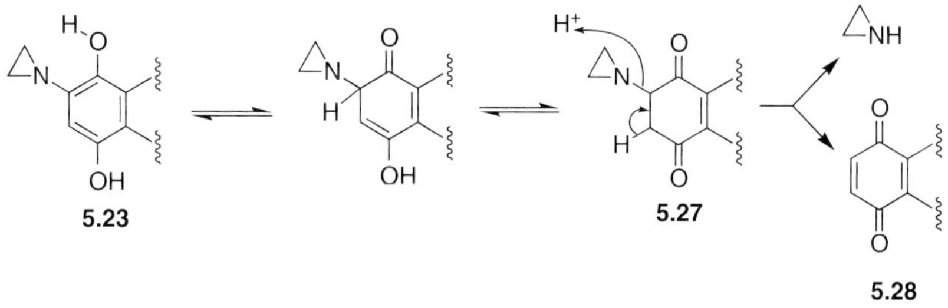

FIGURE 5.18   Inactivation of activation of aziridinylbenzoquinones by loss of the aziridine ring.

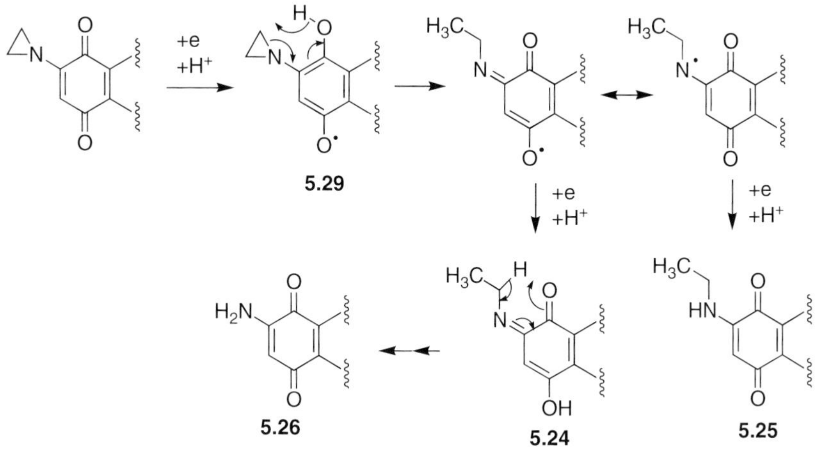

FIGURE 5.19   Inactivation of activation of aziridinylbenzoquinones by one-electron reduction.

the indole nitrogen leads to a low acidity for **5.29**. For instance, the pK_a of the semiquinone derived from EO9 is 9.3, while the corresponding pK_a values of benzosemiquinones are below neutrality. For this reason, benzosemiquinones are mostly deprotonated and the hydrogen sigmatropic shift cannot take place.[36]

Several natural products, including the mitomycins, FR-900482, and FR-69979, among others, contain one fused aziridine ring[37] but, because of their specificity toward the minor groove, these agents will be studied in Chapter 6.

4. EPOXIDES

The high reactivity of the epoxide ring toward nucleophilic groups in biomolecules is the basis of the use of ethylene oxide to sterilize substances that would be damaged by heat, including medical supplies such as bandages, sutures, and surgical implements. It has also become quite common as a substructure in side chains of compounds aimed at alkylating DNA[38] or other macromolecular targets.[39]

Diepoxybutane **5.30** is the simplest epoxide which is able to cross-link DNA. Although this compound is not employed as such, it is nonenzymatically generated from treosulfan, a member of the methanesulfonate family (see Section 5) that can be regarded as its prodrug, since this transformation (Fig. 5.20) is necessary for treosulfan cytotoxicity.[40] Treosulfan alkylates DNA at guanine bases, very similar to nitrogen mustards, and is employed for the treatment of ovarian cancer.

Similarly, mitobronitol, the 1,6-dibromo analog of mannitol, is a bromohydrin prodrug that undergoes a double intramolecular nucleophilic displacement to give diepoxide **5.31**, another DNA cross-linking reagent (Fig. 5.21). It is used for myelosuppression prior to allogeneic bone marrow transplantation in accelerated chronic granulocytic leukemia, showing lower toxicity than other alkylating agents such as busulfan.[41]

Mixed epoxide-aziridine antitumor compounds, such as the azinomycins, are also known. For instance, azinomycin B (carzinophilin), isolated from *Streptomyces*

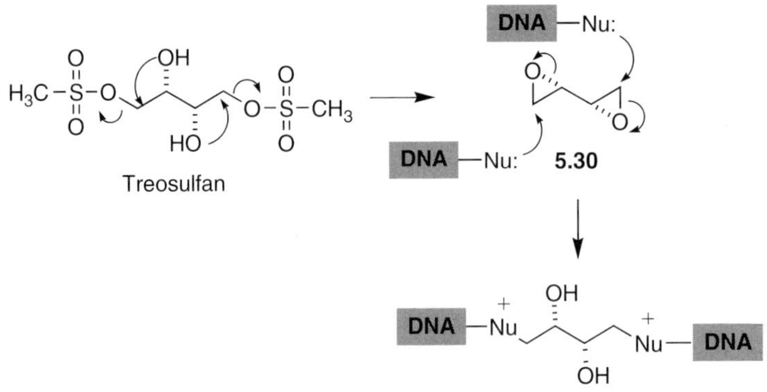

FIGURE 5.20 DNA alkylation by treosulfan.

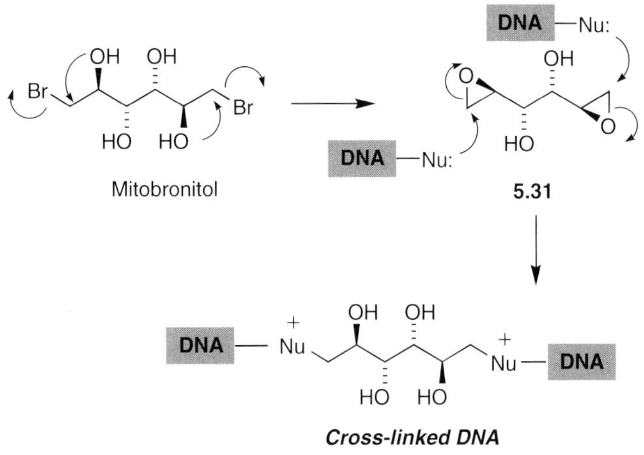

FIGURE 5.21   DNA alkylation by mitobronitol.

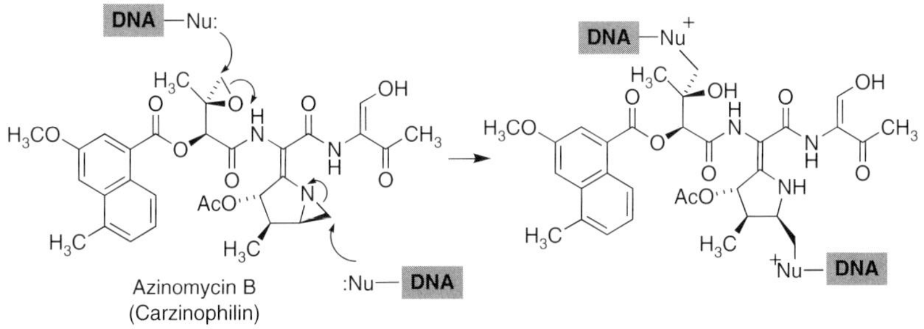

FIGURE 5.22   DNA cross-linking by azinimycin B.

sahachiroi, is capable of DNA intercalation and interstrand cross-linking (Fig. 5.22) and demonstrated submicromolar *in vitro* and *in vivo* cytotoxic activity.

5. METHANESULFONATES

Methanesulfonate is a good leaving group because of the efficient delocalization of negative charge between three oxygen atoms. For this reason, several compounds containing two methanesulfonate groups separated by a polymethylene chain were tested as antitumor agents, finding that the optimal activity corresponded to the compound with four carbon atoms (busulfan). Other members of this family are piposulfan, improsulfan, hepsulfam, and the previously mentioned diepoxide prodrug treosulfan.

Busulfan is used in the treatment of chronic granulocytic leukemia and, in high-dose combination with cyclophosphamide, to condition patients for allogeneic bone marrow transplantation. It is particularly toxic for pulmonary tissue, and this toxicity may be dose-limiting.

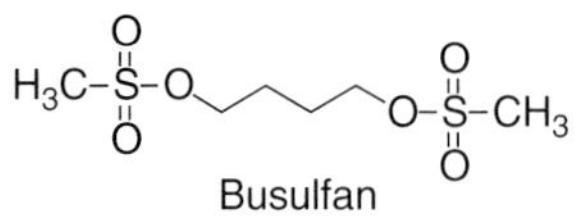

Busulfan

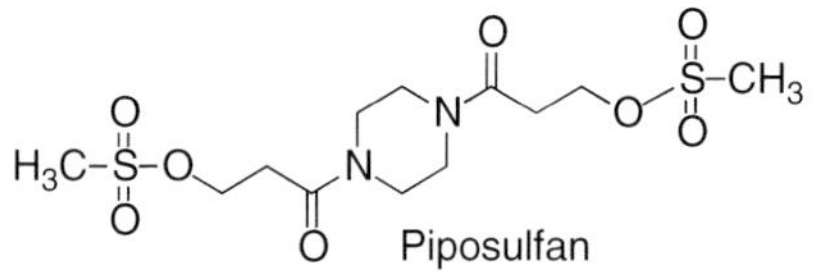

Piposulfan

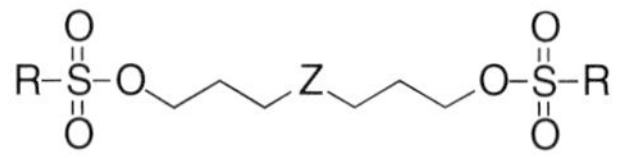

R	Z	Compound
CH_3	NH	Improsufan
NH_2	CH_2	Hepsulfam

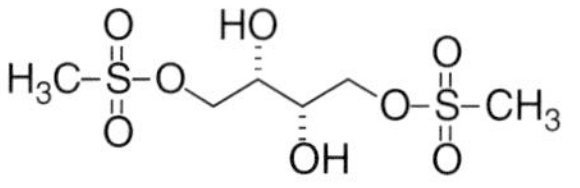

Treosulfan

In contrast with nitrogen mustards, where the rate-limiting step is the unimolecular formation of the aziridinium ion, busulfan reacts with guanine N-7 by an S_N2 mechanism (Fig. 5.23), where the rate-limiting step depends on the concentration of both reaction partners.[42] The formation of interstrand DNA cross-links has been demonstrated for busulfan[43] and treosulfan.[44]

The study of metabolites of busulfan suggests that it is also able to alkylate cysteine residues. Thus, the urinary excretion of compound **5.32** can be explained by the mechanism summarized in Fig. 5.24 and involves a double nucleophilic attack by cysteine.

6. NITROSOUREAS

In a random screen carried out by the NCI in 1959, 1-methyl-3-nitro-1-nitrosoguanidine showed very weak antileukemic activity. Assay of analogs of this compound led to the discovery of the antitumor activity of 1-methyl-1-nitrosourea, the lead compound of the nitrosourea group. It was soon discovered that introduction of a 2-chloroethyl chain on the nitrogen atom bearing the nitroso group (CNUs) led to much increased activity. These chloroethyl derivatives were lipophilic enough to cross the blood–brain barrier and therefore were useful in the treatment

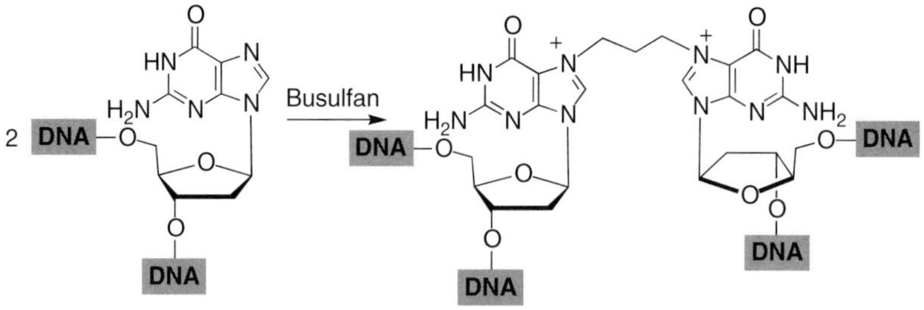

FIGURE 5.23 DNA alkylation by busulfan.

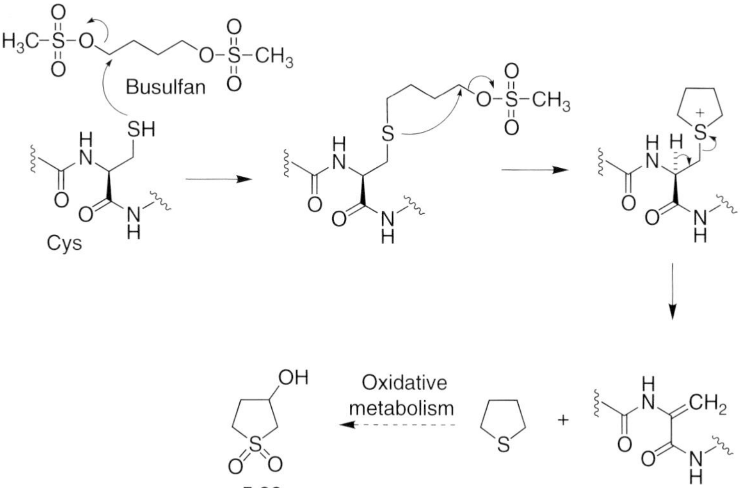

FIGURE 5.24   Alkylation of cysteine residues by busulfan.

of brain tumors, which led to the synthesis of a large number of nitrosoureas, including lomustine (CCNU) and its methyl derivative semustine, carmustine (BCNU), nimustine (ACNU), the water-soluble tauromustine and fotemustine, but toxicity problems have prevented their widespread use. In 1967, streptozoto-cin (streptozocin), a hydrophilic natural nitrosourea, was isolated from a strain of *S. achromogenes*. This compound was chosen as a lead because initial SAR studies suggested that hydrophilic nitrosoureas were more potent and less toxic, and a number of analogs, like chlorozotocin, were prepared. Currently, the most clini-cally important nitrosoureas are CCNU, BCNU, ACNU, and streptozotocin.

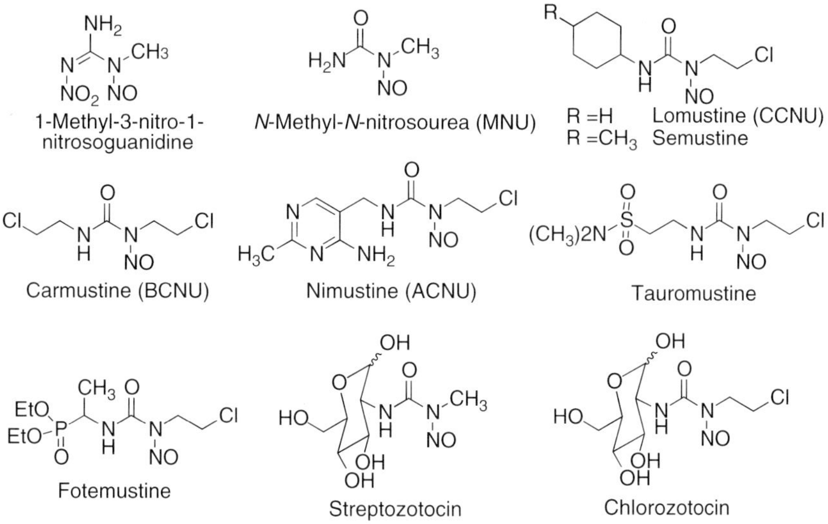

Nitrosoureas have been widely studied from a mechanistic point of view. The presence of the nitroso group labilizes the nitrogen-carbon bond, leading to two electrophiles, an isocyanate **5.33** and a diazene hydroxide **5.34**, which has been detected in some cases by electrospray ionization mass spectroscopy.[45] This intermediate in turn generates a diazonium salt **5.35**[46] (Fig. 5.25). Alkylation seems to be the main reaction responsible for antitumor activity, while carbamoylation takes place primarily on amino groups in proteins, leading to inhibition of several DNA repair mechanisms. N-Nitrosoamides and N-nitrosocarbamates, which can behave as alkylating (but not carbamoylating) agents have also antitumor activity, which supports the above statement.[47]

The above mechanism was based mainly on studies of the thermal decomposition of nitrosoureas under anhydrous conditions,[46] but in water solution the reaction is much more complex and has been explained by the mechanism shown in Fig. 5.26. Addition of a molecule of water to the nitrosourea, in its tautomeric

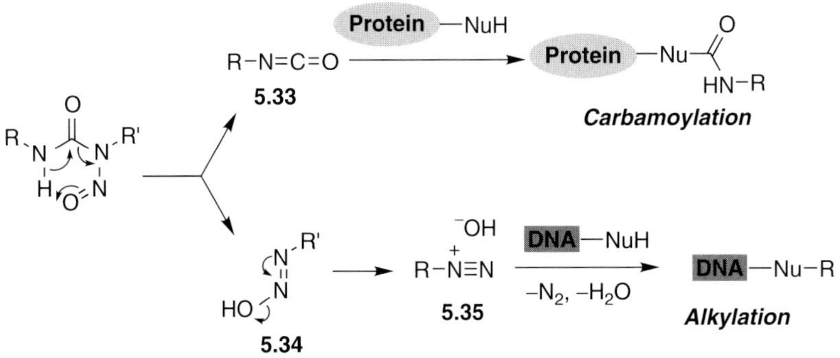

FIGURE 5.25   Thermal decomposition of nitrosoureas.

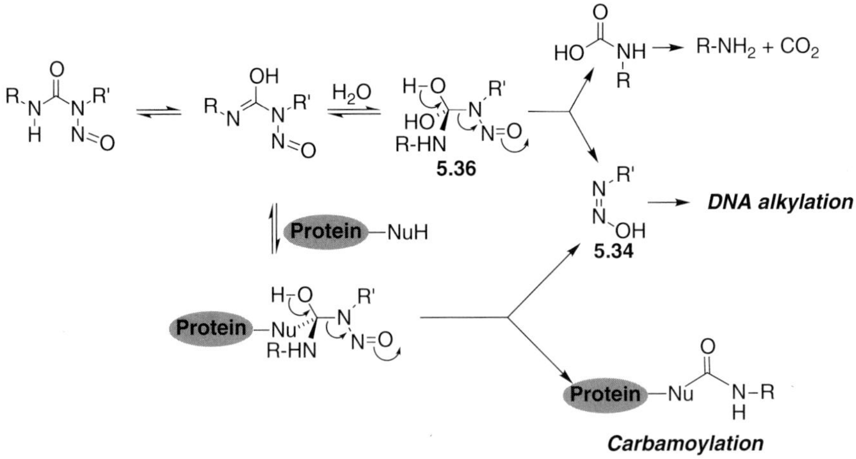

FIGURE 5.26   Decomposition of nitrosoureas in water solution.

form,[48] gives the tetrahedral intermediate **5.36**, which is decomposed into a primary amine, carbon dioxide, and **5.34**. This elimination requires an anti-periplanar conformation for **5.37**. Addition of a nucleophile other than water to the nitrosourea tautomer explains the isolation of carbamoylated products, formed by elimination of **5.34**.

Most nitrosoureas contain one chloroethyl chain on the nitrosated nitrogen, which allows them to act as DNA cross-linking agents. Reaction of electrophilic diazonium species **5.37** with guanine is assumed to take place on O-6 to give **5.38** (see also Section 1). In fact, addition of O^6-alkylguanine-DNA alkyltransferase, an enzyme that breaks O-6 guanine adducts, prevents cross-linking. This monoalkylated product reacts subsequently with the N-3 atom of the cytosine unit in the complementary DNA strand, by anchimeric assistance of the guanine N-1 atom through intermediate **5.39**, giving the cross-linked product **5.40** (Fig. 5.27).

In an alternative mechanism, intact nitrosourea molecules rather than diazonium species can directly alkylate DNA. Thus, nucleophilic attack of guanine O-6 to the nitrosourea tautomer **5.41** gives intermediate **5.42**. Although alternative mechanisms have been proposed, according to labeling experiments it is probable that **5.42** cyclizes to the nitrosoisoxazolidine **5.43**, which is attacked by another O-6 atom of a guanine unit neighboring in the DNA sequence to give **5.44**. In this adduct, the O-6 of the first guanine is carbamoylated and the O-6 of the second guanine is alkylated with a 2-hydroxydiazoethyl group (Fig. 5.28). Diazonium generation and attack of N-3 from a cytosine of the opposite DNA strand, with anchimeric assistance from guanine N-1, finally gives the carbamoylated cross-linked product **5.45**.

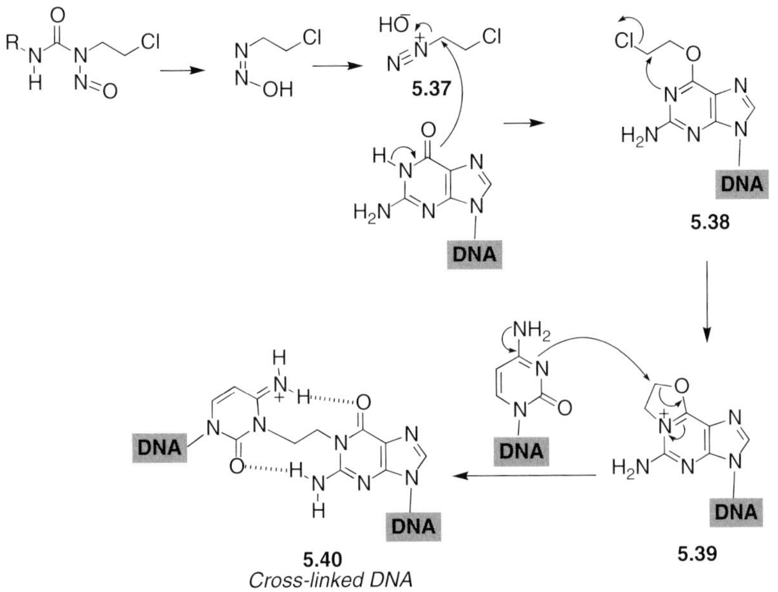

FIGURE 5.27   DNA cross-linking by nitrosoureas.

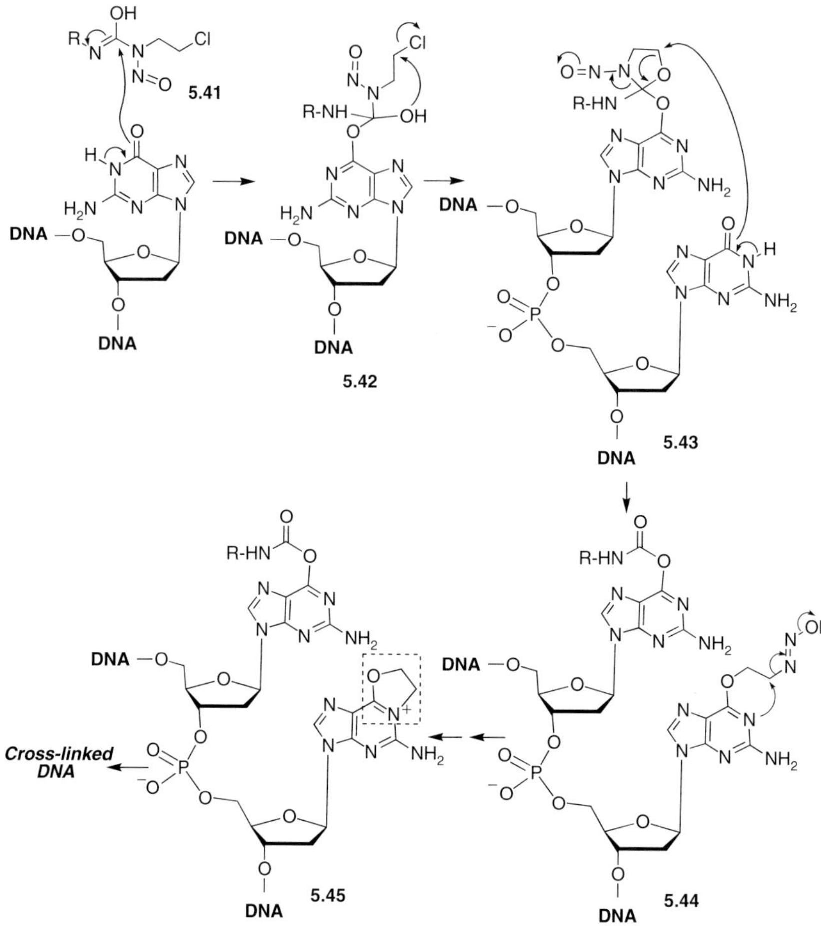

FIGURE 5.28   Alternative mechanisms for DNA cross-linking by nitrosoureas.

Streptozotocin differs from other nitrosoureas in that it does not cross the blood–brain barrier because of its high hydrophilicity, and it also shows a relatively low myelosuppression because of decreased entry into bone marrow cells. Its main cytotoxicity is exerted on the pancreas β cells because their glucose carrier facilitates drug uptake to the islets. Therefore, the main applications of streptozotocin are the induction of diabetes mellitus in experimental animals and treatment of islet cell pancreatic tumors, normally in association with nicotinamide for reasons that will be explained below. As expected from its nitrosourea structure, streptozotocin methylates DNA, specially at the guanine N-7 and O-6 positions,[49] but there is also much evidence that shows that free radicals play an essential role in its cytotoxicity.[50] It has been shown that streptozotocin induces the generation of nitric oxide,[51] superoxide and hydroxyl radicals, and also that association with oxygen radical scavengers, such as nicotinamide, prevents streptozotocin-induced cleavage of islet DNA.[52]

7. TRIAZENES

Dacarbazine (DTIC) is employed in combination therapy for the treatment of meta-static malignant melanoma and Hodgkin's disease. This compound was initially designed as an antimetabolite since it is an analog of 5-aminoimidazole-4-carbox-amide, an intermediate in purine biosynthesis. However, its cytotoxic activity is due to the generation during its metabolism of methyldiazonium, which methylates DNA.[53] Methyldiazonium has a half-life of about 0.4 s in aqueous solution, which is sufficient to allow it to reach its target. A mechanism for this process is summarized in Fig. 5.29, where activation of dacarbazine by metabolic oxidative demethylation to **5.46** (5-methyltriazenoimidazole-4-carboxamide, MTIC) was proved by the isolation of labeled formaldehyde and 5-aminoimidazole-4-carboxamide (AIC) when dacar-bazine was labeled with ^{14}C at one of the methyl groups. Intermediate **5.46** is then transformed by tautomerism into **5.47**, a diazonium precursor. The major methyla-tion reaction takes place at the guanine N-7 atom, and is relatively nontoxic. Meth-ylation at guanine O-6 also occurs, and is thought to be the main cytotoxic mechanism.[54] It is interesting to note that compounds that act as precursors to the ethyldiazonium cation lack any DNA binding properties, which has been explained by the lower stability in aqueous solution of ethyldiazonium with regard to methyl-diazonium,[55] leading to its evolution to ethylene by elimination or to ethanol by reaction with a molecule of water before reaching DNA.

Besides its toxicity, dacarbazine has several drawbacks because of its hydrophilicity, which leads to slow and incomplete oral absorption and therefore intravenous administration becomes necessary. Another disadvantage is its high photosensitivity, with a very short half-life (about 30 min), decomposing to 2-azahypoxanthine via an intermediate diazonium species (Fig. 5.30). For this reason, intravenous infusion bags of dacarbazine must be protected from light.

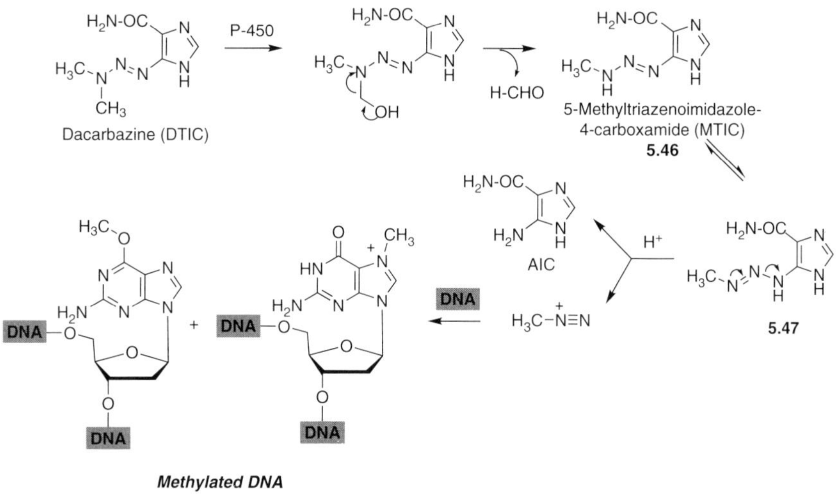

FIGURE 5.29 Generation of methyldiazonium from dacarbazine and subsequent methylation of DNA.

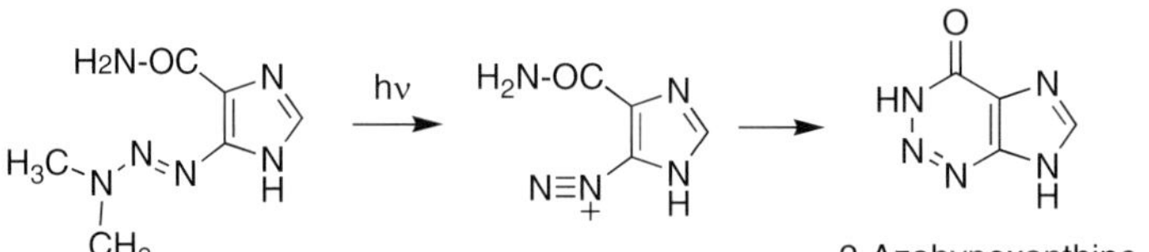

FIGURE 5.30   Photodegradation of dacarbazine.

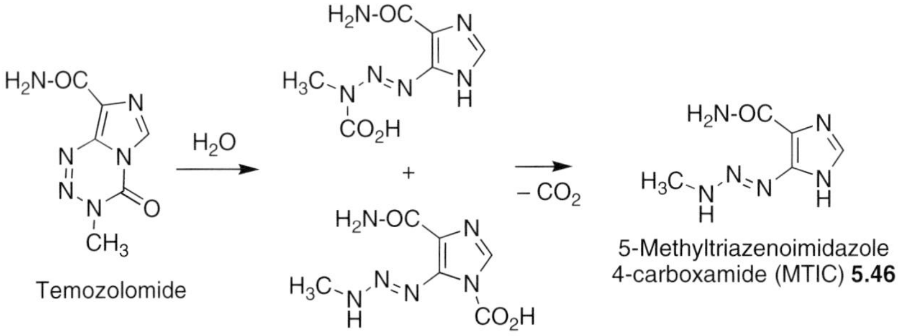

FIGURE 5.31   Temozolomide hydrolysis.

These problems have stimulated the synthesis of dacarbazine analogs, the most important of which is temozolomide. This compound is one of the few drugs specifically approved for a brain tumor, namely anaplastic astrocytoma, and the first that can be administered orally. It is converted into the same intermediate **5.46** (MTIC) generated by dacarbazine, but in the case of temozolomide the bioactivation process involves a non-enzymatic hydrolysis reaction followed by spontaneous decarboxylation (Fig. 5.31). The absence of hepatic activation is an advantage because metabolic individual variation in patient microsomal activity need not be taken into account. The main problem associated with temozolomide administration is bone marrow toxicity. The development of temozolomide is associated to the Universities of Nottingham, Aston, and Strathclyde and started as a purely synthetic project related to the chemistry of imidazotetrazines, but screening studies identified some of the compounds as promising anticancer targets.

8. METHYLHYDRAZINES

When a series of N,N'-dialkylhydrazine derivatives that had been prepared as monoaminooxidase (MAO) inhibitors were routinely submitted to cytotoxicity tests, it was shown that compounds with an N-methyl substituent had anticancer potential. This discovery ultimately led to the development of procarbazine, which was approved for use in combination therapy for advanced Hodgkin's disease. Mechanistically, procarbazine is a unique agent with multiple sites of action that is not cross-resistant with other alkylating agents. It inhibits

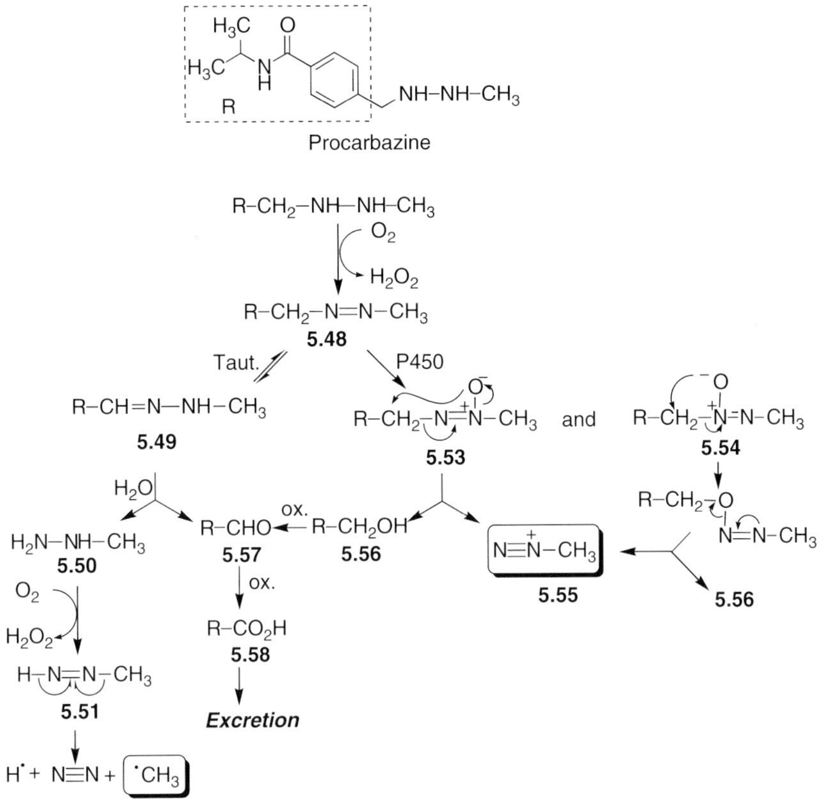

H₃C O
H₃C   N   Procarbazine structure
      R

Procarbazine

R–CH₂–NH–NH–CH₃
        │ O₂
        ↓ → H₂O₂
R–CH₂–N=N–CH₃
     5.48

Taut. ⫽   P450

R–CH=N–NH–CH₃   R–CH₂–N⁺=N–CH₃   and   R–CH₂–N⁺=N–CH₃
     5.49   **5.53**   **5.54**

H₂O   R–CH₂–O
         ox.   N=N–CH₃
H₂N–NH–CH₃   R–CHO ← R–CH₂OH
   5.50   **5.57**   **5.56**   N⁺≡N–CH₃
                                          5.55   **5.56**
O₂
         ox.
H₂O₂   R–CO₂H
        5.58
H–N=N–CH₃
   5.51   *Excretion*

H• + N≡N + •CH₃
      5.52

FIGURE 5.32 Generation of methyldiazonium during procarbazine metabolism.

incorporation of small DNA precursors, as well as RNA and protein synthesis. Procarbazine can also directly damage DNA through a methylation reaction, whose precise mechanism is unclear. The major species found in plasma after administration of procarbazine is azoprocarbazine **5.48**, formed by oxidation by P450 or MAO. This reaction also generates hydrogen peroxide that was initially believed to be responsible for the antitumor activity, although much evidence has accumulated against this hypothesis. Tautomerism can transform **5.48** into hydrazone **5.49**, which gives by hydrolysis aldehyde **5.57**, a precursor of the primary excreted metabolite N-isopropylterephthalamic acid **5.58**, and methylhydrazine **5.50**. Although this route can potentially lead to methylating species such as **5.52**, it appears to lack physiological significance; however, it does explain the low stability of procarbazine in aqueous solution. In contrast, azoprocarbazine (**5.48**) is further metabolized by cytochrome P450 to azoxy derivatives **5.53** and **5.54**. The first of these intermediates is responsible for anticancer activity, DNA methylation being explained by generation of methyldiazonium **5.55**. Liberation of alcohol **5.56** and subsequent oxidative metabolism of this compound explains the excretion of acid **5.58**. Alternatively, a side chain rearrangement in **5.54** to give a diazo

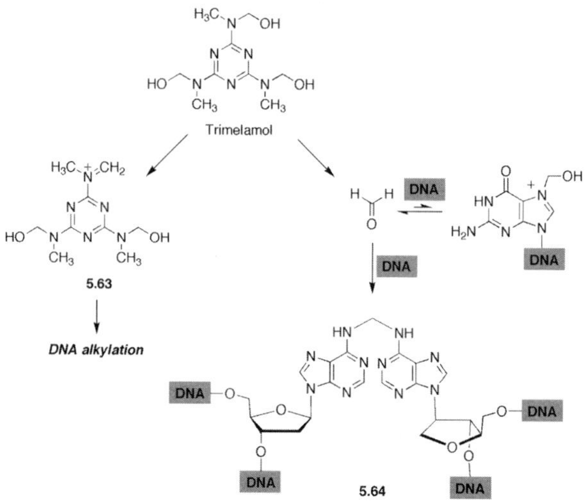

FIGURE 5.33   DNA alkylation by altretamine metabolites.

compound followed by its fragmentation can also explain the generation of methyldiazonium **5.55** and alcohol **5.56** (Fig. 5.32).

9. 1,3,5-TRIAZINES: HEXAMETHYLMELAMINE AND TRIMELAMOL

Hexamethylmelamine (HMM, altretamine) was originally prepared as a resin precursor, but it was studied as an antitumor compound because of its structural analogy with the previously mentioned aziridine derivative TEM. Although it is active in several types of tumors, its main therapeutic role is in the treatment of recurrent ovarian cancer, following first-line treatment with cisplatin. The precise mechanism of altretamine cytotoxicity is unknown, although several proposals have been made. The main metabolic pathway is oxidative cytochrome P450-catalyzed *N*-demethylation, with carbinolamine **5.59** as an intermediate, which yields the pentamethyl derivative **5.62**, formaldehyde, and smaller amounts of inactive compounds arising from further demethylation. Alternatively, elimination of the hydroxy group from **5.59** gives the iminium species **5.60**. In the case of altretamine, the pattern of adduct formation suggests that **5.60** is the alkylating species,[56] reacting with DNA to give **5.61** rather than the formaldehyde generated in the demethylation process (Fig. 5.33).

Trimelamol is a tris(hydroxymethyl) analog of altretamine that has the advantage of not requiring metabolic activation, although it is obviously less stable due to the presence of its carbinolamine moieties. Involvement of formaldehyde in the cytotoxicity of trimelamol has been established,[57] as evidenced by the isolation of adduct **5.64** from reaction of formaldehyde with two adenine amino groups, although participation of iminium species **5.63** cannot be discarded. Reaction with the more nucleophilic guanine N-7 should be easily reversed because of the positive charge at nitrogen in the adduct (Fig. 5.34)

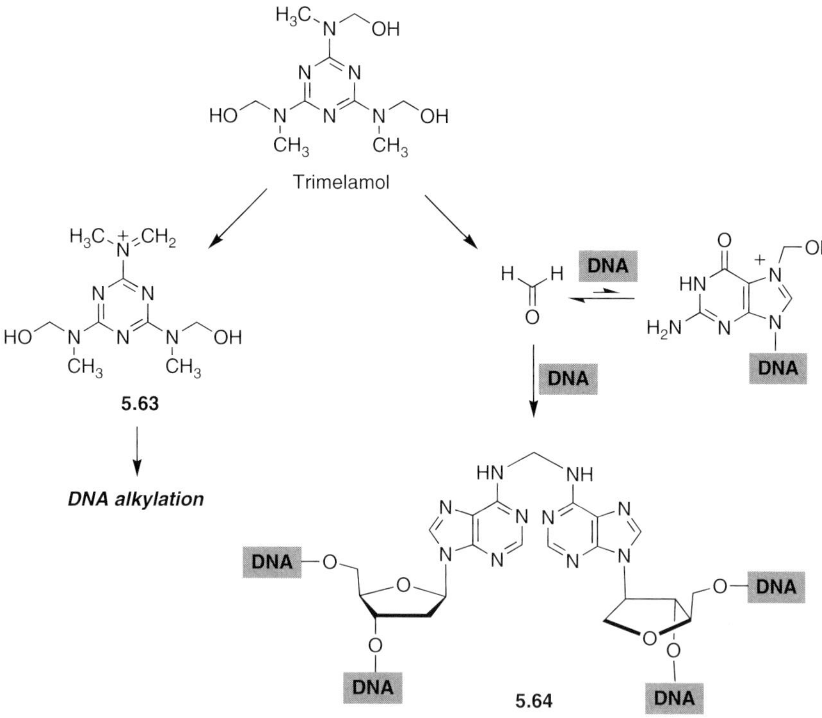

FIGURE 5.34   DNA alkylation by trimelamol.

10. PLATINUM COMPLEXES

Cisplatin (CDDP, *cis*-diamminedichloroplatinum II) provides an excellent example of serendipity in the discovery of antitumor drugs. In the course of the study of the effects of electric currents on cells, it was discovered that *Escherichia coli* cells formed long filaments, but they did not divide. Further research showed that inhibition of bacterial cell division was due to cisplatin, generated from the platinum electrodes and the ammonium chloride present in the media.

Cisplatin is a very effective, but highly toxic, antitumor drug. Its clinical use was initiated in the early 1970s, and it is one of the most widely employed anticancer agents, useful in ovarian, testicular, small cell lung, and other cancers. It is a square-planar complex, containing two labile chlorines and two relatively inert ammonia molecules coordinated to the central Pt (II) atom in a *cis* configuration. In plasma, the high chloride concentration prevents its hydrolysis, but when it enters the cell the much lower chloride concentration prompts its reaction with water to give the positively charged species **5.65** and specially **5.66** (Fig. 5.35).

The active complexes enter the nucleus and become attracted by the negatively charged DNA. This electrostatic interaction is followed by complexation with nitrogen atoms of purine bases, normally the N-7 atoms of two vicinal guanine units[58] that displace the two water molecules leading to intrastrand cross-linking,

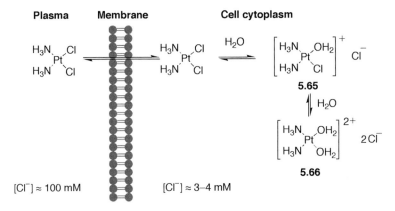

FIGURE 5.35   Intracellular bioactivation of cisplatin.

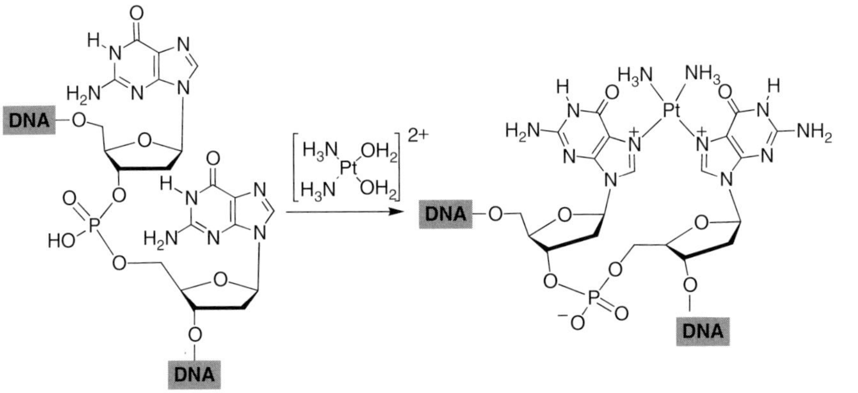

FIGURE 5.36   Coordination complex generated from the cisplatin active species and DNA.

which deforms the DNA tertiary conformation as shown by X-ray crystallography and causes its unwinding at the complexation site (Fig. 5.36).[59] As a consequence, high-mobility group (HMG) domain proteins become attached to DNA by intercalation of a phenylalanine unit at the unwound DNA damage site and the protein lies along a widened minor groove, preventing DNA replication.[60] Although, strictly speaking, Pt coordination with DNA bases cannot be considered an alkylation reaction, cisplatin and its analogs are normally studied among the alkylating agents.

An additional mechanism for prevention of DNA transcription is replacement of Zn by Pt in the so-called zinc-finger protein transcription factor. The existence of the zinc cation is essential to coordinate amino acids of the protein, usually cysteine and histidine, and thus pack together the DNA binding domains into a dense structure. Replacing the zinc ion with platinum disrupts the conformation, and binds the zinc-finger permanently to DNA-polymerase α, which is a transcription enzyme vital for cell replication (Fig. 5.37). Pt-DNA adducts also activate several cellular processes that mediate the cytotoxicity of these anticancer drugs.[61]

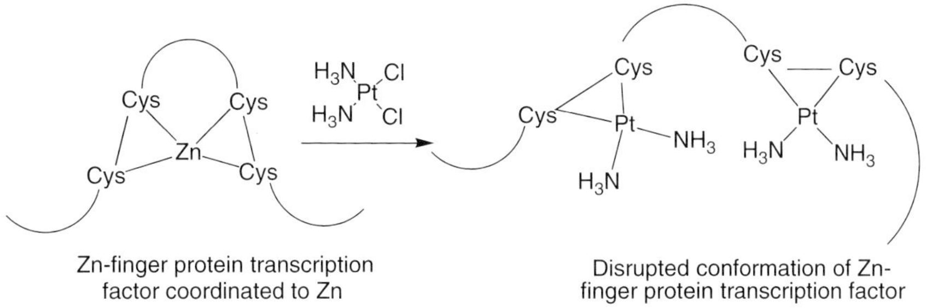

Zn-finger protein transcription
factor coordinated to Zn

Disrupted conformation of Zn-
finger protein transcription factor

FIGURE 5.37   Replacement of Zn by Pt in Zn-finger transcription factors.

Because of the very high toxicity of cisplatin, thousands of analogs have been prepared in an effort to improve its selectivity and therapeutic index. The dose-limiting toxicity is renal and can be attributed to interactions with renal components, leading to tubular necrosis of both proximal and distal renal tubules. Cisplatinum analogs include tetragonal Pt (II) complexes, such as carboplatin, nedaplatin, oxaliplatin, ZD-0473, and SKI-2053R. Octahedral Pt (IV) complexes are also known, including tetraplatin, iproplatin, and satraplatin (JM 216). The development of these cisplatin analogs has revealed common requirements that are necessary for their use as an anticancer drug:

- Electroneutrality, to facilitate transport through cell membranes, although the active form may be charged after ligand exchange.
- Presence of at least two good leaving groups, preferentially *cis* to one another, although *trans* complexes also show activity in some cases (see below).
- Presence of "inert" carrier ligands, usually nontertiary amine groups which increase adduct stabilization through hydrogen bonding with nearby bases.

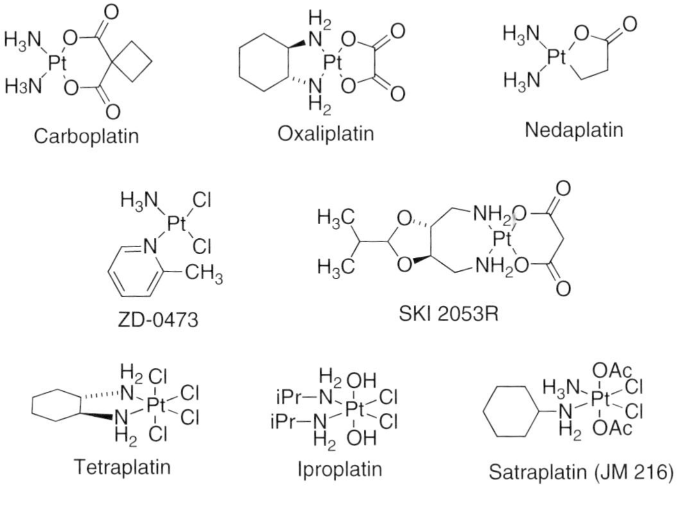

Carboplatin

Oxaliplatin

Nedaplatin

ZD-0473

SKI 2053R

Tetraplatin

Iproplatin

Satraplatin (JM 216)

Carboplatin has a mechanism of action identical to that of cisplatin, forming cross-links with guanine in DNA. At effective doses, carboplatin produces substantially reduced nephrotoxicity because of the dicarboxylate ligands which facilitate its excretion. Oxaliplatin has shown *in vitro* and *in vivo* efficacy against many tumor cell lines, including some that are resistant to cisplatin and carboplatin. The presence of the bulky diaminocyclohexane ring is thought to result in the formation of Pt-DNA adducts more effective at blocking DNA replication than in the case of cisplatin.

Oxaliplatin has a spectrum of activity different from that of either cisplatin or carboplatin and lacks cross-resistance with them, suggesting that it has different molecular targets and/or mechanisms of resistance.[62] Unlike other platinum complexes, oxaliplatinum is useful in the treatment of colorectal cancer, the fourth largest cause for cancer deaths.[63]

Other Pt (II) compounds under clinical trials include nedaplatin, which is less toxic than cisplatin, but only moderately successful in overcoming cisplatin resistance, ZD-0473, which is able to overcome the thiol-dependent resistance with very little nephrotoxicity and neurotoxicity,[64] and SKI-2053R, with considerably less toxicity than the parent molecule.[65]

Pt (IV) complexes appear to act by different mechanism, and evidence suggests that reduction to the corresponding Pt (II) derivatives is necessary for activity. For instance, the active species for JM 216 is believed to be JM 118 (Fig. 5.38).[66]

During the 1990s, it was reported that some *trans*-platinum complexes had activity against tumors resistant to cisplatin, implying differences in the DNA binding of both types of complexes. The *trans* isomer of cisplatin, called TDDP, is unable to form 1,2-intrastrand adducts due to its stereochemistry, but it forms interstrand cross-links between complementary guanine and cytosine and 1,3-intrastrand adducts, causing a different type of conformational distortion of the double helix.[67] Another type of *trans*-platinum antitumor compounds are dinuclear and trinuclear Pt (II) complexes (containing two or three reactive platinum centers), designed to form long-range interstrand and intrastrand DNA cross-links. Two examples are compound **5.67** and the triplatinum complex BBR 3464, which has a broad spectrum of antitumor activity and is currently undergoing clinical trials.[68] BBR 3464 forms DNA interstrand cross-links as well as 1,4- and 1,5-intrastrand cross-links, showing preference for the guanine-guanine sequence.[69]

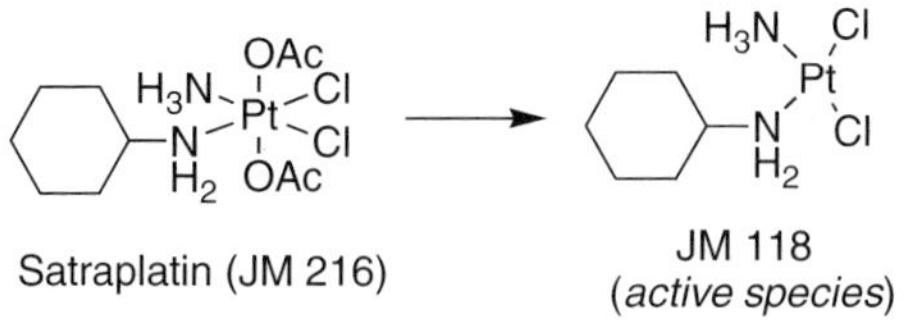

Satraplatin (JM 216)   JM 118
(*active species*)

FIGURE 5.38   Bioactivation of a Pt (IV) complex.

5.67   BBR 3464

11. MISCELLANEOUS ALKYLATING AND ACYLATING ANTITUMOR AGENTS

Pipobroman is used for treatment of polycythemias, like polycythemia vera (Vaquez's disease), a relatively rare chronic disease of the blood in which the red cells are increased in number,[70] and essential thrombocythemia.[71] Pipobroman has a chemical structure close to that of alkylating agents, although its exact mechanism of action has not been demonstrated.

Pipobroman

Among the many DNA-damaging natural cytotoxins, leinamycin is of particular interest because it represents a new structural type of DNA-damaging agent, although it has not been clinically tested.[72] Leinamycin was isolated from a strain of *Streptomyces* found in soil samples collected in Japan.[73] Early *in vitro* experiments revealed that DNA damage by leinamycin is thiol-triggered and due to its unique 1,2-dithiolan-3-one-1-oxide moiety. Leinamycin is relatively stable in water; however, on entering the thiol-rich environment of the cell, a cascade of chemical reactions is initiated that leads to oxidative DNA damage (and perhaps general oxidative stress),[74] as well as DNA alkylation,[75] which is sequence specific.[76] As shown in Fig. 5.39, the initial reaction with thiols gives intermediate **5.68**, which cyclizes to **5.70** with release of hydrodisulfide **5.69** that causes oxidative DNA damage. The spatial arrangement of **5.70** allows nucleophilic attack of the alkene to the electrophilic sulfur to give the highly electrophilic episulfonium ion **5.71**, which alkylates DNA at the N-7 position of guanine residues.

Hydrodisulfides are more easily oxidized than sulfides because of their higher acidity, which leads to complete ionization under physiological pH. Therefore, compound **5.69** liberated from leinomycin can transfer one electron to molecular oxygen, leading to the generation of oxygen radicals. Catalytic amounts of **5.69** are sufficient to cause oxidative DNA damage and subsequent strand breaking by this mechanism because polysulfides **5.72** are transformed back to **5.69** by reaction with thiols **5.73**, which are thus depleted from the cell (Fig. 5.40).

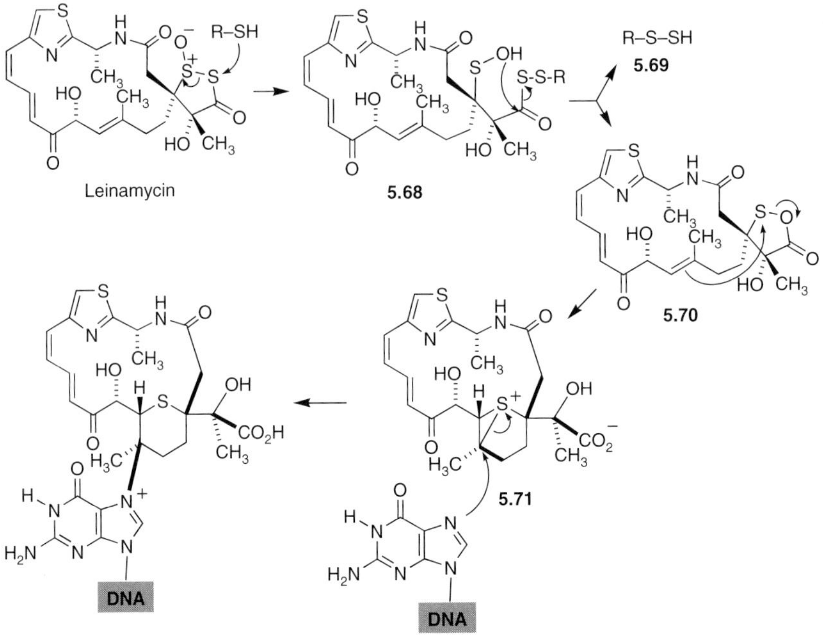

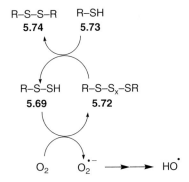

FIGURE 5.39   DNA alkylation by leinamycin.

FIGURE 5.40   Generation of hydroxyl radicals from a hydrodisulfide generated from leinamycin.

REFERENCES

1. Hurley, L. H. (2002). *Nat. Rev. Cancer* **2,** 188.
2. Nelson, S. M., Ferguson, L. R., and Denny, W. A. (2004). *Cell Chromosome* **3,** 2.
3. Blackburn, G. M. (2006). Covalent interactions of nucleic acids with small molecules and their repair. *In* "Nucleic Acids in Chemistry and Biology" (G. M. Blackburn, M. J. Gait, D. Loakes, and D. M. Williams, eds.), 3rd ed. Royal Society of Chemistry, Cambridge.
4. Adair, F. E., and Bagg, H. J. (1931). *Ann. Surg.* **93,** 190.
5. Gilman, A., and Phillips, F. S. (1946). *Science* **103,** 409.
6. Persmark, M., and Guengerich, F. P. (1994). *Biochemistry* **33,** 8662.

7. Greenberg, M. M., Hantosi, Z., Wiederholt, C. J., and Rithner, C. D. (2001). *Biochemistry* **40,** 15856.
8. Werner, W., Letsch, G., Ihn, W., Sohr, R., and Preiss, R. (1991). *Pharmazie* **46,** 113.
9. Wu, Z. Y., Thompson, M. J., Roberts, M. S., Addison, M. S., Cannell, G. R., Grabs, A. J., and Smithers, B. M. (1995). *J. Chromatog.* **673,** 267.
10. Brightman, K., Finlay, G., Jarvis, I., Knowlton, T., and Manktelowa, C. T. (1999). *J. Pharm. Biomed. Anal.* **20,** 439.
11. Urbaniak, M. D., Bingham, J. P., Hartley, J. A., Woolfson, D. N., and Caddick, S. (2004). *J. Med. Chem.* **47,** 4710.
12. Tew, K. D. (1983). *Semin. Oncol.* **10,** 21.
13. Laing, N., Dahlöff, B., Hartley-Asp, B., Ranganathan, S., and Tew, K. D. (1997). *Biochemistry* **36,** 871.
14. Walz, P. H., Bjork, P., Gunnarsson, P. O., Edman, K., and Hartley-Asp, B. (1998). *Clin. Cancer Res.* **4,** 2079.
15. Cox, P. J. (1979). *Biochem. Pharmacol.* **28,** 2045.
16. Palmer, B. D., Wilson, W. R., Cliffe, S., and Denny, W. A. (1992). *J. Med. Chem.* **35,** 3214.
17. Ware, D. C., Palmer, B. D., Wilson, W. R., and Denny, W. A. (1993). *J. Med. Chem.* **36,** 1839.
18. Killian, D., Gharat, L., and Chikhale, P. (2000). *Drug Deliv.* **7,** 21.
19. Hargreaves, R. H. J., Hartley, J. A., and Butler, J. (2000). *Front. Biosci.* **5,** 172.
20. Begleiter, A. (2000). *Front. Biosci.* **5,** 153.
21. Eagan, R. T., Dinapoli, R. T., Cascino, T. L., Scheithauer, B., O'Neill, B. P., and O'Fallon, J. R. (1987). *J. Neurooncol.* **5,** 3009.
22. Obe, G., and Beek, B. (1979). *Mutat. Res.* **65,** 21.
23. Naylor, M. A., and Thomson, P. (2001). *Mini Rev. Med. Chem.* **1,** 17.
24. Moore, H. W. (1977). *Science* **197,** 527.
25. Butler, J., Dzielendziak, A., Lea, J. S., Ward, T. H., and Hoey, B. M. (1990). *Free Radic. Res. Comm.* **8,** 231.
26. Akhtar, H. M., Begleiter, A., Johnson, D., Lown, J. W., McLaughlin, L., and Sim, S. K. (1975). *Can. J. Chem.* **53,** 2891.
27. Beall, H. D., and Winski, S. L. (2000). *Front. Biosci.* **5,** 639.
28. Danson, S., Ward, T. H., Butler, J., and Ranson, M. (2004). *Cancer Treat. Rev.* **30,** 437.
29. Gibson, N. W., Hartley, J. A., Butler, J., Siegel, D., and Ross, D. (1992). *Mol. Pharmacol.* **42,** 531.
30. Begleiter, A. (2000). *Front. Biosci.* **5,** E153.
31. Fourie, J., Guziec, F., Guziec, L., Monterrosa, C., Fiterman, D. J., and Begleiter, A. (2004). *Cancer Chemother. Pharmacol.* **53,** 191.
32. Winski, S. L., Hargreaves, R. H., Butler, J., and Ross, D. (1998). *Clin. Cancer Res.* **4,** 3083.
33. Ward, T. H., Danson, S., McGown, A. T., Ranson, M., Coe, N. A., Jayson, G. C., Cummings, J., Hargreaves, R. H. J., and Butler, J. (2005). *Clin. Cancer Res.* **11,** 2695.
34. Zhou, R., and Skibo, E. B. (1996). *J. Med. Chem.* **39,** 4321.
35. Li, B. B., Gutiérrez, P. L., Amstad, P., and Blough, N. V. (1999). *Chem. Res. Toxicol.* **12,** 1042.
36. Xing, C., and Skibo, E. B. (2000). *Biochemistry* **39,** 10770.
37. Coleman, R. S. (2001). *Curr. Opin. Drug Discov. Devel.* **4,** 435.
38. Eilon, G. F., Gu, J., Slater, L. M., Hara, K., and Jacobs, J. W. (2000). *Cancer Chemother. Pharmacol.* **45,** 183.
39. Xie, X., Lemcke, T., Gussio, R., Zaharevitz, D. W., Leost, M., Meijer, L., and Kunick, C. (2005). *Eur. J. Med. Chem.* **40,** 655.
40. Hartley, J. A., O'Hare, C. C., and Baumgart, J. (1999). *Br. J. Cancer* **79,** 264.
41. Szebeni, J., Barna, K., Uher, F., Milosevits, J., Paloczi, K., Gaal, D., Petranyi, G. G., and Kelemen, E. (1997). *Leukemia* 1769.
42. Farmer, P. B. (1987). *Pharmacol. Ther.* **35,** 301.
43. Bedford, P., and Fox, B. W. (1983). *Biochem. Pharmacol.* **32,** 2297.
44. Hartley, J. A., O'Hare, C. C., and Baumgart, J. (1999). *Br. J. Cancer* **79,** 264.
45. Hayes, M. T., Bartley, J., Parsons, P. G., Eaglesham, G. K., and Prakask, A. S. (1997). *Biochemistry* **36,** 10646.
46. Montgomery, J. A., James, R., McCaleb, G. S., and Johnston, T. P. (1967). *J. Med. Chem.* **10,** 668.
47. Johnston, T. P., and Montgomery, J. A. (1986). *Cancer Treat. Rep.* **70,** 13.
48. Buckley, N. (1987). *J. Org. Chem.* **52,** 484.

49. Murata, M., Takahashi, A., Saito, I., and Kawanishi, S. (1999). *Biochem. Pharmacol.* **57**, 881.

50. Bolzán, A. D., and Bianchi, M. S. (2002). *Mutat. Res.* **512**, 121.

51. Kroncke, K. D., Fehsel, K., Sommer, A., Rodriguez, M. L., and Kolb-Bachofen, V. (1995). *Biol. Chem. Hoppe Seyler* **376**, 179.

52. Bedoya, F. J., Solano, F., and Lucas, M. (1996). *Experientia* **52**, 344.

53. Meer, L., Janzer, R. C., Kleihues, P., and Kolar, G. F. (1986). *Biochem. Pharmacol.* **35**, 3243.

54. Kyrtopoulos, S. A., Souliotis, V. L., Valavanis, C., Boussiotis, V. A., and Pangalis, G. A. (1993). *Environ. Health Perspect.* **99**, 143.

55. Glaser, R., Sik-Cheung Choy, G., and Kirk Hall, M. (1991). *J. Am. Chem. Soc.* **113**, 1109.

56. Ames, M. M. (1991). *Cancer Treat. Rev.* **18**(Suppl. A), 3.

57. Coley, H. M., Brooks, N., Phillips, D. H., Hewer, A., Jenkins, T. C., Jarman, M., and Judson, I. R. (1995). *Biochem. Pharmacol.* **11**, 1203.

58. Lippard, S. J. (1987). *Pure Appl. Chem.* **59**, 731.

59. Takahara, P. M., Rosenzweig, A. C., Frederick, C. A., and Lippard, S. J. (1995). *Nature* **377**, 649.

60. Ohndorf, U., Rould, M. A., He, Q., Pabo, C. O., and Lippard, S. J. (1999). *Nature* **399**, 708.

61. Dong, W., and Lippard, S. J. (2005). *Nat. Rev. Drug Discov.* **4**, 307.

62. Raymond, E., Faivre, S., Woynarowski, J. M., and Chaney, S. G. (1998). *Semin. Oncol.* **25**, 4.

63. Graham, J., Mushim, M., and Kirkpatrick, P. (2004). *Nat. Rev. Drug Discov.* **3**, 11.

64. Hoctin-Boes, G., Cosaert, J., and Koehler, M. (2001). *Proc. Am. Soc. Clin. Oncol.* **20**, 344a.

65. Kim, N. K., Kim, T. Y., and Shin, S. G. (2001). *Cancer* **91**, 1549.

66. Kelland, L. R. (2000). *Expert Opin. Invest. Drugs* **9**, 1373.

67. Radulovic, S., Tesic, Z., and Manic, S. (2002). *Curr. Med. Chem.* **9**, 1611.

68. Jodrell, D. I., Evans, T. R. J., Steward, W., Cameron, D., Prendiville, J., Aschele, C., Noberasco, C., Lind, M., Carmichael, J., Dobbs, N., Camboni, G., Gatti, B., *et al.* (2004). *Eur. J. Cancer* **40**, 1872.

69. Perego, P., Caserini, C., Gatti, L., Carenini, N., Romanelli, S., Supino, R., Colangelo, D., Viano, I., Leone, R., Spinelli, S., Pezzoni, G., Manzotti, C., Farrell, N., and Zunino, F. (1999). *Mol. Pharmacol.* **55**, 528.

70. Kiladjian, J. J., Gardin, C., Renoux, M., Bruno, F., and Bernard, J. F. (2003). *Hematol J.* **4**, 198.

71. Passamonti, F., and Lazzarino, M. (2003). *Leuk. Lymphoma* **44**, 1483.

72. Gates, K. S. (2000). *Chem. Res. Toxicol.* **13**, 953.

73. Hara, M., Takahashi, I., Yoshida, M., Kawamoto, I., Morimoto, M., and Nakano, H. (1989). *J. Antibiot.* **42**, 333.

74. Mitra, K., Kim, W., Daniels, J. S., and Gates, K. S. (1997). *J. Am. Chem. Soc.* **119**, 11691.

75. Asai, A., Hara, M., Kakita, S., Kanda, Y., Yoshida, M., Saito, H., and Saitoh, Y. (1996). *J. Am. Chem. Soc.* **118**, 6802.

76. Zang, H., and Gates, K. S. (2003). *Chem Res Toxicol.* **16**, 1539.

CHAPTER 6

Alkylating and Non-Alkylating Compounds Interacting with the DNA Minor Groove

Contents

1. Introduction   177
2. Netropsin, Distamycin, and Related Compounds   178
3. Mitomycins   182
4. Tetrahydroisoquinoline Alkaloids   189
5. Cyclopropylindole Alkylating Agents   193
6. Pyrrolo[1,4]Benzodiazepines   195
   References   196

1. INTRODUCTION

Besides non-specific electrostatic interaction with phosphate groups, there are two main ways in which a molecule can bind to DNA in a reversible way: (a) groove-binding interactions, which do not require conformational changes in DNA and usually shows high sequence specificity; and (b) intercalation of planar or quasi-planar aromatic ring systems between adjacent base pairs, which requires separation of the latter and normally takes place with low sequence specificity (Fig. 6.1).

Because of the differences in electrostatic potential, hydration, hydrogen bonding ability, and steric hindrance, the major and minor grooves differ in their molecular recognition properties. Thus, the major groove normally binds to large molecules, like proteins and oligonucleotides, and the minor groove has a tendency to bind to small molecules. Because of the curved shape of the minor groove, molecules with torsional freedom interact with it more easily (Fig. 6.1A),

Medicinal Chemistry of Anticancer Drugs
DOI: 10.1016/B978-0-444-52824-7.00006-8

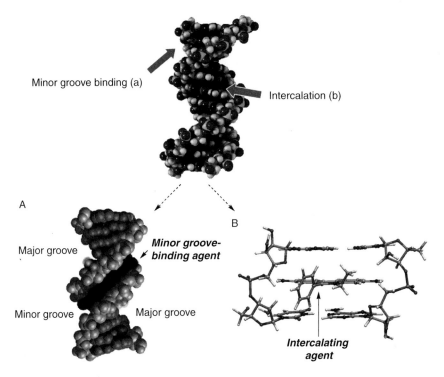

FIGURE 6.1   Main types of reversible interactions with DNA.

and for this reason many of the compounds studied in this chapter contain several simple aromatic or heteromatic rings linked by torsionally free bonds. The interaction with the minor groove of some antitumor agents has been mentioned in previous chapters (anthracyclines in Section 3, bleomycins in Section 7, and enediynes in Section 8 of Chapter 4).

2. NETROPSIN, DISTAMYCIN, AND RELATED COMPOUNDS

Minor groove interaction was first discovered in the natural products netropsin and distamycin A. Although these compounds do not have relevant antitumor activity, they are the prototype minor groove binders (MGBs) and for this reason they will be briefly discussed below. They bind non-covalently to the minor groove of DNA, thereby preventing DNA and RNA synthesis by inhibition of the corresponding polymerase reaction and display a pronounced sequence specificity, leading to much current interest in them.[1]

Netropsin

Distamycin A

Studies on this specificity have been carried out mainly on distamycin and related compounds, which have shown a pronounced specificity for AT sequences.[2] Ligand recognition by the minor groove is governed, in the first place, by hydrogen bonding interactions, involving hydrogen acceptor groups in DNA bases, particularly N_3 and $C_2=O$ of the adenine-thymine or guanine-citosine pairs. As shown in Fig. 6.2, these interactions are hampered in the latter pair, mainly due to steric reasons. Additionally, the minor groove is strongly solvated, and liberation of water molecules into the bulk solvent upon complex formation leads to a favourable binding entropy (hydrophobic effect), since

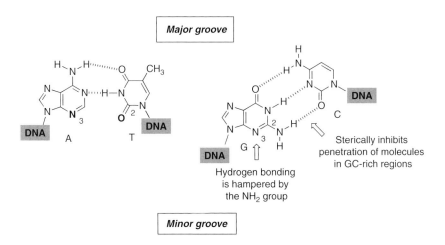

FIGURE 6.2   Adenine-thymine and guanine-cytosine pairs.

AT-rich regions are more hydrated than GC-rich regions and hence they provide a bigger entropic contribution. Finally, the negative electrostatic potential is greater in AT-rich than in GC-rich regions, thus favouring an initial electrostatic interaction with positively charged groups in the ligand. Hydration of the ligand molecules is also an important factor in the understanding of differences in binding affinity.[3]

Hydrogen bonds involve the amido or amidino groups of the drugs as hydrogen donors and the N_3 of adenine and C_2=O groups of thymine as hydrogen acceptors, as shown in Fig. 6.3 for the case of distamycin A.

Theoretical and X-ray diffraction studies suggest the formation of bifurcated (three-centred) hydrogen bonds,[4] where each carboxamide is bound to two acceptor groups belonging to bases in complementary DNA strands (Fig. 6.4). Contrary to

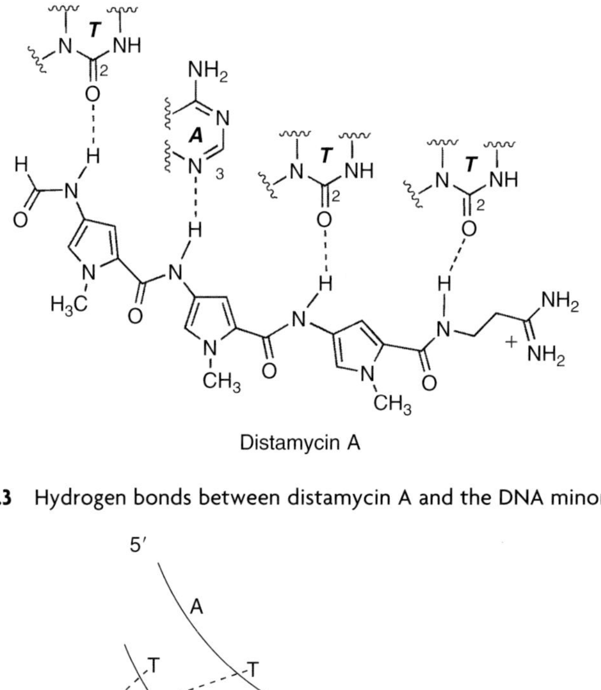

Distamycin A

FIGURE 6.3   Hydrogen bonds between distamycin A and the DNA minor groove.

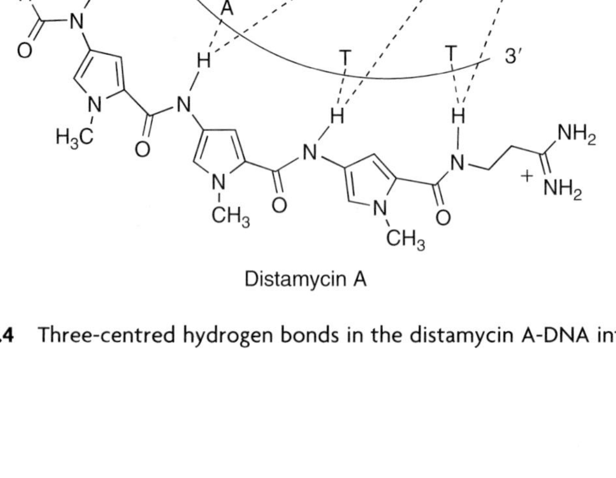

Distamycin A

FIGURE 6.4   Three-centred hydrogen bonds in the distamycin A-DNA interaction.

initial expectations, the protonated guanidine or amidine groups do not bind directly to DNA phosphate groups, but line the floor of the minor groove.

The synthesis of analogues of distamycin A by increasing the number of N-methylpyrrole-2-carboxamide units or replacement of some pyrrole nucleus by an imidazole, and also by preparation of hybrid structures with intercalating or alkylating portions, has led, in some instances, to much enhanced cytotoxicity.[5] Two of the most promising compounds in this area are tallimustine and brostallicin (PNU-166196).

Tallimustine

Brostallicin (PNU-166196)

Tallimustine contains a benzoyl nitrogen mustard unit, which acts as an alkylating moiety, attached to the distamycin A framework. This compound exhibits a most striking DNA sequence specificity of alkylation, which has been studied using the combinatorial selection method known as restriction endonuclease protection, selection, and amplification (REPSA).[6] The highest affinity tallimustine binding sites contain one of two sequences, either the expected distamycin hexamer binding sites followed by a CG base pair (e.g. 5'-TTTTTTC-3' and 5'-AAATTTC-3') or the unexpected sequence 5'-TAGAAC-3'. It was also found that tallimustine preferentially alkylates the N-7 position of guanines located on the periphery of these sequences. These findings suggest a cooperative binding model for tallimustine in which one molecule non-covalently resides in the DNA minor groove and locally perturbs the DNA structure, thereby facilitating alkylation by a second tallimustine of an exposed guanine on another side of the DNA. Tallimustine is a potent antitumor agent, but its severe myelotoxicity led to discontinuing its clinical development.[7] This is a common problem with many minor groove binding agents.[8]

Brostallicin (PNU-166196) is a synthetic α-bromoacrylamido derivative of a four-pyrrole distamycin in which the amidine terminal function is replaced by a guanidine moiety. Unlike tallimustine, this compound showed a tolerable myelotoxicity and is now under clinical investigation.[9]

Brostallicin is inactive *in vitro*, and it requires the presence of glutathione and glutathione-S-transferase (GST) to behave as an alkylating agent.[10] The mechanism of alkylation involves an initial Michael attack of glutathione onto the brostallicin α,β-unsaturated carbonyl system, which uncovers an electrophilic alkyl bromide capable of DNA alkylation (Fig. 6.5). This unique mechanism of action leads to synergism with cisplatin because the latter drug increases the levels of GST in cancer cells.

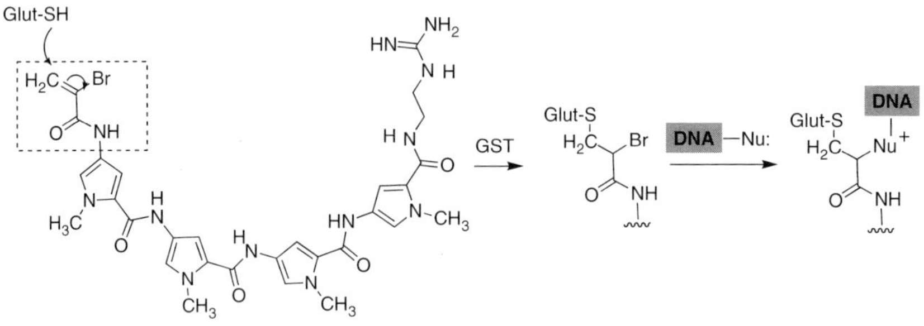

FIGURE 6.5   Bioactivation of brostallicin and DNA alkylation.

Another interesting compound that interacts with DNA in AT-rich sequences is Hoechst 33258 (pibenzimol), initially designed as an antifilarial. Latter studies on this compound showed antitumor activity, leading to Phase I clinical studies, which were discontinued because of the development of hyperglycemia in some patients.[11] This observation led to a Phase II study in patients with advanced carcinoma of the exocrine pancreas, but no relevant activity was observed.[12] When complexed to DNA, this compound exhibits enhanced fluorescence under high ionic strength conditions, which allows its use for DNA quantitation.[13] The N–H groups of the benzimidazole rings in Hoechst 33258 can be considered as bioisosters of the amide N–H groups in distamycin, and have been shown to lead to similar binding to DNA by X-ray diffraction studies.[14]

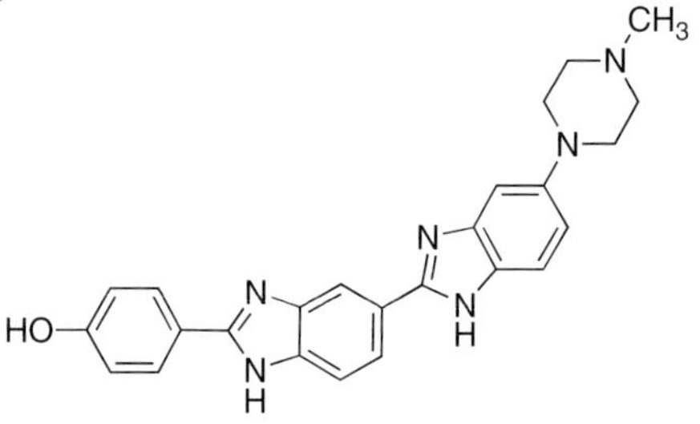

Hoescht-33258 (pibenzimol)

3. MITOMYCINS

Mitomycin C is a naturally occurring antitumor quinone from *Streptomyces caespitosus*, which contains quinone and aziridine units, although not directly linked. It has been used as a cytotoxin since the 1960 decade and is active against a variety of tumors, including breast, stomach, oesophagus, and bladder,[15] as well as non-small cell lung cancer.[16] The N-methyl derivative of mitomycin C is also a natural product called porfiromycin, which has reached Phase III clinical studies for the treatment of head and neck cancer in combination with radiotherapy, with acceptable toxicity and encouraging activity.[17]

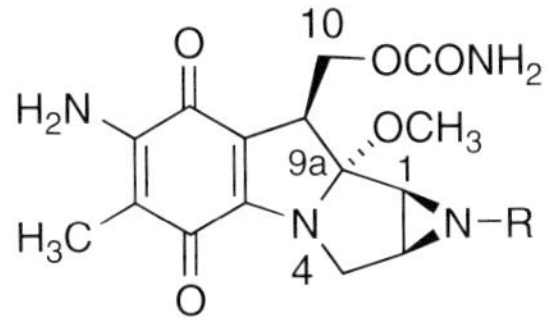

R = H   Mitomycin C
R = Me Porfiromycin

Mitomycin C and porfiromycin can be considered as the prototype of reductively activated alkylating agents. The most common structural motif in these compounds is the quinone, which has reduction potentials similar to the substrates of reductases. These compounds are particularly useful for the treatment of hypoxic tumors because in these environments the bioreduction to hydroquinones is not reversed by oxygen, and can also act as radiosensitizers.[18] Hypoxia-based strategies for tumor-specific prodrug activation are studied in more detail in Section 2.2 of Chapter 11.

The main mechanism of action of mitomycin is a characteristic example of an *in situ* bioreductive activation[19] leading to cytotoxic species (Fig. 6.6). It involves two consecutive one-electron reduction steps to the corresponding semiquinone **6.1** and then to hydroquinone **6.2**. Both forms can initiate the cascade of reactions leading to DNA alkylation, but available evidence points at hydroquinone as the active species.[20] Furthermore, human carcinoma cell lines with high levels of DT-diaphorase, an obligate two-electron reducing enzyme that cannot generate

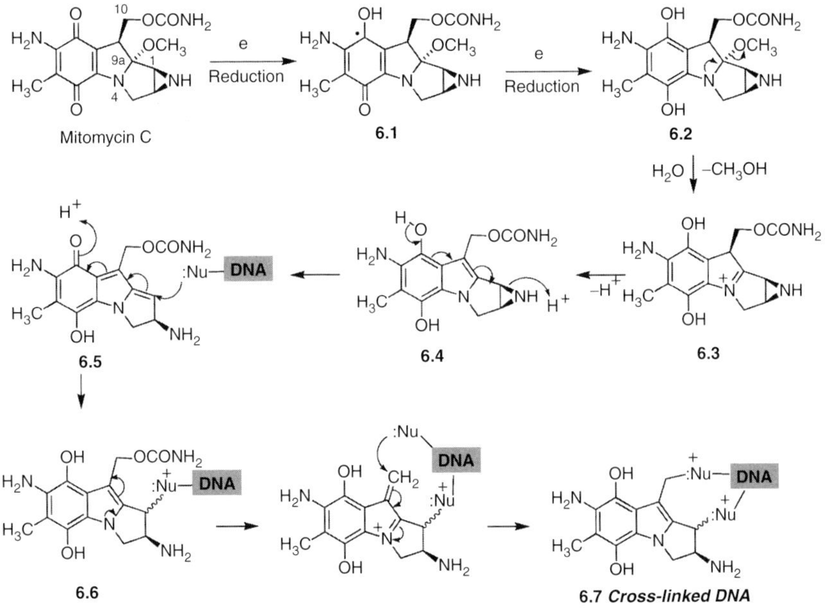

FIGURE 6.6   Bioreductive activation of mitomycin C.

intermediate semiquinones, show greater susceptibility to mitomycin, which is inhibited by treatment with diaphorase inhibitors.[21] Spontaneous elimination of methanol from hydroquinone **6.2** gives the iminium derivative **6.3**; this reaction takes place only in aqueous solution, which suggests that protonation of the leaving group by water is essential.[22] A similar elimination reaction is not possible in mitomycin because the N-4 nitrogen lone pair is conjugated with one of the quinone carbonyls, leading to a vinylogous amide structure. Indole derivative **6.4**, formed by deprotonation of **6.3**, contains two good leaving groups, namely the aziridine ring and the carbamate. Protonation of the aziridine nitrogen of **6.4** and subsequent elimination with concomitant opening of the aziridine ring affords quinone methide **6.5**. This highly reactive intermediate contains an electrophilic position that reacts with nucleophilic groups on DNA through a Michael-type reaction to give the unstable intermediate **6.6**. This reaction proceeds with absolute specificity towards certain sequences at the minor groove (see below), and involves the guanine N-2 amino group or N-7 position as nucleophiles. Elimination of the carbamate group generates an electrophilic iminium species, which undergoes a second alkylation by attack from a guanine 2-amino group, and leads to DNA cross-linking products **6.7**.[23]

Both inter- and intrastrand cross-linking by mitomycin has been observed, although the former is predominant. Inter- and intrastrand cross-linking are specific, respectively, to 5'-CG[24] and 5'-GG[25] sequences in the minor groove.[26] This selectivity arises from the first alkylation event and has been explained in terms of hydrogen bonding between the guanine N-2 amino group[27,28] and one of the carbamate oxygens, as shown in the models in Fig. 6.7, which are based on high-resolution NMR and molecular modelling studies.[28]

Intermediates similar to **6.2** are generated from the aziridine alkaloids FR-900482 and FR-69979, isolated from a culture broth of *S. sandaenis*. These compounds give interstrand cross-linking reactions with the same selectivity as mitomycin.[29] The cascade of reactions is initiated by bioreductive activation involving cleavage of the N–O bond to give the eight-membered ketone **6.8**, which is transformed into **6.9** by intramolecular nucleophilic attack of the amino group thus generated onto the ketone carbonyl. Evolution of this intermediate as described for **6.2** gives quinone methide intermediate **6.11**, which is very similar to mitomycin intermediate **6.5**, and leads to DNA cross-linking products by a similar mechanism involving amino groups at the guanine N-2 position (Fig. 6.8).[30,31] Covalent cross-linking between the DNA minor groove and DNA-binding proteins has also been described.[32]

FR-900482 and FR-69979 are more efficient cross-linking agents than mitomycin. This can be explained in terms of the dual nucleophilic–electrophilic character of the quinone methide **6.5** generated from the latter, which facilitates its protonation at C-1,[33] a reaction that competes with nucleophilic attack from DNA (Fig. 6.9). In spite of their apparent similarity, intermediates **6.11** generated from the FR compounds lack nucleophilic character due to the absence of a C_5–OH group conjugated with the C-1 position.

The unique mechanism of action and clinical success of mitomycin, coupled to its high toxicity, has prompted the preparation of a large number of synthetic

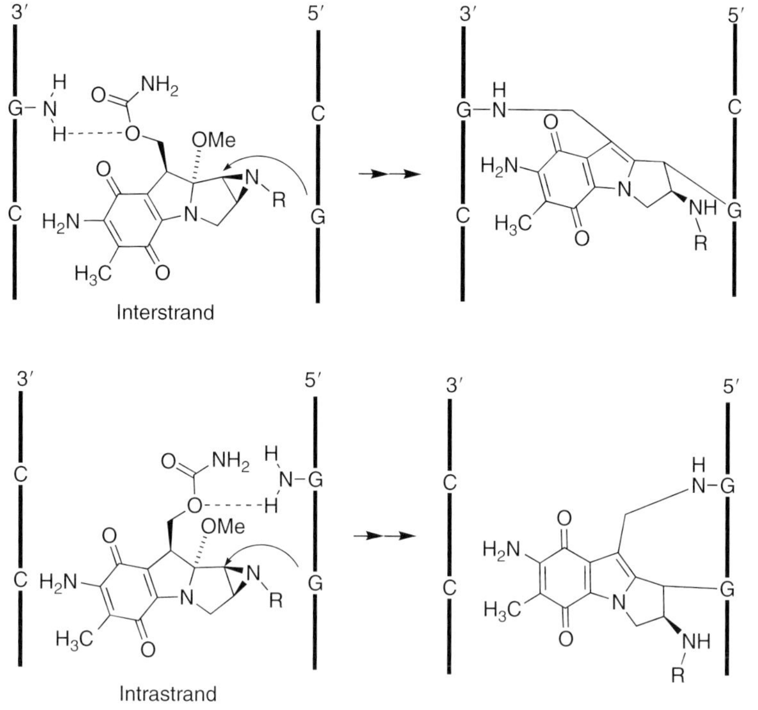

FIGURE 6.7   Inter- and intrastrand DNA cross-linking by mitomycin.

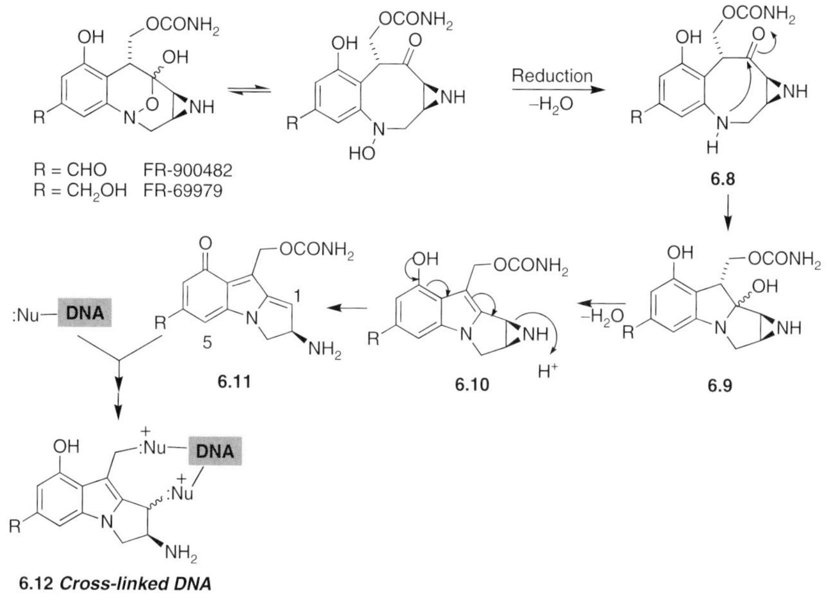

FIGURE 6.8   DNA cross-linking by other aziridine alkaloids.

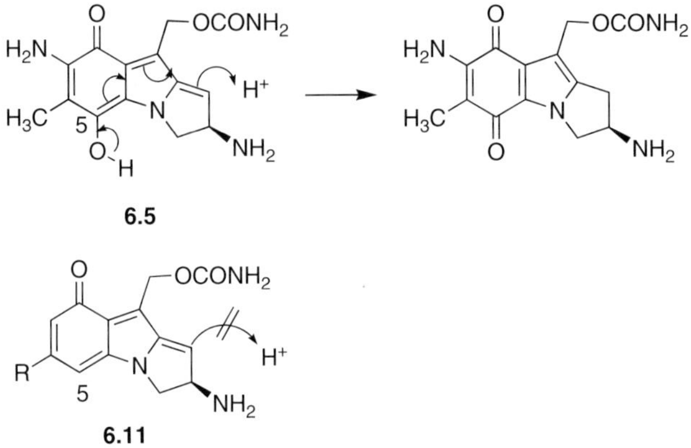

6.5

6.11

FIGURE 6.9   Different chemical reactivity of the quinone methides derived from mitomycin C (**6.5**) and other aziridine alkaloids (**6.11**).

analogues, many of which belong to the mitosene group, with the general structure **6.12**. Some simpler indolequinone derivatives, such as EO4 and EO9, were also designed as mitomycin analogues.

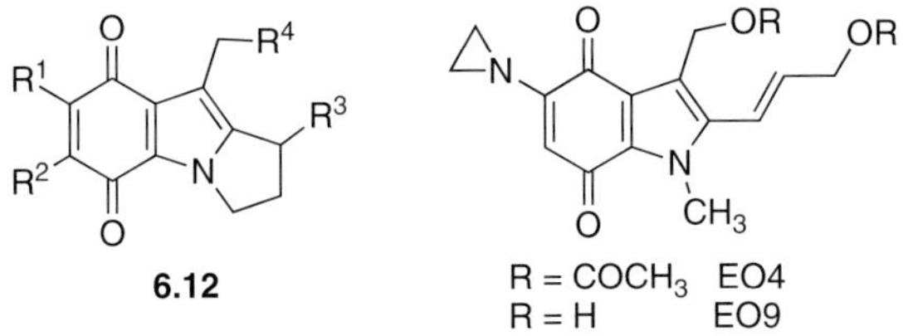

6.12

R = COCH$_3$ EO4
R = H   EO9

The mechanism of DNA alkylation by the mitosenes is shown in Fig. 6.10, using the compound known as WV15 (**6.13**) as an example. After reductive activation to **6.14**, elimination of an acetate generates iminium cation **6.15**, which is able to alkylate DNA to give **6.16**. A second elimination of a benzylic acetate group generates cation **6.17**, which can again act as a DNA alkylating species, leading to the bis-adduct **6.18**. The order of reactivity of the C-1 and C-10 positions of the mitosenes is apparently reversed with regard to that of mitomycin C, and the mitosene C-10 position is covalently bonded to the guanosine 2-amino[34] and adenosine 6-amino positions.[35]

The aziridinylquinone EO9 has undergone extensive clinical trials owing to its good activity against hypoxic cells and its lack of bone marrow toxicity in preclinical models but, in spite of achieving partial responses in Phase I studies, it showed no antitumor activity in Phase II trials for breast, colon, pancreatic, gastric,[36] and non-small lung[37] cancers. The reasons for this failure can be the very short half-life of the drug because of fast elimination following intravenous administration, and its poor tissue penetration. These shortcomings prevent its systemic use but they may actually prove advantageous for local administration. Thus, EO9 is currently being assayed for treatment of early-stage superficial

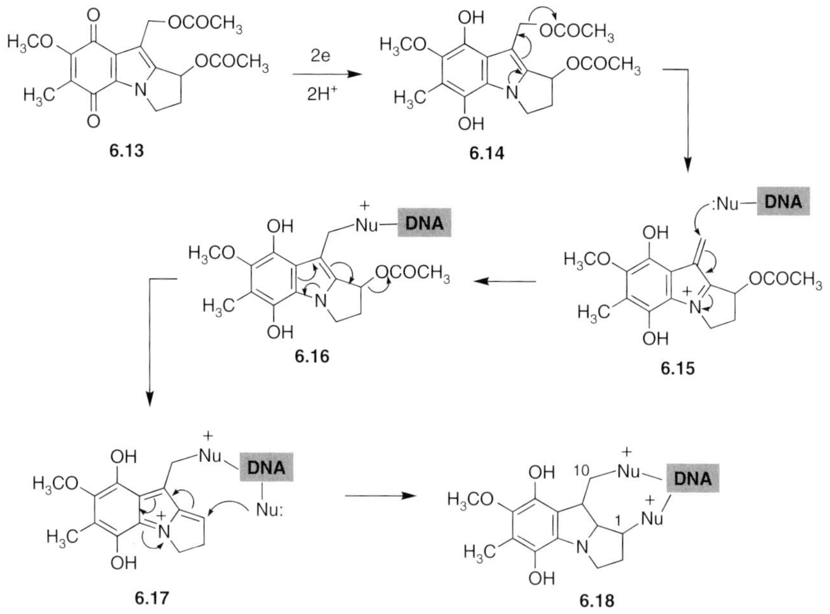

FIGURE 6.10 DNA alkylation by the mitosenes.

bladder cancer by intravesical administration,[38] where it has shown good activity and the absence of major organ toxicity.[39]

The EO compounds were designed to alkylate DNA after reduction via formation of quinone methide species. As shown in Fig. 6.11, reduction of the drug molecule yields the hydroquinone **6.19**, activating the aziridine ring for nucleophilic attack by DNA (**a**). When X is a good leaving group, two elimination reactions afford highly electrophilic quinone methide intermediates **6.20** and **6.21**, allowing two other sites for DNA alkylation (**b** and **c**). EO4 has been shown to give cross-linked DNA adducts involving the **a** and **c** modes of attack,[40] while in the case of EO9 both monoalkylation at the aziridine ring[40] and cross-linking[41] have been described.

One of the main limitations of mitomycin and the mitosenes is the need for reductive activation, which renders them less active in tissues where the bioreduction can be reverted, as for instance in the presence of oxygen. In search for mitomycin analogues with activity in non-hypoxic cells, a number of semisynthetic compounds have been designed that are activated by processes other than reduction. Structurally, these compounds are characterized by the presence of an aminoethylene disulphide side chain as exemplified by KW-2149, which has been examined in clinical trials,[42] although serious pulmonary toxicity was observed.[43] KW-2149 causes interstrand DNA cross-links and DNA–protein cross-links, resulting in single-strand DNA breaks and inhibition of DNA synthesis. The mechanism proposed to account for these observations is summarized in Fig. 6.12, and involves liberation of thiol **6.22** by reaction of the drug with a mercapto group contained in glutathione. Compound **6.22** can be activated by

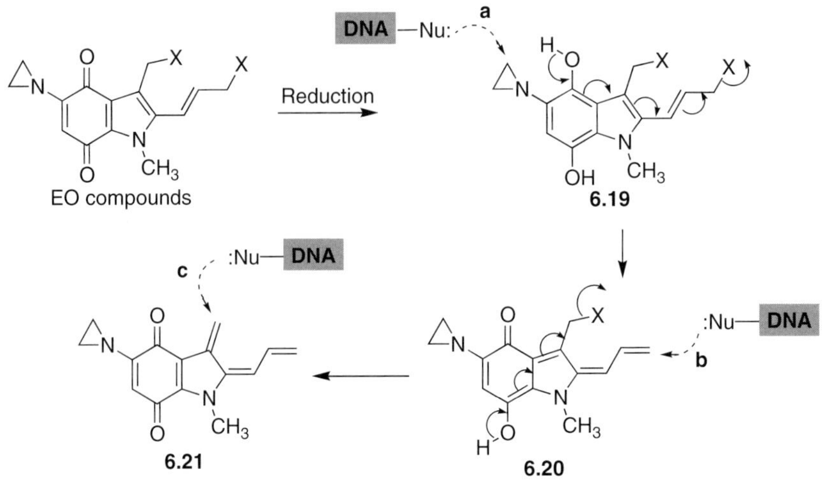

FIGURE 6.11   Bioreductive activation of the EO compounds.

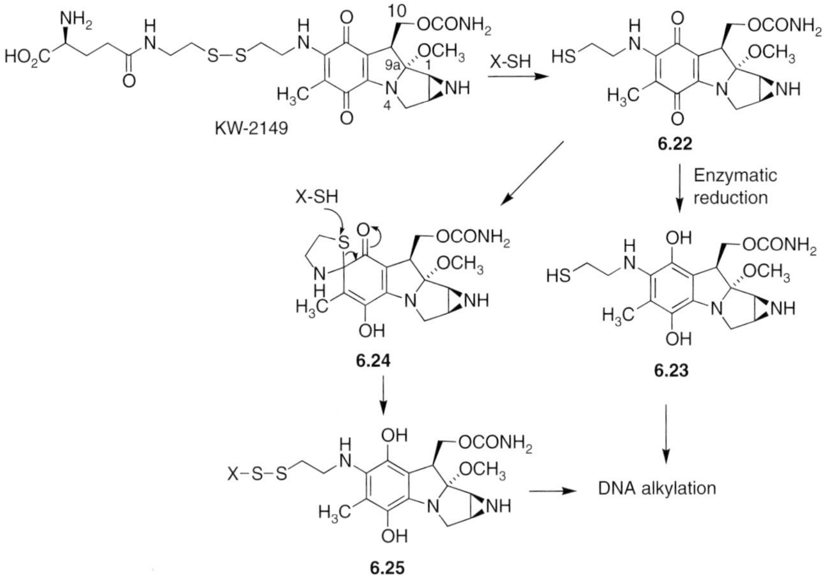

FIGURE 6.12   Non-reductive bioactivation of KW-2149, a mitomycin analogue.

reductases through the standard mechanism, involving the formation of **6.23** and subsequent DNA alkylation by a mechanism related to that proposed for the case of mitomycin. On the other hand, *in vitro* studies have shown that **6.22** exists predominantly as its spiro isomer **6.24**; this intermediate is proposed to react with intracellular thiols to give **6.25**, thus providing an alternative route for hydroquinone generation that is not dependent on reductase activity.[44] Due to this mechanism, KW-2149 is active in non-hypoxic tumor cells and in cell lines that express low levels DT-diaphorase and are therefore resistant to mitomycin.[45]

4. TETRAHYDROISOQUINOLINE ALKALOIDS

Antitumor natural products belonging to the tetrahydroisoquinoline family have been under study for the last 30 years, starting with the isolation of napthyridinomycin.[46] They normally bind to DNA by alkylation of specific nucleotide sequences in the minor groove. Most of these alkaloids contain quinone moieties and act by reductive alkylation mechanisms and also by generation of oxygen radicals via their one-electron reduction to a semiquinone species. The presence of either a nitrile or a hydroxy group on the position of the pyrazine ring α to the isoquinoline nitrogen is essential for DNA alkylation, which involves the generation of an intermediate iminium species.

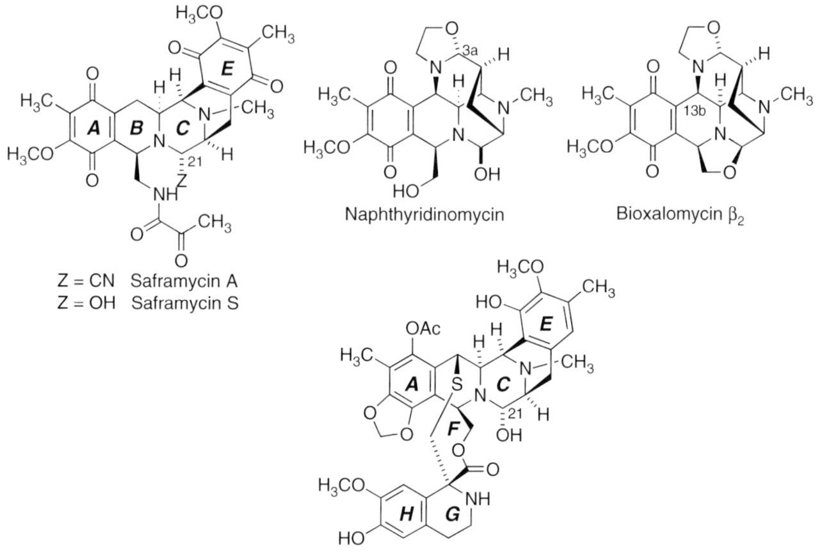

Z = CN   Saframycin A
Z = OH   Saframycin S

Naphthyridinomycin

Bioxalomycin β₂

Ecteinascidin-743 (trabectedin)

Recognition of the saframycins by the DNA minor groove shows some specificity towards 5'-GGG and 5'-GGC sequences,[47] and is followed by alkylation. Saframycin S, one of the most active saframycins, is active in the quinone form, which has been explained through the formation of iminium cation **6.26** and subsequent covalent binding to DNA involving attack by guanine amino groups to give aminal **6.27** [48] (Fig. 6.13).

In the case of saframycin S, there is a second type of covalent binding mechanism involving previous reduction to dihydroquinone, which facilitates the formation of the alkylating iminium species.[49] The less-reactive saframycin A only alkylates DNA in its hydroquinone form,[50] and indeed several hydroquinone analogues of saframycin A have been shown to be up to 20-fold more active than the parent

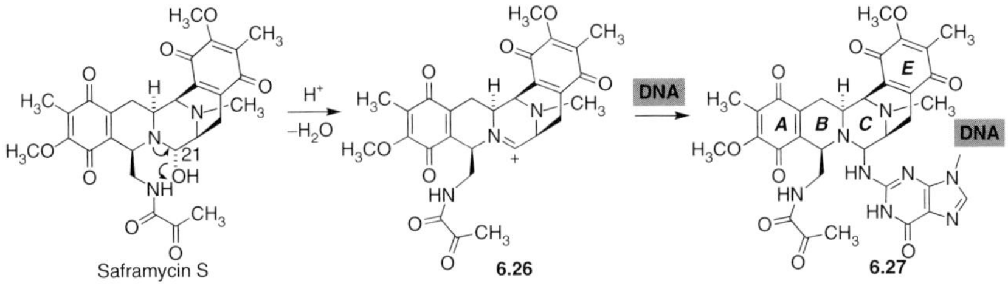

FIGURE 6.13   Iminium ion-mediated DNA alkylation by saframycin S.

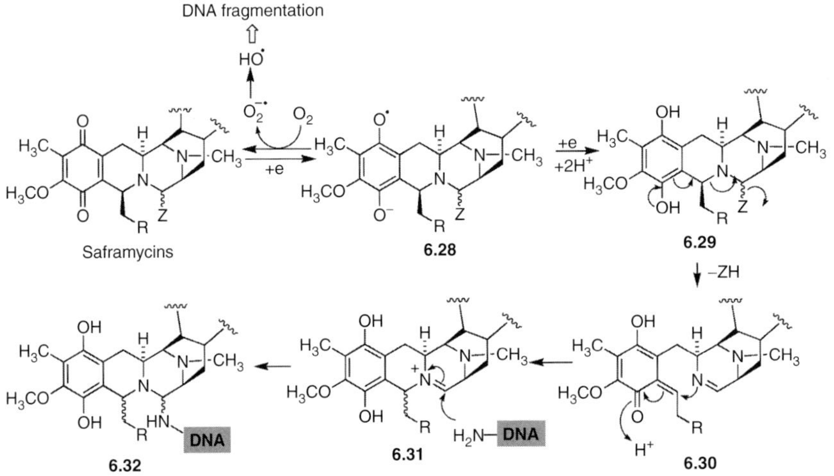

FIGURE 6.14   Bioreductive activation of saframycins.

quinone.[51] The mechanism of DNA alkylation by these hydroquinones (**6.29**) is proposed to involve B-ring opening with assistance from the phenolic hydroxyl group to give quinone methides **6.30**, which subsequently cyclize again to iminium derivatives **6.31**, the actual DNA alkylating agents. The redox equilibrium between the saframycins and their semiquinones **6.28**, as intermediates in the reduction of the natural products to hydroquinones **6.29**, is also involved in the generation of cytotoxic oxygen radicals (Fig. 6.14). Finally, we will mention that glyceralde-hyde-3-phosphate dehydrogenase (GAPDH), a key transcriptional coactivator necessary for entry into S-phase due to its involvement in the maintenance and/or protection of telomeres, has been identified as a protein target of DNA–small molecule adducts of several members of the saframycin class. Additionally, GAPDH is also capable of forming a ternary complex with saframycin-related compounds and DNA that induces a toxic response in cells.[52]

A mechanism very similar to the one summarized in Fig. 6.14 accounts for DNA alkylation by bioxalomycin β_2,[53] although a second mode of alkylation at C-14 in structure **6.33** after quinone reduction and opening of the oxazolidine ring has been suggested following molecular modelling studies.[54] In the case of bioxalomycins, it has been shown that the reduced form yields DNA interstrand

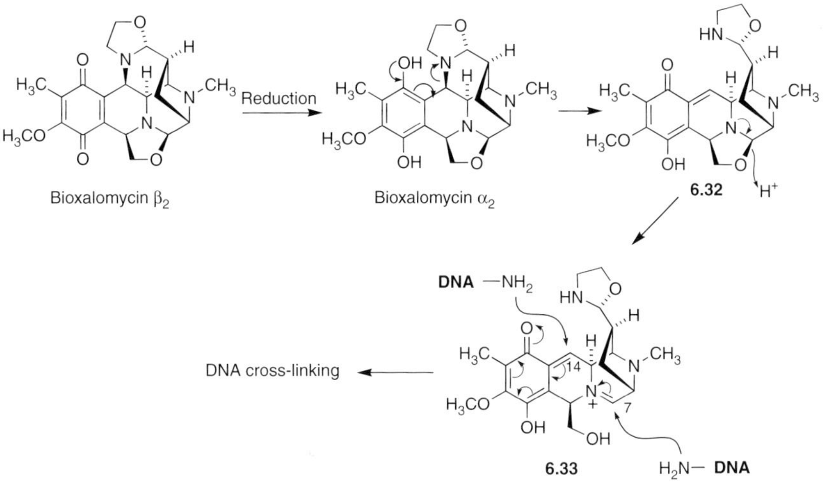

FIGURE 6.15   Bioreductive activation of bioxalomycin β_2.

cross-links with 5'-CpG-3' selectivity,[55] involving alkylation at C-7 following the usual mechanism and also at C-13b, as shown in Fig. 6.15.

The ecteinascidins are broad-spectrum antitumor agents, several orders of magnitude more potent than other tetrahydroisoquinoline alkaloids. Ecteinascidin 743 (ET-743, trabectedin), originally isolated from the marine tunicate *Ecteinascidia turbinata*,[56] has undergone extensive clinical studies[57–59] and is currently being tested in Phase III for several types of cancer. This drug was granted the status of orphan drug for treatment of soft tissue sarcoma and ovarian cancer,[60] and, more recently, it has been approved by the European Medicines Agency (EMEA) for the former indication.

Recognition of ET-743 by the DNA minor groove is specific for certain sequences like 5'-AGC[61] and involves hydrogen bonding with three different base pairs, as shown in Fig. 6.16 (the arrows are oriented from hydrogen donor to hydrogen acceptor groups).[62,63] DNA alkylation involves attack of the guanine amino group onto an iminium species generated at C-21 by loss of the hydroxyl group. NMR studies have shown that the covalent adduct is protonated at N-12, and this has led to the proposal that iminium generation is assisted by proton transfer from N-12 to the hydroxyl acting as a leaving group.[64]

On the basis of gel electrophoresis and ^{1}H NMR experiments, the site selectivity of ET-743 has been shown to depend on the rate of reversibility of the covalent adducts and not on the covalent reaction rate. Minor groove alkylation by ET-743 is reversible, and it has been proposed that the differences in rate of the reverse reaction are responsible for the observed sequence specificity, since non-favoured sequences (e.g. 5'-AGT) are dealkylated at an enhanced rate, allowing migration of ET-743 to the favoured ones (e.g. 5'-AGC). Due to hydrogen bonding, ET-743 forms a stable and tight complex at the 5'-AGC target sequence, where the covalent linkage is less accessible to attack by a water molecule. In the case of ET-743-AGT adducts, the complex is less stable and has more dynamic motion, leading

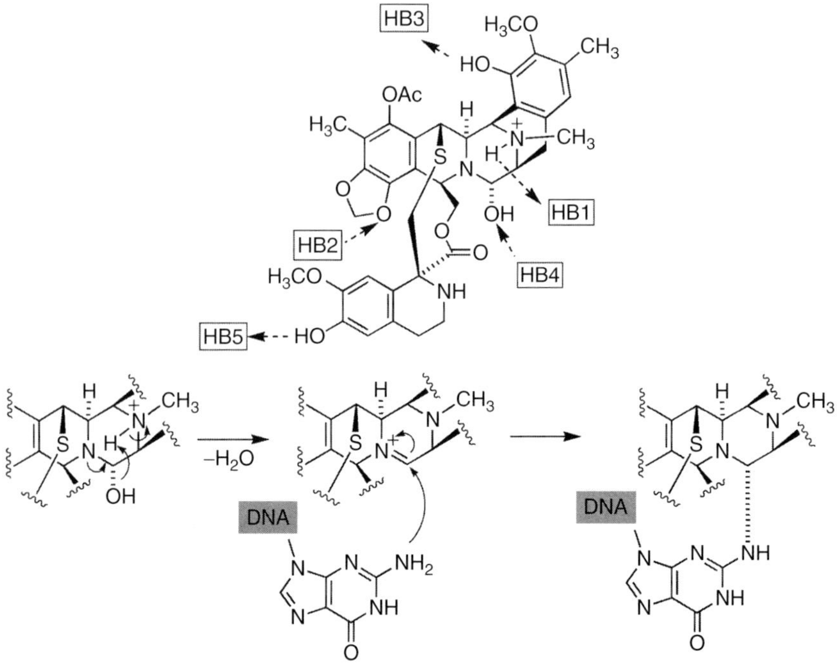

FIGURE 6.16   Significant hydrogen-bond interactions and DNA alkylation by ET-743.

to higher conformational flexibility that renders it more accessible to solvation, with the consequent increase in the rate of the reverse reaction, as shown in Fig. 6.17.

The mechanism of action of ET-743 and related compounds has been the matter of intense investigation in several laboratories.[65] X-ray crystallography and NMR studies show that ET-743 alkylates guanine amino groups in a sequence-specific manner, binding tightly into the minor groove of DNA. This induces widening of the minor groove and bending of the helix towards the major groove,[66,67] a distortion of the helix that would normally trigger nucleotide excision repair (NER) in which the damaged part of sequence is cut out by endonuclease and repaired by DNA polymerase (see Section 4.4.3 of Chapter 10). However, ET-743, in a unique mechanism of action, reverses NER, causing the endonuclease components to create lethal single-strand breaks in the DNA rather than repairing it.[68,69] At biological concentrations, the ET-743-DNA adduct also interacts with some DNA transcription factors, specially the NF-Y factor.[70] A molecular modelling study has shown that the DNA-ET-743 complex is superimposable with the minor groove of DNA bound to the zinc finger of the transcription regulator EGR-1, suggesting that ET-743 may target chromosome sites where zinc fingers of transcription factors interact with DNA.[71] Other studies have revealed that, like taxol, ET-743 disrupts the microtubule network of tumor cells,[72] and, at doses higher than therapeutic, it forms a cross-link between DNA and topoisomerase I by interaction of its spirotetrahydroisoquinoline subunit with the protein.[73]

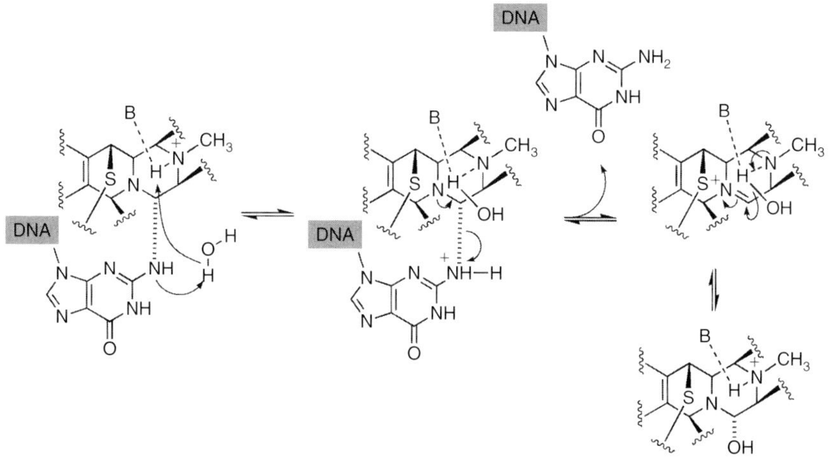

FIGURE 6.17   Reversibility of the covalent DNA-ET-743 complex.

Because of the complexity of the ET-743 structure, extensive studies have been carried out on the preparation of simpler analogues. Among them, the most important is phthalascidin,[74] with an activity similar to that of the natural product, where the phthalimino group plays a similar role to the spirotetrahydroisoquino-line unit in ET-743.[75] Another related compound is PM00104/50, which has recently begun Phase I clinical trials for the treatment of solid tumors.[76]

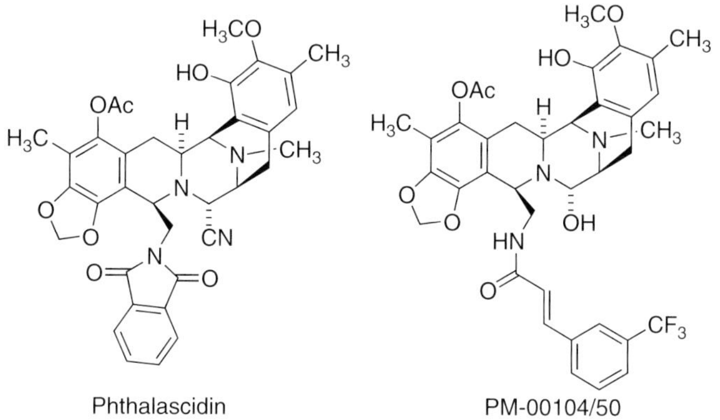

Phthalascidin

PM-00104/50

5. CYCLOPROPYLINDOLE ALKYLATING AGENTS

This name, although incorrect from the point of view of chemical nomenclature, is usually employed to design a number of antitumor compounds that contain a cyclopropane ring fused to an indole system. The first member of this class was the natural product CC-1065, an extremely potent cytotoxic agent isolated in trace quantities from the culture of *S. zelensis* in 1978, whose unique structure was confirmed by single-crystal X-ray diffraction in 1981. In spite of its very high *in vitro* antitumor activity, CC-1065 cannot be used in humans because it caused deaths in experimental animals due to its delayed hepatotoxicity.[77] In the search for compounds with better antitumor selectivity and DNA sequence specificity, many CC-1065 analogues have been synthesized in an attempt to avoid the undesired side effects while retaining its potency against tumor cells. Among them, the duocarmycins,[78,79] adozelesin, and halomethyl analogues such as bizelesin,[80] U-80224,[81] and KW-2189[82] may be mentioned. Among these compounds, the water-soluble prodrug KW-2189, which is activated by carboxyl esterases, is the most advanced one, having undergone Phase II clinical trials in patients with advanced malignant melanoma.[83] Hybrid compounds containing the cyclopropylindole fragment or its precursors and minor groove binding distamycin portions have also been prepared.[84]

CC-1065 · Duocarmycin A · Adozelesin · Bizelesin · KW-2189 · U-80224

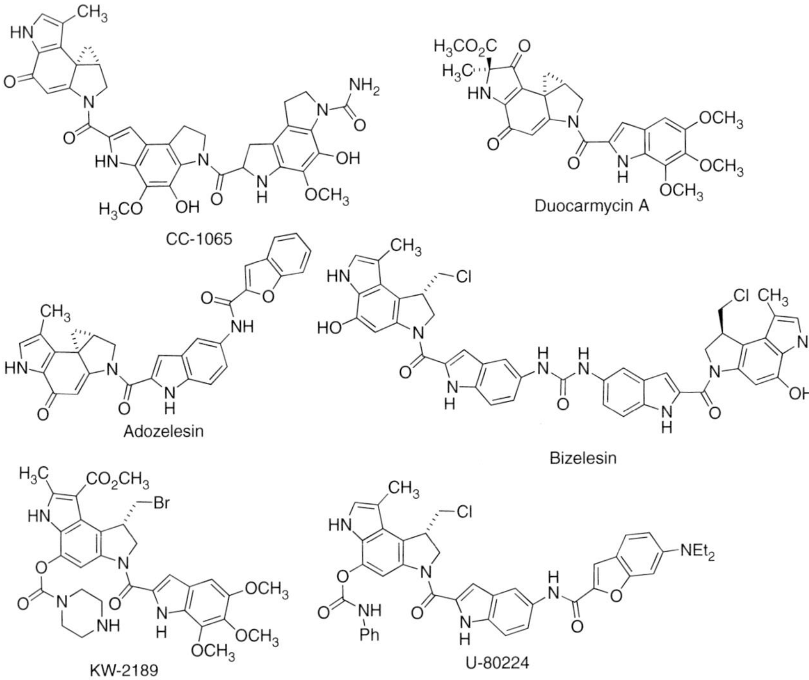

The structure of CC-1065 and their analogues fits the DNA minor groove curvature, where they bind specifically to AT-rich sequences, followed by irreversible alkylation of adenine N-3 (Fig. 6.18A). The halomethyl compounds are activated by cyclization to a cyclopropane derivative after hydrolysis of any protection on the phenolic hydroxyl (Fig. 6.18B).

As shown in Fig. 6.18A, cyclopropane ring opening needs to be assisted by the electron-withdrawing effect of the carbonyl group. Prior to interaction with DNA, this assistance is prevented by the conjugation between the carbonyl and the indole nitrogen atom, which form a vinylogous amide. However, the twist that the drug molecule needs to undergo in order to be accommodated into the deep and narrow minor groove AT regions forces the nitrogen atom out of the plane of the unsaturated carbonyl system and therefore out of conjugation (Fig. 6.19).

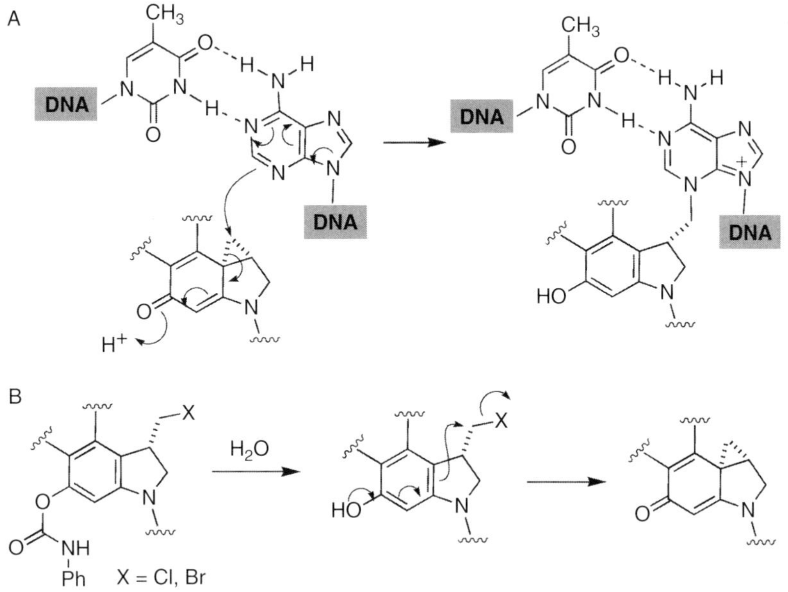
A
CH3
DNA
DNA
DNA
CH3
DNA
DNA
HO
H+
B
X
H2O
HO
X
NH
Ph
X = Cl, Br

FIGURE 6.18 A. DNA alkylation by cyclopropylindoles. B. *In vivo* generation of the cyclopropane ring from halomethyl precursors.

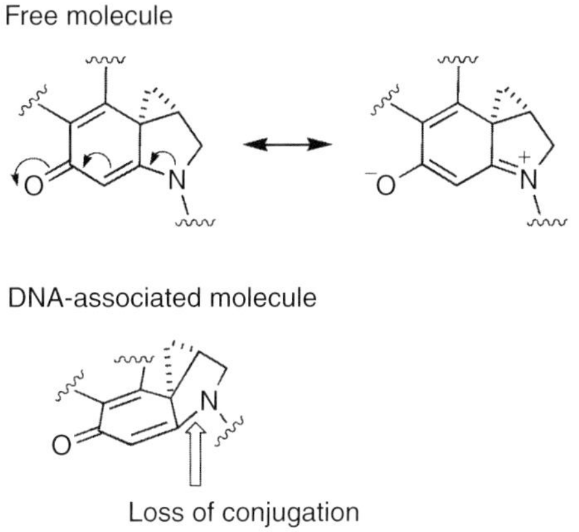
Free molecule
DNA-associated molecule
Loss of conjugation

FIGURE 6.19 Conjugative effects in cyclopropylindoles.

6. PYRROLO[1,4]BENZODIAZEPINES

Anthramycin, tomaymycin, and sibiromycin are natural pyrrolo[1,4]benzodiazepine antitumor antibiotics that react with the minor groove of DNA to form covalently bound complexes. They show activity towards several tumors, but their clinical use is limited by their cardiotoxicity and tissue necrosis induction.

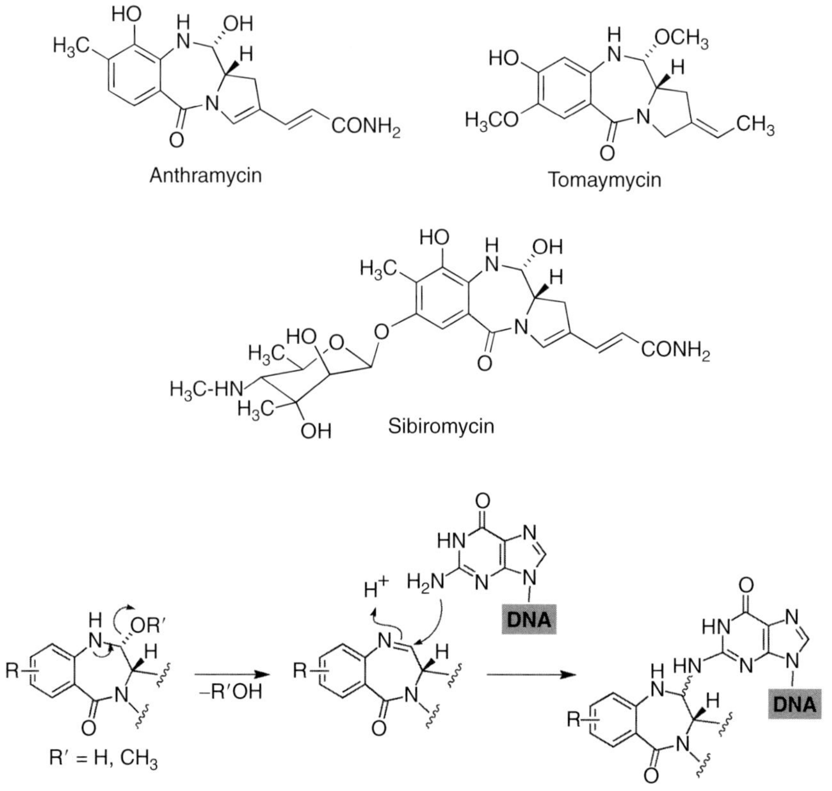

Anthramycin

Tomaymycin

Sibiromycin

R' = H, CH₃

FIGURE 6.20   DNA alkylation by pyrrolo[1,4]benzodiazepines.

These compounds form a covalent bond with the 2-amino group of guanine, as shown by X-ray diffraction,[85] through the formation of an intermediate iminium cation (Fig. 6.20).

REFERENCES

1. Ren, J., and Chaires, J. B. (1999). *Biochemistry* **38**, 16067.
2. (a) Wartell, R. M., Larson, J. E., and Wells, R. D. (1974). *J. Biol. Chem.* **249**, 6719. (b) Van Dyke, M. W., Hertzberg, R. P., Dervan, P. B. *Proc. Natl. Acad. Sci. USA* **1982**, *79*, 5470.
3. Dolenc, J., Oostenbrink, C., Koller, J., and van Gusteren, W. F. (2005). *Nucl. Acid Res.* **33**, 725.
4. Uytterhoeven, K., Sponer, J., and Van Meervelt, L. (2002). *Eur. J. Biochem.* **269**, 2868.
5. Baraldi, P. G., Núñez, A. C., Espinosa, A., and Romagnoli, R. (2004). *Curr. Top. Med. Chem.* **4**, 231.
6. Sunavala-Dossabhoy, G., and Van Dyke, M. W. (2005). *Biochemistry* **44**, 2510.
7. Viallet, J., Stewart, D., Shepherd, F., Ayoub, J., Cormier, Y., Di Pietro, N., and Steward, W. (1996). *Lung Cancer* **15**, 367.
8. D'Incalci, M., and Sessa, C. (1997). *Expert Opin. Investing. Drugs.* **6**, 875.
9. Ten Tije, A. J., Verweij, J., Sparreboom, A., van der Gaast, A., Fowst, C., Fiorentini, F., Tursi, J., Antonellini, A., Mantel, M., Hartman, C. M., Stoter, G., Planting, A. S. T., *et al.* (2003). *Clin. Cancer Res.* **9**, 2957.

10. Fedier, A., Fowst, C., Tursi, J., Geroni, C., Haller, U., Marchini, S., and Fink, D. (2003). *Br. J. Cancer* **89,** 1559.
11. Kraut, E., Malspeis, L., Balcerzak, S., and Grever, M. (1988). *Proc. Am. Soc. Clin. Oncol.* **7,** 62.
12. Kraut, E., Fleming, T., Segal, M., Neidhart, J., Behrens, B. C., and MacDonald, J. (1991). *Invest. New Drugs* **9,** 95.
13. Hard, T., Fan, P., and Kearns, D. R. (1990). *Photochem. Photobiol.* **51,** 77.
14. Teng, M., Usman, N., Frederik, C. A., and Wang, A. H.-J. (1988). *Nucleic Acid Res.* **16,** 2671.
15. Teicher, B. A. (1997). *In* "Cancer: Principles and Practice of Oncology," (V. T. DeVita, S. Hellman, and S. A. Rosenberg, eds.) 5th ed. p. 405. Lippincott-Raven, Philadelphia.
16. Spain, R. C. (1993). *Oncology* **50,** 35.
17. Haffty, B. G., Son, Y. H., Wilson, L. D., Papac, R., Fischer, D., Rockwell, S., Sartorelli, A. C., Ross, D., Sasaki, C. T., and Fischer, J. J. (1997). *Radiat. Oncol. Investig.* **5,** 235.
18. Workman, P., and Stratford, I. J. (1993). *Cancer Metastasis Rev.* **12,** 73.
19. Wolkenberg, S. E., and Boger, D. L. (2002). *Chem. Rev.* **102,** 2477.
20. Kumar, G. S., Lipman, R., Cummings, J., and Tomasz, M. (1997). *Biochemistry* **36,** 14128.
21. (a) Siegel, S., Gibson, N. W., Preusch, P. C., and Ross, D. (1990). *Cancer Res.* **50,** 7483. (b) Mikami, K., Naito, M., Tomida, A., Yamada, M., Sirakusa, T., and Tsuruo, T. (1996). *Cancer Res.* **56,** 2823.
22. Danishefsky, S. J., and Ciufolini, M. (1984). *J. Am. Chem. Soc.* **106,** 6425.
23. Tomasz, M., Chawla, A. K., and Lipman, R. (1988). *Biochemistry* **27,** 3182.
24. Sastry, M., Fiala, R., Lipman, R., Tomasz, M., and Patel, D. J. (1995). *J. Mol. Biol.* **247,** 338.
25. Bizanek, M., McGuinness, B. F., Nakanishi, K., and Tomasz, M. (1992). *Biochemistry* **31,** 3084.
26. Norman, D., Live, D., Sastry, M., Lipman, R., Hingerty, B. E., Tomasz, M., Broyde, S., and Patel, D. J. (1990). *Biochemistry* **29,** 2861.
27. Li, V.-S., and Kohn, H. (1991). *J. Am. Chem. Soc.* **113,** 275.
28. Kumar, S., Lipman, R., and Tomasz, M. (1992). *Biochemistry* **31,** 1399.
29. Williams, R. M., Rajski, S. R., and Rollins, S. B. (1997). *Chem. Biol.* **4,** 127.
30. Paz, M. M., and Hopkins, P. B. (1997). *J. Am. Chem. Soc.* **119,** 5999.
31. Paz, M. M., Sigursson, S. T., and Hopkins, P. B. (2000). *Bioorg. Med. Chem.* **8,** 173.
32. Rajski, S. R., and Williams, R. M. (2000). *Bioorg. Med. Chem.* **8,** 1331.
33. Kohn, H., and Zein, N. (1983). *J. Am. Chem. Soc.* **105,** 4105.
34. Maliepaard, M., de Mol, N. J., Tomasz, M., Gargiulo, D., Janssen, L. H. M., Duynhoven, J. P. M., van Velzen, E. J. J., Verboom, W., and Reinhoudt, D. N. (1997). *Biochemistry* **36,** 9211.
35. Ouyang, A., and Skibo, B. (2000). *Biochemistry* **39,** 5817.
36. Dirix, L. Y., Tonnesen, F., Cassidy, J., Epelbaum, R., ten Bokkel Huinink, W. W., Pavlidis, N., Sorio, R., Gamucci, T., Wolff, I., te Velde, A., Lan, J., and Verweij, J. (1996). *Eur. J. Cancer* **32a,** 2019.
37. Pavlidis, N., Hanauske, A. R., Gamucci, T., Smyth, J., Lehnert, M., te Velde, A., Lan, J., and Verweij, J. (1996). *Ann. Oncol.* **7,** 529.
38. Choudry, G. A., Stewart, P. A. H., Double, J. A., Krul, M. R. L., Naylor, B., Flannigan, G. M., Shah, T. K., Brown, J. E., and Phillips, R. M. (2001). *Brit. J. Cancer* **85,** 1137.
39. Aamdal, S., Lund, B., Koier, I., Houten, M., Wanders, J., and Verweij, J. (2000). *Cancer Chemother. Pharmacol.* **45,** 85.
40. Phillips, R. M. (1996). *Biochem. Pharmacol.* **52,** 1711.
41. Bailey, S. M., Wyatt, M. D., Friedlos, F., Hartley, J. A., Canox, R. J., Lewis, A. D., and Workman, P. (1997). *Br. J. Cancer* **76,** 1596.
42. Saijo, N. (1998). *Chest* **113,** 17S.
43. Schrijvers, D., Catimel, G., Highley, M., Hopponer, F. J., Dirix, L., De Bruijn, E., Droz, J. P., and Van Oesterom, A. T. (1999). *Anticancer Drugs* **10,** 633.
44. Na, Y., Wang, S., and Kohn, H. (2002). *J. Am. Chem. Soc.* **124,** 4666.
45. Dirix, L., Catimel, G., Koier, I., Prove, A., Schrijvers, D., Joossens, E., de Bruijn, E., Ardiet, C., Evene, E., Dumortier, A., Clavel, M., and van Oosterom, A. (1995). *Anticancer Drugs* **6,** 53.
46. Scott, J. D., and Williams, R. M. (2002). *Chem. Rev.* **102,** 1669.
47. Rao, K. E., and Lown, J. W. (1990). *Chem. Res. Toxicol.* **3,** 262.
48. Lown, J. W., Joshua, A. V., and Lee, J. S. (1982). *Biochemistry* **21,** 419.
49. Ishiguro, K., Takahashi, K., Yazawa, K., Sakiyama, S., and Arai, T. (1981). *J. Biol. Chem.* **256,** 2162.
50. Hill, G. C., and Remers, W. A. (1991). *J. Med. Chem.* **34,** 1990.

51. Myers, A. G., and Plowright, A. T. (2001). *J. Am. Chem. Soc.* **123,** 5114.
52. Xing, C., LaPorte, J. R., Barbay, J. K., and Myers, A. G. (2004). *Proc. Natl. Acad. Sci.* **101,** 5862.
53. Zmijewski, M. J., Miller-Hatch, K., and Mikolajczak, M. (1985). *Chem. Biol. Interact.* **52,** 361.
54. Hill, G. C., Wunz, T. P., McKenzie, N. E., Gooley, P. R., and Remers, W. A. (1991). *J. Med. Chem.* **34,** 2079.
55. Williams, R. M., and Herberich, B. (1998). *J. Am. Chem. Soc.* **120,** 10272.
56. Rinehart, K. L., Holt, T. G., Fregeau, N. L., Stroh, J. G., Kieffer, P. A., Sun, F., Li, L. H., and Martin, D. G. (1990). *J. Org. Chem.* **55,** 4512.
57. D'Incalci, M., Erba, E., Damía, G., Galliera, E., Carrasa, L., Marchini, S., Mantovani, R., Tognon, G., Fruscio, R., Jimeno, J., and Faircloth, G. T. (2002). *Oncologist* **7,** 210.
58. Schwartsmann, G., Da Rocha, A. B., Mattei, J., and Lopes, R. (2003). *Expert Opin. Investig. Drugs* **12,** 1367.
59. D'Incalci, M., and Jimeno, J. (2003). *Expert Opin. Investig. Drugs* **12,** 1843.
60. http://www.pharmamar.es/es/pipeline/yondelis.cfm
61. Zewail-Foote, M., and Hurley, L. H. (2001). *J. Am. Chem. Soc.* **123,** 6485.
62. Seaman, F. C., and Hurley, L. H. (1998). *J. Am. Chem. Soc.* **120,** 13028.
63. Marco, E., García Nieto, R., Mendieta, J., Manzanares, I., Cuevas, C., and Gago, F. (2002). *J. Med. Chem.* **45,** 871.
64. Moore, R. M., Seman, F. C., Wheelhouse, R. T., and Hurley, R. H. (1998). *J. Am. Chem. Soc.* **120,** 2490.
65. Manzanares, I., Cuevas, C., García-Nieto, R., and Gago, F. (2001). *Curr. Med. Chem. Anticancer Agents* **1,** 257.
66. Zewail-Foote, M., and Hurley, L. H. (1999). *J. Med. Chem.* **42,** 2493.
67. García-Nieto, R., Manzanares, I., Cuevas, C., and Gago, F. (2000). *J. Am. Chem. Soc.* **122,** 7172.
68. Takebayashi, K., Pourquier, P., Zimonjic, D. B., Nakayama, K., Emmert, S., Ueda, T., Urasaki, Y., Kanzaki, A., Akiyama, S., Popescu, N., Kraemer, K. H., and Pommier, Y. (2001). *Nat. Med.* **7,** 961.
69. Zewail-Foote, M., Ven-Shun, L., Kohn, H., Bearss, D., Guzmán, M., and Hurley, L. H. (2001). *Chem. Biol.* **135,** 1.
70. Bonfanti, M., La Valle, E., Fernández-Sousa, J.-M., Faircloth, G., Caretti, G., Mantovani, R., and D'Incalci, M. (1999). *Anticancer Drug Des.* **14,** 179.
71. García-Nieto, R., Manzanares, I., Cuevas, C., and Gago, F. (2000). *J. Med. Chem.* **43,** 4367.
72. García-Rocha, M., García-Grávalos, M. D., and Ávila, J. (1996). *Br. J. Cancer* **73,** 875.
73. Takebayashi, K., Pourquier, P., Yoshida, A., Kohlhagen, G., and Pommier, Y. (1999). *Proc. Natl. Acad. Sci. USA* **96,** 7196.
74. Martínez, E. J., Owa, T., Schreiber, S. L., and Corey, E. J. (1999). *Proc. Natl. Acad. Sci. USA* **96,** 3496.
75. Martínez, E. J., Corey, E. J., and Owa, T. (2001). *Chem. Biol.* **8,** 1151.
76. http://www.pharmamar.es/es/pipeline/zalypsis.cfm
77. McGovren, J. P., Clarke, G. L., Pratt, E. A., and DeKoning, T. F. (1984). *J. Antibiot.* **37,** 63.
78. Boger, D. L. (1994). *Pure Appl. Chem.* **66,** 837.
79. Boger, D. L., Boyce, C. W., Garbaccio, R. M., and Golberg, J. A. (1997). *Chem. Rev.* **97,** 787.
80. Schwartz, G. H., Patnaik, A., Hammond, L. A., Rizzo, J., Berg, K., von Hoff, D. D., and Rowinsky, E. K. (2003). *Ann. Oncol.* **14,** 775.
81. Li, L. H., DeKoning, T. F., Kelly, R. C., Krueger, W. C., McGovern, J. P., Padbury, G. E., Petzold, G. L., Wallace, T. L., Ouding, R. J., Prairie, M. D., and Gebhard, I. (1992). *Cancer Res.* **52,** 4904.
82. Ogasawara, H., Nishio, K., Takeda, Y., Ohmori, T., Kubota, N., Funayama, Y., Ohira, T., Kuraishi, Y., Isogai, Y., and Saijo, N. (1994). *Jpn. J. Cancer Res.* **85,** 418.
83. Markovic, S. N., Suman, V. J., Vukov, A. M., Fitch, T. R., Hillman, D. W., Adjei, A. A., Alberts, S. R., Kaur, J. S., Braich, T. A., Leitch, J. M., and Creagan, E. T. (2002). *Am. J. Clin. Oncol.* **25,** 308.
84. Baraldi, P. G., Tabrizi, M. A., Preti, D., Fruttarolo, F., Avitabile, B., Bovero, A., Pavani, G., Núñez-Carretero, M. C., and Romagnoli, R. (2003). *Pure Appl. Chem.* **75,** 187.
85. Kopka, M. L., Goodsell, D. S., Baikalov, I., Grzeskowiak, K., Cascio, D., and Dickerson, R. E. (1994). *Biochemistry* **33,** 13593.

CHAPTER 7

DNA Intercalators and Topoisomerase Inhibitors

Contents

1. DNA Intercalation and Its Consequences   200
2. Monofunctional Intercalating Agents   201
    2.1. Ellipticine and its analogues   201
    2.2. Actinomycins   204
    2.3. Fused quinoline compounds   204
    2.4. Naphthalimides and related compounds   205
    2.5. Chartreusin, elsamicin A, and related compounds   206
    2.6. Other monofunctional intercalating agents   206
3. Bifunctional Intercalating Agents   206
4. DNA Topoisomerases   209
    4.1. Topoisomerase I mechanism   209
    4.2. Topoisomerase II mechanism   211
5. Topoisomerase II Poisons   213
    5.1. Acridine derivatives   213
    5.2. Anthracyclines and related compounds   214
    5.3. Non-intercalating topoisomerase II poisons   216
6. Topoisomerase II Catalytic Inhibitors   218
    6.1. Inhibitors of the binding of topoisomerase II to DNA: Aclarubicin   219
    6.2. Merbarone   219
    6.3. Bis(dioxopiperazines)   219
7. Specific Topoisomerase I Inhibitors   220
    7.1. Camptothecins   221
    7.2. Non-CPT topoisomerase I inhibitors   223
References   225

Medicinal Chemistry of Anticancer Drugs
DOI: 10.1016/B978-0-444-52824-7.00007-X

199

1. DNA INTERCALATION AND ITS CONSEQUENCES

Many anticancer drugs in clinical use (e.g. anthracyclines, mitoxantrone, dactinomycin) interact with DNA through intercalation, which can be defined as the process by which compounds containing planar aromatic or heteroaromatic ring systems are inserted between adjacent base pairs perpendicularly to the axis of the helix and without disturbing the overall stacking pattern due to Watson–Crick hydrogen bonding. Since many typical intercalating agents contain three or four fused rings that absorb light in the UV–visible region of the electromagnetic spectrum, they are usually known as chromophores. Besides the chromophore, other substituents in the intercalator molecule may highly influence the binding mechanism, the geometry of the ligand–DNA complex, and the sequence selectivity, if any.

The intercalation process[1] starts with the transfer of the intercalating molecule from an aqueous environment to the hydrophobic space between two adjacent DNA base pairs. This process is thermodynamically favoured because of the positive entropy contribution associated to disruption of the organized shell of water molecules around the ligand (hydrophobic effect). In order to accommodate the ligand, DNA must undergo a conformational change involving an increase in the vertical separation between the base pairs to create a cavity for the incoming chromophore. The double helix is thereby partially unwound,[2] which leads to distortions of the sugar–phosphate backbone and changes in the twist angle between successive base pairs (Fig. 7.1). Once the drug has been sandwiched

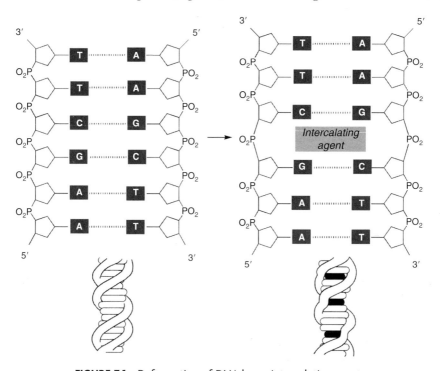

FIGURE 7.1   Deformation of DNA by an intercalating agent.

between the DNA base pairs, the stability of the complex is optimized by a number of non-covalent interactions, including van der Waals and π-stacking interactions,[3] reduction of coulombic repulsion between the DNA phosphate groups associated with the increased distance between the bases because of helix unwinding, ionic interactions between positively charged groups of the ligand and DNA phosphate groups, and hydrogen bonding. Generally speaking, cationic species are more efficient DNA intercalators because they interact better with the negatively charged DNA sugar–phosphate backbone in the initial stages and also because intercalation releases counterions associated to phosphate group, such as Na^+, leading to the so-called polyelectrolyte effect. This is a very important driving force for intercalation, since it diminishes repulsive interactions between the closely spaced charged counterions. In fact, most intercalating agents are either positively charged or contain basic groups that can be protonated under physiological conditions.

DNA intercalators are less sequence selective than minor groove binding agents, and, in contrast with them, show a preference for G-C regions. This selectivity is mainly due to complementary hydrophobic or electrostatic interactions, which are due to substituents attached to the chromophore within the major or minor grooves. DNA intercalation is also governed by the nearest-neighbour exclusion principle, which states that both neighbouring sites on each site of the intercalation remain empty, that is, they bind, at most, between alternate base pairs.[4] This is an example of a negative cooperative effect, whereby binding to one site induces a conformational change that hampers binding to the adjacent base pair.

Intercalation of a drug molecule into DNA is only the first step in a series of events that eventually lead to its biological effects.[5] Structural changes induced in DNA by intercalation lead to interference with recognition and function of DNA-associated proteins such as polymerases, transcription factors, DNA repair systems, and, specially, topoisomerases. The role of these enzymes in the design of antitumor drugs will be discussed in Sections 4 and 5.

2. MONOFUNCTIONAL INTERCALATING AGENTS

2.1. Ellipticine and its analogues

Ellipticine, an alkaloid isolated from the leaves of *Ochrosia elliptica* and other *Apocynaceae* plants, is the prototype of intercalators based on the pyridocarbazole system and displays a broad spectrum of antitumor activity.[6] Although at physiological pH values it can exist both as a neutral species and as a monocation (Fig. 7.2), it is the latter form that seems responsible for DNA intercalation, which leads to RNA polymerase inhibition. Other DNA-related enzymes that are inhibited by ellipticine include DNA polymerase, RNA methylase, and topoisomerase II, although it is not known whether these effects are a consequence of intercalation.

Ellipticine is also known to lead to cytochrome P450 (CYP)-dependent metabolites that are able to bind covalently to DNA.[7] *In vitro* experiments employing a peroxidase–H_2O_2 oxidizing system have shown that one of the metabolites from ellipticine, namely its 9-hydroxy derivative **7.1**, oxidizes to quinonimine **7.2**[8] but,

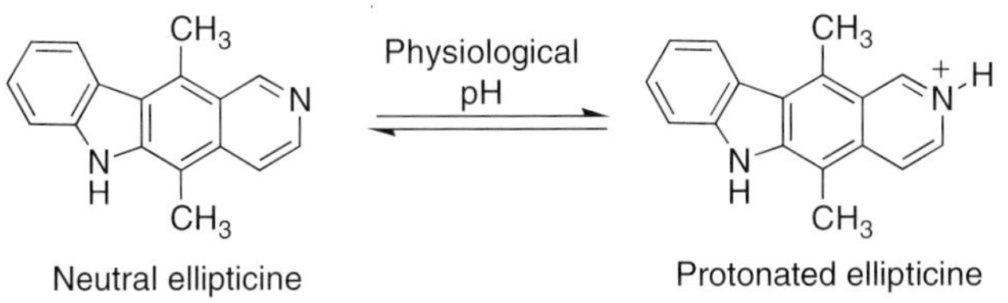

FIGURE 7.2   Neutral and protonated forms of ellipticine.

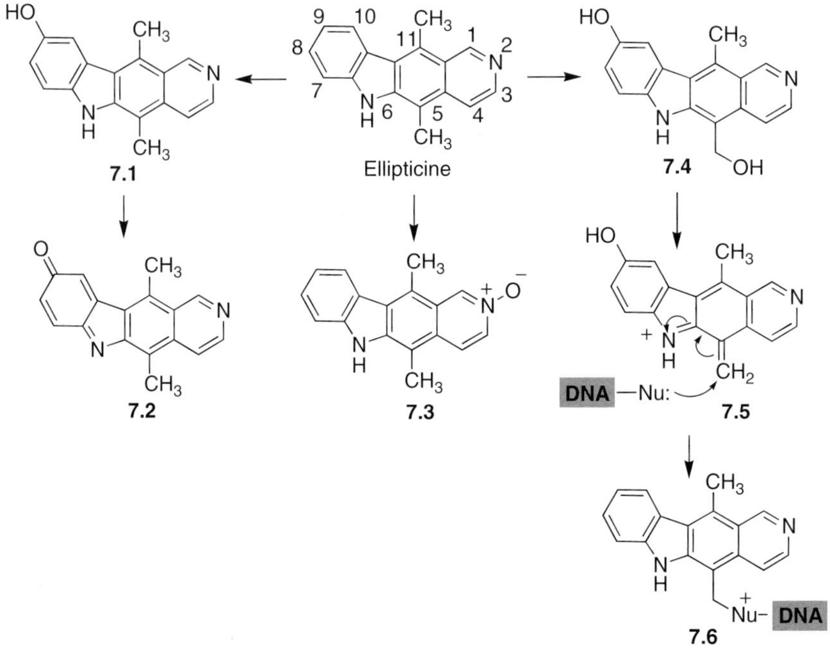

FIGURE 7.3   Ellipticine metabolites and their binding to DNA

in spite of its high electrophilicity, this intermediate seems not to be covalently bonded to DNA. More recent studies have proved that DNA binding is associated to other metabolites, including the N-oxide **7.3** and the hydroxymethyl derivative **7.4**, which can be tentatively assumed to react through the intermediacy of stabilized cation **7.5** to give the DNA-alkylated product **7.6**, as shown in Fig. 7.3.[9]

Because of the higher efficiency of cations as intercalating agents, some N-2 quaternized ellipticine analogues were assayed, among which the most interesting was N-methyl-9-hydroxyellipticinium (NMHE). Its quinonimine **7.7** is more reactive than its previously mentioned analogue from ellipticine (**7.2**) because of the presence of the strongly electron-withdrawing cationic heterocyclic nitrogen atom, and has been shown to react with a variety of biologically relevant nucleophiles at its C-10 position to give adducts **7.9** (Fig. 7.4). However, a correlation between the *in vivo* antitumor activity of NMHE and the formation of covalent adducts has not been established; in fact, it has been shown that the extent of

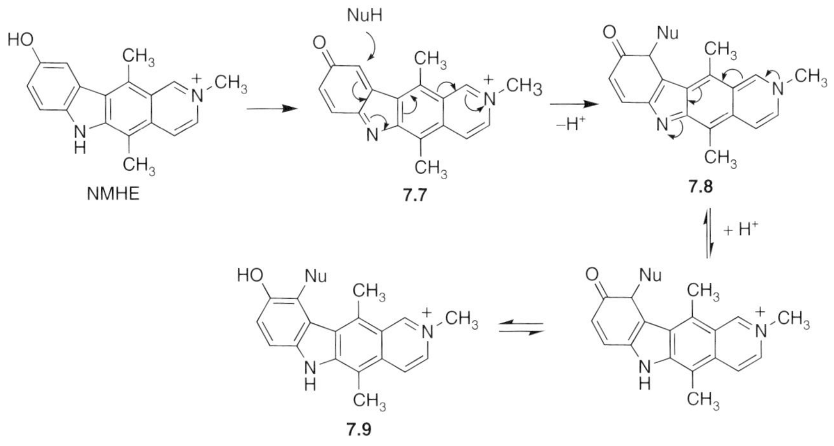

FIGURE 7.4   Reaction of *N*-metylhydroxyellipticinium with nucleophilic biomolecules.

irreversible binding to DNA is similar in NMHE-sensitive and NMHE-resistant cell lines.[10] Compounds related to NMHE have been employed as the basis for the design of bis-intercalating compounds (see Section 4).

S-16020 is another important antitumor pyridocarbazole derivative, bearing a (dimethylamino)ethylcarboxamide side chain that increases its DNA intercalating ability. This drug is a potent stimulator of topoisomerase II-mediated DNA cleavage and is not affected by resistance mediated by P-gp. Despite its close similarity with ellipticine, both compounds show little cross-resistance. Phase I clinical trials have indicated limited antitumor activity in head and neck cancer.[11]

Intoplicine is an intercalating compound that can be considered as structurally related to the ellipticines. It behaves as a dual topoisomerase I and II at cleavage sites different to those of other known topoisomerase inhibitors.[12] From spectroscopic results two types of DNA complexes have been proposed accounting for topoisomerase I- and II-mediated cleavages, involving a 'deep intercalation mode' or an 'outside binding mode', respectively.[13] Because of the high activity of intoplicine in preclinical cancer models, original mechanism of action and acceptable toxicity profile, it was further evaluated in several Phase I studies.[14] In these trials, patients developed serious liver toxicity at dose levels below the one believed to be necessary for antitumor activity. This toxicity was considered to be dose-limiting.

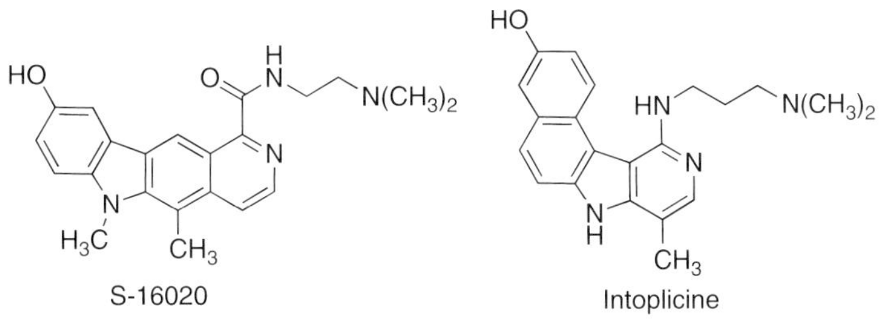

S-16020

Intoplicine

2.5. Chartreusin, elsamicin A, and related compounds

Chartreusin and elsamicin A are structurally related antitumor antibiotics that were isolated from *Streptomyces chartreusis* and from an unidentified actinomycete strain, respectively. Chartreusin suffered from unfavourable pharmacokinetic properties (slow oral absorption and biliar excretion) which prevented its clinical development. Semi-synthetic chartreusin analogues with improved pharmacokinetics have been developed. One of them, IST-622, is under Phase II clinical trials for the oral treatment of breast cancer.[27]

On the other hand, elsamicin A, one of the most potent known inhibitors of topoisomerase II, has entered Phase I clinical studies for relapsed or refractory non-Hodgkin's lymphoma. The activity was modest, but the compound was nevertheless considered promising because of the absence of myelosuppression.[28]

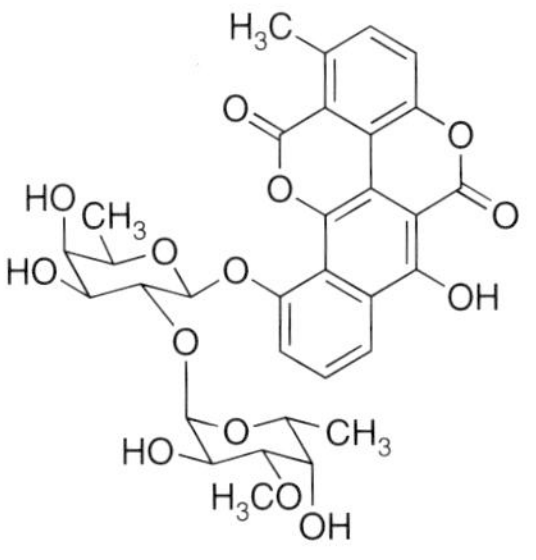

Chartreusin

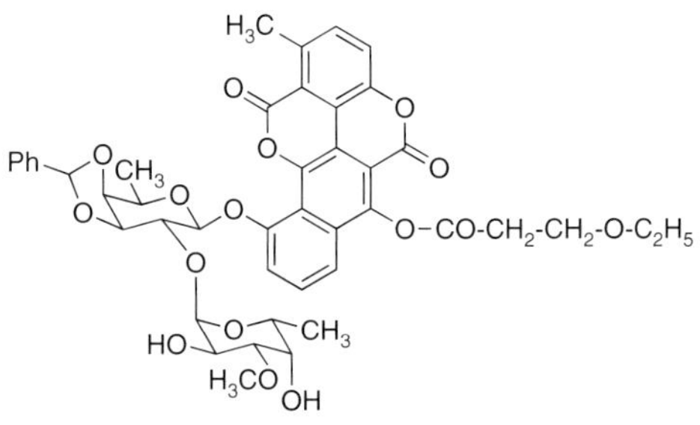

IST-622

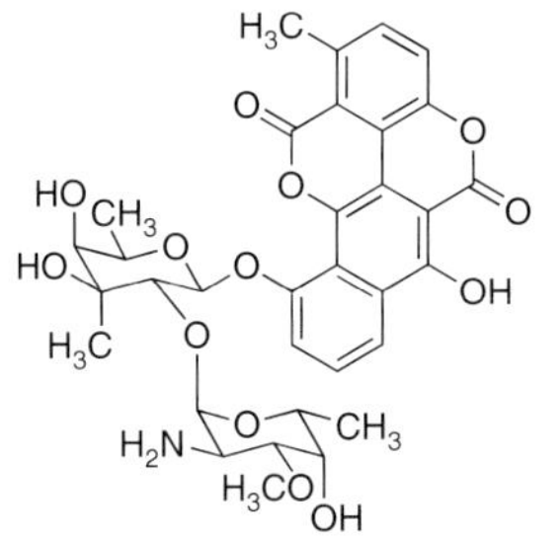

Elsamicin A

2.6. Other monofunctional intercalating agents

Some other intercalating agents (acridines and anthracyclines) are discussed in Section 5.

3. BIFUNCTIONAL INTERCALATING AGENTS

In efforts to increase the binding constant of intercalating compounds, bifunctional or even polyfunctional compounds have been designed. Bifunctional intercalators (bis-intercalators) contain two intercalating units, normally cationic, separated by a spacer chain that must be long enough to allow double intercalation taking into account the neighbour exclusion principle (Fig. 7.6).

Ditercalinium is an interesting bis-intercalator derived from ellipticinium with a novel mechanism of action different from that of its monomer, since topoisomerase II inhibition is not involved. Ditercalinium causes inhibition of enzymes that locate and repair damaged DNA sites, specially the nucleotide excision repair (NER) system,[29] due to the unstacking and bending that it induces on DNA because of the rigidity of the linker chain.[30]

Elinafide is a bis-intercalator derived from the naphthalimide pharmacophore[31] that exhibited excellent antitumor activity and reached Phase I clinical trials,[32] showing anti-neoplastic activity in ovarian cancer, breast cancer, and mesothelioma. Mechanistic studies on elinafide and its analogues are still in progress,[33] but this drug suffers from neuromuscular dose-limiting toxicity that has halted its clinical development.

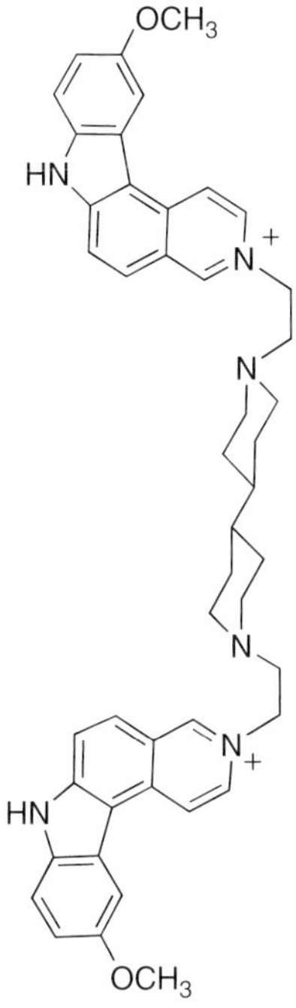

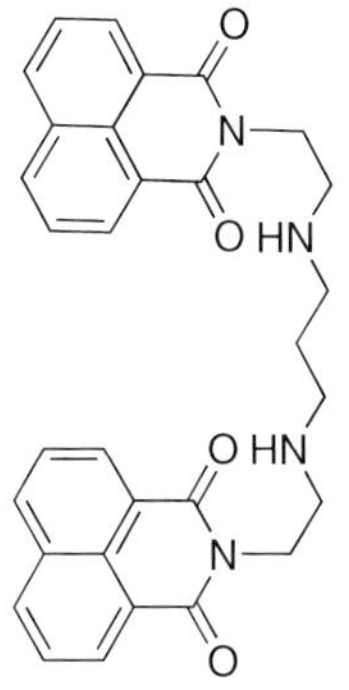

Elinafide

Ditercalinium

Echinomycin is an antitumor antibiotic isolated from *S. echinatus*, which consists of two quinoxaline chromophores attached to a cyclic octadepsipeptide ring, with a thioacetal cross-bridge. Because of its potent antitumor activity, this compound has been advanced to several Phase II clinical studies,[34,35] although it was eventually withdrawn from further clinical trials because it showed a high toxicity without any marked therapeutic benefit. More recently, echinomycin has been characterized as a very potent inhibitor of the binding of HIF-1 (hypoxia-inducible factor 1) to DNA. This is an interesting feature because HIF-1 is a transcription

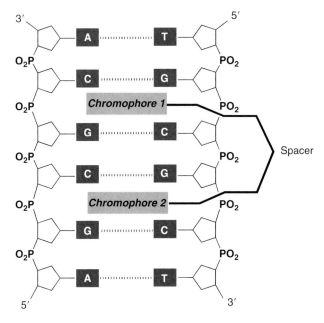

FIGURE 7.6   Schematic interaction between a bis-intercalator and DNA.

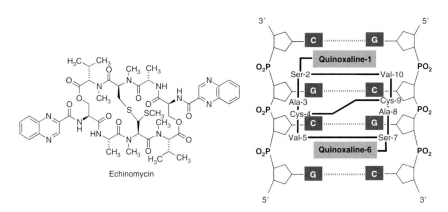

FIGURE 7.7   Schematic interaction between echinomycin and DNA.

factor that controls genes involved in processes important for tumor progression and metastasis, including angiogenesis, migration, and invasion.[36]

Several studies have proved that both echinomycin quinoxaline rings bis-intercalate into DNA, with CG selectivity, while the inner part of the depsipeptide establishes hydrogen bonds with the DNA bases of the minor groove region of the two base pairs comprised between the chromophores (Fig. 7.7).[37] A calorimetric study has proved that the binding reaction is entropically driven, showing that the complex is predominantly stabilized by hydrophobic interactions, although direct molecular recognition between echinomycin and DNA, mediated by hydrogen bonding and van der Waals contacts, also plays an important role in stabilizing the complex.[38]

4. DNA TOPOISOMERASES

Identical loops of DNA having different numbers of twists are topoisomers, that is, molecules with the same formula but different topologies, and their interconversion requires the breaking of DNA strands. DNA topoisomerases are enzymes that regulate the three-dimensional geometry (topology) of DNA, leading to the interconversion of its topological isomers and to its relaxation. This is related to the regulation of DNA supercoiling, which is essential to DNA transcription and replication, when the DNA helix must unwind to permit the proper function of the enzymatic machinery involved in these processes.

Topoisomerase I breaks a single DNA strand while topoisomerase II breaks both strands and requires ATP for full activity. In both cases, the enzyme is covalently attached to the DNA through tyrosine residues in the active site. These are transient, easily reversible linkages, and for this reason this covalently bound structure is known as the 'cleavable complex'. Afterwards, another DNA strand passes through the transient break in the DNA, and finally the DNA break is resealed. The end result of the reaction is a DNA molecule which is chemically unchanged, but closed in a different topology. The normal catalytic cycle of both types of topoisomerases involves two transesterification steps, one for the cleavage and other for the religation process. In the cleavage reaction, nucleophilic attack of an active site tyrosine forms a covalent bond with DNA by nucleophilic attack of its hydroxy group to a phosphate group of the phosphodiester DNA backbone. In the religation step, the 5'-hydroxyl group from deoxyribose attacks the previously formed tyrosine phosphate.

Topoisomerases are crucial for the several DNA functions (e.g. replication and transcription) that require the DNA to be unravelled, a process that generates tension and entanglement in DNA. Drugs that inhibit the topoisomerases include some of the most widely used anticancer drugs.[39] On the other hand, topoisomerase poisons may trigger chromatid breakage to inactivate the ataxia telangiectasia (AT) gene function, disable cell cycle control, and induce genetic instability.[40] In this connection, some alarming studies have been published, suggesting that maternal exposure to low doses of dietary topoisomerase II poisons, including bioflavonoids such as genistein or quercetin, may contribute to the development of infant leukaemia.[41]

4.1. Topoisomerase I mechanism

In the case of eukaryotic topoisomerase I, a single strand is attacked and a 3'-phosphotyrosyl linkage is formed. Religation takes place through attack of the 5' hydroxyl to the previously formed phosphate group (Fig. 7.8).

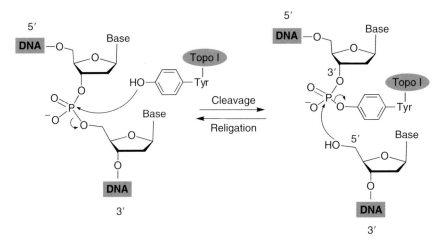

FIGURE 7.8   Transesterification reactions involved in topoisomerase I (topo I) activity.

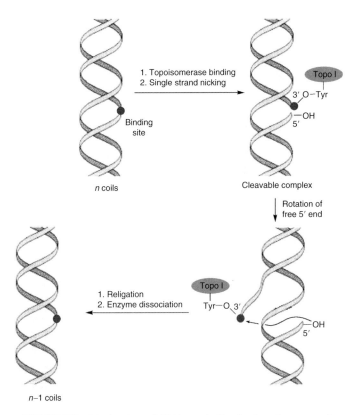

FIGURE 7.9   Mechanism of DNA unwinding by topoisomerase I.

Topoisomerase I acts by making a transient break (nick) of a single strand of DNA, catalyzing the passage of DNA strands through one another and allowing release of the superhelical tension. Topoisomerase I enzymes have been sub-divided into type IA and type IB sub-families based on their reaction mechanism. Type I topoisomerases of the type IA sub-family form covalent linkages to the 5′ end of the DNA break, while type IB sub-family enzymes form covalent linkages to the 3′ end of DNA break (Fig. 7.9). Eukaryotic DNA topoisomerase I is attached to the 3′ DNA end of the break site, and is therefore a type IB topoisomerase. This enzyme is located in areas of active RNA transcription to release superhelical stress generated during mRNA synthesis.

4.2. Topoisomerase II mechanism

Eukaryotic topoisomerase II is a homodimeric enzyme that requires ATP to function. It makes a transient double strand break, where the tyrosines from the active sites of both monomers attack the phosphodiester bond to the 5′-side of the phosphate, leading to a covalent 5′-phosphotyrosyl linkage in each strand (Fig. 7.10).

After binding of the enzyme to DNA, a double strand DNA break is produced by nucleophilic attack of both tyrosine residues. These breaks between the strands are not directly opposite to each other; instead, they are separated by a four base pair overhang, generating a space through which another region of intact DNA can be passed. The final steps involve religation of the DNA break, dissociation, and release of DNA from the topoisomerase (Fig. 7.11). Several of these steps require the binding and hydrolysis of ATP.

The catalytic cycle of topoisomerase II is complex and is summarized in Fig. 7.12, together with the names of some drugs that have steps of this cycle as targets.[42] The enzyme assumes two different conformations, resembling an open

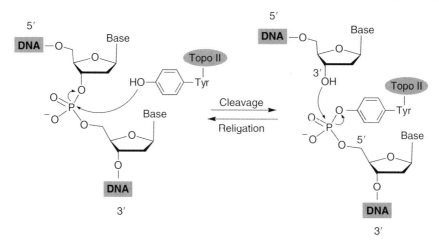

FIGURE 7.10 Transesterification reactions involved in topoisomerase II (topo II) activity.

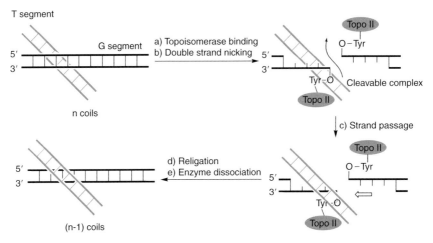

FIGURE 7.11   Mechanism of DNA unwinding by topoisomerase II.

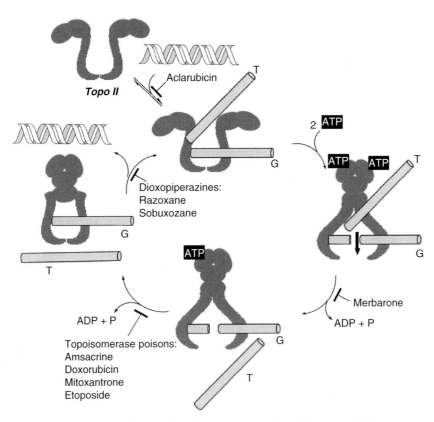

FIGURE 7.12   Catalytic cyclic of topoisomerase II and its main inhibitors.

clamp in the absence of ATP and a closed clamp in the presence of ATP. The open conformation can bind two segments of DNA, forming the pre-cleavage complex. One of these segments will be nicked by the enzyme (G segment) and another that will be transported (T segment). Afterwards, two ATP molecules are bound, leading to the dimerization of the ATPase domains and hence to a conformational change from the open- to the closed-clamp structure. The nucleophilic reactions that break both strands of the G segment of DNA then take place, generating the post-cleavage complex. This allows the passage of the T segment through the gap thus produced, which requires the hydrolysis of one molecule of ATP. The broken ends of the G segment are then ligated and the remaining ATP molecule is hydrolyzed. Upon dissociation of the two ADP molecules from ATP hydrolysis, the T segment is transported through the opening at the C-terminal part of the enzyme, which is then closed. Finally, the enzyme returns to the open clamp conformation, liberating the G segment.

Some antitumor drugs acting at the topoisomerase level have inhibition of enzymatic activity as their primary mode of action, and are known as 'catalytic topoisomerase inhibitors'.[43–45] Other drugs targeting the topoisomerases, including intercalating drugs, interfere with the enzyme's cleavage and rejoining activities by trapping the cleavable complex and thereby increasing the half-life of the transient topoisomerase catalyzed DNA break. Some of the most clinically useful anticancer drugs are of the latter type and are normally referred to as 'topoisomerase poisons' because they convert the topoisomerase enzyme into a DNA-damaging agent.

Because the level and time-course of expression of these enzymes vary in different cell types, and the development of resistance to one type of inhibitor is often accompanied by a concomitant rise in the level of the other enzyme, there is an increasing interest in drugs that can act as dual topoisomerase I and II poisons.[46,47] Finally, it is important to mention that topoisomerase inhibitors are among the most efficient inducers of apoptosis.[48]

5. TOPOISOMERASE II POISONS

This class of topoisomerase II inhibitors act by trapping the G strand enzyme intermediate, thus blocking religation and enzyme release and leaving the DNA with a permanent double strand break. Besides the compounds discussed here, many intercalating agents previously mentioned in Section 2 have this property.

5.1. Acridine derivatives

The intercalation concept was first introduced to explain the non-covalent binding of some acridine derivatives to DNA. Interest in these intercalators has led to the development of amsacrine (mAMSA), a drug used in the treatment of malignant lymphomas and acute non-lymphocytic leukaemia.[49,50] The main mechanism of action of mAMSA is the formation of a ternary complex with DNA and topoisomerase II, trapping the cleavable complex, and inhibiting the religation step.[51] Besides amsacrine, a large number of natural and synthetic acridines have been tested as anticancer agents and, so far, a few molecules have entered clinical trials and have been approved for chemotherapy.[52] For instance, asulacrine is a close analogue with a broader spectrum of activity in experimental tumors but without improved clinical antitumor activity. DACA (XR5000) is an acridinecarboxamide and a mixed topoisomerase I and II poison that has undergone extensive clinical trials.[53] Hybrid compounds have also been designed which combine the acridine intercalating moiety with other groups that provide secondary interactions with the DNA minor groove.

Amsacrine

Asulacrine

DACA

The pyrazoloacridone KW-2170 is a topoisomerase II inhibitor of synthetic origin that has entered Phase II clinical trials.[54] On the other hand, the related pyrazoloacridine PD-115934 is a dual topoisomerase I and II inhibitor, and has also entered Phase II clinical trials.[55]

KW-2170

PD-115934

5.2. Anthracyclines and related compounds

The anthracycline antibiotics, which were studied in Section 3 of Chapter 4, also intercalate with DNA. The tetracyclic A-D chromophore of these compounds is oriented with its long axis perpendicular to the long axis of adjacent base pairs at the intercalation site. The daunorubicin–DNA complex is stabilized by the stacking interactions of rings B and C and by hydrogen bonding involving the hydroxyl group at C-9 of ring A, which acts as a donor to N-3 of guanine and as an acceptor from the amino group of the same guanine. Ring D protrudes into the major groove and the amino sugar moiety lies in the minor groove and does not take part in the interaction with DNA, although it is crucial for antitumor activity (see below).

As other antitumor intercalating agents, anthracyclines are topoisomerase II poisons because of the formation of a stable drug–DNA–topoisomerase II ternary complex and consequent inhibition of replication and transcription. The sugar unit is crucial for the stabilization of this complex, and suppression of the C-4 methoxy and C-3′ amino groups increases topoisomerase II inhibition.[56] The formation of topoisomerase-mediated DNA breaks seem to be too modest to explain the activity of the anthracyclines unless other mechanisms are taken into account (see Chapter 4), but some of these mechanisms are enhanced by anthracycline intercalation and minor groove binding; for instance, intercalation is known to favour DNA propenylation by malondialdehyde.[57]

In the case of nogalamycin, the presence of two sugar residues at both ends of the chromophore leads to a special way of interaction with DNA, called threading intercalation[58] in which one of the sugar units is located at the minor groove and the other at the major groove. The structure of the nogalamycin–DNA complex has been studied by X-ray diffraction.[59]

Other anthracyclines that act primarily as topoisomerase II catalytic inhibitors, such as aclarubicin, will be mentioned in Section 6.1.

R = OH Doxorubicin
R = H   Daunorubicin (daunomycin)

Nogalamycin

Mitoxantrone is a simplified analogue of the anthracyclines which has also been discussed in Chapter 4. It has a complex mechanism of action that includes generation of a stable drug–DNA–topoisomerase II ternary complex. Isosteric substitution of one or more carbons of the benzene rings by nitrogen atoms has been employed as a strategy for the design of mitoxantrone analogues with geometries similar to those of the parent compounds, but with increased affinity for DNA due to the presence of sites suitable for hydrogen bonding or ionic interactions. This increased affinity allows the suppression of the phenolic hydroxyls of mitoxantrone, which are responsible for its chelating properties and therefore for its cardiotoxicity through oxygen radicals generated through Fenton chemistry. Based on this idea, some aza-bioisosters related to the anthracene-9, 10-diones have been synthesized and screened *in vitro* and *in vivo* against a wide spectrum of tumor cell lines.[60,61]

Among these compounds, pixantrone has a high level of activity in blood-related tumors and is currently being studied in Phase III trials for the treatment of non-Hodgkin's lymphoma.[62,63] Interestingly, pixantrone was curative in some models of lymphoma and leukaemia where currently marketed anthracyclines only prolonged survival, but it showed no measurable cardiotoxicity compared to them at equi-effective doses in animal models.[64] Another potential application of this drug is as an immunosuppressant in multiple sclerosis patients.[65]

The mechanism of action of pixantrone involves intercalation with DNA and interaction with topoisomerase II, causing breaks in DNA strands.[66]

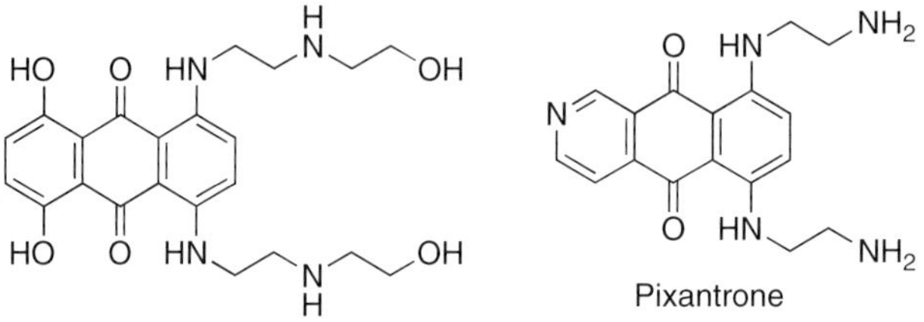

Mitoxantrone

Pixantrone

5.3. Non-intercalating topoisomerase II poisons

5.3.1. Etoposide and its analogues

Podophyllin resin derivatives have been used as folk medicines for centuries, its main active ingredient being podophyllotoxin. In the 1950s, a search began to identify a more effective podophyllotoxin derivative[67] that eventually resulted in the development of a new class of anti-neoplastic agents which target topoisomerase II. The most important compounds are etoposide and teniposide, two semi-synthetic derivatives of 4-epipodophyllotoxin. Etoposide (VP-16)[68] is used mainly to treat testicular cancer which does not respond to other treatment and as a first-line treatment for small cell lung cancers. It is also used to treat chorionic carcinomas, Kaposi's sarcoma, lymphomas, and malignant melanomas. A phosphate pro-drug of etoposide (etopophos) has been used for ADEPT therapy and will be discussed in Section 3 of Chapter 11. Teniposide is used less frequently, especially to treat lymphomas.

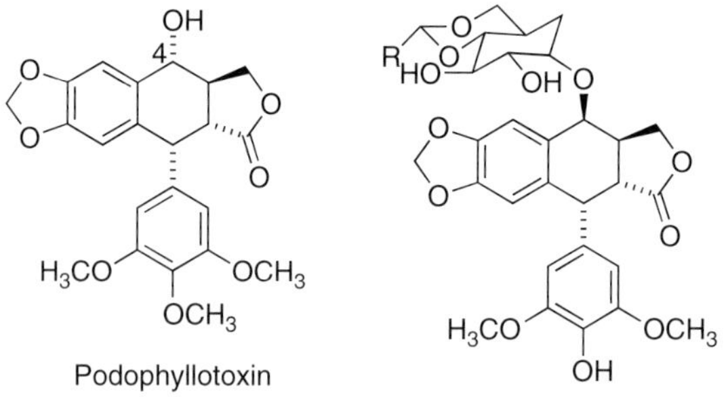

Podophyllotoxin

R = CH₃   Etoposide
R = 2-Thienyl Teniposide

Etoposide and teniposide activity is cell cycle dependent and phase specific, with maximum effect on the S and G2 phases of cell division. They cause DNA damage through inhibition of topoisomerase II, and their mechanism of action has been studied specially for the case of etoposide. DNA religation inhibition by this compound seems to be due to inhibition of the release of ADP from the hydrolysis of ATP[69] and to its activation through oxidation–reduction reactions to produce derivatives that bind directly to DNA. It has been shown that the O-demethylated metabolite of etoposide **7.10** has the same potency as the parent drug. This etoposide catechol is subsequently oxidized to an *ortho*-quinone metabolite **7.12** which is also a potent inhibitor of the topoisomerase II–DNA cleavable complex.[70] It has been proposed that the presence of free radical intermediates such as semi-quinone **7.11** contribute to DNA strand breakage, which seems to be supported by the fact that the 4'-OH group of etoposide is essential for its activity as shown by the inactivity of its 4'-OMe derivative. On the other hand, etoposide is a substrate of myeloperoxidase, an enzyme with tyrosinase activity that catalyses a one-electron oxidation to form the phenoxyl radical **7.13** (Fig. 7.13). However, the formation of radicals **7.11** and **7.13** has been proposed to be related to the increased risk of secondary myeloid acute leukaemia induced by long-term etoposide treatment.[71,72]

Other interesting epipodophyllotoxins under clinical assay are TOP-53 and tafluposide. TOP-53,[73] which bears a basic aminoalkyl side chain that improves its solubility while allowing its association with phosphatidylserine resulting in selective accumulation in lung and is in Phase I trials. The phosphate pro-drug tafluposide[74] is a lipophilic perfluorinated epipodophyllotoxin that has a dual topoisomerase I and II inhibitory activity, has shown high *in vivo* activity and has entered Phase I clinical trials for solid tumours.

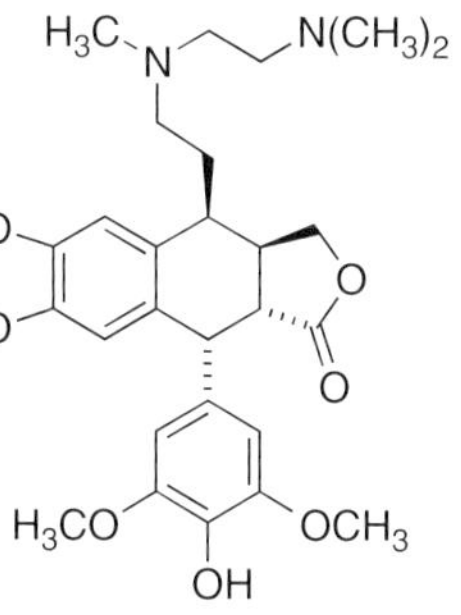

TOP-53

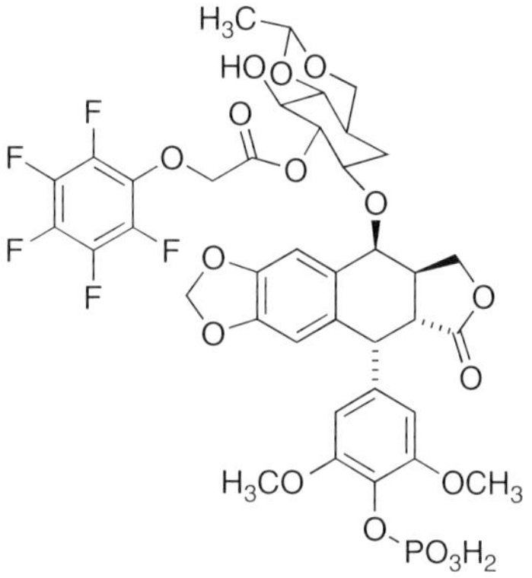

Tafluposide

5.3.2. Salvicine

Salvicine is a semi-synthetic diterpenoid quinone compound obtained by structural modification of a natural lead isolated from the Chinese medicinal herb *Salvia prionitis*. This compound is a non-intercalative topoisomerase II poison with a potent, broad spectrum *in vitro* and *in vivo* antitumor activity, and is currently in Phase II clinical trials. Salvicine is also an inhibitor of several resistance mechanisms (see Chapter 12), including multi-drug resistance (MDR) by down-regulating the expression of MDR-1 mRNA via the activation of c-jun, and DNA repair by the DNA protein kinase (DNA-PK) enzyme.

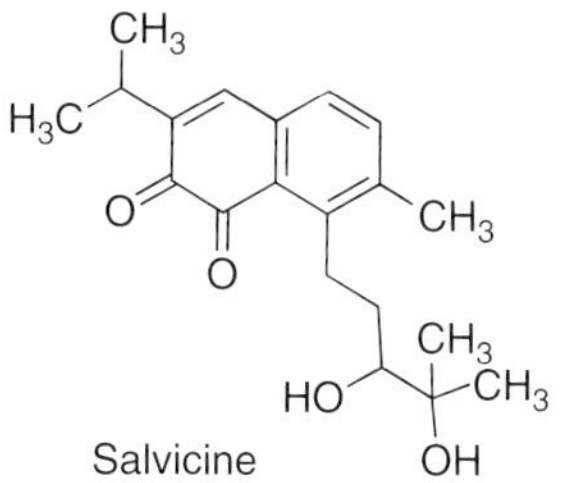

Salvicine

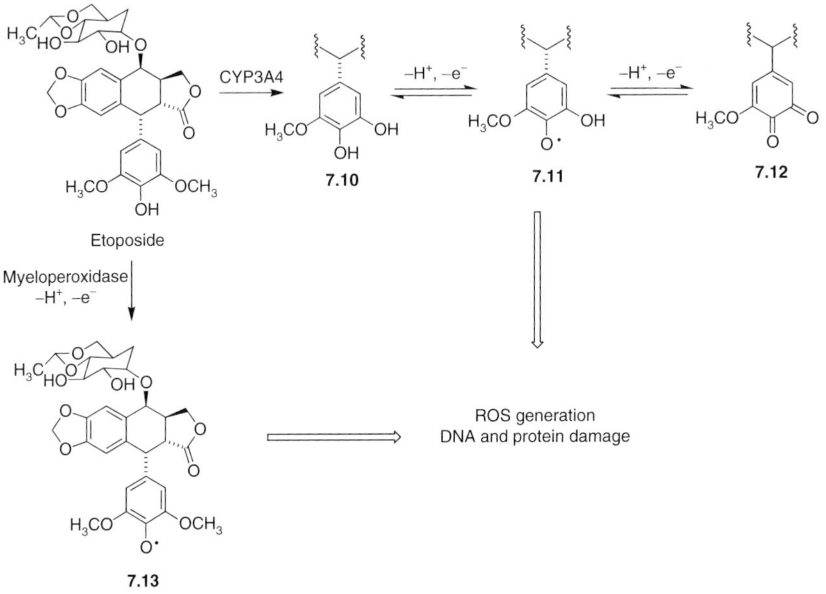

FIGURE 7.13   Reactive species generated in etoposide metabolism.

Salvicine inhibits the catalytic activity of topoisomerase II with weak DNA cleavage action in contrast to the classic topoisomerase II poison etoposide. It stabilizes DNA strand breaks through interactions with the enzyme by trapping the DNA–topoisomerase II complex.[75] Molecular modelling studies predicted that salvicine binds to the ATP pocket in the ATPase domain and superimposes on the phosphate and ribose groups, while competition with ATP was confirmed experimentally.[76]

6. TOPOISOMERASE II CATALYTIC INHIBITORS

This group of topoisomerase II inhibitors differ from topoisomerase poisons in that they do not stabilize the cleavable complex, but act on other steps of the catalytic cycle. Catalytic inhibitors and topoisomerase II poisons can exert synergic or antagonistic effects, depending on the treatment schedule. When cells are treated with high concentrations of drugs for short periods of time, competition is observed between both types of inhibitors because all available enzyme molecules are occupied by one of them, which brings about competition for the other. On the other hand, synergistic effects are observed after continuous exposure of cells to low concentrations of both types of inhibitors because under these conditions not all the available enzyme molecules are occupied by one of the drugs, and some of them are therefore available to the other. These results resemble those observed under clinical conditions and for this reason additive or synergistic effects are normally observed for both types of inhibitors under clinical settings. The therapeutic use of catalytic topoisomerase II inhibitors as anticancer agents is limited to aclarubicin and sobuzoxane.[44]

6.1. Inhibitors of the binding of topoisomerase II to DNA: Aclarubicin

Although most anthracyclines act as specific topoisomerase II poisons, some of them, such as aclarubicin (aclacinomycin A), can act by different mechanisms. This drug is clinically used in the treatment of acute myelocytic leukaemia and it behaves as a strong intercalating agent that prevents the binding of topoisomerase II to DNA and hence as a topoisomerase II catalytic inhibitor. Subsequent studies have shown that aclarubicin is also a topoisomerase I inhibitor at biologically relevant concentrations.[77]

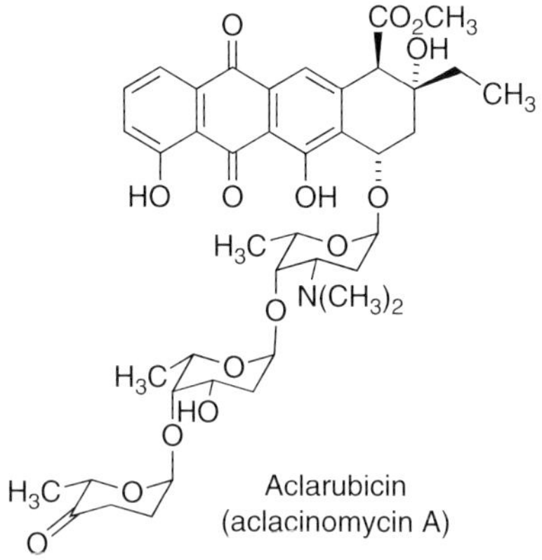

Aclarubicin
(aclacinomycin A)

6.2. Merbarone

Merbarone is a derivative of thiobarbituric acid that was discovered in the course of a study of a large number of barbituric acid analogues by the NCI. This compound has been shown to inhibit the induction of DNA–topoisomerase II cleavable complexes and has been tested clinically against a large number of tumors,[78] although it showed nephrotoxicity and poor anticancer activity.

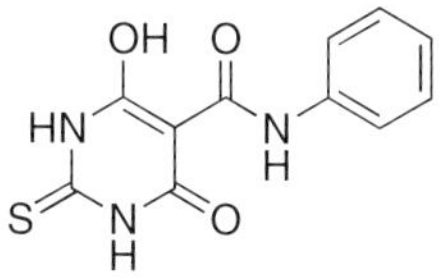

Merbarone

6.3. Bis(dioxopiperazines)

As mentioned in Section 3 of Chapter 4, this class of drugs were introduced as chelating agents, since they behave as pro-drugs to EDTA amides, and are useful as cardioprotectors when associated with anthracyclines. They have subsequently been shown to inhibit topoisomerase II at a point upstream to the formation of the cleavable DNA–enzyme complex by stabilizing the closed-clamp form of topoisomerase II as a post-passage complex. This is achieved by inhibiting the ATPase activity of the enzyme after interaction with its N-terminal domain. The main bis(dioxopiperazines)[79] are shown below.

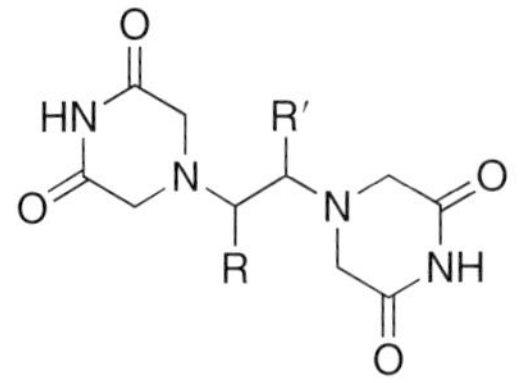

Compound	R	R′
ICRF-154	H	H
ICRF-159 (dexrazoxane)	H	CH₃
ICRF-193	CH₃	CH₃

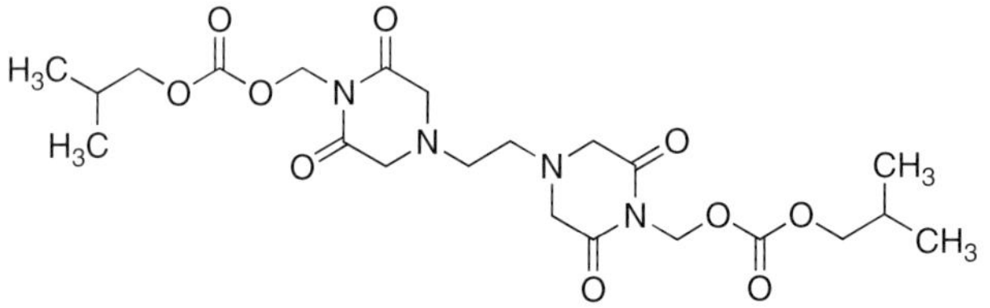

Sobuzoxane (MST-16)

7. SPECIFIC TOPOISOMERASE I INHIBITORS

Compounds that inhibit topoisomerase I can be divided into following two categories:[80]

a. Topoisomerase I suppressors, which are those compounds that inhibit the enzyme but do not stabilize the intermediate DNA–topoisomerase I covalent complex.

b. Topoisomerase I poisons, which act after DNA cleavage by inhibiting religation. This can be achieved through three different mechanisms, involving (1) binding of the enzyme to the previously formed drug–DNA binary complex, (2) recognition of the enzyme–DNA binary complex by the drug, and (3) interaction of DNA with the drug–enzyme complex.[81]

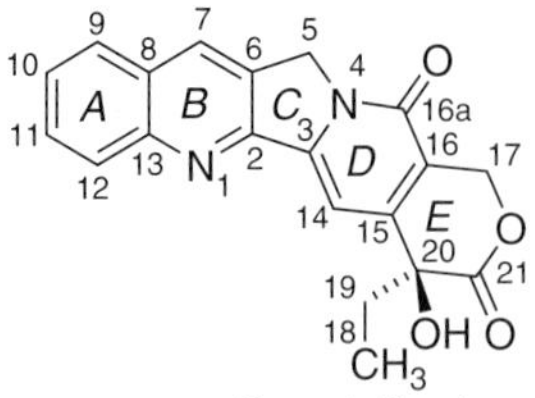

Camptothecin

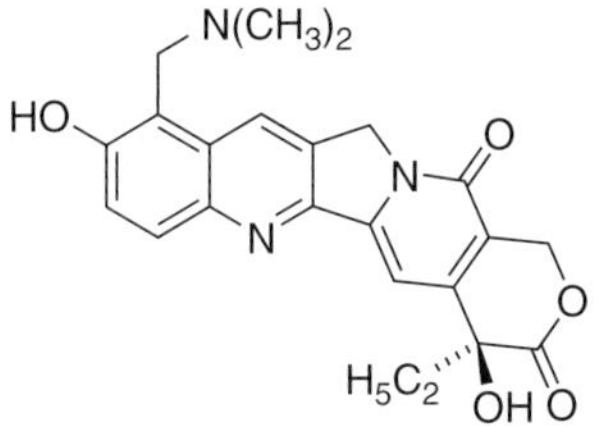

Topotecan

7.1. Camptothecins

Topoisomerase I was validated as a target for cancer chemotherapy when it was identified as the sole target of camptothecin (CPT). This compound was isolated in 1966 from the Chinese tree *Camptotheca acuminata* and its therapeutic development was initially limited by its poor solubility and unacceptable toxicity. The identification of topoisomerase I as its target prompted the search for water-soluble, more active, less toxic analogues. Structure–activity relationship studies showed that substituents at ring A and at the C-7 position of ring B were allowed, whereas the ring E lactone was essential for activity. Two of these compounds are widely used in the clinic, namely topotecan for the treatment of fluoropyrimidine-refractory ovarian and small cell lung cancers[82] and irinotecan (CPT-11). Irinotecan is a prodrug that needs to be hydrolysed by carboxylesterase[83] to its active metabolite SN-38 (Fig. 7.14). It is used in colorectal cancer, showing synergism with cisplatin,[84] and several studies have underscored the importance of pharmacogenetic considerations in its clinical application.[85]

Other second-generation CPT analogues (e.g. lurtotecan, rubitecan,[86] exatecan,[87] gimatecan, karenitecin) are currently undergoing clinical trials[88,89] and belotecan (CKD-602) has been recently launched for the treatment of ovarian and small cell lung cancer.[90] These topoisomerase I targeted drugs are S-phase specific and therefore adequate for tumors with a high proportion of proliferating cells but unsuitable for those tumors that have high numbers of non-cycling cells in the G1 phase, such as prostate and kidney cancer.

These drugs share the unstable six-membered lactone ring of CPT, which is essential for activity. This ring is rapidly converted under physiological conditions into the inactive hydroxyacid, which readily binds to serum albumin and thus becomes unavailable to cells (Fig. 7.15).[91] The higher activity of topotecan and irinotecan with regard to CPT has been attributed to interference of their substituents with binding to albumin.[92] Homocamptothecins,[93] with a seven-membered lactone ring, have enhanced plasma stability and reinforced inhibition of topoisomerase I compared with conventional six-membered CPTs. The most promising of these compounds are elomotecan and diflomotecan, which are undergoing clinical trials for colon, breast, and prostate cancer and lung cancer, respectively.[94]

CPT and its analogues act as topoisomerase poisons by targeting the cleavable DNA–topoisomerase I complex, as shown for the cases of CPT[95,96] and

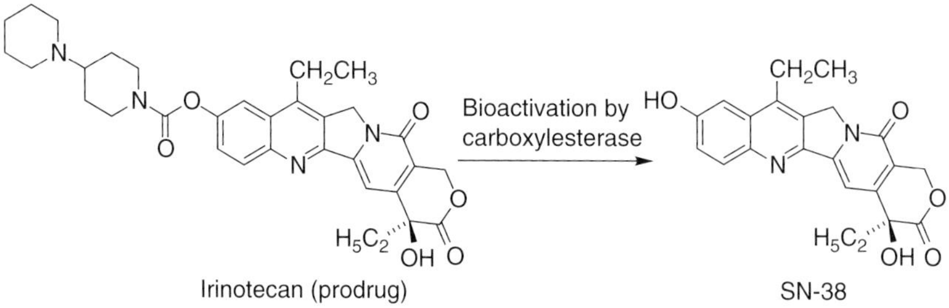

FIGURE 7.14 Bioactivation of irinotecan.

topotecan.[97] The high stability of the cleavable complex is essential for antitumor activity and is due to the unfavourable activation entropy of the reversal process.

A model of this complex has been proposed, based on protein–DNA and protein–drug–DNA crystal structures, where most of the CPT molecule is included in the protein–DNA complex while the region of the C_7-C_{10} positions is outside, associated with water molecules from the first hydration layer of the DNA–topoisomerase I complex. The ternary complex corresponding to topotecan is shown in Fig. 7.16.[98,99]

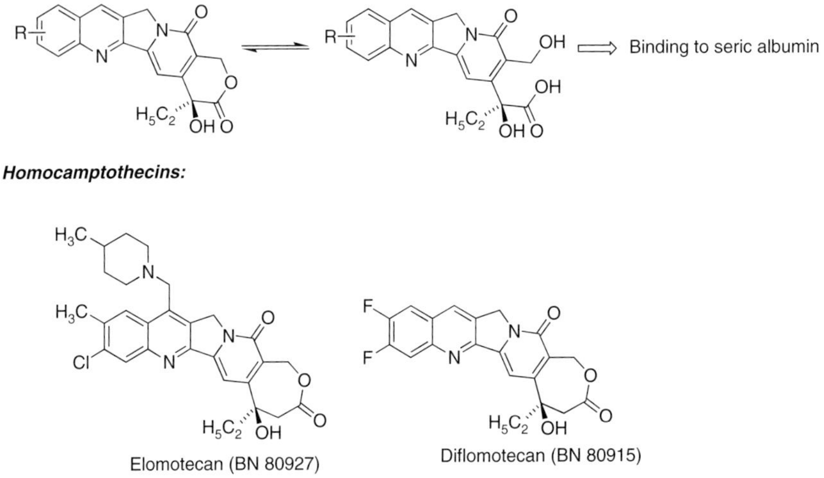

Homocamptothecins:

Elomotecan (BN 80927)   Diflomotecan (BN 80915)

FIGURE 7.15   Basis for the design of homocaptohecins.

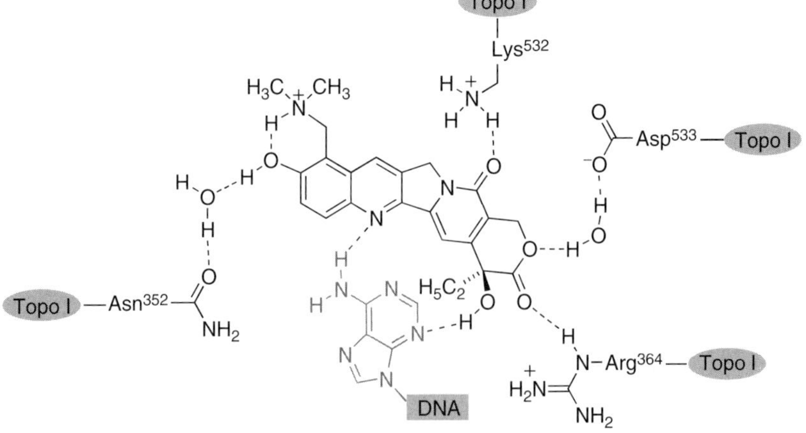

FIGURE 7.16   Key interactions in the topotecan-DNA-topo I complez.

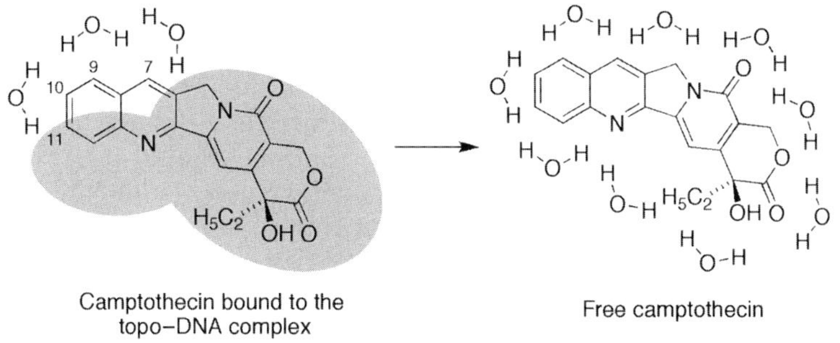

Camptothecin bound to the
topo–DNA complex

Free camptothecin

FIGURE 7.17   Unfavourable activation entropy for the dissociation of the camptothecin ternary complex.

In this model, the very high activation entropy associated with the reversal process is due to the need for the CPT derivative to accumulate an ordered layer of water molecules around itself, as shown in Fig. 7.17 for the case of CPT.[100]

7.2. Non-CPT topoisomerase I inhibitors

Indolocarbazoles are the more advanced class of non-CPT topoisomerase I inhibitors.[101] This ring system is present in several structurally related families of compounds that can target DNA, topoisomerase I, and several protein kinases.[102] The first of these compounds was staurosporine, a natural product originally isolated in 1977 from *S. staurosporeus* that has a wide range of biological activities but is best known as an ATP-competitive kinase inhibitor. The related UCN-01, also a natural product isolated from *Streptomyces* cultures, is currently undergoing clinical studies as an antitumor agent and will be studied in Chapter 9.[103]

Rebeccamycin is also a natural product, isolated from the actinomycete *Saccharothrix aerocolonigenes*, with a dual topoisomerase I and II inhibiting activity. This compound showed an impressive cytotoxicity *in vitro* but could not be further developed because of poor water solubility. Among the many water-soluble rebeccamycin analogues that have been developed, compound NSC-655649 (BMY-27557–14, XL-119) has entered Phase II clinical trials for renal cancer.[104] Interestingly, the presence of the aminoethyl side chain in this compound led to specific topoisomerase II inhibitory activity.

NB-506 has been characterized as a topoisomerase I inhibitor that enhances DNA cleavage mediated by this enzyme. Since it shows cross-resistance with CPT, it has been suggested that they share a common binding site in the topoisomerase I–DNA complex, although NB-506 probably targets other additional cellular processes.[105] Although this compound is an intercalating agent, intercalation is apparently not required to stabilize the topoisomerase I–DNA complex, and in fact a regioisomer of NB-506 without capacity to intercalate into DNA is an extremely potent topoisomerase I poison.[106] Clinical studies on NB-

506 started in 1994, and it has shown a particular good activity in ovarian and breast cancer. The related hydroxy derivative J-107088 is more active *in vitro* than NB-506 or CPT in the induction of topoisomerase I cleavage complexes.[107] This compound is being studied clinically and has shown potent activity against lung and prostate cancers, and a wider therapeutic window than many established drugs.[108] Its glycoside edotecarin has shown activity in clinical trials for colon, breast, and other cancers. The larger size of the imide nitrogen substituent hampers imide ring opening and glucuronidation and leads to an increased half-life.

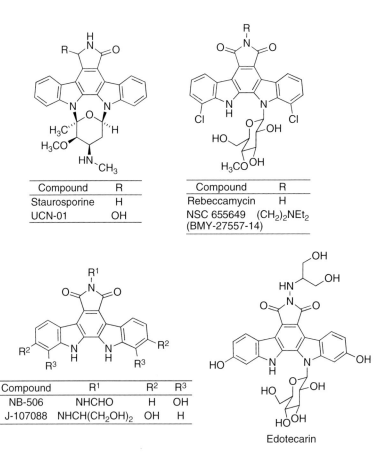

Compound	R
Staurosporine	H
UCN-01	OH

Compound	R
Rebeccamycin	H
NSC 655649 (BMY-27557-14)	(CH$_2$)$_2$NEt$_2$

Compound	R^1	R^2	R^3
NB-506	NHCHO	H	OH
J-107088	NHCH(CH$_2$OH)$_2$	OH	H

Edotecarin

Another promising class of topoisomerase I inhibitors are the lamellarins,[109] isolated from marine organisms such as mollusks from the *Lamellaria* genus and *Didemnum* ascidians. The lamellarins are weak intercalating agents, although their cationic derivatives are more potent in this regard, as expected; nevertheless, no correlation exists in these compounds between their intercalating activity and their cytotoxicity. Several members of the family, especially lamellarin I, reverse MDR by direct inhibition of the P-gp-mediated efflux.[110] This pharmacological profile opens the possibility of their use as antitumor agents in resistant cells as well as using them as modulators of the MDR phenotype in combination with other antitumor compounds.

Lamellarin D, one of the most potent compounds of the series, promotes DNA cleavage through statilization of DNA–topoisomerase I cleavable complexes.[111] Since it displays potent cytotoxic activities against multi-drug-resistant tumor cell lines and is highly cytotoxic to prostate cancer cells, it is being considered for clinical development, together with other analogues. Structure–activity relationship studies in the lamellarins[112] showed little tolerance towards changes in the substitution pattern in the natural products and underscored the importance of the methoxy and hydroxyl groups. A molecular modelling study of the binding of lamellarin D to the DNA–topoisomerase I complex has revealed the presence of hydrogen bonding interactions of the hydroxyls at C-8 and C-20 with the Glu-356 and Asn-722 residues of the enzyme.[113]

Topoisomerase I is probably not the only target of the lamellarins, as deduced from cross-resistance studies with CPT.

Lamellarin D

REFERENCES

1. Graves, D. E., and Velea, L. M. (2000). *Curr. Org. Chem.* **4**, 915.
2. Berman, H. M., and Young, P. R. (1981). *Annu. Rev. Biophys. Bioeng.* **10**, 87.
3. Gago, F. (1998). *Methods* **14**, 277.
4. Kapur, A., Beck, J. L., and Sheil, M. M. (1999). *Rapid Commun. Mass Spectrom.* **13**, 2489.
5. Braña, M. F., Cacho, M., Gradillas, A., de Pascual-Teresa, B., and Ramos, A. (2001). *Curr. Pharm. Des.* **7**, 1745.
6. Garbett, N. C., and Graves, D. E. (2004). *Curr. Med. Chem. Anticancer Agents* **4**, 149.
7. Stiborová, M., Breuer, A., Aimová, D., Stiborová-Rupertová, M., Wiessler, M., and Frei, E. (2003). *Int. J. Cancer* **107**, 885.
8. Auclair, C., and Paoletti, C. (1981). *J. Med. Chem.* **24**, 289.
9. Stiborová, M., Sejbal, J., Borek-Dohalská, L., Aimová, D., Poljaková, J., Forsterová, K., Rupertová, M., Wiesner, J., Husecek, J., Wiessler, M., and Frei, E. (2004). *Cancer Res.* **64**, 8374.
10. Auclair, C. (1987). *Arch. Biochem. Biophys.* **259**, 1.
11. Awada, A., Giacchetti, S., Gerard, B., Eftekhary, P., Lucas, C., De Valeriola, D., Poullain, M. G., Soudon, J., Dosquet, C., Brillanceau, M.-H., Giroux, B., Marty, M., *et al.* (2002). *Ann. Oncol.* **13**, 1925.
12. Poddevin, B., Riou, J. F., Lavelle, F., and Pommier, Y. (1993). *Mol. Pharmacol.* **44**, 767.
13. Nabiev, I., Chourpa, I., Riou, J. F., Nguyen, C. H., Lavelle, F., and Manfait, M. (1994). *Biochemistry* **33**, 9013.
14. Abigerges, D., Armand, J. P., Chabot, G. G., Bruno, R., Bissery, M. C., Bayssas, M., Klink-Alakl, M., Clavel, M., and Catimel, G. (1996). *Anticancer Drugs* **7**, 166.
15. Gallego, J., Ortiz, A. R., de Pascual-Teresa, B., and Gago, F. (1997). *J. Comput. Aided Mol. Des.* **11**, 114.

98. Kerrigan, J. E., and Pilch, D. S. (2001). *Biochemistry* **40,** 9792.
99. Stewart, L., Staker, B., Hjerrild, K., Burgin, A., and Kim, H. (2001). *Proc. Am. Assoc. Cancer Res.* **42,** 80.
100. Wadkins, R. M., Bearss, D., Manikumar, G., Wani, M. C., Wall, M. E., and Von Hoff, D. D. (2004). *Curr. Med. Chem. Anticancer Agents* **4,** 327.
101. Meng, L., Liao, Z., and Pommier, Y. (2003). *Curr. Top. Med. Chem.* **3,** 305.
102. Prudhomme, M. (2004). *Curr. Med. Chem. Anticancer Agents* **4,** 509.
103. Ruegg, U. T., and Burgess, G. M. (1989). *Trends Pharmacol. Sci.* **10,** 218.
104. Goel, S., Wadler, S., Hoffman, A., Volterra, F., Baker, C., Nazario, E., Ivy, P., Silverman, A., and Mani, S. (2003). *Invest. New Drugs* **21,** 103.
105. Urasaki, Y., Laco, G., Takebayashi, Y., Bailly, C., Kohlhagen, G., and Pommier, Y. (2001). *Cancer Res.* **61,** 504.
106. Bailly, C., Dassonneville, L., Colson, P., Houssier, C., Fukasawa, K., Nishimura, S., and Yoshinari, T. (1999). *Cancer Res.* **59,** 2853.
107. Yoshinari, T., Ohkubo, M., Fukasawa, K., Egashira, S., Hara, Y., Matsumoto, M., Nakai, K., Arakawa, H., Morishima, H., and Nishimura, S. (1999). *Cancer Res.* **59,** 4271.
108. Ohkubo, M., Nishimura, T., Honma, T., Nishimura, I., Ito, S., Yoshinari, T., Suda, H. A., Morishima, H., and Nishimura, S. (1999). *Bioorg. Med. Chem. Lett.* **9,** 3307.
109. Bailly, C. (2004). *Curr. Med. Chem. Anticancer Agents* **4,** 363.
110. Quesada, A. R., García-Grávalos, M. D., and Fernández-Puentes, J. L. (1996). *Br. J. Cancer* **74,** 677.
111. Facompré, M., Tardy, C., Bal-Mahieu, C., Colson, P., Pérez, C., Manzanares, I., Cuevas, C., and Bailly, C. (2003). *Cancer Res.* **63,** 7392.
112. Ishibashi, F., Tanabe, S., Oda, T., and Iwao, M. (2002). *J. Nat. Prod.* **65,** 500.
113. Marco, E., Laine, W., Tardy, C., Lansieaux, A., Iwao, M., Ishibashi, F., Bailly, C., and Gago, F. (2005). *J. Med. Chem.* **48,** 3796.

CHAPTER 8

Anticancer Drugs Targeting Tubulin and Microtubules

Contents

1.	Introduction	229
2.	Drugs That Inhibit Microtubule Polymerization at High Concentrations	231
	2.1. Compounds binding at the *Vinca* site	231
	2.2. Compounds binding at the colchicine site	236
3.	Microtubule-Stabilizing Agents: Compounds Binding at the Taxane Site	237
	3.1. Taxanes	237
	3.2. Epothilones	241
	3.3. Miscellaneous marine compounds that bind to the taxane site	243
4.	Miscellaneous Anticancer Drugs Acting on Novel Sites on Tubuline	245
5.	Antivascular Effects of Microtubule-Targeted Agents	245
6.	Mitotic Kinesin Inhibitors	246
	References	247

1. INTRODUCTION

Microtubules are filamentous intracellular structures that are responsible for several aspects of the cell morphology since they form the cytoskeleton in eukaryotic cells and are also responsible for various kinds of cell movements because they are part of the cilia and flagella.

Microtubules are hollow structures formed by 13 parallel protofilaments that grow and shorten by the reversible, noncovalent addition of tubulin dimers at their ends. Tubulin is a protein that contains two subunits called α and β in a head to tail arrangement. Microtubules and free tubulin dimers are involved in a highly dynamic equilibrium, which is very sensitive to external factors (Fig. 8.1).

Medicinal Chemistry of Anticancer Drugs
DOI: 10.1016/B978-0-444-52824-7.00008-1

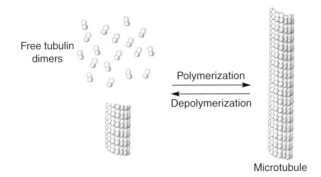

FIGURE 8.1 Dynamic equilibrium between microtubules and tubulin dimers.

A very important structure generated from microtubules is the mitotic spindle, used by eukaryotic cells to segregate their chromosomes correctly during cell division and allow the transfer of the chromosomes of the original cell to the daughter cells. During cell division, microtubules in the cytoplasmic network depolymerize, and the tubulin thus liberated is again polymerized to give the mitotic spindle.

Several important antitumor drugs exert their action by disrupting these equilibria, either by binding to tubulin and inhibiting polymerization or by binding to the microtubules and inhibiting depolymerization by stabilizing them.[1,2] This leads to inhibition of the formation of the mitotic spindle and therefore these compounds behave as antimitotic agents.

Microtubules are the main target of cytotoxic natural products, and most of the drugs discussed in this chapter have been discovered in large-scale screens of natural materials. These compounds are highly successful in cancer treatment,[3] and it has been argued that microtubules represent the best known cancer target.

Drugs acting on microtubules bind to several sites of tubulin and at different positions of the microtubules but they all suppress microtubule dynamics, thereby blocking mitosis at the metaphase/anaphase transition and inducing cell death. The spindle microtubules are much more dynamic than the cytoskeletal ones, and exchange their tubulin units with the soluble pools with half-times of about 15 s, explaining why drugs that interfere with microtubule dynamics are so effective against dividing cells.

Based on their behavior at high concentrations, antitumor drugs acting on microtubules have been traditionally classified into two groups: (1) drugs that inhibit microtubule polymerization (microtubule-destabilizing agents) and (2) drugs that stimulate microtubule polymerization (microtubule-stabilizing agents). Although we will adopt this time-sanctioned classification for organizing this chapter, it is probably overly simplistic as it has been recently shown that at low concentrations both types of drugs act similarly by stabilizing spindle microtubule dynamics.[4,5]

An interesting feature of drugs acting on microtubules is the synergistic effects that can often be found among them that potentially allow their combination, avoiding high doses of any individual drug.

2. DRUGS THAT INHIBIT MICROTUBULE POLYMERIZATION AT HIGH CONCENTRATIONS

There are three main binding sites of drugs to tubulin, which are designed according to their best known ligands as the *Vinca*, colchicine, and taxol sites. For some of them, further research has uncovered the existence of different subsites corresponding to different ligand-structural families.

2.1. Compounds binding at the *Vinca* site

2.1.1. *Vinca* alkaloids and their synthetic analogs

Vincristine and vinblastine are complex molecules produced by the leaves of the rosy periwinkle plant *Catharanthus roseus* (*Vinca rosea*), whose potent cytotoxicity was discovered in 1958. They were introduced in cancer chemotherapy in the late 1960s and remain in widespread clinical usage to this day. Despite their very similar structures and common mechanism of action, they have widely different toxicological properties and antitumor spectra. Thus, vinblastine is currently used in the treatment of Hodgkin's disease and metastatic testicular tumors, where it is combined with bleomycin and cisplatin, while vincristine is used in the treatment of leukemia and lymphomas.

Several semisynthetic analogs of these alkaloids[6] are also in clinical use, most notably vindesine, used mainly to treat melanoma and lung carcinomas and, associated with other drugs, to treat uterine cancers, and the nor-derivative vinorelbine, used for non-small cell lung cancer, metastatic breast cancer, and ovarian cancer. The fluorinated analog vinflunine is in clinical development.[7]

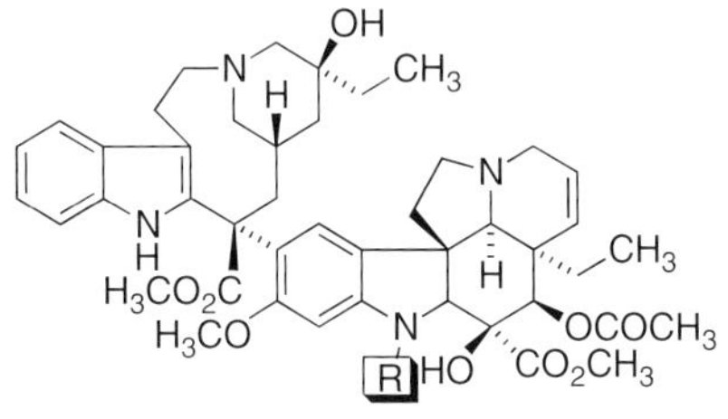

R = CHO Vincristine
R = CH₃ Vinblastine

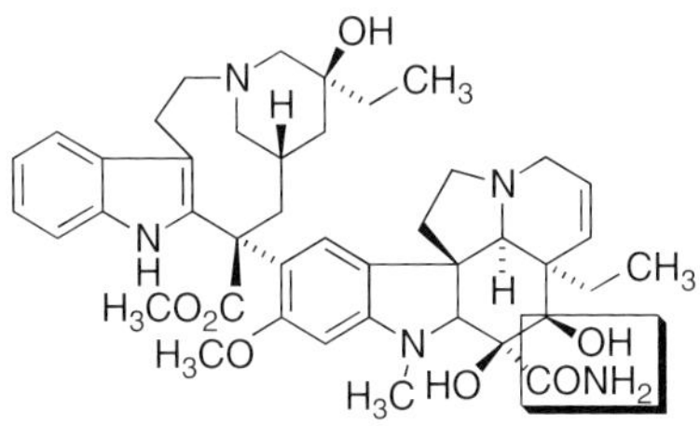

Vindesine

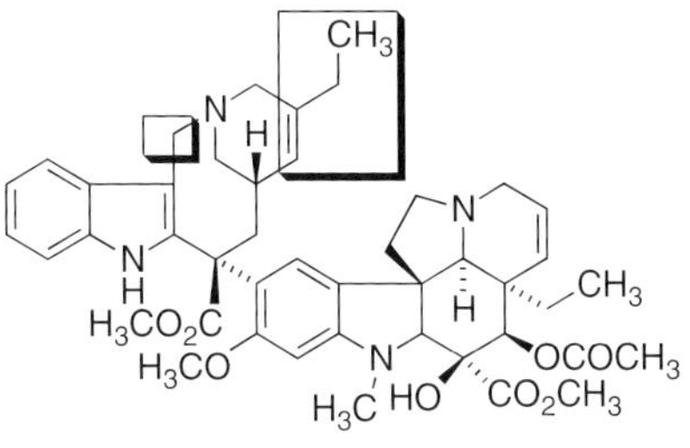

Vinorelbine

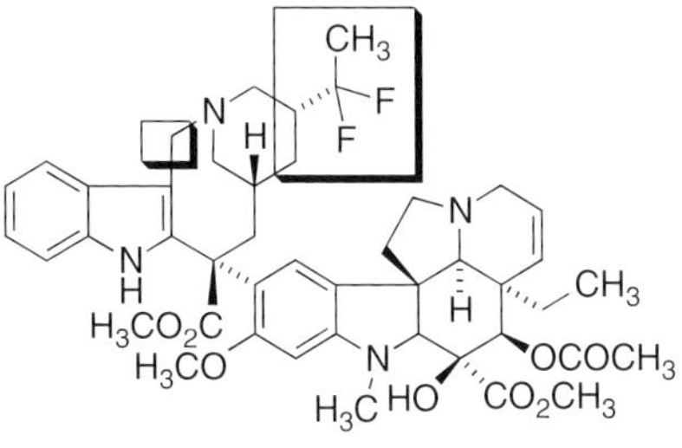

Vinflunine

The *Vinca* alkaloids specifically block cells in mitosis with metaphase arrest, and hence are antimitotic drugs. Their biological activity is explained by their specific binding to the β subunit of tubulin dimers, in a region called the *Vinca* domain. Binding is fast and reversible, but it induces a conformational change in tubulin, increasing its affinity for itself and leading to the formation of paracrystalline aggregates. This decreases the pool of free tubulin dimers available for microtubule assembly, resulting in a shift of the equilibrium toward disassembly and microtubule shrinkage. These phenomena result in microtubule depolymerization and destruction of the mitotic spindles, as verified in HeLa cells at high (10–100 nM) concentrations (Fig. 8.2). As a consequence, dividing cells are blocked in mitosis with condensed chromosomes.

The mechanism described above led to the *Vinca* alkaloids being thought for many years to act solely as microtubule-depolymerizing agents. However, recent observations have shown that, at concentrations that are low but clinically relevant (0.8 nM in HeLa cells), the spindle microtubules are not depolymerized but mitosis is still blocked and cells die by apoptosis. This suggests that the block is due to suppression of microtubule dynamics rather than to microtubule depolymerization.

One of the drawbacks of *Vinca* alkaloids and their analogs is their neurotoxicity, which is probably related to the fact that microtubules are a key component of neurons. Another problem associated with the use of *Vinca* alkaloids is the easy development of resistance, normally mediated by the overexpression of the Pgp-170 transport protein (see Chapter 12).

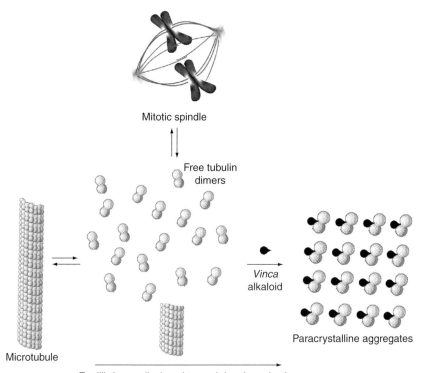

FIGURE 8.2 Depoymerization of microtubules following binding of *Vinca* alkaloids.

2.1.2. Marine natural products binding at the *Vinca* domain and their analogs

Marine organisms are a rich source of antitumor compounds that have probably evolved as defense mechanisms in the highly competitive marine environment. Many of these compounds are in advanced preclinical or clinical stage of development.[8] Those acting on microtubules by binding at the *Vinca* domain include the halichondrins, the dolastatins, the hemiasterlins, the cryptophycins, and the spongistatins, among others.

Halichondrin B is a complex polyether macrolide isolated from the marine sponge *Halichondria okadai*, with an extraordinarily high potency as an antitumor agent and a high therapeutic index. Although its scarcity in natural sources has hampered efforts to develop halichondrin B as a new anticancer drug, the existence of a route allowing its total synthesis[9] has paved the way for the preparation of structurally simpler analogs that retain the remarkable potency of the parent compound, specially the closely related E7389 (ER0865) and ER-086526.[10] Besides the deletion of a large region of the molecule, the readily biodegradable lactone group in the natural compounds has been replaced with a ketone. Although available evidence points to a mechanism of action involving tubulin binding and microtubule depolymerization, the reasons for the high potency and broad therapeutic indexes of these compounds are unclear. The more active of the synthetic compounds, E-7389, is under clinical trials for breast[11] and prostate[12] cancers.

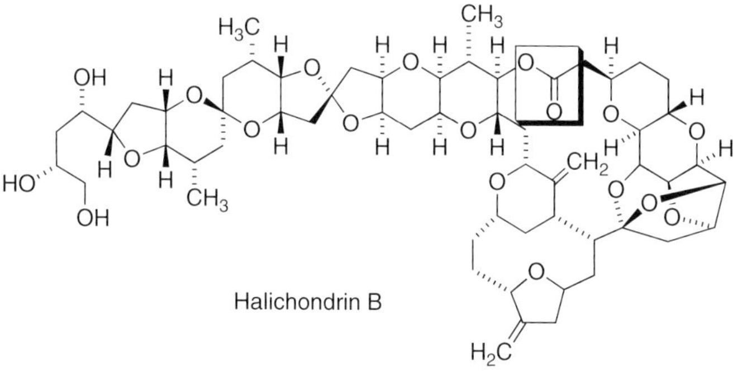

Halichondrin B

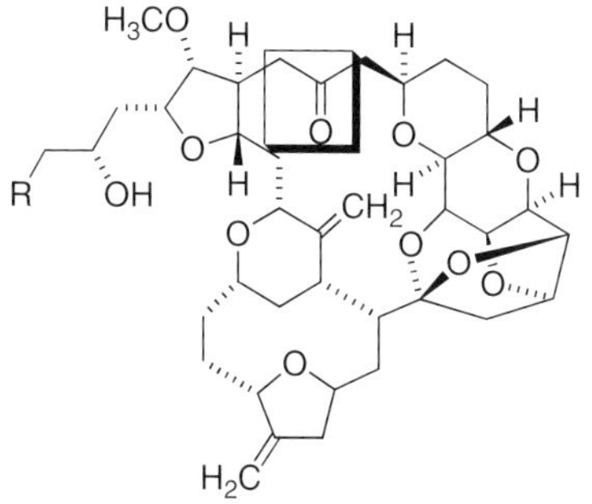

R = NH$_2$ E7389 (ER-086526)
R = OH   ER-076349

Dolastatin 10, a linear peptide, was isolated in 1987 from an Indian Ocean mollusc, the sea hare *Dolabella auricularia*. Although this compound progressed through to Phase II trials as a single agent, it did not demonstrate significant antitumor activity against prostate cancer[13] or metastatic melanoma.[14] Many synthetic derivatives of the dolastatins have been prepared, among which TZT-1027 (auristatin PE, soblidotin),[15] cemadotin, and synthadotin have entered clinical trials. The latter compound has the advantage of being orally active and seems to be promising for the treatment of non-small lung cell cancer and refractory prostate cancer.[16]

Dolastatin 10 was shown to bind to a site close to the *Vinca* domain where other peptidic agents bound.[17] In connection with this finding, it has recently been shown that the *Vinca* domain in tubulin may be composed of a series of overlapping domains rather than being a single entity, as different levels and types of competition were found when selected tubulin interactive agents were used to investigate the binding characteristics of a tritium-labeled dolastatin probe.[18]

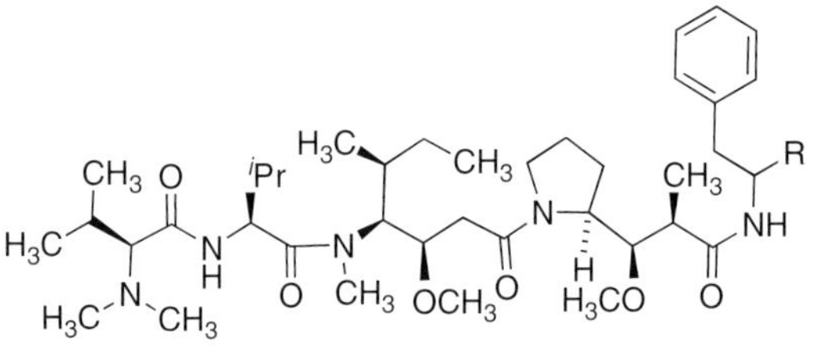

Dolastatin 10 R =

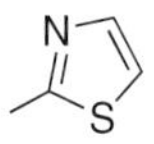

TZT-1027 R = H
(auristatin PE, soblidotin)

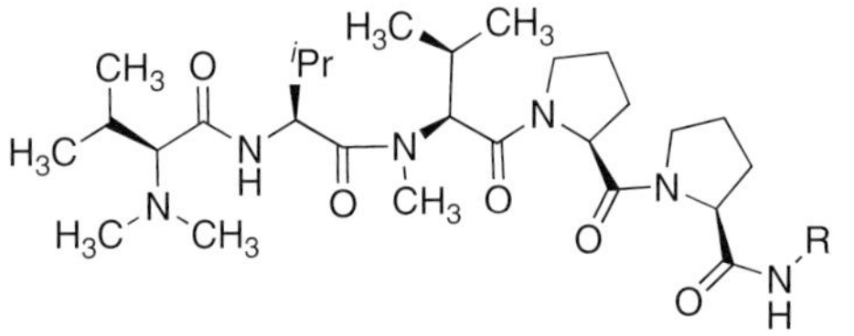

R = PhCH₂ Cemadotin
R = C(CH₃)₃ Synthadotin

Hemiasterlin was originally reported from the South African sponge *Hemiasterella minor*, although it was soon also isolated from sponges of the genus *Cymbastela*, together with the related hemiasterlins A and B. These agents inhibit tubulin assembly and probably bind at the "peptide binding site" shared with the dolastatins and cryptophycins.[19] Many synthetic analogs of the hemiasterlins have also been developed, and HTI-286 is under clinical trials.[20]

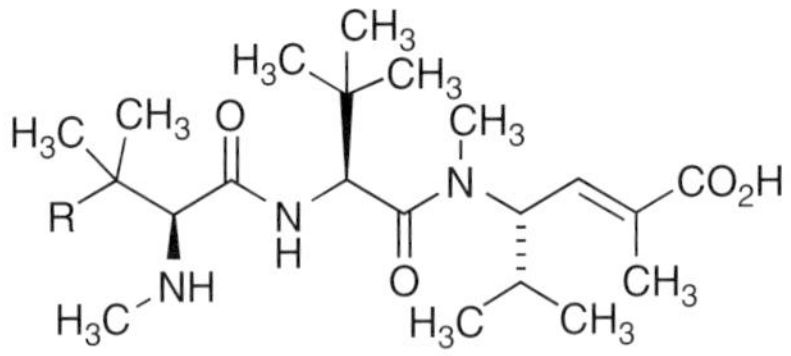

Hemiasterlin R = 1-methyl-3-indolyl
HTI-286 R = Ph

Cryptophycin-1 is a depsipeptide isolated from the cyanobacterium *Nostoc sp.* that was initially described as an antifungal agent[21] and was later shown to have antimitotic and cytotoxic activity. Subsequently many cryptophycins have been isolated and prepared by synthesis, the most important one being cryptophycin 52

(LY-355703), which is in advanced clinical trials for the treatment of solid tumors.[22] The cryptophycins are among the most potent antimitotic agents described, and their binding is very strong and poorly reversible, making them relatively exempt from efflux by the Pgp-170-mediated multidrug (MDR)-resistance mechanism.[23] The somewhat related natural product maytansine 1 is another inhibitor of tubulin polymerization, about 1,000-fold more potent than vincristine. Although its toxicity led to abandoning clinical trials, it is now being considered as a candidate for antibody-drug conjugates (Chapter 11).

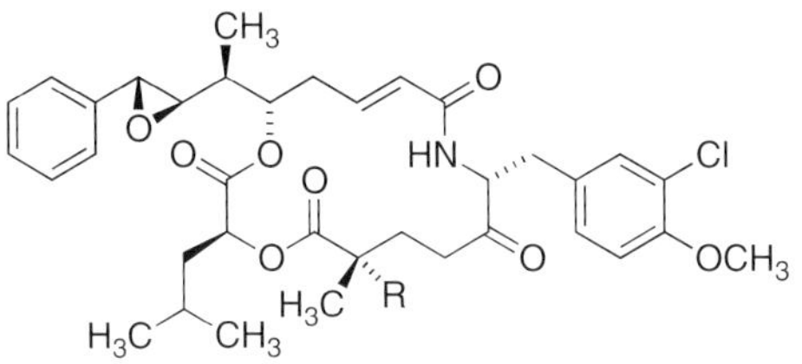

Cryptophycin 1   R = H
Cryptophycin 52   R = CH3
(LY-355703)

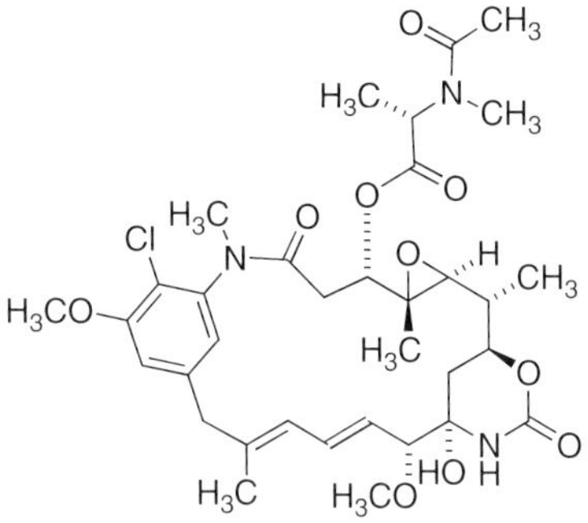

Maytansine 1

Spongistatins are macrocyclic lactones containing six pyran rings, four of which are incorporated into two spiroketal moieties that were isolated from sponges of the *Hytrios* genus. The spongistatins elicit extraordinarily potent (10^{-11} M) cytotoxic responses, especially in solid tumors, and are being examined in Phase I clinical trials.[24] Spongistatin 1 is a noncompetitive inhibitor of the binding of [^{3}H]vinblastine and [^{3}H]dolastatin to tubulin, in contrast to competitive patterns obtained with vincristine versus [^{3}H]vinblastine and with a stereoisomer of dolastatin 10 versus [^{3}H]dolastatin 10. Since dolastatin 10 is itself a noncompetitive inhibitor of *Vinca* alkaloid binding to tubulin, this implies the existence of at least three distinct binding sites in the *Vinca* domain.[25] Molecular modeling studies of the binding of the spongistatins led to the discovery of a hydrophobic pocket containing an unusual cluster of 10 aromatic amino acids, which allowed the rational design of simplified analogues containing a single spiroketal system that are known as SPIKET compounds. One of them, SPIKET-P, inhibited the division of human breast cancer cells at low-nanomolar concentrations.[26]

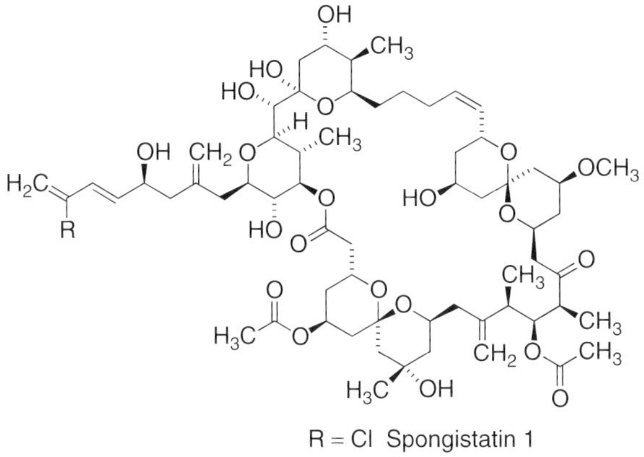

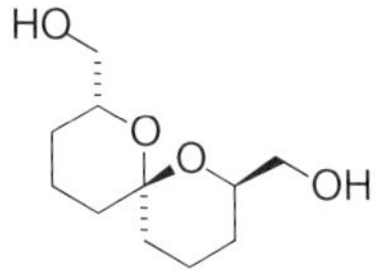

SPIKET-P

R = Cl Spongistatin 1
R = H   Spongistatin 2

2.2. Compounds binding at the colchicine site

The colchicine site is named from the well-known tropolone alkaloid isolated from *Colchicum autumnale*, a plant widely employed in traditional medicine and still used in the treatment of gout. Several compounds binding in the colchicine site, including the combretastatins, 2-methoxyestradiol, and ABT-751, are now under clinical investigation. Besides their antimitotic properties, some of these compounds are receiving much attention because of their vascular actions (Section 5).

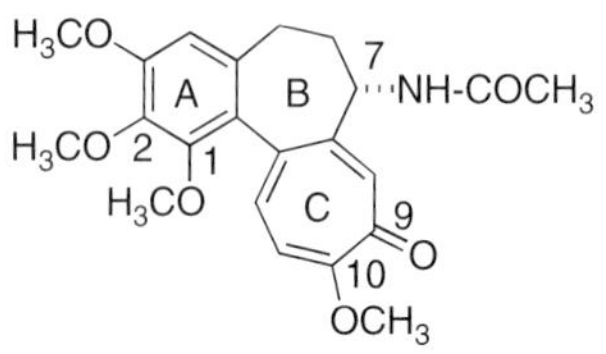

Colchicine 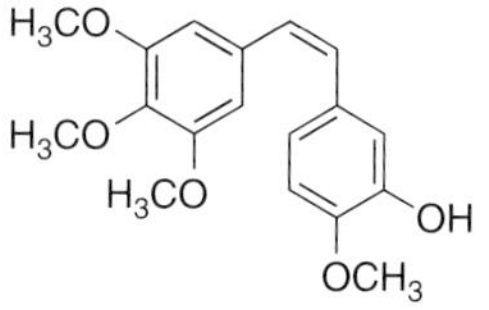   Combretastatin A-4 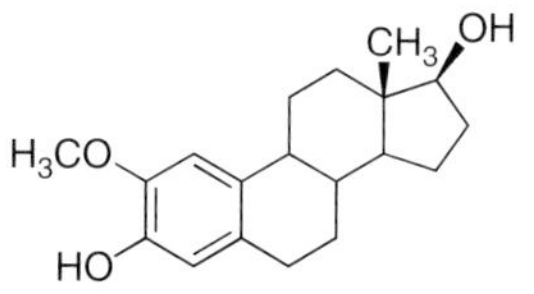   2-Methoxyestradiol

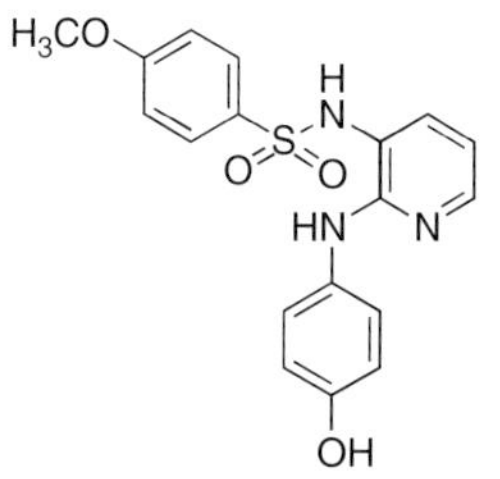

ABT-751 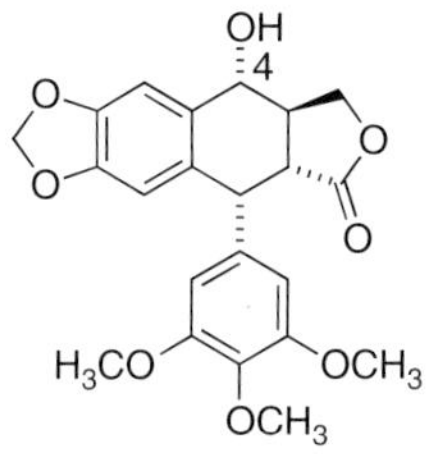   Podophyllotoxin

Colchicine played a fundamental role in studies of mitosis, but it has not found significant use in cancer treatment perhaps because of its toxicity. Similarly to *Vinca* alkaloids, colchicine depolymerizes microtubules at high concentrations and stabilizes microtubule dynamics at low concentrations. It first binds to soluble tubulin, leading to a complex that copolymerizes into the ends of the microtubules and suppresses their dynamics because it binds more tightly to its tubulin neighbors than free tubulin. The structural features required for this binding were elucidated by extensive structure–activity relationships (SAR) studies that showed the importance of the 9-keto function and the methoxy groups at C-1, C-2, and C-10. The 7-acetamido function is not required for binding to tubulin and may be replaced by other substituents, although the stereochemistry of this center is critical for antimitotic activity probably because of the effect of this substituent in the overall conformation of the colchicine molecule. Ring B appears to be responsible for the irreversible nature of colchicine binding to tubulin, although it may also contribute to its toxic effects. Finally, the tropolone ring C may be replaced by a suitably substituted benzene ring with retention of the antimitotic activity.

The combretastatins[27] are natural products isolated from the African willow tree *Combretum caffrum*.[28] They bear structural similarities with colchicine, since both possess a trimethoxyphenyl ring and the aromatic tropone ring of colchicine relates to the isovanillinyl group in the combretastatins. The most active is combretastatin A-4, a very effective antimitotic agent due to its rapid binding to tubulin at the colchicine site. SAR studies showed that the *cis* configuration of its stilbene moiety is a critical structural feature for its activity. Its low water solubility stimulated the preparation of a number of prodrugs,[29] the most studied of which is its 4-*O*-phosphate (CA4P). Combretastatin A-4 and its phosphate have striking vascular effects, which will be discussed in Section 5.

Two other compounds that bind tubulin at the colchicine domain and are undergoing clinical trials are 2-methoxyestradiol, which is being studied for the treatment of solid tumors,[30] and the methoxybenzenesulfonamide derivative ABT-751,[31] investigated in solid tumors and refractory hematological malignancies.[32] The lignan derivative podophyllotoxin, mentioned in Section 5.3 of Chapter 7 as the lead compound in the development of a family of topoisomerase II inhibitors, is also a ligand of the colchicine site.[33] Its tubulin binding is greatly reduced by epimerization at C-4 (epipodophyllotoxin) and completely abolished by the presence of sugar molecules, as found in etoposide.

3. MICROTUBULE-STABILIZING AGENTS: COMPOUNDS BINDING AT THE TAXANE SITE

The primary ligand for this site in tubulin is the natural terpene taxol, although several structurally dissimilar natural products (epothilones, eleutherobin, discodermolide, and others) were found to share the same mechanism of action. Based on extensive SAR studies and molecular modeling, a plausible common pharmacophore for those microtubule-stabilizing agents has been proposed.

3.1. Taxanes

Paclitaxel (taxol) is the most important natural product in cancer chemotherapy and one of the most successful cancer drugs ever produced, being widely employed in the treatment of breast, ovarian, and lung carcinomas. It was isolated from the Pacific yew *Taxus brevifolia*, and its anticancer activity was discovered in the 1960s during a large-scale plant-screening program sponsored by the National Cancer Institute (NCI). Enormous supply problems were found initially because the location of taxol in the bark required to sacrifice the tree to extract it, the concentration of the compound in yew bark is low, its extraction is complex and expensive, and the Pacific yew is a limited resource that grows very slowly. About 4,000 trees were required to provide 360 g of taxol for the early clinical trials, and 38,000 trees were necessary to isolate 25 kg of taxol to treat 12,000 cancer patients after approval of the use of taxol for treating advanced ovarian cancer in 1992. Fortunately, it was subsequently discovered that the twigs and needles of the European yew, *Taxus baccata*, were a high-yielding (1 g/kg) and renewable source of a related compound, 10-deacetylbaccatin III, lacking the C-13 side chain and the C-10 acetyl group, that could be transformed through a relatively simple semisynthetic route into paclitaxel and also into its more soluble and potent analog docetaxel, which was approved for advanced breast cancer in 1996 (Fig. 8.3). Some other suitable baccatin derivatives have been subsequently discovered in different *Taxus* species that can serve as alternative starting materials in the semisynthesis of taxoids. Biotechnological approaches are also being considered.[34]

Paclitaxel arrests cells at the G_2/M stage of the cell cycle by stabilizing the spindle microtubules and thus arresting mitosis. It binds specifically at the 1–31 and the 217–233 sequences of the β-tubulin subunit, at the inner surface of the microtubule lumen, and it shows much higher affinity for tubulin in microtubules than for free tubulin in solution. Paclitaxel also increases the microtubule polymer mass, a phenomenon known as microtubule "bundling."

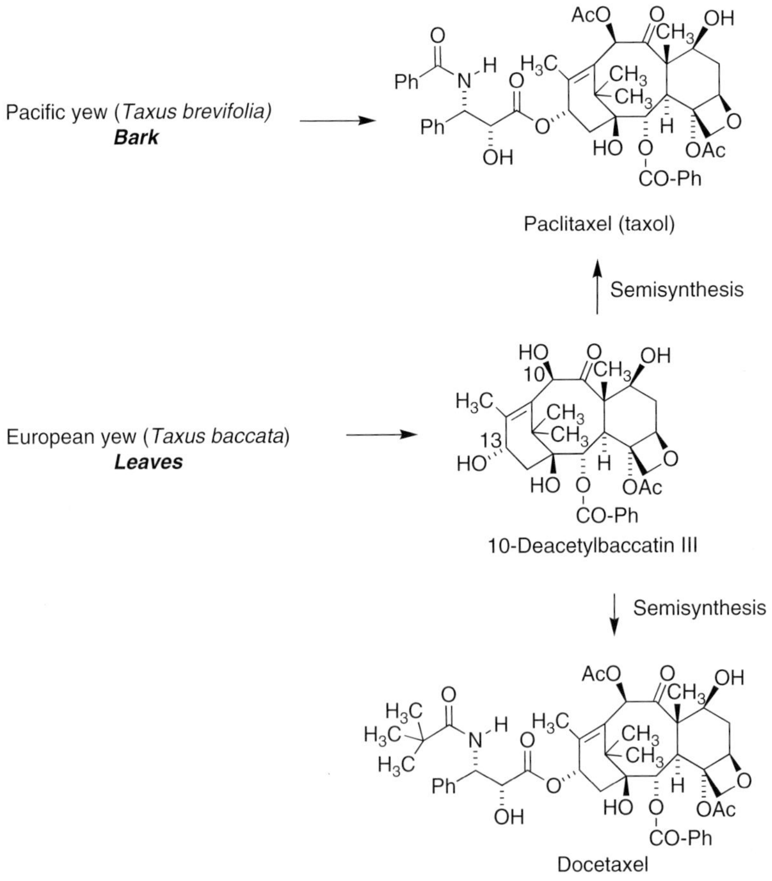

FIGURE 8.3   Semisynthesis of taxanes.

Although paclitaxel and docetaxel are widely used for the therapy of a variety of solid tumors and are being investigated clinically for numerous other cancers, they have some limitations. The main ones are the impossibility of oral administration and the frequent development of resistances mediated by tubulin mutation, leading to weaker interactions, or by overexpression of the Pgp-170 transport pump, leading to efflux from the cell. Another problem is the need to associate them with formulation vehicles to allow their administration. Thus, paclitaxel, very insoluble in water, is generally formulated using polyoxyethylated castor oil (Cremophor EL) while docetaxel, more soluble in water, is formulated using Tween 80 and ethanol. Cremophor EL is responsible for many hypersensitivity reactions and Tween 80, albeit less toxic than Cremophor, may also be responsible of some toxic effects.[35] These problems have stimulated the search for new taxoids, several of which are under clinical evaluation.[36] Among the first-generation analogs, we will mention BMS-188797 and BMS-184476, which have improved pharmacokinetic properties. More substantial variations can be observed in ortataxel, where the aromatic rings of paclitaxel have been replaced by other lipophilic substituents and the hydroxyl at the bridgehead position is part of a cyclic carbonate structure. Ortataxel shows increased potency with respect to paclitaxel and is the first orally active taxoid. Another structurally related, orally active, semisynthetic taxane is BMS-275183. Both ortataxel[37] and BMS-275183[38] have reached clinical trials for solid tumors.

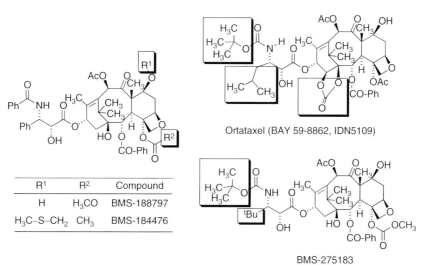

Ortataxel (BAY 59-8862, IDN5109)

BMS-275183

R[1]	R[2]	Compound
H	H_3CO	BMS-188797
$H_3C-S-CH_2$	CH_3	BMS-184476

The large number of taxol analogs that have been synthesized has allowed the establishment of several structure-activity relationships (SAR)[34] that can be summarized as follows:

a. The hydroxyl group **1** is not essential and can be removed, epimerized, or esterified.
b. The oxetane ring **2** (or a small-ring analog) is essential for activity.

c. The presence of acyl substituents **3**, **4**, and **8** is essential. Other acetoxy and benzoyloxy groups present in the natural product may be replaced by other acyls or removed.

d. Removal of the hydroxyl **5** leads only to a slight decrease in activity.

e. A free hydroxyl group in the side chain (**6**) is required. Esterification is possible if the ester group is easily hydrolyzable, leading to a variety of water-soluble and cell-specific paclitaxel prodrugs.

f. The phenyl group at the end of the side chain (**7**), or a close analog, is required for activity.

g. Reduction of the carbonyl **10** leads to slightly improved activity.

  In summary, the northern half of the molecule allows more structural variations than the southern portion. The 2′R-3′S-isoserine side chain is also a key element in the antitubulin activity.

  Structural and molecular modeling studies, as well as the evaluation of conformationally restricted analogs, have been undertaken to explain these SAR. The taxane core has a rigid conformation, and the side chain is the only portion of the molecule with rotational freedom. It can adopt a variety of conformations, two of which were identified as the potential active conformations and differ only in the value of the H2′-C2′-C3′-H3′ dihedral angle. Further research based on electron crystallographic analysis of tubulin sheets has led to evidence showing that taxol adopts a T-shaped conformation when it is bound to tubulin.[39] This binding model has been confirmed by the synthesis of a macrocyclic analog that adopts the T-taxol conformation and is significantly more active than paclitaxel in both cytotoxicity and tubulin polymerization assays.[40] The model is being used in the design of new taxanes.[41]

  The clinical success of taxanes, many of which are under clinical development,[42] has prompted an intensive search for drugs with a related mechanism of action. This search has led to the identification of several families of natural products that bind to the taxane site and share the ability of taxol to promote microtubule assembly and induce mitotic arrest, and will be discussed in Sections 3.2 and 3.3.

3.2. Epothilones

The epothilones A and B (a name derived from its molecular features: epoxide, thiazole, and ketone) are naturally occurring 16-membered macrolides that were isolated in 1993 from the myxobacterium *Sorangium cellulosum* and first employed as agrochemical antifungal agents. In 1995, their taxol-like mechanism of action was discovered,[43] and subsequently they have been shown to have a number of advantages over taxoids, including a higher potency in some cases, activity against taxol-resistant cell lines because they seem to be poor P-170 substrates, higher aqueous solubility, and simpler structures, leading to easier access to analogs.[44,45,46] Epothilone B (EPO906, patupilone) has been granted orphan designation by the European Commission for the treatment of ovarian cancer. Epothilone D, also known as deoxyepothilone B, KOS-862, or NSC-703147, displays a much more promising therapeutic index than epothilone B despite its slightly decreased *in vitro* cytotoxicity,[47] and is under clinical assays as second-line therapy in non-small cell lung cancer.[48] Resistances to epothilone are known, but their mechanism seems to involve mutations in tubulin rather than upregulation of drug efflux pumps.[49]

One of the limitations of the natural epothilones is their metabolic lability, resulting from the easy hydrolysis of their lactone ring by esterases. This led to the design of metabolically more stable lactam analogs, among which ixabepilone (BMS-247550) is under clinical trials in paclitaxel-resistant colorectal, metastatic breast, and non-small-cell lung cancers.[50,51] Although early Phase II data seemed to indicate that ixabepilone and patupilone could be useful in taxane-refractory tumors, this expectation has turned out to be unfounded.

Another limitation of the epothilones is their poor water solubility, which requires their formulation with cosolubilizers. For instance, ixabepilone is formulated in Cremophor, leading to hypersensitivity reactions that require the prophylactic administration of oral histamine blockers.[52] This has stimulated the development of water-soluble analogs like the amino-derivative of epothilone B, known as BMS-310705, which is under clinical assays in patients with advanced solid cancer.[53] Another compound modified at the thiazole substituent is ABJ879, which also shows the replacement of the epoxide oxygen by a methylene group. ABJ879 is slightly more potent than epothilone B or paclitaxel at inducing tubulin polymerization, but much more potent as an antiproliferative agent, and has recently entered clinical studies.[54]

ZK-Epothilone (ZK-EPO) is a promising, fully synthetic epothilone that was designed to overcome MDR resistance.[55] This compound, currently under clinical assays,[56] exhibited significant activity across a broad spectrum of preclinical tumor models, including those resistant to widely used chemotherapeutic agents, because it is not recognized by cellular efflux pumps. It is also more water-soluble than taxanes and does not require a formulating agent such as Cremophor.

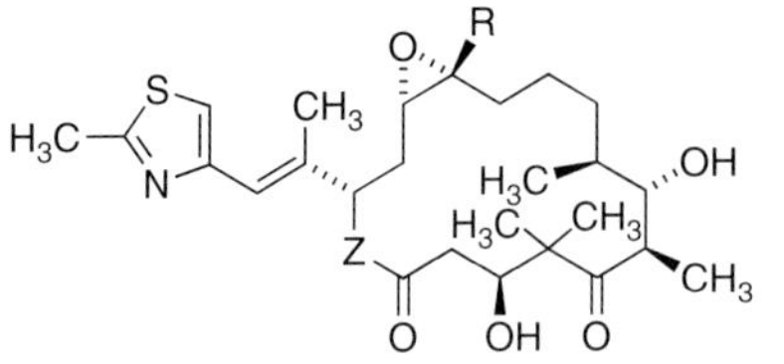

Compound	Z	R
Epothilone A	O	H
Epothilone B (EPO906, patupilone)	O	CH_3
Ixabepilone (BMS-247550)	NH	CH_3

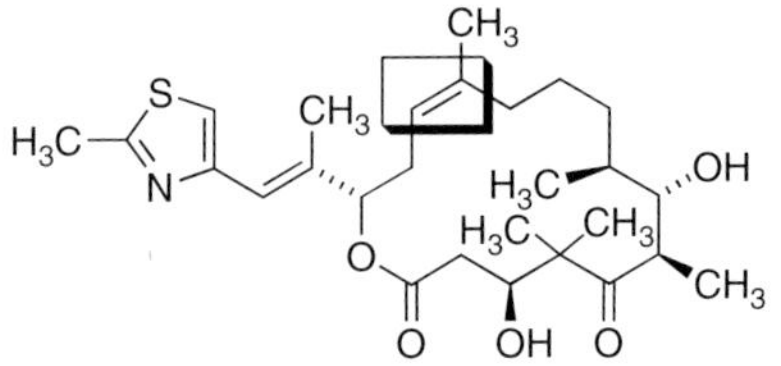

Epothilone D (KOS-862, NSC-703147)

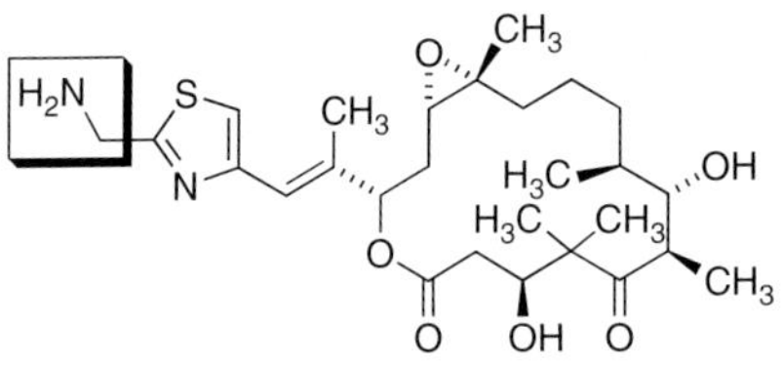

BMS-310705

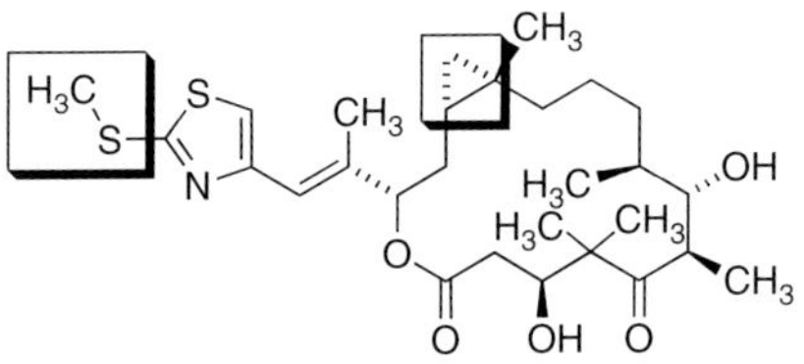

ABJ879

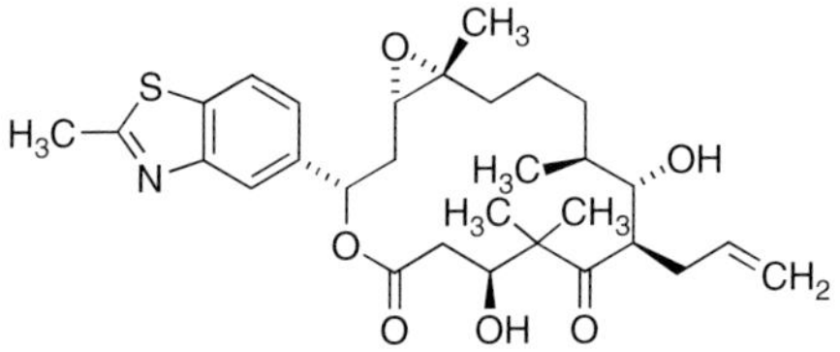

ZK-EPO

Hundreds of epothilone analogs have been prepared using conventional solution chemistry or combinatorial strategies. Their screening has allowed to establish a detailed SAR profile,[49,57,58] which is summarized below:

a. The configuration at the stereocentres C-6, C-8, C-13, and C-15 is important and must be that of the natural products (**1**).

b. The epoxide function is not essential, and it may be replaced by a C_{12}–C_{13} double bond or a cyclopropane ring (**2**). Analogs incorporating a *trans* epoxide or *trans* olefin structure at C_{12}–C_{13} appear to be almost equipotent with the corresponding *cis* isomers.

c. A methyl group at C-12 enhances activity (**3**).

d. Expansion to a 17-membered ring, created by the presence of a *trans* C_{11}–C_{12} double bond and an additional methylene, leads to a compound where antiproliferative activity is substantially maintained (**4**).

e. Z can be O or NH. In the latter case, the molecule is metabolically more stable.

f. A correct location for the nitrogen in the side chain at C-15 is significant for activity. However, the replacement of the thiazole ring either by an oxazole or various pyridine moieties is well tolerated (**6**).

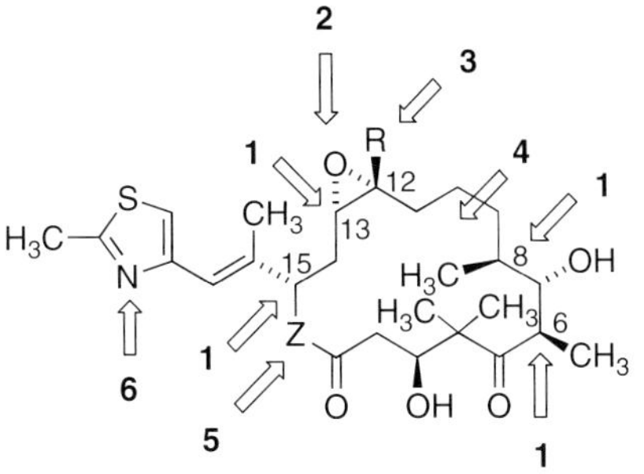

The epothilone binding site in tubulin has been studied by 3D quantitative structure–activity relationship (QSAR) models[59] and by electron crystallography, which has allowed to identify a common binding site on tubulin for paclitaxel, epothilone-A, and eleutherobin.[60] Prior to these studies, a common pharmacophore had been proposed for the taxanes, the epothilones, and the sarcodictyines.[61]

3.3. Miscellaneous marine compounds that bind to the taxane site

Eleutherobin is a natural product isolated from an *Eleutherobia* marine soft coral that is extremely potent for inducing tubulin polymerization *in vitro* and is cytotoxic *in vitro* for cancer cells with an IC_{50} lower than that of paclitaxel.[62] The same as paclitaxel, eleutherobin is a substrate for Pgp and both compounds show cross-resistance in *MDR1*-expressing lines. The related sarcodictyins were also isolated from the mediterranean coral *Sarcodictyon roseum* and seem more promising than eleutherobin, in spite of their lower activities, because of the MDR sensitivity of the latter.

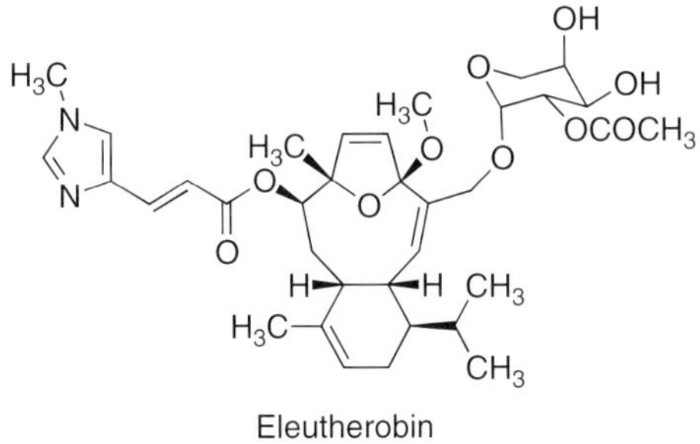

Eleutherobin

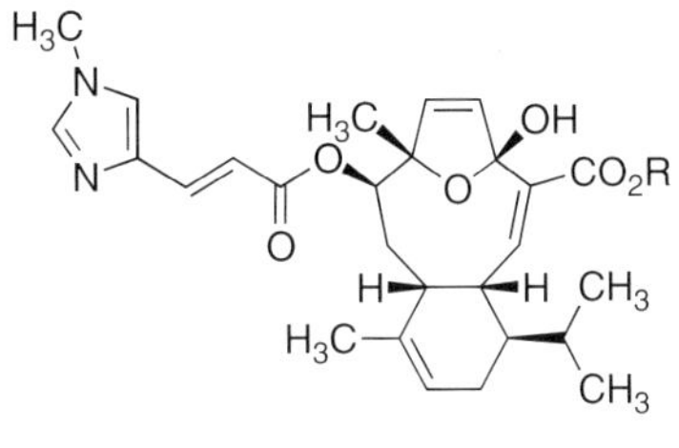

R = CH₃   Sarcodictyin A
R = C₂H₅ Sarcodictyin B

The eleutherobins and sarcodictyins have been extensively modified using conventional and combinatorial chemistry techniques, which have also allowed the formation of hybrid molecules of the two base structures. These studies have led to several conclusions regarding their structure-activity relationships.[44,63]

a. The side chain is essential for activity. Both nitrogen atoms of the imidazole ring are important (**1**).
b. Both OH (hemiketal) and OCH_3 (ketal) R^1 groups are tolerated, with little difference in activity.
c. In eleutherobin, removal or modification of the sugar moiety (R^2) alters the cytotoxicity and resistance pattern. In the sarcodictyins, esters are more active than amides (**3**).

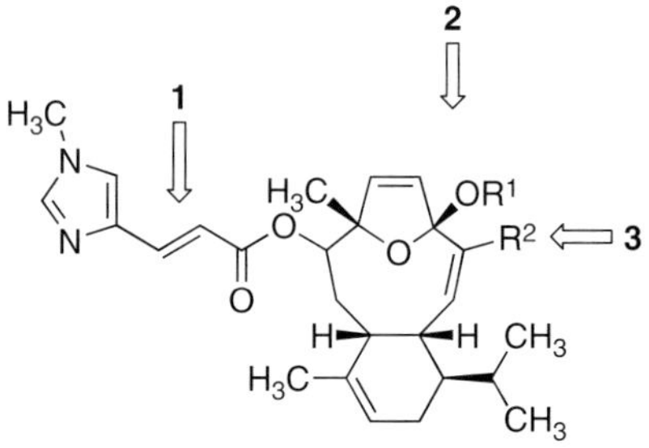

Discodermolide is a polyketide from the sponge *Discodermia dissoluta* with a mechanism of action similar to both paclitaxel and the epothilones. Discodermolide has several promising features such as its broad-spectrum antitumor activity, its potent inhibition of taxane and epothilone-resistant tumors in cell cultures and in animal models, and its synergic effect when combined with paclitaxel.[64] Early clinical evaluations with discodermolide have begun in patients with various advanced solid malignancies,[65] but because only small amounts are available from natural sources, all discodermolide used for preclinical activities as well as for the ongoing clinical trials has been supplied by total synthesis.[66,67] This has required developing an impressive 39-step process that has been described by a leading synthetic chemist as "probably the best piece of synthetic work to come out from an industrial company."[68]

The Okinawan ocean sponge *Fasciospongia rimosa* and other Pacific sponges produce a potent microtubule stabilizing agent named laulimalide or figianolide B. Although laulimalide is less potent than paclitaxel in drug-sensitive laboratory cell lines, it is up to 100 times more potent in MDR-resistant cell lines, again because it is a very poor substrate of Pgp-170. Another similarity of laulimalide with discodermolide is its synergistic action with paclitaxel.[69]

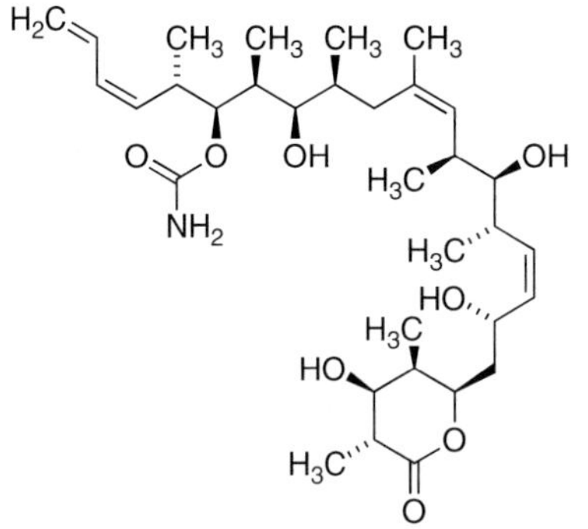

Discodermolide

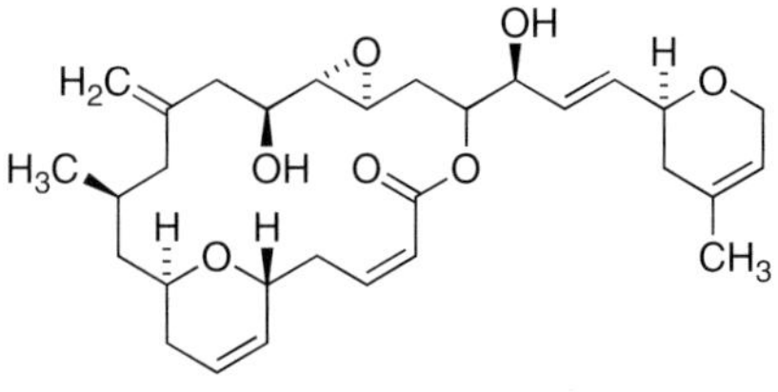

Laulimalide

4. MISCELLANEOUS ANTICANCER DRUGS ACTING ON NOVEL SITES ON TUBULINE

Estramustine phosphate, mentioned in Section 2.4, is used in the treatment of advanced metastatic prostate cancer, alone or in combination with other antitubulin agents such as vinblastine, paclitaxel, or ixabepilone.[70] It is administered as a phosphate prodrug, which is inactive because it does not enter the cells but is rapidly metabolized to the active species. Estramustine depolymerizes microtubule networks, inhibiting cell growth and inducing mitotic arrest, by binding to a site different from other drugs.[71]

NSC-639829 is a representative of the benzoylphenylurea (BPU) class of compounds,[72] which were developed initially as insecticides but showed antitumor activity in random screening. It inhibits tubulin polymerization by binding to a novel site and is being evaluated in clinical trials in patients with refractory metastatic cancer.[73] NSC-639829 is also a potent inhibitor of DNA polymerase.

NSC-639829

Estramustine phosphate

5. ANTIVASCULAR EFFECTS OF MICROTUBULE-TARGETED AGENTS

The tumor vasculature is an attractive target for tumor therapy.[74] The main approach to inhibiting vascular function in tumors is antiangiogenic therapy, which will be discussed in Chapters 9 and 10. However, it has been shown more recently that some compounds, especially microtubule-targeted agents, have the ability to shut down the existing vasculature at tumors because of depolymerization of the microtubule cytoskeleton at the endothelial cells [vascular-targeting agents (VTAs)].[75,76] Furthermore, the compounds of this group that are under development seem to damage the tumor vasculature with preference to normal tissues. This selectivity for the microvessels of tumors may reflect, in part, variability in the cytoskeletal makeup of rapidly proliferating endothelial cells inherent to microvessels feeding tumor cells versus the normally proliferating endothelial cells of microvessels serving healthy cells.[77]

Among the tubulin-targeted agents previously discussed, the most efficient at harming tumor vasculature are the ones targeting the colchicine site.[78] Several compounds of this type have entered clinical trials, including some derivatives of the combretastatins such as combretastatin A-4-3-O-phosphate, combretastatin A-2 phosphate, AVE8062A[79] the N-acetylcolchinol phosphate ZD6126,[80,81] and the flavonoid 5,6-dimethylxanthenone acetic acid (DMXAA, AS-1404). The previously mentioned TZT-1027, which binds in the *Vinca* domain, is also in clinical trials as a small-molecule vascular disrupting agent.

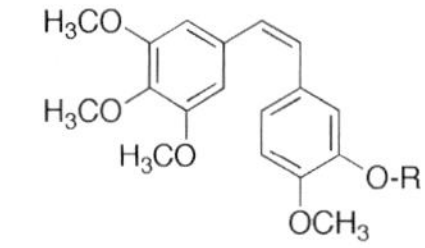

R = H   Combretastatin A-4
R = PO₂Na₂   CA-4P

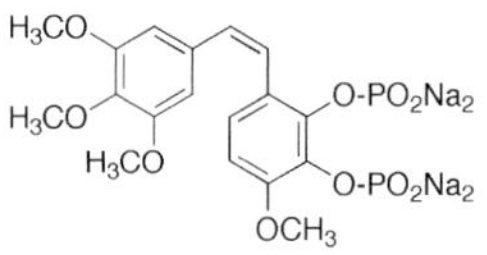

OXI-4503

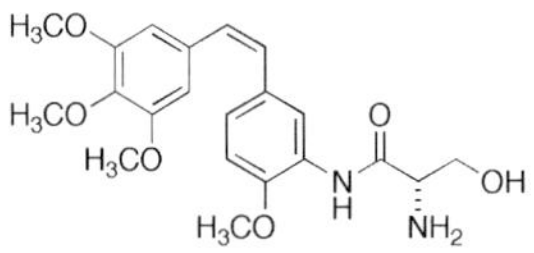

AVE-8062 (AC-7700)

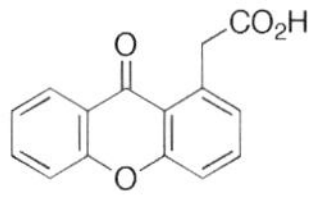

DMXAA (AS-1404)

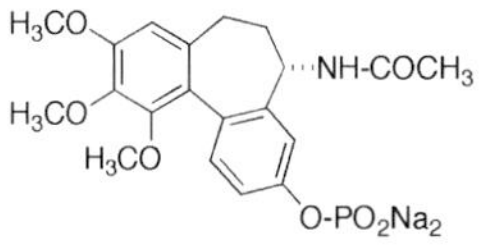

ZD-6126

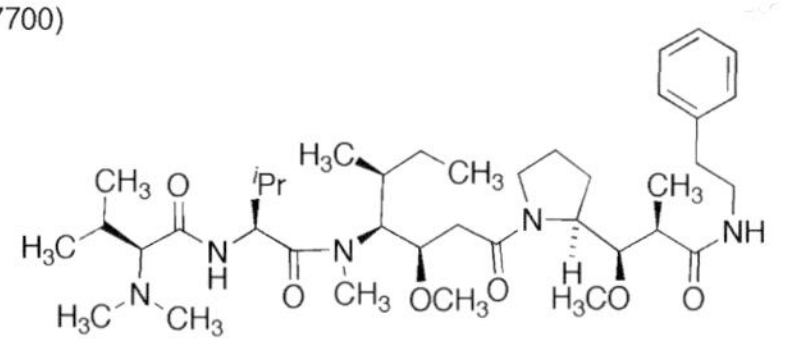

TZT-1027

Another field of interest for these drugs that is also under clinical evaluation is the therapy of various retinopathies such as the wet form of age-related macular degeneration (AMD), where inhibition of the formation of eye vasculature is beneficial, and other vascular diseases.

6. MITOTIC KINESIN INHIBITORS

Despite the diverse array of essential spindle proteins that could be exploited as targets for the discovery of novel cancer therapies, all spindle-targeted drugs in clinical use today that we have mentioned in this chapter act on only one protein, tubulin. Kinesins are motor proteins that function to transport organelles within cells, and one group of them (mitotic kinesins) move chromosomes along microtubules during cell division, playing essential roles in assembly and function of the mitotic spindle. Mitotic kinesins have an ATPase site that allows them to convert chemical energy into mechanical energy for the transport of DNA. They represent the first novel class of drug targets within mitosis to emerge in nearly 20 years.[82]

The most studied mitotic kinesin is the so-called kinesin spindle protein (KSP, Eg5), which functions at the earliest stages of mitosis to mediate centrosome separation and formation of a bipolar mitotic spindle. Eg5 interacts with microtubules in mitosis, but not with interphase microtubules, suggesting that its inhibitors may specifically target proliferating tumor tissue, thereby avoiding dose-limiting neuropathy observed with other antimicrotubule agents like taxanes or *Vinca* alkaloids. The first characterized small-molecule inhibitor of the motor protein Eg5 was monastrol, which is an allosteric inhibitor of the ATPase function of Eg5 that prevents ADP release by forming a ternary complex. The β-carboline derivative monastroline (HR22C16) was identified through a high-throughput microscopy-based forward-chemical-genetic screen.[83] Another class of inhibitors of Eg5 function are quinazoline derivatives, which function via an allosteric mechanism similar to that of monastrol. Among them, ispinesib (SB-715992) has reached clinical trials in patients with a variety of refractory solid tumors.[84]

| Monastrol | Monastroline (HR22C16) | Ispinesib (SB-715992, CK0238273) |

REFERENCES

1. Hamel, E. (1996). *Med. Res. Rev.* **16**, 207.
2. Wood, K. W., Cornwell, W. D., and Jackson, J. R. (2001). *Curr. Opin. Pharmacol.* **1**, 370.
3. Kuppens, I. E. L. M. (2006). *Curr. Clin. Pharmacol.* **1**, 57.
4. Jordan, M. A., and Wilson, L. (2004). *Nat. Rev. Cancer* **4**, 253.
5. Jordan, M. A. (2002). *Curr. Med. Chem. Anticancer Agents* **2**, 1.
6. Fahy, J. (2001). *Curr. Pharm. Des.* **7**, 1181.
7. Hill, B. T. (2001). *Curr. Pharm. Des.* **7**, 1199.
8. Newman, C. J., and Cragg, G. M. (2004). *Curr. Med. Chem.* **11**, 1693.
9. Aicher, T. D., Buszek, K. R., Fang, F. G., Forsyth, C. J., Jung, S. H., Kishi, Y., Matelich, M. C., Scola, P. M., Spero, D. M., and Yoon, S. K. (1992). *J. Am. Chem. Soc.* **114**, 3162.
10. Towle, M. J., Salvato, K. A., Budrow, J., Wels, B. F., Kuznetsov, G., Aalfs, K. K., Welsh, S., Zheng, W., Seletsky, B. M., Palme, M. H., Habgood, G. J., Singer, L. A., *et al.* (2001). *Cancer Res.* **61**, 1013.
11. Silberman, S., O'Shaughnessy, J., Vahdat, L., *et al.* (2005). Proceedings from the 28th annual San Antonio Breast Cancer Symposium, Abstract 1063.
12. Molife, R., Cartwright, T. H., Loesch, D. M., Garbo, L. E., Sonpavde, G., Calvo, E., Das, A., Wanders, J., Petrylak, D. P., and de Bon, J. (2007). *J. Clin. Oncol.* **25**(18S), 15513.
13. Vaishampayan, H., Glode, M., Du, W., Kraft, A., Hudes, G., Wright, J., and Hussain, M. (2000). *Clin. Canc. Res.* **6**, 4205.
14. Margolin, K., Longmate, J., Synold, T. W., Gandara, D. R., Weber, J., González, R., Johansen, M. J., Newman, R., and Doroshaw, J. H. (2001). *Invest. New Drugs* **19**, 335.
15. Schöffski, P., Thate, B., Beutel1, G., Bolte, O., Otto, D., Hofmann, M., Ganser, A., Jenner, A., Cheverton, P., Wanders, J., Oguma, T., Atsumi, R., *et al.* (2004). *Ann. Oncol.* **15**, 671.
16. Ebbinghaus, S., Hersh, E., Cunningham, C. C., O'Day, S., McDermott, D., Stephenson, J., Richards, D. A., Eckardt, J., Haider, O. L., and Hammond, L. A. (2004). *J. Clin. Oncol.* **22**, 7530.
17. Hamel, E. (2002). *Biopolymers* **66**, 142.
18. Cruz-Monserrate, Z., Mullaney, J. T., Harran, P. G., and Pettit, G. R. (2003). *Eur. J. Biochem.* **270**, 3822.
19. Bai, R., Durso, N. A., Sackett, D. L., and Hamel, E. (1999). *Biochemistry* **38**, 14302.
20. Loganzo, F., Discafani, C. M., Annable, T., Beyer, C., Musto, S., Hari, M., Tan, X., Hardy, C., Hernández, R., Baxter, M., Singanallore, T., Khafizova, G., Poruchynsky, M. S., Fojo, T.,

Nieman, J. A., Ayral-Kaloustian, S., Zask, A., Andersen, R. J., and Greenberger, L. M. (2003). *Cancer Res.* **63,** 1838.

21. Subbaraju, G. V., Golakoti, T., Patterson, G. M. L., and Moore, R. E. (1997). *J. Nat. Prod.* **60,** 302.
22. Shih, C., and Teicher, B. A. (2001). *Curr. Pharm. Des.* **7,** 1259.
23. Panda, D., Ananthnarayan, V., Larson, G. S., Shih, C., Jordan, M. A., and Wilson, L. (2000). *Biochemistry* **39,** 14121.
24. Uckun, F. M., Mao, C., Jan, S.-T., Wanh, H., Vassilev, A. O., Navara, C. S., and Narla, R. K. (2001). *Curr. Pharm. Des.* **7,** 1291.
25. Bai, R., Taylor, G. F., Cichacz, Z. A., Herald, C. L., Kepler, J. A., Pettit, G. R., and Hamel, E. (1995). *Biochemistry* **34,** 9714.
26. Uckun, F. M. (2001). *Curr. Pharm. Des.* **7,** 1627.
27. Hsieh, H. P., Liou, J. P., and Mahindroo, N. (2005). *Curr. Pharm. Des.* **11,** 1655.
28. Cirla, A., and Mann, J. (2003). *Nat. Prod. Rep.* **20,** 558.
29. Hadimani, M. B., Hua, J., Jonklaas, M. D., Kessler, R. J., Sheng, Y., Olivares, A., Tanpure, R. P., Weiser, A., Zhang, J., Edvardsen, K., Kanea, R. R., and Pinneya, K. G. (2003). *Bioorg. Med. Chem. Lett.* **13,** 1505.
30. Lakhani, N. J., Sarkar, M. A., Venitz, J., and Figg, W. D. (2003). *Pharmacotherapy* **23,** 165.
31. Galmarini, C. M. (2005). *Curr. Opinion Invest. Drugs* **6,** 623.
32. Yee Karen, W. L., Hagey, A., Verstovsek, S., Cortes, J., García-Manero, G., O'Brien, S. M., Faderl, S., Thomas, D., Wierda, W., Kornblau, S., Ferrajoli, A., Albitar, M., *et al.* (2005). *J. Clin. Cancer Res.* **11,** 6615.
33. Desbène, S., and Giorgi-Renault, S. (2002). *Curr. Med. Chem. Anticancer Agents* **2,** 71.
34. Guéritte, F. (2001). *Curr. Pharm. Des.* **7,** 1229.
35. Immordino, M. L., Brusa, P., Arpicco, S., Stella, B., Dosio, F., and Cattel, L. (2003). *J. Control Release* **91,** 417.
36. Bissery, M. C. (2001). *Curr. Pharm. Des.* **7,** 1251.
37. Gurtler, J. S., Von Pawel, J., Spiridonidis, C. H., Grossi, F., Larriba, J. L., Moscovici, M., Markovitz, E., Voliotis, D., and Gottfried, M. (2004). *J. Clin. Oncol.* **22,** 7136.
38. Broker, L. E., De Vos, F. Y., Gall, H., Gietema, J. A., Voi, M., Cohen, M. B., De Vries, E. G., and Giaccone, G. (2004). *J. Clin. Oncol.* **22,** 2029.
39. Ganesh, T., Guza, R. C., Bane, S., Ravindra, R., Shanker, N., Lakdawala, A. S., Snyder, J. P., and Kingston, D. G. I. (2004). *Proc. Nat. Acad. Sci. USA* **101,** 10006.
40. Ganesh, T., Guza, R. C., Bane, S., Ravindra, R., Shanker, N., Lakdawala, A. S., Snyder, J. P., and Kingston, D. G. I. (2004). *Proc. Natl. Acad. Sci. USA* **101,** 10006.
41. Ganesh, T., Norris, A., Sharma, S., Bane, S., Alcaraz, A. A., Snyder, J. P., and Kingston, D. G. I. (2004). *Bioorg. Med. Chem.* **14,** 3447.
42. Cragg, G. M., and Newman, D. J. (2004). *J. Nat. Prod.* **67,** 232.
43. Bollag, D. M., McQueney, P. A., Zhu, J., Hensens, O., Koupal, L., Liesch, J., Goetz, M., Lazarides, E., and Woods, C. M. (1995). *Cancer Res.* **55,** 2325.
44. Stachel, S. J., Biswas, K., and Danishefsky, S. J. (2001). *Curr. Pharm. Des.* **7,** 1277.
45. Nicolau, K. C., and Snyder, S. A. (2003). "Classics in Total Synthesis II". Wiley-VCH, Weinheim Chapter 7.
46. Watkins, E. B., Chittiboyina, A. G., Jung, J.-C., and Avery, M. A. (2005). *Curr. Pharm. Des.* **11,** 1615.
47. Chou, T. C., O'Connor, O. A., Tong, W. P., Guan, Y., Zhang, Z.-G., Stachel, S. J., Lee, C., and Danishefsky, S. J. (2001). *Proc. Nat. Acad. Sci. USA* **98,** 8113.
48. Yee, L., Lynch, T., Villalona-Calero, M., Rizvi, N., Gabrail, N., Sandler, A., Cropp, G., and Palmer, G. (2005). *J. Clin. Oncol.* **23,** 7127.
49. Wartmann, M., and Altmann, K.-H. (2002). *Curr. Med. Chem. Anticancer Agents* **2,** 123.
50. Kolman, A. (2004). *Curr. Opin. Investig. Drugs* **5,** 657.
51. Low, J. A., Wedam, S. B., Lee, J. J., Berman, A. W., Brufsky, A., Yang, S. X., Poruchynsky, M. S., Steinberg, S. M., Mannan, N., Fojo, T., and Swain, S. M. (2005). *J. Clin. Oncol.* **23,** 2726.
52. De Jonge, M., and Verweeij, J. (2005). *J. Clin. Oncol.* **23,** 9048.
53. Höfle, G., Glaser, N., Leibold, T., Karama, U., Sasse, F., and Steinmetz, H. (2003). *Pure Appl. Chem.* **75,** 167.

54. Wartmann, M., Loretan, J., Reuter, R., Hattenberger, M., Muller, M., and Vaxelaire, J. (2004). *Proc. Am. Assoc. Cancer Res.* **45,** abstract #5440.
55. Klar, U., Buchmann, B., Schwede, W., Skuballa, W., Hoffmann, J., and Lichtner, R. B. (2006). *Angew. Chem. Int. Ed.* **45,** 7942.
56. Schmid, P., Kiewe, P., Kuehnhardt, D., Korfel, A., Lindemann, S., Giurescu, M., Reif, S., Thiel, E., and Possinger, K. (2005). *J. Clin. Oncol.* **23,** 2051.
57. Altmann, K. H. (2004). *Org. Biomol. Chem.* **2,** 2137.
58. Altmann, K. H. (2005). *Curr. Pharm. Des.* **11,** 1595.
59. Manetti, F., Maccari, L., Corelli, F., and Botta, M. (2004). *Curr. Topics Med. Chem.* **4,** 203.
60. Nettles, J. H., Li, H., Cornett, B., Krahn, J., Snyder, J. P., and Downing, K. H. (2004). *Science* **305,** 866.
61. Giannakakou, P., Gussio, R., Nogales, E., Downing, K. H., Zaharevitz, D., Bollbuck, B., Poy, G., Sackett, D., Nicolaou, K. C., and Fojo, T. (2000). *Proc. Nat. Acad. Sci. USA* **97,** 2904.
62. Long, B. J., Carboni, J. M., Wasserman, A. J., Cornell, L. A., Casazza, A. M., Jensen, P. R., Lindel, T., Fenical, W., and Fairchild, C. R. (2000). *Cancer Res.* **58,** 1111.
63. Kingston, D. G. I., and Newman, D. J. (2002). *Curr. Opin. Drug. Discov. Devel.* **5,** 304.
64. Giannakakou, P., and Fojo, T. (2002). *Clin. Cancer Res.* **6,** 1613.
65. Mani, S., Macapinlac, M., Goel, S., Verdier-Pinard, D., Fojo, T., Rothenberg, M., and Colevas, D. (2002). *Anticancer Drugs* **15,** 553.
66. Mickel, S. J., Niederer, D., Daeffler, R., Osmani, A., Kuesters, E., Schmid, E., Schaer, K., Gamboni, R., Chen, W., Loeser, E., Kinder, F. R., Konigsberger, K., *et al.* (2002). *Org. Process Res. Dev.* **8,** 122 and four preceeding papers.
67. Mickel, S. J. (2002). *In* ''Strategies and Tactics in Organic Synthesis,'' (M. Harmata, ed.) vol. 6, Elsevier, Amsterdam Chapter 9.
68. Freemantle, M. (2004). *Chem. Eng. News* **82,** 33.
69. Gapud, E. J., Bai, R., Ghosh, A. K., and Hamel, E. (2004). *Mol. Pharmacol.* **66,** 113.
70. Smaletz, O., Galsky, M., Scher, H. I., De la Cruz, A., Slovin, S. F., Morris, M. J., Solit, D. B., Davar, U., Schwartz, L., and Kelly, W. K. (2004). *Ann. Oncol.* **14,** 1518.
71. Panda, D., Miller, H. P., Islam, K., and Wilson, L. (2004). *Proc. Natl. Acad. Sci. USA* **94,** 10560.
72. Hallur, G., Jimeno, A., Dalrymple, S., Zhu, T., Jung, M. K., Hidalgo, M., Isaacs, J. T., Sukumar, S., Hamel, E., and Khan, S. R. (2006). *J. Med. Chem.* **49,** 2357.
73. Messerschmith, W. A., Baker, S. D., Donehower, R. C., Dolan, S., Zabelina, Y., Zhao, M., Carducci, M. A., and Wolff, A. C. (2003). *Proc. Am. Soc. Clin. Oncol.* **22,** 203.
74. Thorpe, P. E. (2004). *Clin. Cancer Res.* **10,** 415.
75. Marx, M. A. (2002). *Exp. Opin. Ther. Pat.* **12,** 769.
76. Dhanabal, M., Jeffers, M., and LaRochelle, W. J. (2005). *Curr. Med. Chem. Anticancer Agents* **5,** 115.
77. Kanthou, C., and Tozer, G. M. (2002). *Blood* **99,** 2060.
78. Lawrence, N. J., and McGown, A. T. (2005). *Curr. Pharm. Des.* **11,** 1679.
79. Hori, K., and Saito, S. (2003). *Br. J. Cancer* **89,** 1334.
80. Davis, P. D., Dougherty, G. J., Blakey, D. C., Galbraith, S. M., Tozer, G. M., Holder, A. L., Naylor, M. A., Nolan, J., Stratford, M. R., Chaplin, D. J., and Hill, S. A. (2002). *Cancer Res.* **62,** 7247.
81. Soltau, J., and Drevs, J. (2004). *IDrugs* **7,** 380.
82. Wood, K. W., and Bergnes, G. (2004). *Annu. Rep. Med. Chem.* **39,** 173.
83. Hotha, S., Yarrow, J. C., Yang, J. C., Garrett, S., Renduchintala, K. V., Mayer, T. U., and Kapoor, T. M. (2003). *Angew. Chem. Int. Ed.* **42,** 2379.
84. http://www.clinicaltrials.gov/ct/show/NCT00097409.

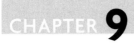

Drugs That Inhibit Signalling Pathways for Tumor Cell Growth and Proliferation

Contents

1. Introduction: The Role of Protein Kinases in Cancer 252
2. Signalling Pathways Related to Kinases 254
3. Inhibitors of Tyrosine Kinases (TKs) 254
   3.1. Inhibitors of EGFRs (HER-1) 258
   3.2. Inhibitors of other receptors of the EGFR family: HER-2 264
   3.3. Inhibitors of insulin-like growth factor receptors: IGFR-1 265
   3.4. Inhibitors of TKs with pro-angiogenic activity: VEFGR and related kinases 265
   3.5. Inhibitors of FLT-3 270
   3.6. Inhibitors of BCR-ABL TK (Abelson kinase) 271
   3.7. Dual Inhibitors of BCR-ABL and Src TKs 274
4. Inhibitors of Serine-Threonine Kinases 275
   4.1. Cyclin-Dependent Kinases 275
   4.2. PDK1, AKT, and mTOR kinases 279
   4.3. Aurora kinases 283
   4.4. PKC modulators 284
5. Inhibitors of the RAS–RAF–MEK Signalling Pathway and Farnesyl Transferase 286
   5.1. Inhibitors of Ras protein expression 288
   5.2. Inhibitors of Ras processing by farnesyltranferase 289
   5.3. Inhibitors of downstream effectors of Ras function 294
6. Inhibitors of Farnesyldiphosphate Synthase and Geranylgeranyldiphosphate Synthase 295
7. Anticancer Drugs Acting on Apoptotic Signalling Pathways 296
   7.1. BCL-2 proteins 296
   7.2. p53 proteins 298

Medicinal Chemistry of Anticancer Drugs
DOI: 10.1016/B978-0-444-52824-7.00009-3

7.3. Death receptors   298
7.4. Nuclear factor κB   298
8.   Inhibitors of Heat-Shock Proteins (HSP 90)   299
References   302

1. INTRODUCTION: THE ROLE OF PROTEIN KINASES IN CANCER

Intra- or inter-cellular communication disorders are a major cause of pathogenic mechanisms. For this reason, modern drug research has become increasingly focused on signal transduction therapy and many of the recently validated targets are transduction-related macromolecules, especially kinases.

Protein kinases (PTKs) are enzymes that regulate the biological activity of proteins by phosphorylation of specific amino acids with ATP as the source of phosphate, thereby inducing a conformational change from an inactive to an active form of the protein. There are three main types of PTKs, which are classified according to the amino acid side chain that they phosphorylate:

a. Tyrosine kinases (TKs) that phosphorylate the Tyr phenolic hydroxyl (Fig. 9.1).
b. Serine-threonine kinases that phosphorylate the hydroxy group of these two amino acids.
c. Histidine kinases, recently discovered, that phosphorylate the nitrogen of His residues.

Protein phosphorylation is one of the most significant signal transduction mechanisms by which inter-cellular signals regulate crucial intra-cellular processes such as ion transport, cellular proliferation and differentiation, and hormone responses. Recently, the human genome project has revealed that 20% of the approximately 32,000 human genes encode proteins involved in signal transduction. Among these proteins are more than 500 PTK enzymes and around 150 protein phosphatases exerting tight control on protein phosphorylation. Preclinical and clinical data strongly support the involvement of specific PTKs in the formation and progression of a subset of tumors, with around 16 PTKs being considered as possible therapeutic targets.

Many PTKs are cytoplasmic enzymes, but others, known as receptor protein kinases (RPTKs), transverse the cell membrane and have dual roles as enzymes and as receptors. The latter proteins have an extracellular domain that recognizes an external messenger (growth hormones, growth factors)[1] and an intracellular kinase active site that becomes activated upon binding of the messenger, triggering a signalling cascade that ultimately controls the transcription of specific genes related to

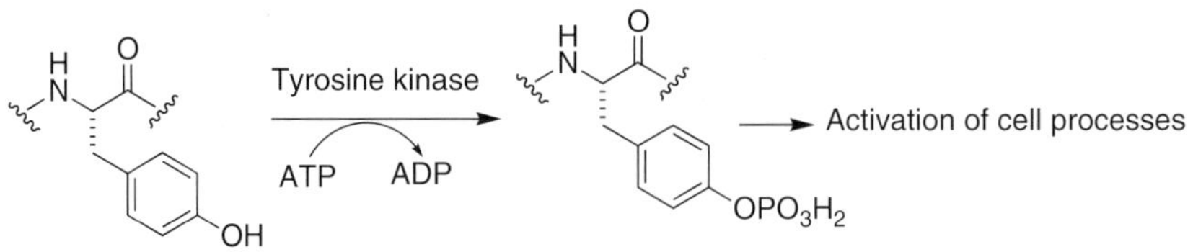

FIGURE 9.1   Role of tyrosine kinases.

cellular proliferation and differentiation. Non-receptor PTKs have no extra-cellular domain, and are activated by upstream signalling molecules such as G-protein–coupled receptors and immune system receptors, and also by receptor TKs.

Targeting PTKs is a compelling approach to cancer chemotherapy because in many cancers there is an overexpression of PTKs or their associated messengers.[2–4] In fact, following the discovery in the early 1980s that the protooncogene Src was in fact a PTK, it has subsequently been proved that most PTKs are related to oncogenes.

All PTKs have a region in their active site that recognizes ATP, which is the phosphorylating agent in all cases, as well as another for their substrates. Most clinically used inhibitors act in the ATP recognition site. Because, in spite of having a common substrate, the ATP binding sites are relatively different for different kinases, some selectivity in the inhibition is possible.

A number of substructures related to kinase inhibitors have reached clinical investigation status. These include compounds identified from screening studies and they include 4-aminoquinazolines, oxindoles, ureas, and 2-phenylaminopyrimidines, natural products and their analogues such as flavonoids, staurosporine, and structural analogues of ATP like roscovitine (seliciclib). Some representative examples of these structural families are given in Fig. 9.2.

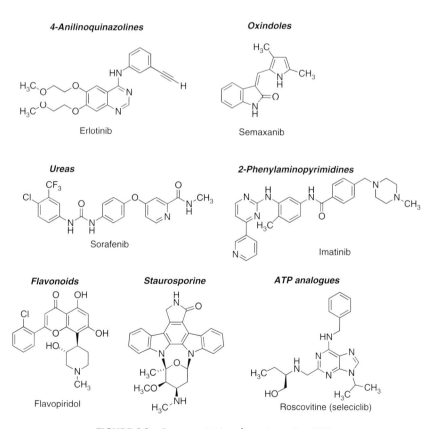

FIGURE 9.2   Representative drugs targeting PTKs.

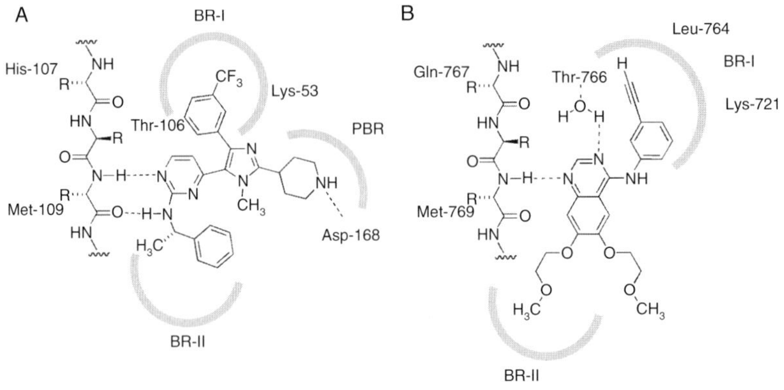

FIGURE 9.3 Binding modes of inhibitors at the ATP-site of PTKs.

These pharmacophores target a highly conserved structural determinant of the ATP binding site in the kinase family, namely an alternating hydrogen bonding pattern present in the so-called hinge peptide portion that connects the N- and C-terminal domain of kinases. Inhibitors form hydrogen bonds with the protein backbone and peripheral groups are oriented towards two hydrophobic pockets called BR-I (binding region-I) and BR-II or towards the phosphate-binding region (PBR). There are two typical inhibitor binding modes, shown in Fig. 9.3, and very often structurally close compounds bind to the ATP site in different topologies and are able to recognize different kinases. For this reason, chemical similarity between kinase inhibitors often fails to correlate with target specificity.

2. SIGNALLING PATHWAYS RELATED TO KINASES

A brief pictorial summary of the main signalling pathways targeted by drugs described in this chapter is given in Fig. 9.4. For a more detailed explanation, see the individual sections.

A summary of the main kinase inhibitors that will be studied in this chapter is given in Table 9.1. Since most of them are not completely selective for a particular kinase, their classification has been made according to their main target.

3. INHIBITORS OF TYROSINE KINASES (TKs)

The development of specific tyrosine kinase (TK) inhibitors started by the synthesis of hydroxyphenyl compounds as tyrosine mimics. Some of them were derivatives of itaconic acid, a compound that inhibited the insulin receptor with no effect on serine-threonine kinases. Another source of inspiration was the natural product erbstatin, an inhibitor of epidermal growth factor receptor (EGFR) and

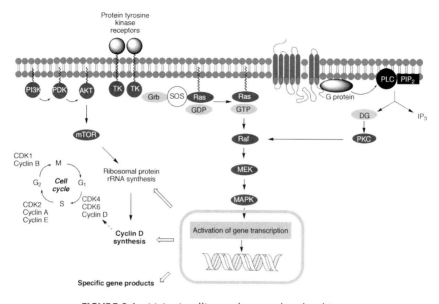

FIGURE 9.4   Main signalling pathways related to kinases.

TABLE 9.1   Selected kinase inhibitors in the market or in clinical development

Type	Target	Agents
Tyr kinases	EGFR (HER-1)	*Small-molecule inhibitors*
		4-Anilinoquinazolines
		Gefitinib (ZD-1839)
		Erlotinib (OSI-774)
		Lapatinib (GW-2016)
		Canertinib (CI-1003)
		EKI-785
		EKB-569
		HKI-272
		Monoclonal antibodies
		Cetuximab (IMC-C225)
		ABX-EGF
		EMB-72000
		RH-3
		MDX-447
		Panitumumab
	EGFR (HER-2)	*Monoclonal antibodies*
		Trastuzumab
	IGFR-1	*Small-molecule inhibitors*
		AEW-541

(continued)

TABLE 9.1   (*continued*)

Type	Target	Agents
	VEGFR	*Small-molecule inhibitors*
		Oxindoles
		Semaxanib (SU-5416)
		SU-6668
		Sunitinib (SU-11248)
		Quinoxalines
		Vatalanib (PTK-787, ZK-222584)
		Anthranilamides
		AAL-993 (ZK-260255)
		Quinazolines
		Vandetanib (ZD-6474)
		AZD-2171
		Indazoles
		Axitinib (AG-013736)
		Staurosporine analogues
		Cephalon (CEP-7055)
		Monoclonal antibodies
		Bevacizumab
		PRO-001
		Ribozymes
		Angiozyme
	PDGF	*Small-molecule inhibitors*
		Suramin
	FLT-3	*Small-molecule inhibitors*
		4-Anilinoquinazolines
		Tandutinib (MLN-518, CT-53518)
		Staurosporine analogues:
		CEP-701
		PKC-412
	BCR-ABL	*Small-molecule inhibitors*
		ATP mimics
		Imatinib (STI-571)
		Nilotinib (AMN-107)
		Tyrosine mimics
		Adaphostin
		ON-012380
	BCR-ABL/Src	*Small-molecule inhibitors*
		BMS-354825
		SKI-606
		AZD-0530

(*continued*)

TABLE 9.1   (*continued*)

Type	Target	Agents
Serine-threonine kinases	CDKs	*Small-molecule inhibitors*
		Alvocidib (flavopiridol, HMR-1275)
		Seleciclib (roscovitine, CYC-202)
		BMS-387032
		Indisulam (E-7070)
	PDK1	*Small-molecule inhibitors*
		UCN-01
	AKT	*Small-molecule inhibitors*
		A-443654
		Perifosine
	AKT via HSP 90	*Small-molecule inhibitors*
		Geldanamycin analogues
		17-AAG
		17-DMAG
	PDK-1	*Small-molecule inhibitors*
		UCN-01
	MTOR	*Small-molecule inhibitors*
		Rapamycin analogues
		Tensirolimus (CCI-779)
		Everolimus (RAD-001)
		AP-23573
	Aurora kinases	*Small-molecule inhibitors*
		VX-680
	PKCs	*Small-molecule inhibitors*
		Staurosporine analogues
		UCN-01
		CGP-41251
		Ruboxistaurin (LY-333531)
		Enzastaurin (LY-317615)
		PKC-412
		Bryostatin 1
		Antisense oligonucleotides
		ISIS-3521 (CGP-64128[a])
		ISIS-5132
Ras–Raf–MEK pathway	Ras	*Antisense oligonucleotides*
		ISIS-2503
		Farnesyltransferase inhibitors
		AZD-3409
		BMS-214662

(*continued*)

TABLE 9.1   (*continued*)

Type	Target	Agents
		Tipifarnib (R-115777)
		L-778123
		Lonafarnib (SCH-66366)
		SCH-226374
	Raf	*Small-molecule inhibitors*
		Sorafenib (BAY43–9006)
		Antisense oligonucleotides
		ISIS-5132
	MEK	*Small-molecule inhibitors*
		PD-184352
		ARRY-142886 (AZD-6244)

other kinases. The first potent inhibitor to arise from this work was tyrphostin (AG-213). Conformational restriction strategies by cycle formation in this compound eventually led to the identification of the quinoxaline system as a very useful pharmacophore in the design of TK inhibitors (Fig. 9.5). Interestingly, they act as ATP mimics rather than as substrate analogues, which was the original rationale behind this work.[5]

3.1. Inhibitors of EGFRs (HER-1)

The epidermal growth factor (EGF) was one of the first isolated growth factors. Its receptor (EGFR) is overexpressed or mutated in several cancers due to a mutation of a normal gene to an oncogene, and many tumors that overexpress this receptor also overexpress its ligands. Among several types of EGFRs, the best understood are HER-1 (normally used as a synonym to EGFR) and HER-2. An added complication is that the active form of the receptor is actually a dimer of two HER types, and they seem to be able to mix-and-match.

EGFR is considered as a suitable target for lung cancer, colorectal cancer, myeloid leukaemia, and hormone-dependent or independent breast cancer.[6] It is a 170-kDa membrane TK that is activated by EGF, but in cancer cells is also stimulated by the transforming growth factor α (TGF-α), which is overexpressed in tumors. Ligand binding leads to activation of its kinase activity through homo-dimerization of two protein receptors (or heterodimerization with a receptor belonging to the same family) followed by autophosphorylation at the Tyr-1068 residue, which in turn leads to the activation of a range of cell signalling pathways (e.g. BTAT3, MAPK, and AKT). Transduction of signals to the nucleus and the activation of gene transcription by several factors lead to the induction of several

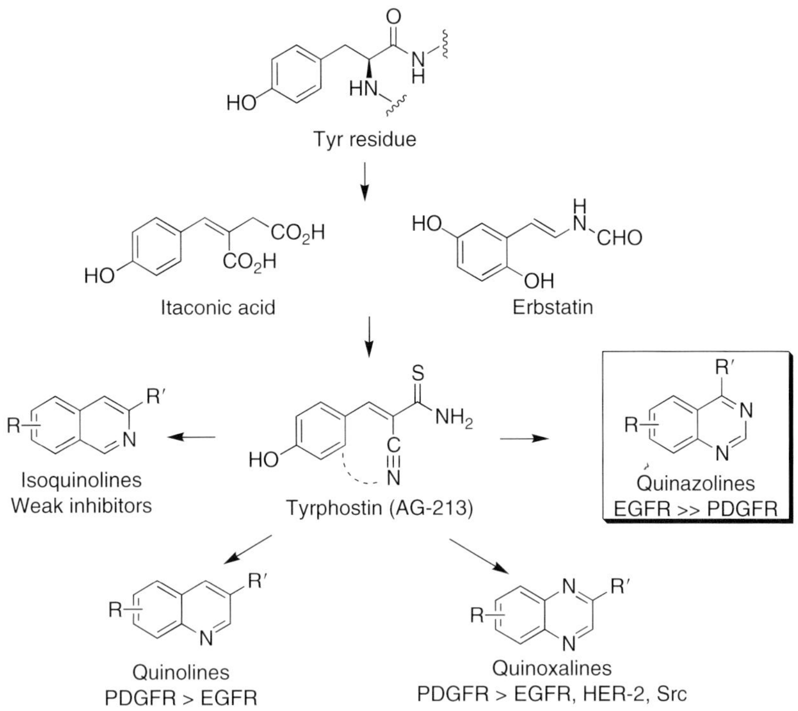

FIGURE 9.5   Representative tyrosine kinase inhibitors.

processes that are essential for tumor cell growth, including cell proliferation, survival, angiogenesis, invasion, and metastasis. Small-molecule inhibitors of this kinase inhibit ATP binding to its site at the TK domain (Fig. 9.6). Many anti-EGFR agents are known, some of which are used in clinical practice or are under clinical development. They can be classified in following two groups:

a. Small molecules that compete with ATP binding to the TK domain of the receptor, inhibiting autophosphorylation and blocking signal transduction.
b. Monoclonal antibodies (mAbs) that are directed at the extra-cellular portion of the EGFR. These antibodies compete with the receptor ligands, EGF and TGF-α, and also inhibit receptor dimerization.

3.1.1. Small-molecule EGFR inhibitors

During studies aimed at characterizing the catalytic domain of EGFR-TK using high-throughput techniques, it was discovered that 4-anilinoquinazolines were promising inhibitors.[7] Investigation of substituent effects on biological activity led to the conclusions summarized in Fig. 9.7.[8]

Among 4-anilinoquinazolines, gefitinib (ZO-1839) was the first small-molecule anti-EGFR agent, and the first non-cytotoxic compound, to be approved for

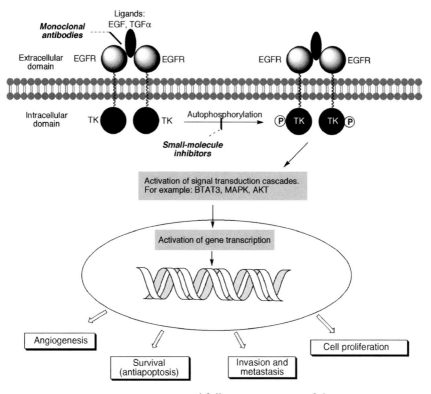

FIGURE 9.6   Events triggered following activation of the EGFRs.

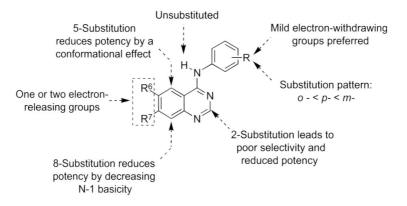

FIGURE 9.7   Structure-activity relationships in 4-anilinoquinazolines as EGFR inhibitors.

clinical use as a monotherapy for the treatment of patients with locally advanced non-small lung cell cancer (NSCLC) following failure of platinum and docetaxel treatments.[9,10] A subsequent large randomized study failed to demonstrate a survival advantage for gefitinib in the treatment of this cancer. However, gefitinib response has been shown to be primarily linked to the presence of EGFR mutations and for this reason it has been suggested that EGFR-TK inhibitors should be tested in clinical trials of first-line treatment of lung adenocarcinomas harbouring EGFR mutations.[11]

These limitations, together with the report of lethal pulmonary toxicity from studies in Japan, led to the replacement of gefitinib by the closely related erlotinib (OSI-774). This compound is indicated for patients with advanced or metastatic NSCLC after failure of prior chemotherapy. As in the case of gefitinib, its combination with platinum agents did not show any clinical benefit.[12,13] Another quinazoline derivative that inhibits EGFR with similar efficacy is lapatinib (GW-2016), a dual inhibitor of EGFR and the closely related receptor ErbB2 (or HER-2). The latter receptor has been identified as an important therapeutic target in a number of cancers as it is overexpressed in around 20–30% of patients with aggressive breast cancer and other tumors. For this reason, lapatinib is under clinical assays for several solid tumors.[14]

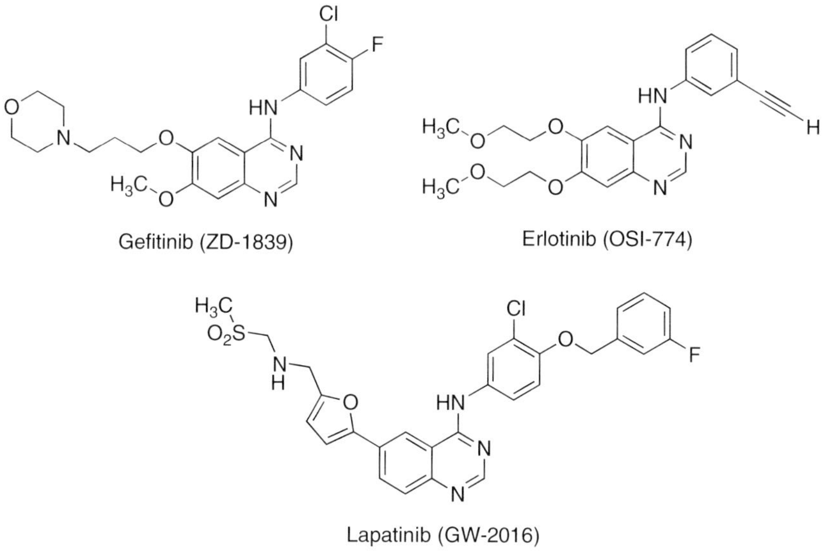

Gefitinib (ZD-1839)   Erlotinib (OSI-774)

Lapatinib (GW-2016)

The binding of ATP to its site at the TK domain of EGFR was initially studied by molecular modelling techniques, based on the X-ray crystal structure of the complex between the related cAMP-dependent PTK, an inhibitor, Mg, and ATP. This binding involves two hydrogen bonds at the Gln-767 and Met-769, among other interactions. The ribose unit binds to its own pocket, and the triphosphate chain is placed in a cleft that leads to the surface of the enzyme (Fig. 9.8A). This active site also contains unoccupied spaces, especially a hydrophobic pocket opposite to the place where the ribose binds. This pocket shows slight differences

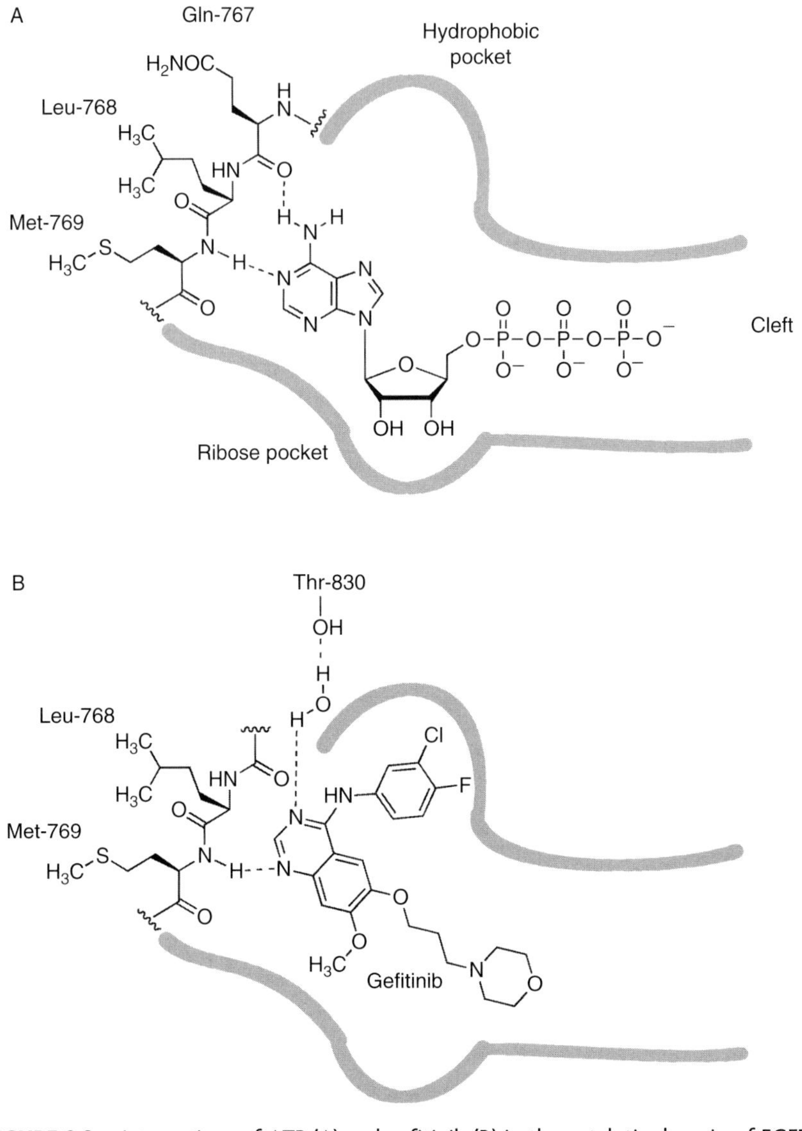

FIGURE 9.8.   Interactions of ATP (A) and gefitinib (B) in the catalytic domain of EGFR.

between the different kinases, allowing relatively selective inhibitors, and is normally occupied by the above-discussed drugs, which thus act as ATP mimics. For instance, the interaction between gefitinib and the EGFR catalytic domain has been studied by X-ray crystallography[15] and can be found in Fig. 9.8B. In the case of gefitinib, where the N-1 atom of the quinazoline ring acts as a hydrogen bond acceptor in an interaction with Met-769, the N-3 atom interacts with Thr-830 through a bridging water molecule, and the aniline ring occupies the normally empty hydrophobic pocket.

Since the ATP binding site is quite spacious, other orientations are possible for inhibitors, even belonging to the same structural class. The substitution of the Met-790 residue for Thr leads to resistance to gefitinib and erlotinib due to steric hindrance to binding of the inhibitor.[16]

ATP-competitive inhibitors need to prevail over the high endogenous concentrations of ATP. For this reason, ATP-competitive EGFR inhibitors are rapidly cleared from tumors. To overcome this problem, intensive efforts have been directed towards the development of irreversible EGFR inhibitors. Some of them are canertinib (CI-1003), a dual EGFR-HER-2 inhibitor,[17] EKI-785, EKB-569, and HKI-272, which are under clinical evaluation.[2,5] In some of these compounds, like EKB-569 and HKI-272, the traditional quinazoline ring has been replaced by a 3-cyanoquinoline.

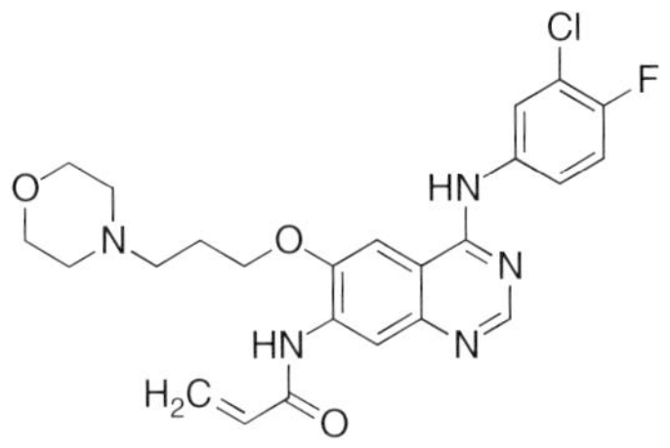

Canertinib (CI-1003)

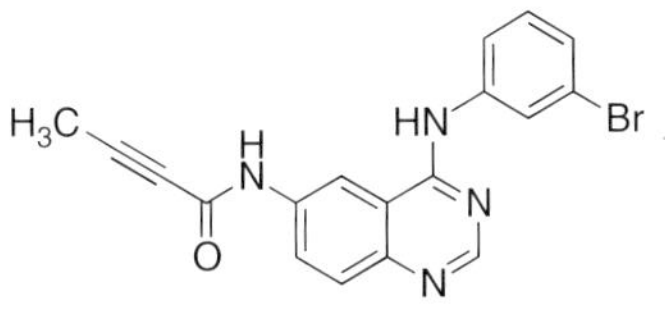

EKI-785

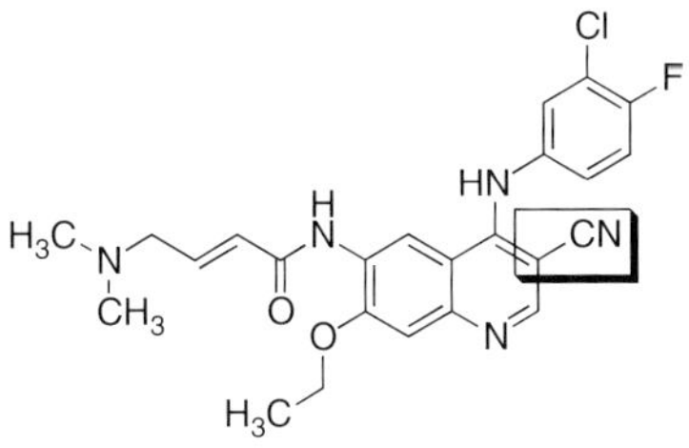

EKB-569

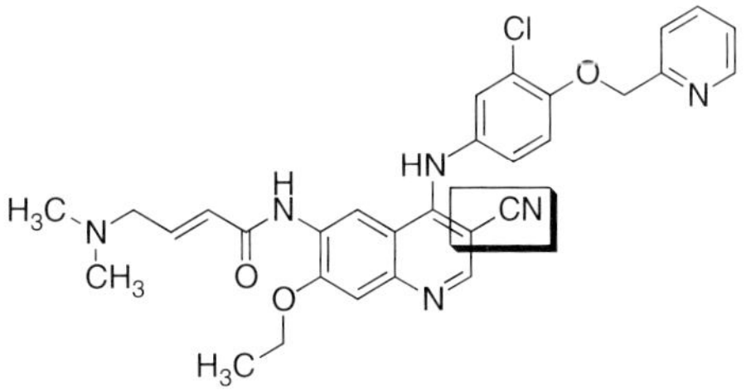

HKI-272

The last four compounds can be considered as active site-directed irreversible inhibitors, since they contain a 4-anilinoquinazoline structural fragment that can be recognized by the ATP site and also an electrophilic α,β-unsaturated carbonyl moiety, responsible for covalent binding to the enzyme. The conserved cysteine residue Cys-773 within the ATP binding pocket seems to be responsible for the nucleophilic attack to this Michael substrate[18] (Fig. 9.9).

3.1.2. Monoclonal antibodies

Because antibodies recognize specific proteins with high specificity, they can be used as antagonists of the binding of an overexpressed protein to its ligands, although they show toxic effects (ADCC, antibody-dependent cell-mediated cytotoxicity). Antibodies for EGFR prevent the binding of EGF or TGF-α, and hence receptor dimerization and signal transduction, in addition to causing receptor internalization and proteosomal degradation.

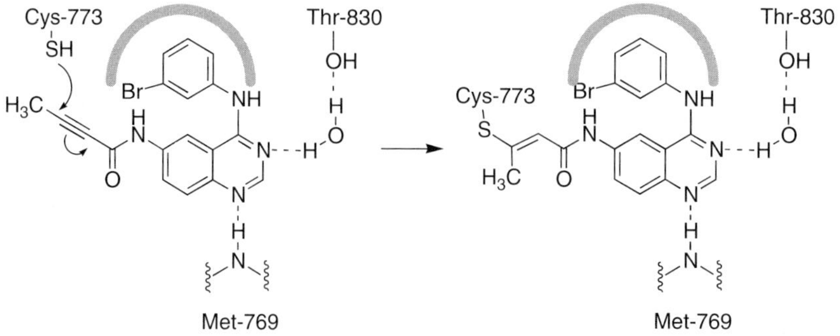

FIGURE 9.9   Irreversible EGFR inhibitors.

Cetuximab (IMC-C225) is a chimeric monoclonal antibody* that has been approved for clinical use as a second-line treatment for EGF-expressing colorectal cancer. Despite not having demonstrated an improvement in survival it is being tested in combination therapies. Other antibodies directed to the same receptor that are under clinical evaluation are ABX-EGF, EMD-72000 (humanized), RH3, MDX-447, and panitumumab (fully human).[2]

3.2. Inhibitors of other receptors of the EGFR family: HER-2

As previously mentioned, HER-2 is a member of the EGFR family of receptors that has been identified as an important therapeutic target because it is overexpressed in around 20–30% of patients with aggressive breast cancer.

Besides the previously mentioned EGFR-HER-2 dual inhibitors such as lapatinib and canertinib, some monoclonal antibodies are directed at this receptor. The most important is trastuzumab, a humanized monoclonal antibody that targets the extra-cellular region of the HER-2 receptor, leading to its internalization and degradation. Interaction of trastuzumab with the human immune system via its human immunoglobulin G1 Fc domain may potentiate its antitumor activities. *In vitro* studies demonstrate that trastuzumab is very effective in mediating antibody-dependent cell-mediated cytotoxicity against HER-2-overexpressing tumor targets. In summary, the mechanism of action of trastuzumab includes antagonizing the constitutive growth-signalling properties of the HER-2 system, enlisting immune cells to attack and kill the tumor target, and augmenting chemotherapy-induced cytotoxicity.[19]

Trastuzumab has been approved for the treatment of metastatic breast cancer in women that have had at least two chemotherapy treatments for this type of cancer, in combination with paclitaxel. It is also being studied in combination with other chemotherapeutic agents. Other related antibodies that are under clinical evaluation are MCX-210 and 2C4.

---

* A chimeric protein can be defined as one that is encoded by a nucleotide sequence made by a splicing together of two or more complete or partial genes, which can even be from different species.

3.3. Inhibitors of insulin-like growth factor receptors: IGFR-1

The insulin-like growth factors (IGFs) are peptides with a high sequence homology with insulin. They are part of a complex system (often referred to as the IGF 'axis') that has a role in the promotion of cell proliferation and in the inhibition of apoptosis. The IGFR-1 is another membrane TK that is inhibited by several families of compounds. The most relevant one is AEW-541, an inhibitor of the receptor autophosphorylation, is being developed against musculoskeletal tumors and multiple myeloma.[20]

AEW-541

3.4. Inhibitors of TKs with pro-angiogenic activity: VEFGR and related kinases

Angiogenesis can be defined as the growth of new blood vessels from pre-existing microvasculature and will be discussed in more detail in Section 2 of Chapter 10. Since angiogenesis has a key role in tumor growth and metastasis because tumors cannot grow beyond a certain size unless they induce angiogenesis in order to establish a blood supply, it is an important source of anticancer drug targets. In adults, it is triggered only locally and transiently in processes such as wound healing, and changes in the equilibrium between pro- and anti-angiogenic factors are associated with a number of disease states. The receptors of some pro-angiogenic growth factors such as the vascular endothelial growth factor (VEGF) family, including VEGFR-1 (FLT-1), VEGFR-2 (KDR), and VEGFR-3 (FLT-4); the platelet-derived growth factor (PDGF); and the fibroblast growth factor (FGF) are TKs, and will be discussed here. The previously mentioned EGF also has activity as a pro-angiogenic growth factor. VEGFs bind to and activate the above-mentioned cell surface receptors (VEGFR).

VEGF signalling is critical for blood vessel formation and is involved in all stages of angiogenesis. Inhibition of VEGF signalling, therefore, is an attractive therapy target in a wide range of tumor types, and disruption of the VEGF has become one dominant strategy for the angiogenesis-related treatment of cancer.

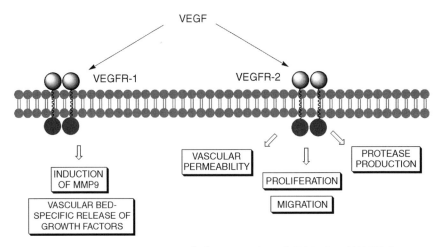

FIGURE 9.10   Events triggered after activation of VEGFR-1 and VEGFR-2.

VEGFR-1 was the first receptor TK to be identified and its signalling can be important in tumor growth and metastasis, including the induction of matrix metalloproteinases (MMPs). VEGFR-2 is expressed in endothelial cells and is the principal receptor through which VEGFs exert their mitogenic, chemotactic, and vascular permeabilizing effects on the host vasculature (Fig. 9.10). Activation of VEGFR-3 promotes lymphangiogenesis.

3.4.1. VEGFR inhibitors

Indolinone derivatives have in common the presence of a hydrogen bond between the C-2 carbonyl and a hydrogen donor in a side chain, generally a pyrrole ring. The first of them was semaxanib (SU-5416), identified in a high-throughput library screening as an inhibitor of VEGF- and PDGF-induced tyrosine autophosphorylation. This compound reached Phase III clinical trials for colorectal cancer, but it was discontinued at that stage.[21] SU-6668[22] and sunitinib (SU-11248)[23] were obtained by introduction of a propionic acid and a (diethylaminoethyl)carmaboyl chain, respectively, at the C-4' position of the latter compound. Sunitinib has been approved by the FDA for gastrointestinal and renal cancer.

Semaxanib
(SU-5416)

SU-6668

Sunitinib (SU-11248)

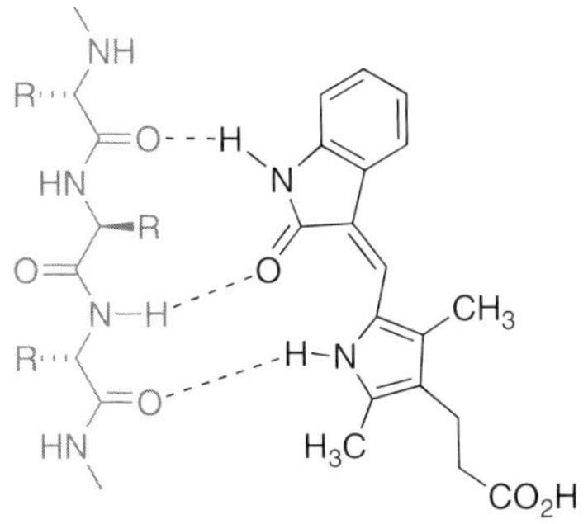

FIGURE 9.11   Binding of the indolinone SU-6668 to VEGFR-1.

X-ray crystallographic studies of some oxindole derivatives co-crystallized with VEGFR-1 showed that they occupy the same region as ATP (Fig. 9.11).

Vatalanib (PTK787, ZK-222584), an orally available aminophthalazine derivative, was identified through a screen of a chemical library against FLT-1.[24] It potently inhibits several VEGFR kinases, and also the TK activity of c-KIT and PDGF. This compound is currently under Phase III studies for metastatic colorectal cancer, with results that suggest a positive effect.[25]

Vatalanib was used as a starting point for the development of second-generation VEGFR inhibitors. Based upon its binding mode to the receptors, an anthranilamide scaffold was selected for optimization leading to the identification of AAL-993 as a potent and selective VEGFR-2 inhibitor.

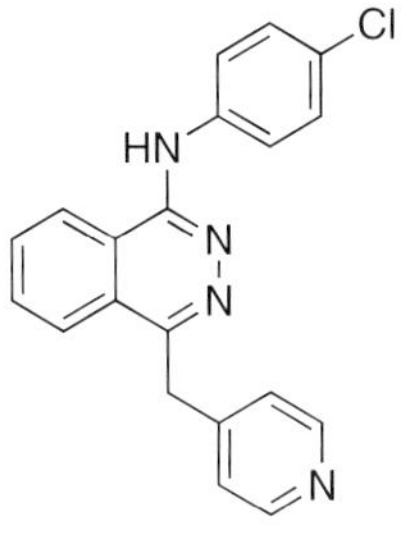

Vatalanib (PTK787,
ZK-222584)

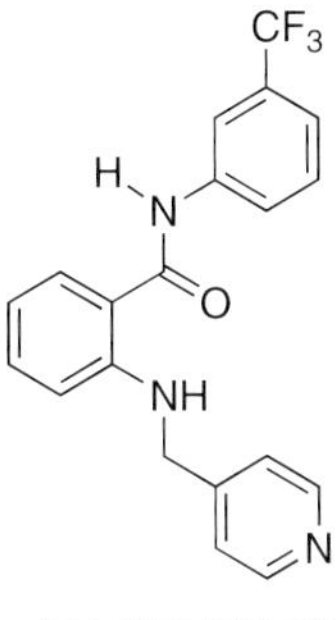

AAL-993 (ZK-260255)

The crystal structure of the drug–protein complex showed that, similar to imatinib, AAL-993 targets the inactive conformation of the enzyme. The binding involves three hydrogen bond interactions (Fig. 9.12) and several hydrophobic interactions. Thus, the phenyl ring of the anthranilamide unit is sandwiched between the hydrophobic side chains of Val-916 and Lys-868, and the trifluoro-methylphenyl substituent fits a lipophilic pocket.[26]

Vandetanib (ZD6474) belongs to the quinazoline family and is being evaluated in several Phase II clinical trials. Quinazolines were initially developed as EGFR-TK

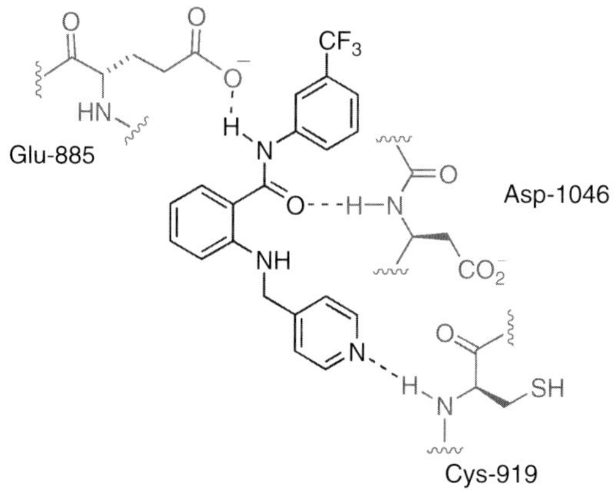

FIGURE 9.12   Binding of AAL-993 to VEGFR-2.

inhibitors and later refined to give VEGFR-2 (KDR)-selective compounds. Vandetanib occupies the ATP adenine binding site, where it forms a single hydrogen bond involving its N-1 nitrogen and the Cys-912 residue of the protein. Several structure–activity relationships have been deduced for this family, including an increased activity for the 2-fluoro and 5-hydroxy derivatives, the latter effect being attributed to the formation of an additional hydrogen bond.[27]

Other promising quinazoline derivatives that act on VEGFR are AZD-2171 (ZD-2171), which demonstrated >800- to 5000-fold *in vitro* selectivity for VEGFR-2 inhibition, compared with a range of tyrosine and serine-threonine kinases. It is undergoing a number of clinical trials (Phase I, Phase II/III) to evaluate its role in a range of solid tumors.[28] GW-786034 is another orally active quinazoline that is also in clinical trials.[29]

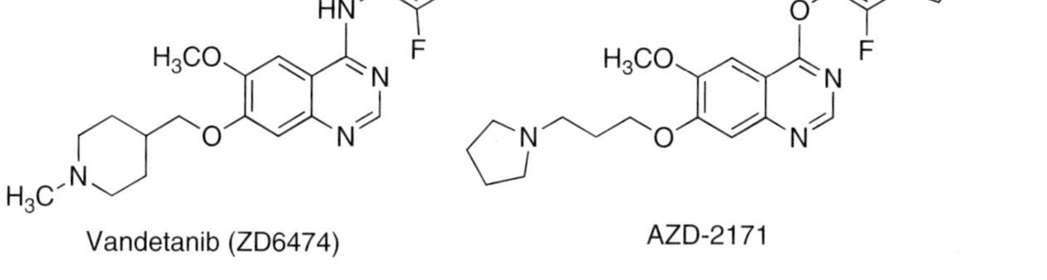

Vandetanib (ZD6474)   AZD-2171

The indazole derivative axitinib (AG-013736) is an orally available inhibitor of VEGFR, and also of the related PDGF and CSF-1 receptor TKs. This agent is in clinical development for head and neck and breast cancers, among others.[30,31]

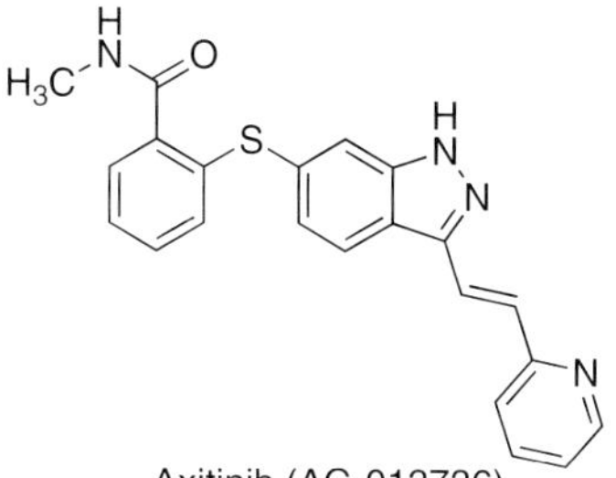

Axitinib (AG-013736)

Other VEGFR inhibitors have been designed as analogues of the natural product staurosporine, a non-selective kinase inhibitor. For instance, CEP-5214, which was identified as the best candidate from SAR studies of about 2000 analogues, has a potent pan-VEGFR kinase inhibitory activity. Its *N,N*-dimethyl-glycine ester CEP-7055 is a water-soluble prodrug that can be orally administered and is undergoing clinical trials.[32]

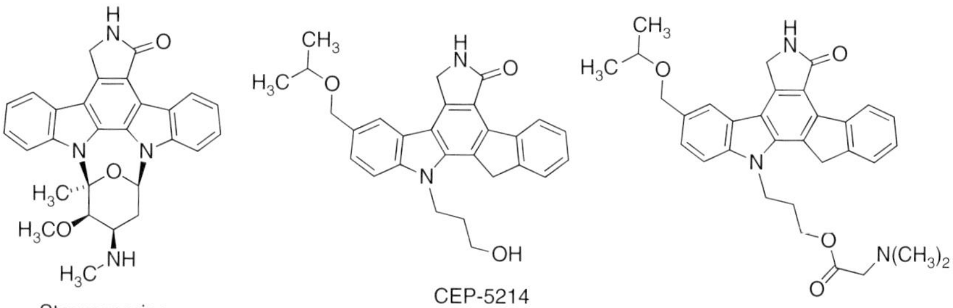

Staurosporine   CEP-5214   CEP-7055

3.4.2. Other types of anti-VEGF therapy

Bevacizumab is a recombinant humanized monoclonal IgG1 antibody against all isoforms of VEGF-A, which are ligands of the VEGFR-1 and VEGFR-2. Bevacizumab was the first approved agent to inhibit tumor angiogenesis, in 2004 by the FDA and in 2005 in Europe. It is used in combination with other drugs such as 5-fluorouracil or irinotecan for the first-line treatment of patients with metastatic colorectal cancer, and is expected to be approved for other tumors such as NSCLC and renal cell cancer.[33] Cytotoxic monoclonal antibodies for related kinases such as PRO-001, an antibody for FGFR-3, are also being developed for the treatment of FGFR-3-expressing myeloma.[34]

Inhibition of the VEGFR activity can also be accomplished using catalytic RNA molecules known as ribozymes, which down-regulate VEGFR function by specifically cleaving the mRNAs for the primary VEGFRs. Angiozyme[35] is one of these ribozymes, which is under clinical studies for the treatment of solid tumors.

3.4.3. Inhibitors of platelet-derived growth factor (PDGF)

Suramin is a polysulphonated naphthylurea originally developed for the treatment of trypanosomiasis and onchocerciasis. Recent studies have shown that suramin possess a variety of biological effects, including anti-AIDS activity due to its capacity to inhibit reverse transcriptase and to prevent HIV entry into the cell. More recently, suramin is also been used in the treatment of cancer and it is being evaluated in clinical trials in combination with several other chemotherapeutic agents in patients with a variety of solid tumors.[36] Suramin blocks the activity of several angiogenic factors, especially PDGF and FGF, and is also an inhibitor of heparanase (see Section 2.2.2 of Chapter 10). It is also internalized into the cell where it may affect the activity of various key enzymes involved in the intracellular transduction of mitogenic signals including protein kinase C (PKC).

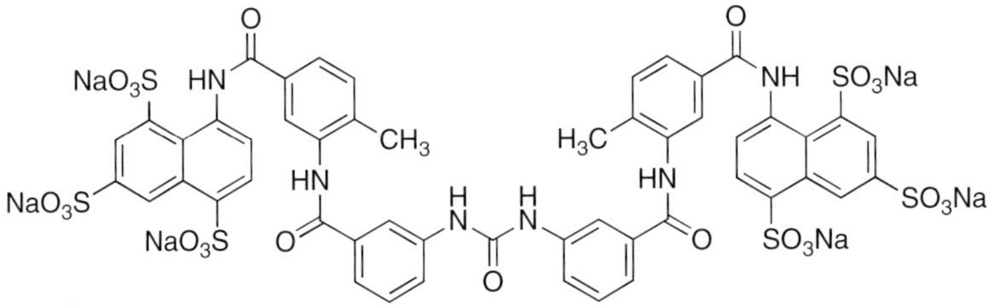

Suramin

3.5. Inhibitors of FLT-3

FLT-3 is a membrane TK structurally related to PDGFR. Activating mutations of FLT-3 are present in about 30% of acute myeloid leukaemia (AML) patients and are associated with lower cure rates from standard chemotherapy. For this reason, this kinase has become a very popular target for the design of drugs against AML.

Tandutinib[37] (MLN-518, CT-53518) is a quinazoline derivative that selectively inhibits FLT-3 and PDGFR and is under clinical trials for AML[38] and other cancers. Other FLT-3 inhibitors belong to the indolocarbazole family of compounds because they have been designed as analogues of staurosporine. The most studied compounds of this group are CEP-701[39] and PKC-412,[40] both of which inhibit several kinases besides FLT-3 and are under clinical evaluation for AML and other tumors.

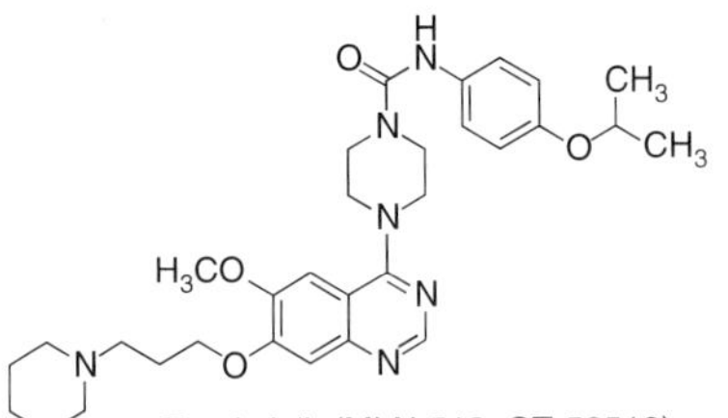

Tandutinib (MLN-518, CT-53518)

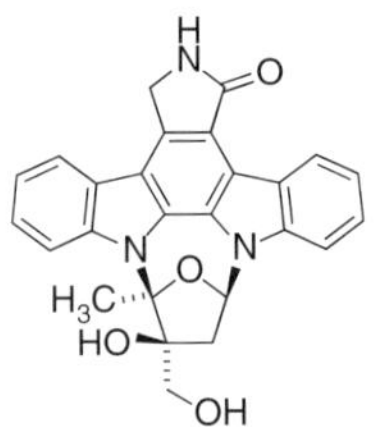

CEP-701

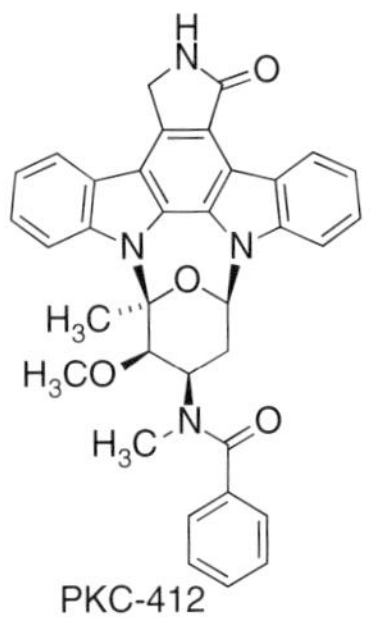

PKC-412

3.6. Inhibitors of BCR-ABL TK (Abelson kinase)

In normal cells, the *bcr* and *abl* genes are in different chromosomes and code different proteins. Chronic myeloid leukaemia (CML) is associated to the exchange of genetic material between the chromosomes 9 and 22, whereby the latter is altered and becomes the so-called Philadelphia chromosome. This transfer leads to a hybrid gene (*bcr-abl*), formed by transfer of one of the normal genes. This hybrid chromosome harbours the oncogenic protein BCR-ABL, a hybrid PTK with deregulated and high ABL kinase activity, resulting in a high leukocyte count. The TK domain is contained in the ABL portion of the hybrid protein, also known as the Abelson TK, which is therefore the natural target for the design of drugs for the treatment of CML.[41]

3.6.1. Compounds acting as ATP mimics

Imatinib (STI-571, from 'signal transduction inhibitor') is an inhibitor of BCR-ABL, and the first protein kinase inhibitor to be approved for cancer treatment after a particularly rapid clinical development phase.[42] It is effective in about 90% of patients with CML, although resistance is increasingly being encountered.

The lead compounds in the development of imatinib were 2-anilinopyrimidine derivatives **9.1**, identified by random screening as inhibitors of PKC, a serine-threonine kinase. All attempts to modify the guanidine portion, shown in bold in Fig. 9.13, were unsuccessful, which was later explained by its involvement in two hydrogen bonds with the active site of kinases. Optimization work led to compound **9.2**, bearing a 3-pyridyl substituent, as a potent inhibitor of PKC, and to the discovery that the addition of an amide group to the anilino substituent led to compounds that are dual inhibitors of PKC and ABL, such as **9.3**. One potential problem with these compounds is their hydrolysis *in vivo* to aniline derivatives, which are known to be mutagens. For this reason, the amide moiety had to be optimized for resistance to hydrolysis, and the benzamido group shown in compound **9.4** was chosen for this purpose. In efforts to eliminate the PKC inhibitory activity, a number of analogues were prepared, and it was found that an *ortho*-methyl substituent led to a selective ABL inhibitor (CGP-53716), which can be explained by assuming that the conformational restriction imposed by this substitution forces the molecule into a conformation that is suitable only for the ABL active site. Finally, further modifications were carried out in order to improve aqueous solubility by the introduction of basic side chains that would allow the preparation of salts, leading to the preparation of STI-571 (imatinib).[43] Unexpectedly, it was later shown that the piperazine ring added for this purpose also contributed to binding at the active site (see below). Nilotinib is an imatinib analogue with an imidazole ring replacing the piperidine moiety and a reverse amide function.

X-ray crystallography of a simplified model compound[44] and of imatinib itself[45] in the active site of ABL and related kinases[46] has shown that imatinib binds at the ATP binding site of ABL, showing specificity for an inactive conformation of the kinase. This inactive form contains the N-terminus of the

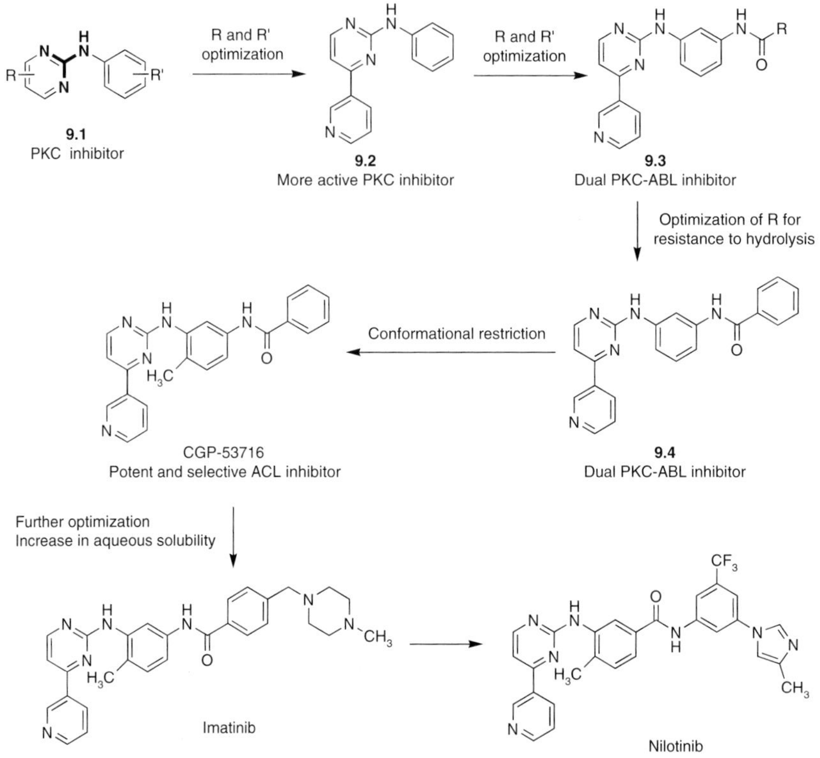

FIGURE 9.13 Development of imatinib and analogues.

kinase activation loop folded into the ATP binding site and mimics a bound peptide sustrate. The fact that imatinib binds to an unusual conformation of the kinase may explain its high selectivity.

The drug is sandwiched between the N- and C-lobes of the kinase domain and penetrates through the central region of the protein. In this arrangement, the pyridine and pyrimidine rings of imatinib occlude the region where the adenine ring of ATP binds. The rest of the compound wedges itself between the activation loop and helix αC, whereby the kinase is maintained in an inactive conformation. The piperazine ring lies along a hydrophobic pocket on the surface, making van der Waals interactions reinforced by hydrogen bonds with the carbonyl oxygen atoms of Ile-360 and His-361. All together, imatinib makes six hydrogen bond contacts (Fig. 9.14), with a large number of complementary van der Waals interactions.

Besides BCR-ABL, imatinib inhibits other kinases including c-KIT, a member of the type III group of receptor kinases. This protein is mutated in a rare subset of gastrointestinal soft-tissue sarcomas known as gastrointestinal stromal tumors (GISTs), and imatinib inhibits this mutated c-KIT. On the basis of a series of Phase II studies, the FDA approved the use of imatinib for GISTs in 2002. Another target for imatinib is the PDGF-receptor TK, which has an important role in

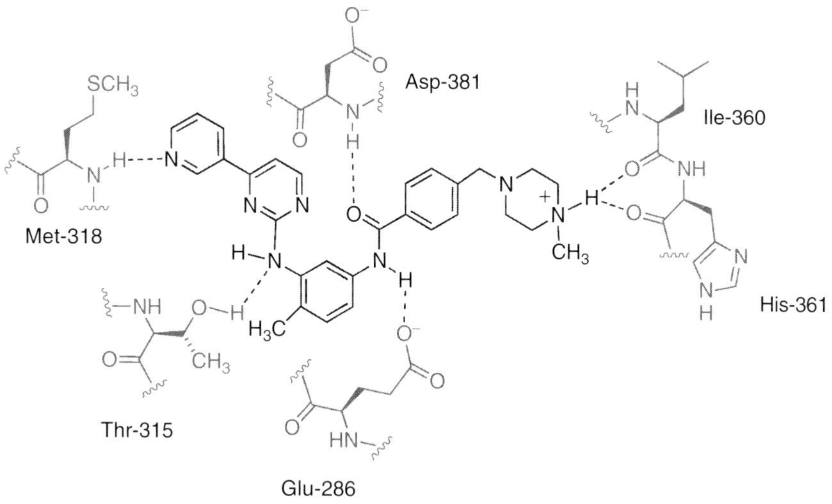

FIGURE 9.14   Binding of imatinib to ABL kinase.

tumorigenesis, specially in chronic myeloproliferative diseases. On this basis, the activity of imatinib in tumors such as glioma, prostate cancer, and small cell lung cancer is under active research.

Together with other mechanisms involving transport by Pgp-170 and others, resistance to imatinib has been associated to mutations in the BCR-ABL[47] and c-KIT[48] kinase domains, which impair the ability of the kinase to adopt the specific conformation to which imatinib binds.

Nilotinib (AMN-107)[49] is an imatinib analogue which has a high affinity and specificity for BCR-ABL. In addition to being more potent than imatinib against wild-type BCR-ABL, nilotinib is also significantly active against most imatinib-resistant BCR-ABL mutants, and is expected to be superior to imatinib in terms of the development of resistance.[50] In Phase I/II clinical trials, nilotinib has produced haematological and cytogenetic responses in CML patients who either did not initially respond to imatinib or developed imatinib resistance. The FDA has granted both fast track designation and orphan drug status to nilotinib, which also received orphan drug status from the European Medicines Evaluation Agency (EMEA).

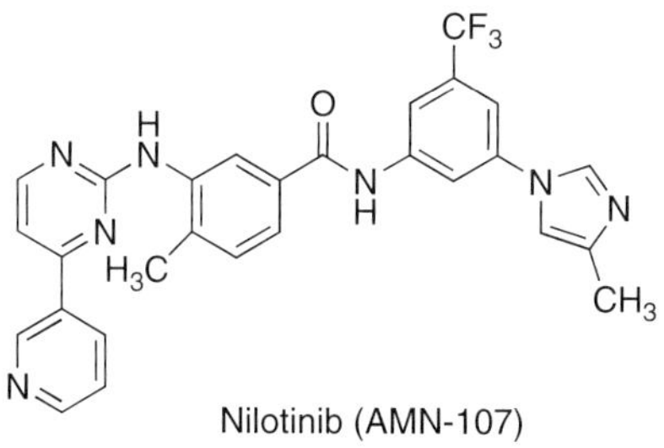

Nilotinib (AMN-107)

3.6.2. Compounds acting as tyrosine mimics

In contrast with the ATP-competitive compounds mentioned so far, another approach to the design of BCR-ABL inhibitors has been analogy to substrate, that is, tyrosine. Some of these compounds that are being developed for use in the clinic for BCR-ABL mutants resistant to imatinib are adaphostin and ON-012380.[5]

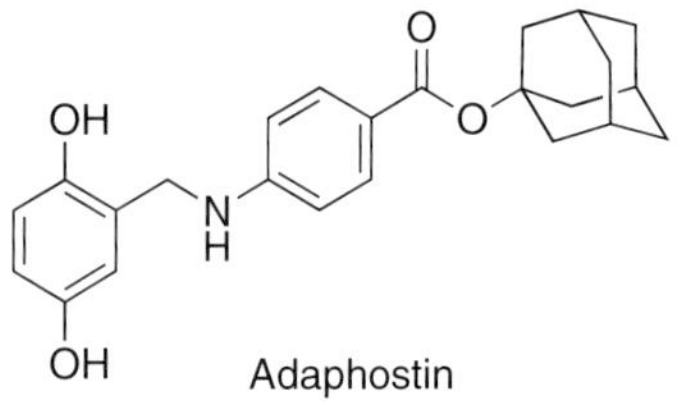

Adaphostin

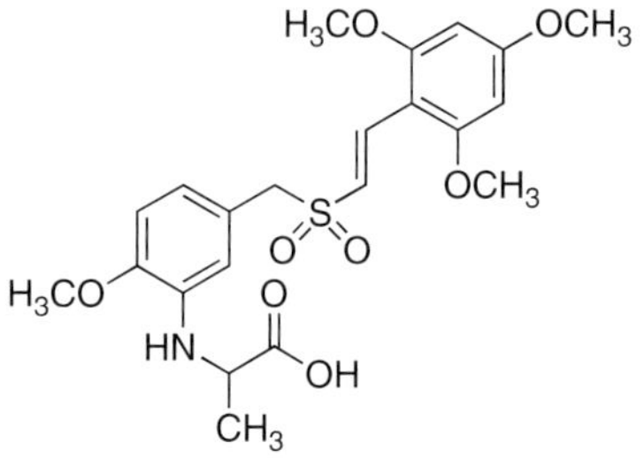

ON-012380

3.7. Dual Inhibitors of BCR-ABL and Src TKs

Src kinases are a family of non-receptor TKs that modulate intracellular signal transduction and whose kinase domain is about 47% identical in sequence with BCR-ABL. Src kinases are highly regulated in most normal cells but are deregulated in several human tumors, including metastatic colon and breast cancers. Elevated Src kinase activity has been linked with poor prognosis. Src kinases cannot recognize imatinib although they have most of the amino acids involved in the binding to BCR-ABL, perhaps due to differences in the inactive conformations of both proteins. Some dual inhibitors of BCR-ABL and Src kinases are known, among which we will mention dasatinib (BMS-354825), SKI-606, and AZD-0530.

In contrast to imatinib, dasatinib binds to both the open and closed conformations of BCR-ABL kinase, although in an opposite orientation and with the inhibitor in different conformations in both cases.[51] As a result, this compound inhibits not only the wild type of BCR-ABL, but also 14 of the 15 reported imatinib-resistant BCR-ABL mutations.[52] Dasatinib is currently undergoing Phase I clinical trials in imatinib-resistant CML patients.[53] Another dual inhibitor is SKI-606, which is a 4-anilinoquinoline-3-carbonitrile structurally related to the previously mentioned EKB-569 and HKI-272. This compound shows potent anti-proliferative activity against chronic myelogenous leukaemia[54] and is in Phase I clinical trials.[55] A structurally related quinazoline derivative, AZD-0530, is also in early clinical studies.[56]

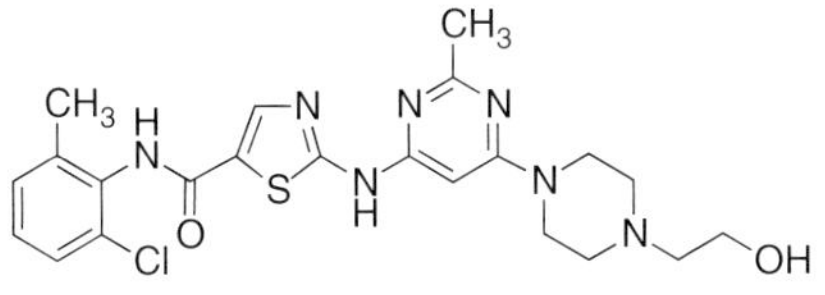

Dasatinib (BMS-354825)

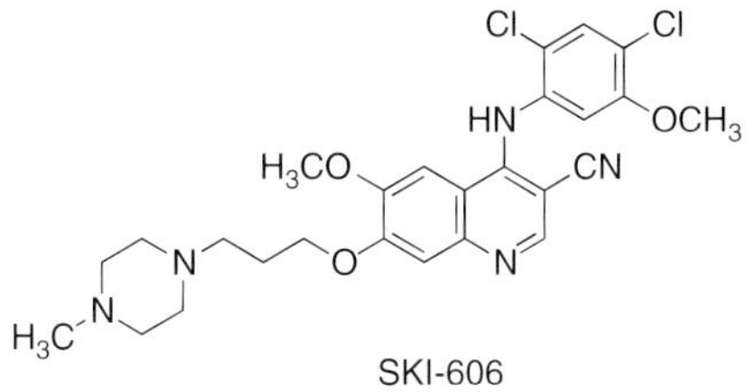

SKI-606

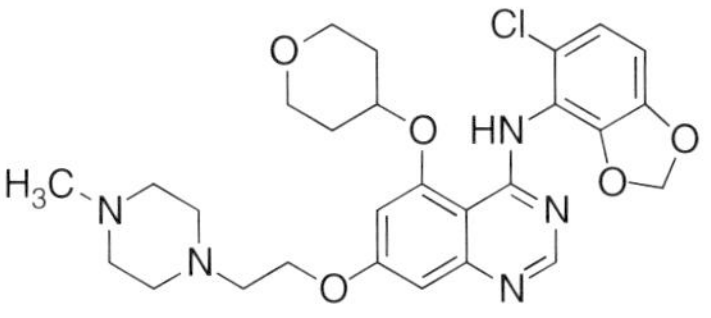

AZD-0530

4. INHIBITORS OF SERINE-THREONINE KINASES

4.1. Cyclin-Dependent Kinases

Cyclin-dependent kinases (CDKs) are involved in the control of the cell cycle, being in charge of moving the cell cycle from one phase to the next. CDKs are activated by complexation with a group of associated proteins called cyclins. There are several types of cyclins and CDKs that play their roles at different stages of the cell cycle. For instance, in the G1 phase, an increase in cyclin D followed by its binding to CDK4 and CDK6 leads to the phosphorylation of the tumor suppressor protein known as retinoblastoma (pRB). This molecule is normally bound to the transcription factor, E2F which is thereby inactivated. Phosphorylation of pRB prevents this binding, leaving the transcription factor free to bind to DNA, leading to the synthesis of several proteins, including cyclin E, which binds to CDK2 and the complex is necessary for the progression from the G1 to the S phase. Other complexes that are required for the progression of the cell cycle through subsequent stages are cyclin E-CDK2 and cyclin B-CDK1 (Fig. 9.15). On the other hand, the cell cycle is down-regulated by CDK inhibitors, also known as CKIs (p15, p21), which are proteins that restrain the activity of CDKs. Over-activity of cyclins or CDKs or insufficient activity of CKIs is associated with several tumors, making these processes attractive anticancer[57] and antiviral[58] targets.

Several structurally varied competitive inhibitors of CDKs have been developed, and some of them are in clinical trials, including flavopiridol, roscovitine, BMS-387032, and indisulam (E-7070).

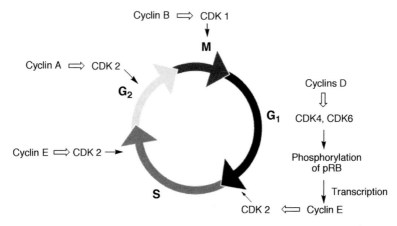

FIGURE 9.15 Control of cell cycle by cyclins and CDKs.

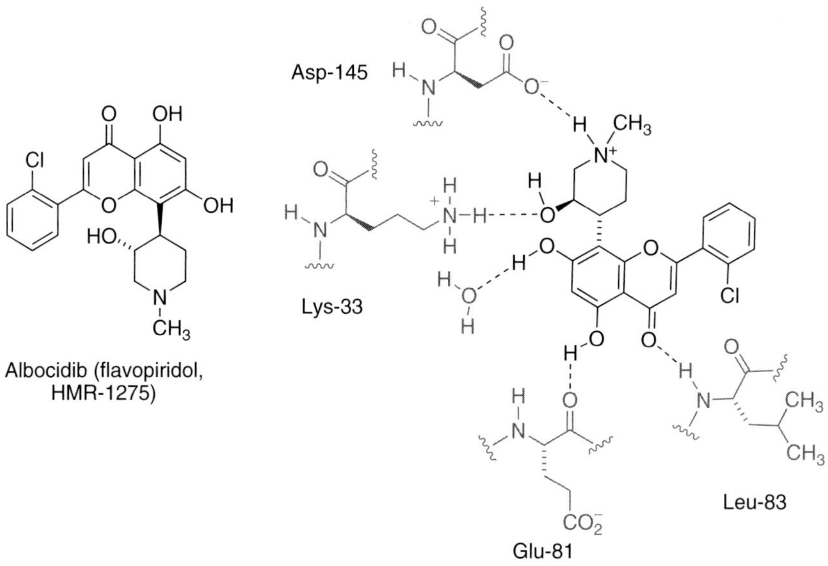

FIGURE 9.16 Binding of flavopiridol to CDKs.

Alvocidib (flavopiridol, HMR-1275) is a semi-synthetic flavone related to a natural product extracted from two Indian plants (*Amoora rohituka* and *Dysoxylum binectariferum*), and was the first CDK inhibitor to reach human clinical trials in patients with NSCLC, in combination with paclitaxel. Flavopiridol is a non-selective CDK inhibitor, thus explaining G1 and G2 arrest, and is also an inhibitor of transcription.[59] In spite of highly promising Phase I trials in a variety of cancers, the results of Phase II studies were rather disappointing in most cases, although encouraging results found in one of these studies[60] have prompted a Phase III study for the treatment of metastatic lung carcinoma, in combination with other chemotherapeutic agents. Flavopiridol binds to the ATP site, with the benzopyran ring lying in the adenine binding region, establishing the hydrogen bonds shown in Fig. 9.16.[61]

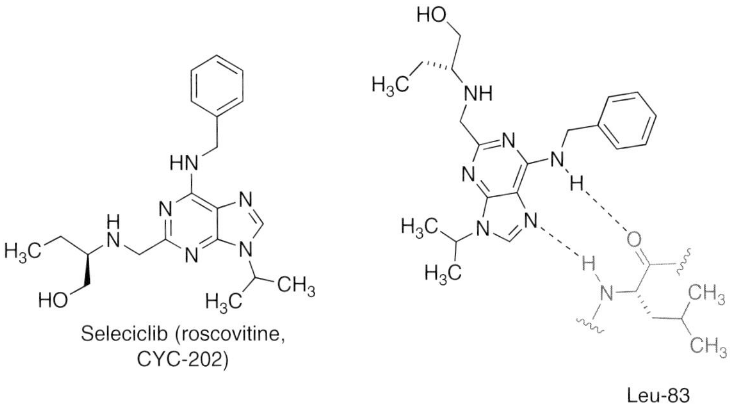

FIGURE 9.17   Binding of seleciclib to CDK2.

Seleciclib (roscovitine, CYC-202) was identified from a study of heterocycles with close analogy to the purine of ATP and is under clinical studies for lung and B-cell malignancies.[62] (*R*)-Roscovitine is rather selective for CDKs, especially CDK2, where it binds as shown in Fig. 9.17, and does not affect most other kinases. However, it binds a non-PTK target, pyridoxal kinase, the enzyme responsible for phosphorylation and activation of vitamin B_6, where, unexpectedly, it recognizes the pyridoxal rather than the ATP site.[63]

BMS-387032 is also a CDK2 inhibitor, and is currently in Phase I clinical trials for anti-cancer therapy. This compound was developed from a lead identified as a selective CDK2 inhibitor by high-throughput screening (BC-2626). However, it was inactive *in vitro*, and it was speculated that this was due to facile hydrolysis of the ester group. BMS-239091 was designed as a metabolically stable bioisoster, and it showed the expected cytotoxic activity against cancer cells. Replacement of the ethyl group by a *tert*-butyl in order to enhance hydrophobic interactions with the enzyme and introduction of a piperidine moiety to improve pharmacokinetic properties led to BMS-387032 (Fig. 9.18).[64] Unfortunately, this compound appears to be a substrate of the P-glycoprotein efflux pump, which limits its absorption.[65]

X-ray crystallographic studies showed that this inhibitor binds to the active site of CDK2 by two hydrogen bonds involving Leu-83 and the aminothiazole moiety and also through hydrophobic interactions of the thiomethylene and *tert*-butyl groups and two hydrophobic pockets (Fig. 9.19).[64]

The sulphonamide indisulam (E-7070) has a complex mechanism of action, partially involving interaction with CDKs. This compound decreases the expression of several cell cycle proteins (cyclins A and B1, CDK2, and CDC2). It also suppresses CDK2 catalytic activity with the induction of p53 and p21 proteins in lung cancer cells, disturbing the cell cycle at multiple points, including both the G1/S and the G2/M transition.[66] Indisulam is also a potent carbonic anhydrase IX inhibitor (see Section 4 of Chapter 12).[67] Subsequent research has located other potential targets for this drug such as of cytosolic malate dehydrogenase, which is inhibited by preventing the binding of its cofactor NADP,[68]

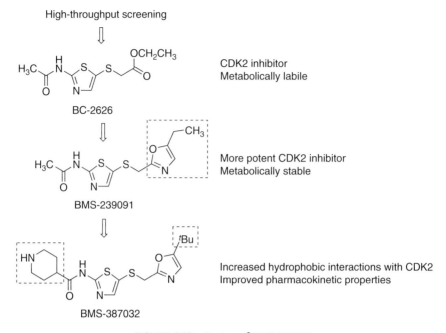

FIGURE 9.18   Design of BMS-387032.

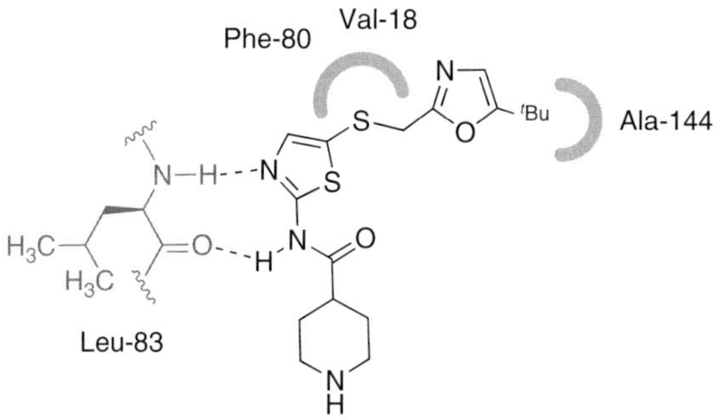

FIGURE 9.19   Binding of BMS-387032 to CDK2.

and leucine and uracil transporters.[69] Indisulam has reached Phase II studies in patients with metastatic melanoma[70] and other solid tumours.[71]

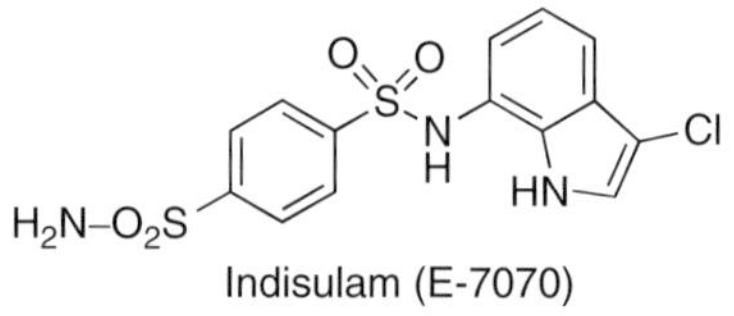

Indisulam (E-7070)

4.2. PDK1, AKT, and mTOR kinases

The PI3K–AKT–mTOR pathway controls many cellular processes that are important for the formation and progression of cancer, including apoptosis, transcription, translation, metabolism, angiogenesis, and cell cycle progression. Genetic alterations and biochemical activation of the pathway are frequent events in pre-neoplastic lesions and advanced cancers and often portend a poor prognosis. Thus, inhibition of this pathway is an attractive concept for cancer prevention and/or therapy.[72,73]

The sequence of events in the pathway starts by activation of PDK1, a serine-threonine kinase. When phosphatidylinositol-3-kinase (PI3K) is activated, it phosphorylates inositol-containing membrane lipids like phosphatidylinositol. The phosphorylation product PIP_3 binds to AKT, another serine-threonine kinase, and cause its translocation to the membrane where it contacts PDK1, which is responsible for at least one of the two phosphorylations necessary to activate AKT, namely the phosphorylation of Thr-308 in its T-loop. AKT then phosphorylates several substrates, leading to the activation, among others, of the so-called mammalian target of rapamycin (mTOR). This kinase, through its effects on other proteins, increases the translation efficiency of growth-regulatory gene products, increasing ribosomal RNA and nucleoprotein synthesis and elaboration of cyclin D. As previously mentioned, this is followed by activation of CDKs (Fig. 9.20).

4.2.1. AKT inhibitors

AKT exists in three isoforms, called AKT-1, 2, and 3. While the kinase domain is highly conserved among these isoforms, the PH domain, where phosphatidylinositol-3-phosphate binds, provides a target for allosteric AKT inhibitors with potential isoform selectivity.

Two types of AKT inhibitors[74] are known, namely ATP-competitive and allosteric inhibitors. The first group is exemplified by A-443654, a pan-AKT inhibitor with particular activity on AKT-1. *In vivo*, it slows the progression of tumors when used as monotherapy or in combination with paclitaxel or rapamycin. Tumor growth inhibition was observed during the dosing interval, and the tumors re-grew when compound administration was ceased.[75] Among allosteric inhibitors, perifosine is a lipophilic choline analogue that disrupts AKT membrane localization and activation, possibly by interference with the interaction of natural phosphatidylinositol phosphate groups with the PH domain of AKT. This compound shows selectivity for other kinases of the same pathway, and has entered Phase II clinical trials for solid tumours.[76] Perifosine is the prototype of a new group of anti-cancer drugs referred to as alkylphosphocholines.

A-443654

Perifosine

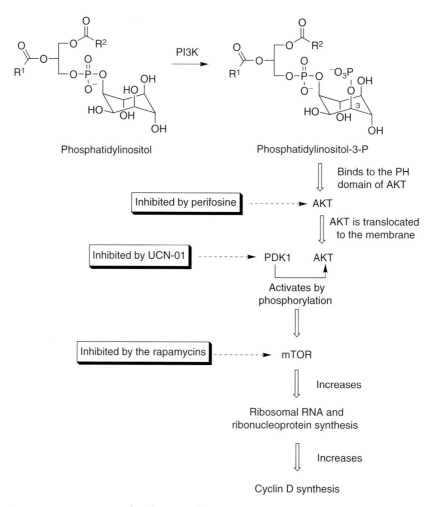

FIGURE 9.20   Activation of cyclin D synthesis involving PI₃K, PDK₁, AKT and mTOR kinases.

Association of these inhibitors with compounds targeting AKT-associated kinases, such as CSNK1G3 and/or IPMK has been suggested as a way to achieve increased efficacy and improved therapeutic index.[77]

Inhibition of heat-shock protein 90 (HSP 90) provides a third, indirect way to achieve AKT inhibition,[74] and will be discussed in Section 7.

4.2.2. PDK1 inhibitors

UCN-01 is a natural staurosporine derivative that was originally described as a selective inhibitor of PKC, but further research showed that it is non-specific; for instance, it is a potent inhibitor of CDKs, checkpoint kinase 1 (CHK-1) and PKC. However, its antitumor activity seems to be related to CHK-1 inhibition[78] and to disruption of the PI3K–AKT pathway through inhibition of PDK1.[79] UCN-01 is currently under clinical development.[80]

UCN-01

The binding of UCN-01 to the active site of PDK1 has been studied by X-ray crystallography and compared with that of staurosporine, showing the importance of the hydroxy group in the former.[81] The inhibitor is located in the ATP-binding site and the heterocyclic moiety is sandwiched with hydrophobic residues Leu-88, Val-96, Ala-109, and Leu-98 of the *N*-terminal lobe, and Thr-222 and Leu-212 of the *C*-terminal lobe. The lactam group mimics the adenine interactions in ATP and shows two hydrogen bonds with the backbone Ser-160 and Ala-162 residues. The key hydroxyl group interacts with side chains of Gln-220 and Thr-222, the latter with the intermediacy of a molecule of water. An additional hydrogen bond, similar to the one formed by the ATP ribose, is formed between the methylamino group and Glu-166. A second hydrogen bond of the methylamino group involves Glu-211 (Fig. 9.21).

4.2.3. mTOR inhibitors

The previously mentioned downstream serine-threonine kinase known as the 'mammalian target of rapamycin' (mTOR) is another cancer target related to the PI3K–AKT–mTOR pathway that acts as a regulator of the translation of specific mRNA sub-populations that are important for cell proliferation and survival.[82–84] mTOR inhibition results in the suppression of growth and proliferation of lymphocytes and certain tumor cell lines.

The parent compound, the macrolide rapamycin (sirolimus), is a natural product isolated from a *Streptomyces hygroscopicus* found in soil samples from Easter Island (*Rapa Nui*). This compound has been approved as an immunosuppressor for the prevention of rejection following cancer transplantation, and the experience gained in this setting has proved that it is well tolerated. Some rapamycin derivatives[85] are being clinically assayed as antitumor agents. They include the water-soluble rapamycin ester prodrug tensirolimus (CCI-779) and the *O*-hydroxyethyl derivative everolimus (RAD-001), both of which are in Phase III clinical evaluation, as well as AP-23573.[82] Rapamycin and its derivatives do not bind directly to mTOR, but to an immunophilin of the FK-506 family, called

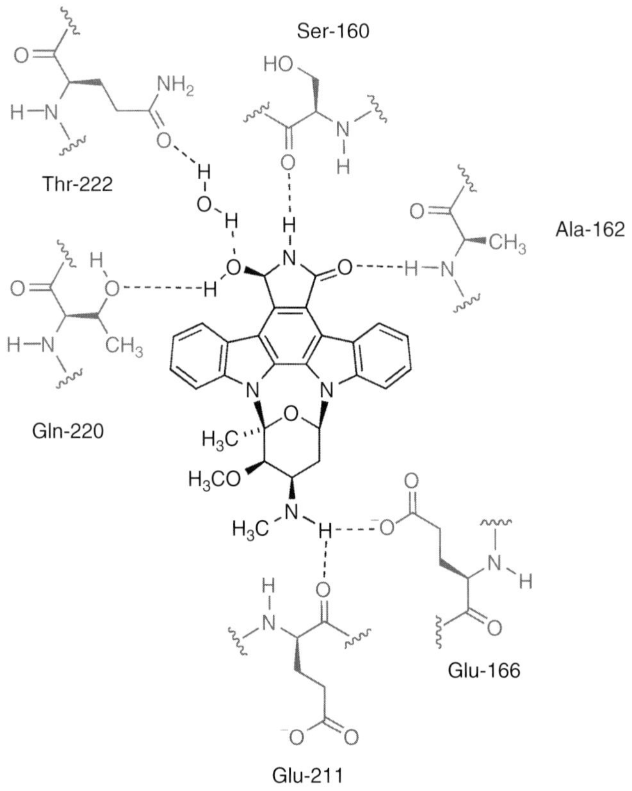

FIGURE 9.21 Binding of UCN-01 to PDK1.

FKBP-12, and this complex then interacts with mTOR at a region adjacent to its kinase domain, thereby preventing the interaction of mTOR with its kinase substrates.

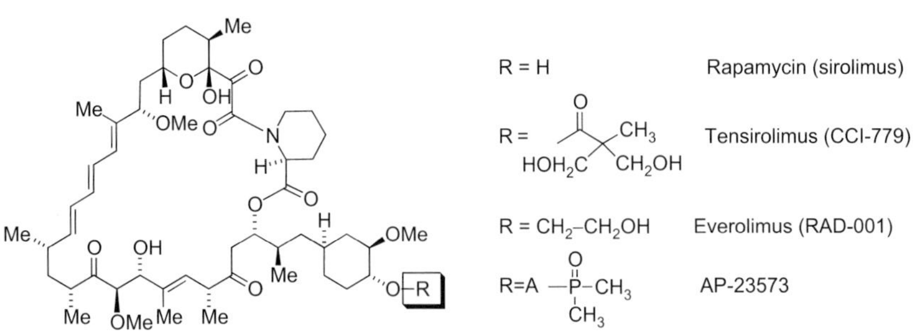

R = H   Rapamycin (sirolimus)

R = (structure)   Tensirolimus (CCI-779)

R = CH$_2$–CH$_2$OH   Everolimus (RAD-001)

R=A (structure)   AP-23573

4.3. Aurora kinases

Aurore kinases are a small family formed by three serine-threonine kinases (Aurora A, B, and C). They play a crucial role in mitosis because they are important for centrosome maturation, chromosome segregation, and cytokinesis. Aurora kinases are implicated in the onset and progression of many human cancers by dysregulating the phosphorylation of histone H3 and the tumor suppressor p53. They are overexpressed in a wide range of human tumors, including 50% of colorectal, ovarian, and gastric cancers, and this over-expression transforms microblasts giving rise to cells containing multiple centrosomes and multipolar spindles, and the resulting genetic instability contributes to tumorigenesis.[86] For these reasons, Aurora kinases are an emerging target in cancer chemotherapy.[87,88] The main difference between Aurora kinase inhibitors and other antimitotic drugs is that the former push the cells through aberrant and irreversible rounds of the cell cycle, resulting in a delayed but sustained response in animal models.[88]

Only a few inhibitors of Aurora kinases are known, which belong to well-known classes of ATP-competitive kinase inhibitors.[88] Among them, VX-680 also inhibits FLT-3 and entered Phase I clinical trials for haematological cancers in 2005. It was designed using the 4-aminopyrimidine template, on the basis of the crystal structures of the ATP binding sites of the three Aurora kinases.[89] Another compound that has recently entered Phase I clinical studies is AZD-1152, which was designed by manipulation of the 4-aminoquinazoline structure, a well-known template for kinase inhibition, particularly at the 4, 6, and 7 positions.

VX-680   AZD-1152

Another compound that has been reported to be moderately selective against Aurora A is PHA-739358, which is in Phase I clinical studies. The structure or pharmacological profile of PHA-739358 has not been divulged, but it could be related to other Aurora analogues derived from the tetrahydropyrrolo[3,4-c] pyrazole framework reported by the same company as an adenine mimetic in the ATP site of Aurore kinases (Fig. 9.22).[90]

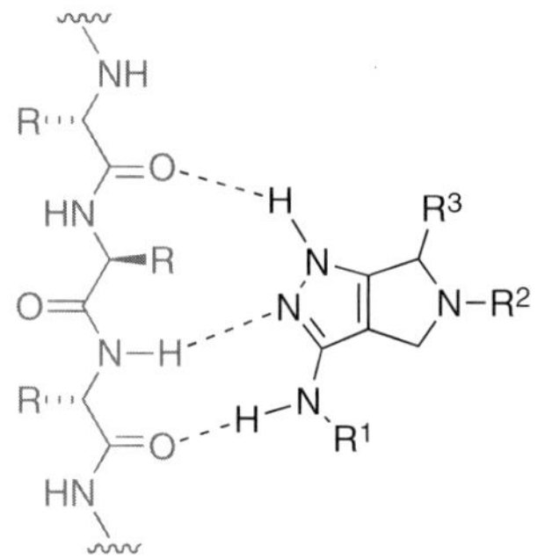

FIGURE 9.22   Binding of PHA-739358 to Aurora kinases.

4.4. PKC modulators

PKC is a family of closely related serine-threonine kinases. They can be activated by G-protein–coupled proteins that contain seven transmembrane domains. Activation of the G-protein–coupled receptor also activates phosphoplipase C (PLC), which catalyses the hydrolysis of phosphatidylinositol diphosphate (PIP_2), which is integrated into the membrane. This hydrolysis generates two secondary messengers, namely inositol triphosphate (IP_3) and diacylglycerol (DG). The latter compound is lipophilic and remains in the cell membrane, where it activates PKC. Once back in the cytoplasm, PKC activates Raf by phosphorylation of serine-threonine residues, thereby providing input into the MAPK pathway (Fig. 9.23). For this reason, PKC is an attractive anti-cancer target.[91]

Some analogues of the natural kinase inhibitor staurosporine have been developed as PKC inhibitors with anti-cancer activity. They include the previously mentioned multi-kinase inhibitor UCN-01, CGP-41251,[92] ruboxistaurin (LY-333531), which is specific for the PKC-β isoform, enzastaurin (LY-317615), in Phase II for recurrent malignant glioblastomes,[93] and PKC-412[94]. All these compounds are under clinical trials as anticancer agents (Fig. 9.24). These compounds have other applications, and thus CGP-41251 is also being evaluated as a multi-drug resistance reversal agent.[95] An important mechanism that may mediate the development of hyperglycemia-induced vascular abnormalities in the retina is mediated by the activation of the PKC pathway, and for this reason LY-333531 is under clinical study for the treatment of microvascular complications of diabetes.[96,97]

Bryostatin 1 is one of a series of cyclic macrolides isolated from the marine bryozoan *Bugula neritina* that is in clinical development as an anti-leukaemic agent and is also in Phase II clinical trials against melanomas, lymphomas, and renal cancer.[98] The mechanism of activity of the bryostatins is not completely understood, but it may be related to their ability to modulate the PKC activity. Human clinical trials have been less promising than *in vitro* studies, but suggest that bryostatins have a synergistic action with other chemotherapeutic agents such as paclitaxel.

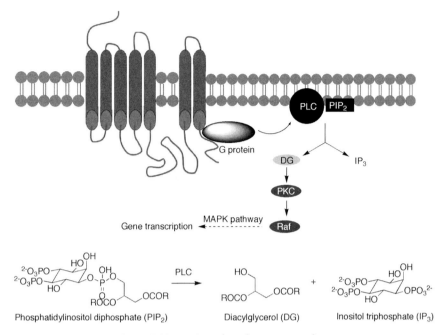

FIGURE 9.23   PKC-mediated activation of RAF.

Bryostatin 1

ISIS 3521 (CGP 64128A) and ISIS 5132 are two phosphorothioate antisense oligonucleotides which hybridize to the PKC mRNA and have undergone clinical trials in patients with locally advanced or metastatic colorectal cancer.[99]

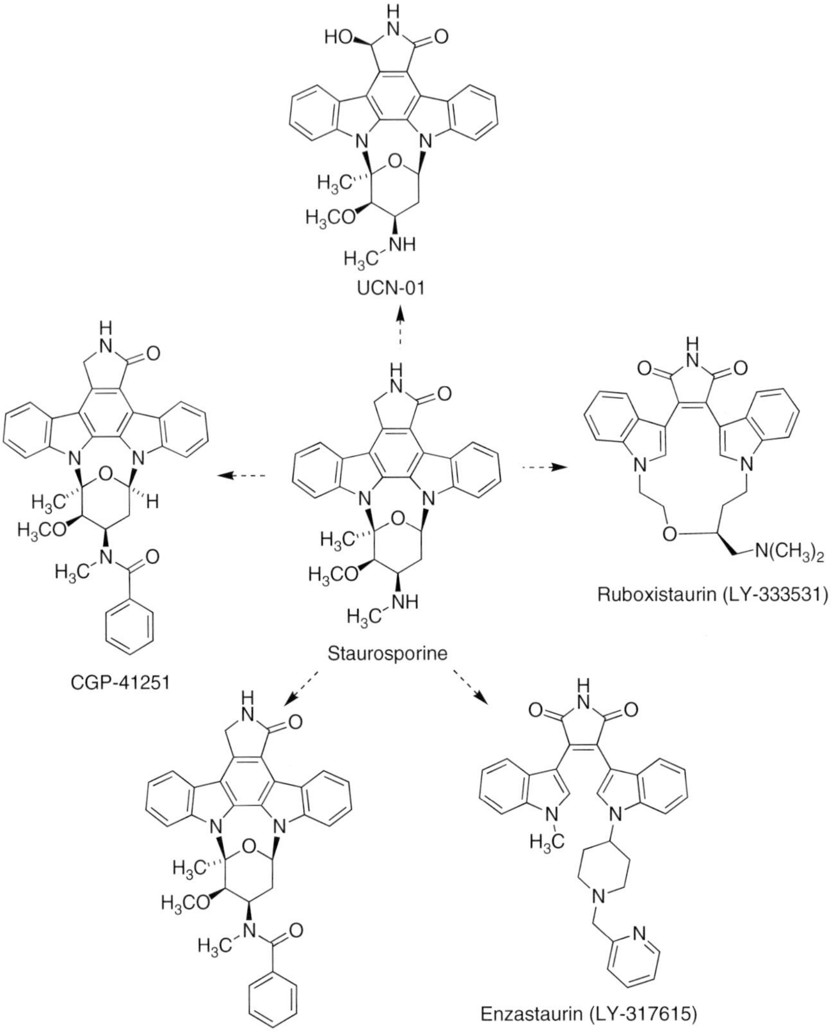

FIGURE 9.24   Staurosporine-related PKC modulators in clinical trials.

5. INHIBITORS OF THE RAS–RAF–MEK SIGNALLING PATHWAY AND FARNESYL TRANSFERASE

The Ras proteins belong to a large family of GTP-binding proteins (GTPases), and were among the first proteins identified as cell growth regulators. In normal cells, the Ras activity is controlled by the GTP/GDP ratio. About 25% of human tumors, including nearly all pancreatic cancers and at least 30% of colon, thyroid, and lung tumors, have undergone an activating mutation in one of the *Ras* genes that leads to proteins remaining locked in an active state, especially those corresponding to three members of the family known as H-Ras, K-Ras, and N-Ras. Because of this large percentage of human tumors containing *Ras* mutants and their key role in maintaining the malignant phenotype, interruption of the Ras signalling pathway is an important focus of anticancer drug development,[100–102] which has resulted in more than 20 new antitumor agents in clinical trials.

The Ras proteins need to be translocated to the membrane inner side in order to be able to recruit their target enzymes. Newly synthesized Ras is a cytoplasmatic protein that requires a post-transtational structural modification to render them sufficiently lipophilic to allow their anchoring in the membrane. This modification involves several steps (Fig. 9.25):

a. Prenylation, that is, the addition of farnesyl residues by farnesyltransferase (FTase), which recognizes the terminal CAAX sequence of Ras, where C represents cysteine, A is an aliphatic amino acid (Leu, Ileu, Val), and X is Met, Ser, Leu, or Gln. Depending on the X residue, some Ras proteins may be geranylgeranylated by other transferases (GGTases).
b. Proteolysis by an endoprotease that removes the last three amino acids of the C-terminus.
c. Esterification of the new C-terminus by a methyltransferase.
d. Introduction of two palmitoyl groups by acylation of the thiol groups of two Cys residues by a palmitoylCoA transferase. This reaction does not take place in K-Ras, whose interaction with the plasma membrane is promoted by electrostatic bonding between a group of charged lysine residues and the charged phospholipid head groups.

Membrane-bound Ras cycles between the quiescent GDP-bound and the activated GTP-bound forms. This activation is triggered by alteration of the affinity of Ras for GDP, allowing exchange for GTP, by a multi-protein scaffold formed by adaptor molecules such as growth factor receptor bound (Grb), which binds to phosphorylated tyrosine receptors to recruit effectors such as the so-called Son of Sevenless (SOS). The main targets recruited by the active, membrane-bound Ras are the Raf family kinases, which in turn activate mitogen activated protein kinase kinases (MEK) to phosphorylate mitogen activated protein kinases (MAPK, also known as ERK) that then influence gene expression (Fig. 9.26).

While the above mechanism promotes GTP binding to Ras, a competing process that involves the so-called GTPase activating proteins (GAPs) prevents it by activating GTP hydrolysis ('Ras switch', Fig. 9.27). A single amino acid change at codons 12 (the most common in human cancer), 13, or 61 results in mutant Ras proteins that are not sensitive to control by GAPs and hence Ras is maintained in a GTP-bound (on) state.

The major approaches that have yielded clinically useful compounds acting at the Ras pathway can be summarized as follows:

a. Inhibitors of Ras protein expression.
b. Inhibitors of Ras processing by farnesyltranferase.
c. Inhibitors of downstream effectors of Ras function.

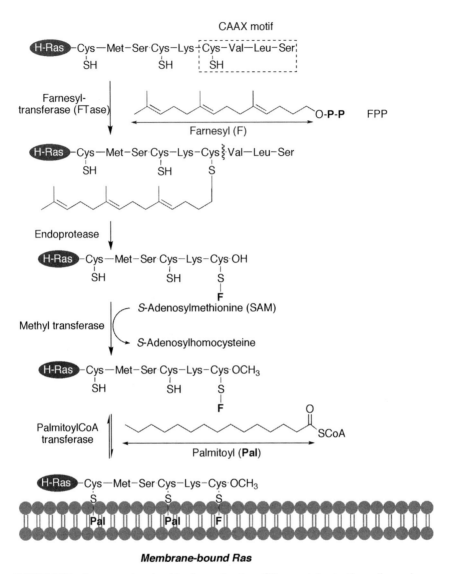

FIGURE 9.25   Processes involved in the anchoring of Ras proteins to the cell membrane.

5.1. Inhibitors of Ras protein expression

Antisense nucleotides targeted at H-Ras mRNA have been developed. The most relevant is the phosphorothioate oligodeoxynucleotide ISIS-2503, containing 20 nucleotides (5′-TCCGTCATCGCTCCTCAGGG-3′) that is under clinical assay for pancreatic carcinoma in combination with gemcitabine.[103]

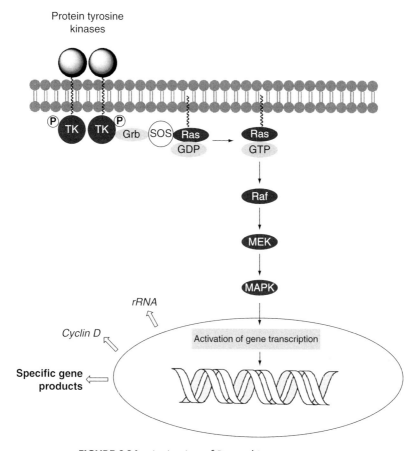

FIGURE 9.26   Activation of Ras and its consequences.

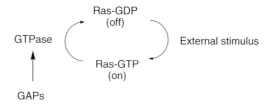

FIGURE 9.27   Control of Ras activation by GTPase activating proteins.

5.2. Inhibitors of Ras processing by farnesyltranferase

Farnesylation is critical for Ras maturation and function, and is therefore an important target for drug development.[104] Farnesylation is carried out by the previously mentioned FTase, a heterodimeric zinc metalloprotein formed by

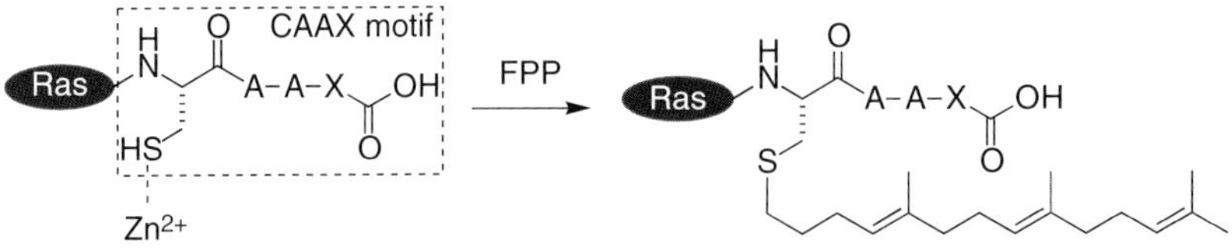

FIGURE 9.28 Farnesylation of Ras.

α and β sub-units that binds to the 'CAAX box' of the Ras protein, which adopts an extended conformation with the cysteine sulphur coordinated to the zinc ion in the active site. This coordination apparently lowers the pK_a of the thiol, increasing the local concentration of thiolate anion and facilitating its farnesylation (Fig. 9.28)

Design of inhibitors of this enzyme has been achieved using three approaches:[105-107]

a. Analogues that compete with the substrate, farnesyl pyrophosphate (FPP).
b. Peptide or non-peptide peptidomimetic compounds targeted at the terminal CAAX sequence of Ras.
c. Bisubstrate analogues that combine both structural features.

5.2.1. FPP mimics

This class of inhibitors has attracted less interest because of their potential lack of selectivity due to the fact that FPP is a substrate for other enzymes such as squalene synthase. Although some of these compounds (e.g. **9.1** and **9.2**) are potent inhibitors of the enzyme, they have failed to show *in vivo* activity.

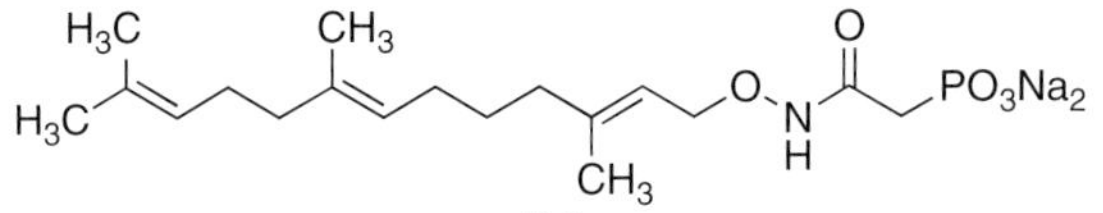

9.1

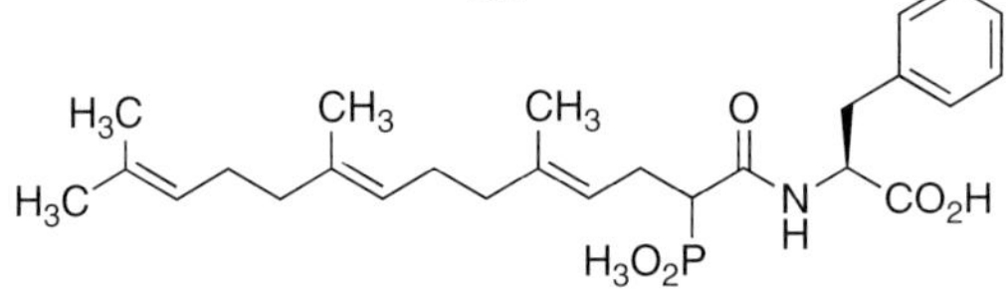

9.2

5.2.2. Peptides and peptidomimetics that mimic the CAAX motif

Initial reports about the FTase inhibitory activity of CAAX tetrapeptides led to the identification of Cys-Val-Phe-Met as a lead for systematic structural modification. Most of these analogues were aimed at achieving suitable pharmacokinetic properties while retaining the thiol group, important for coordination to zinc. Some of the changes consisted of replacing the labile peptide bonds by stable methylenamino or methylenoxy links (e.g. L-739750) or the use of non-proteinogenic

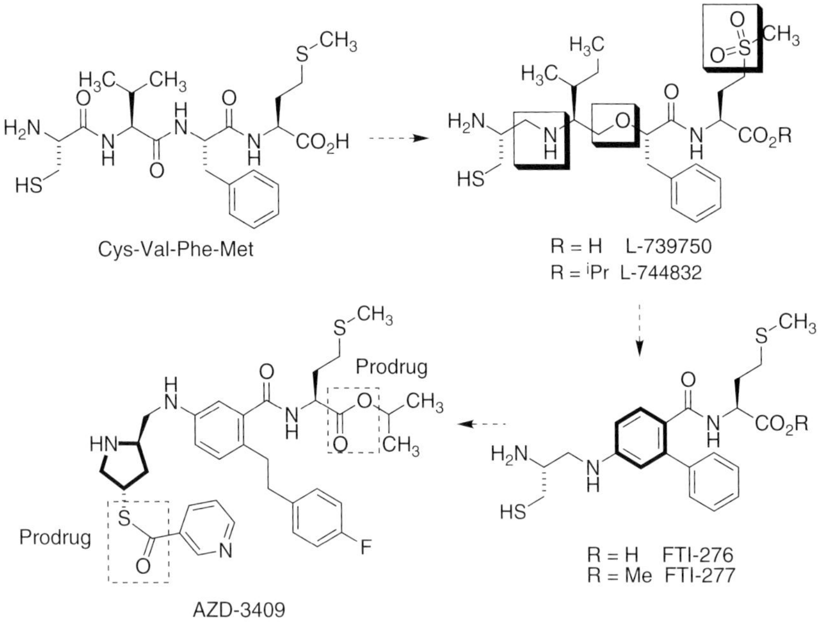

FIGURE 9.29 Peptide-like compounds that mimic the CAAX motif in FTase.

amino acids like aminobenzoic acid derivatives (e.g. FTI-276). L-739750 and FTI-276 were normally employed as ester prodrugs (L-744832 and FTI-277, respectively) in order to enhance their absorption (Fig. 9.29). Despite the encouraging *in vivo* data obtained for these peptidomimetics, there were reservations regarding their clinical use because of their potential thiol-related toxicity; nevertheless, L-744832 has reached clinical trials.[108] A combination of the modifications used for the design of L-739750 and FTI-276, with the additional modifications of the replacement of the reduced cysteine moiety by a mercaptoproline and having both the thiol and the carboxylic groups masked as esters, has led to the design of the double pro-drug AZD-3409, which has reached clinical trials.

The main FTase inhibitors under clinical development[109] are non-peptidic, heterocyclic compounds such as BMS-214662, tipifarnib (R-115777), L-778123, lonafarnib (SCH-66336), and SCH-226374 that have normally been discovered through screening approaches. BMS-214662, tifiparnib (initially developed as an antifungal agent) and L-778123 contain imidazole rings that are able to co-ordinate the catalytic zinc cation competing with the cysteine unit at the CAAX motif in Ras. Lonafarnib was discovered through library screening and it does not have a group able to act as a zinc ligand, which led to the design of its imidazole-bearing analogue SCH-226374.

Both tipifarnib and lonafarnib are orally bioavailable, while BMS-24662 and L-7781123 have been studied as intravenous formulations. BMS-24662, tipifarnib[110,111] L-778123,[112] and lonafarnib[113] are under clinical studies against a variety of cancers.

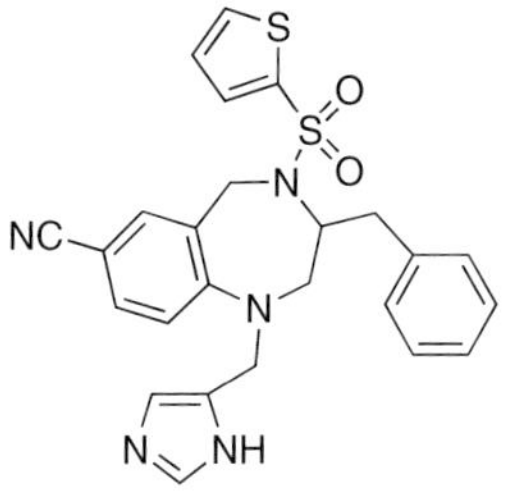

BMS-214662

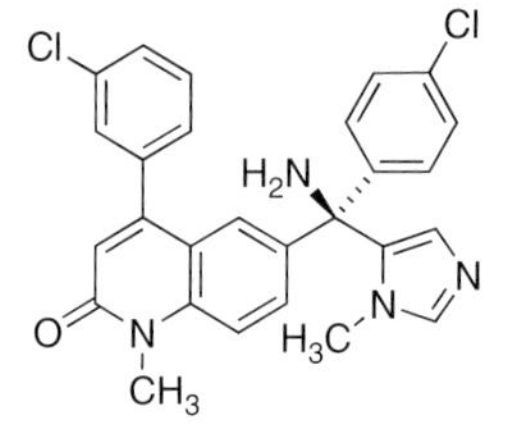

Tipifarnib (R-115777)

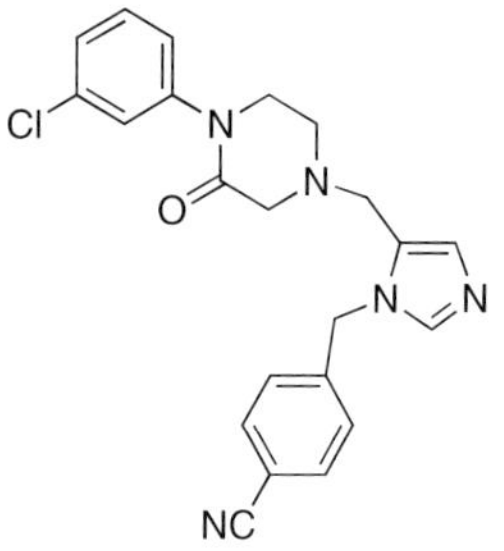

L-778123

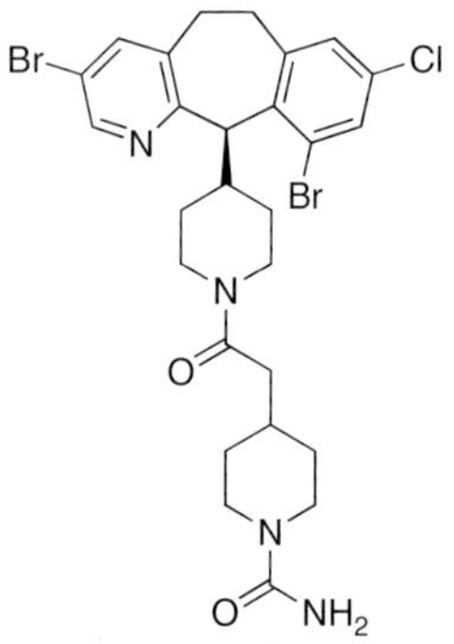

Lonafarnib (SCH-66336)

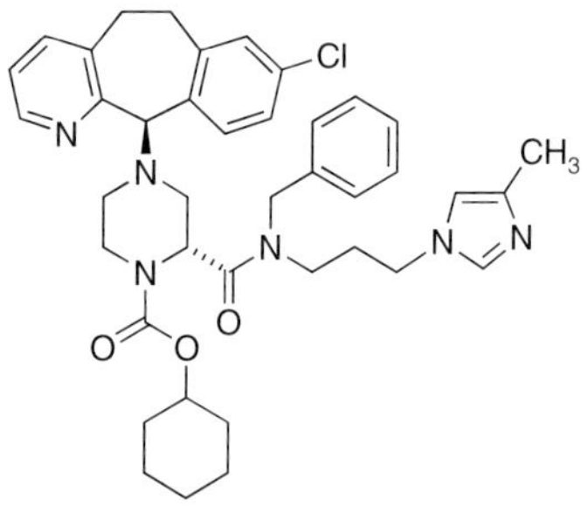

SCH-226374

X-ray diffraction studies of BMS-214662 and tipifarnib complexed with farnesyl transferase show that they bind to a hydrophobic cleft formed at the interface of the α and β sub-units, forming a ternary complex with the FPP substrate and the enzyme, binding the catalytic zinc cation at the rim of the active site. Therefore, they act by a peptide-competitive mechanism.[114] This interaction is exemplified in Fig. 9.30 for the case of tipifarnib, which adopts a U shape stabilized by π-stacking interactions between the two chlorophenyl rings. Other aromatic stacking interactions are important, including those between the 4-chlorophenyl unit and the farnesyl moiety, the quinoline unit and Tyr-361β, and the 3-chlorophenyl ring and Trp-102β and Trp-106β. The imidazole nitrogen coordinates with the zinc cofactor at the catalytic centre, and water-mediated hydrogen bonds are established between the quinolone carbonyl oxygen and the Phe-360β at the protein backbone, as well as between the amino group and the FPP α-phosphate moiety. Similarly, the imidazole ring in BMS-214662 binds to the zinc cation in the active site and the union is stabilized by several π-stacking interactions.[114]

L-778123 was designed to selectively compete with the binding of the CAAX fragment of Ras in FTase, but *in vivo* studies showed that it also inhibited GGTase I in the presence of anions such as sulphate and phosphate by unexpectedly competing with the GGPP substrate rather than with the peptide. The inhibitor

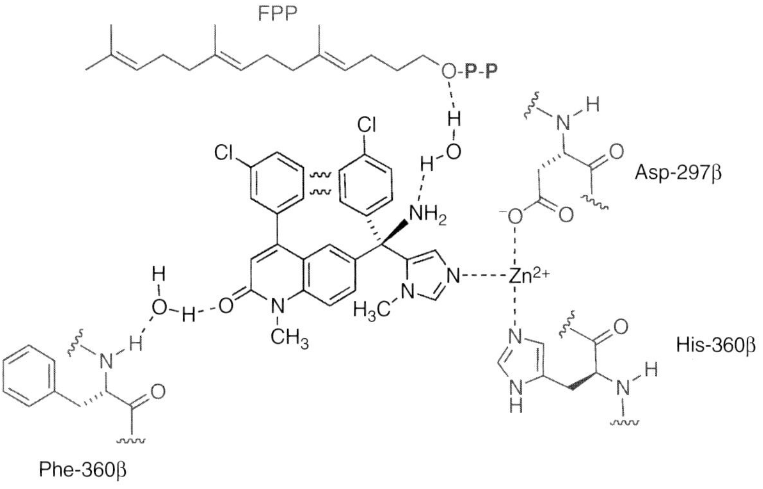

FIGURE 9.30   Ternary complex formed by tifiparnib, FPP and FTase.

adopts a U shape by van der Waals stacking between the cyanophenyl and piperazine units, with the imidazole unit occupying the apex of the structure and coordinating with the zinc cation. In FTase, FPP binds adjacently at the corresponding site, with the pyrophosphate group occupying a positively charged pocket (Fig. 9.31A). However, in GGTase I the inhibitor does not form a ternary complex with geranylgeraniol pyrophosphate and instead it occupies the lipid substrate binding pocket and a portion of the peptide substrate binding pocket. The cationic site is occupied by a sulphate anion, which is placed where the pyrophosphate of GGPP normally binds (Fig. 9.31B).[115]

5.2.3. Bisubstrate analogues

Some FTase inhibitors incorporate structural motifs from both FPP and the CAAX sequence. One example is compound **9.3**, where the thiol moiety of CAAX was substituted by a carboxylic group and the farnesyl chain was covalently attached to the peptide through an amide linkage.

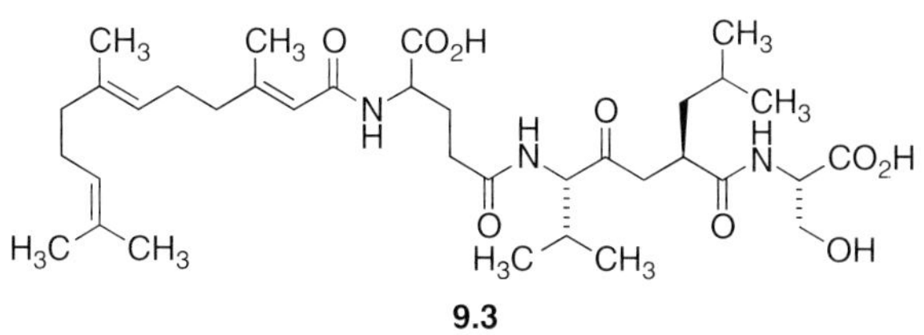

9.3

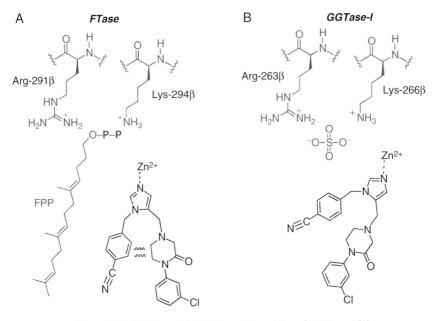

FIGURE 9.31 Binding of L-778123 to FTase (A) and GGTase-I (B).

5.3. Inhibitors of downstream effectors of Ras function

Multiple Ras effectors are known, the best known of which is the c-Raf kinase–MEK–ERK pathway (Fig. 9.26). Inappropriate activation of this pathway through mutations induced via oncogenes is present in many cancers.

5.3.1. Raf inhibitors

Three Raf proteins are known, namely c-Raf (Raf-1), b-Raf, and a-Raf. Sorafenib (BAY43–9006) is a multi-targeted TK inhibitor, which acts on c-raf/b-raf as well as several TKs including VEGFR-2 and PDGFR-β, among others, by binding to their ATP site. It shows activity against renal cell and hepatocellular carcinomas and it was approved by the FDA at the end of 2005, being the first drug to be approved for this indication since 1992. The diarylurea scaffold found in sorafenib was initially proposed in a *de novo* approach to CDK4 inhibitors.[61,116]

Sorafenib (BAY43-9006)

ISIS-5132 is a 20-mer phosphothiorate antisense oligonucleotide that is complementary to c-Raf kinase mRNA and hence it down-regulates the expression of Raf kinase. This oligonucleotide is in Phase II clinical trials for colorectal cancer.[117]

5.3.2. MEK inhibitors

MEK inhibitors were the first selective inhibitors of the MAPK pathway to enter the clinic. Among them, CI-1040 (PD-184352)[118] is an orally active, potent, and selective inhibitor of MEK that targets a non-ATP site of the kinase. This compound is undergoing clinical studies in patients with advanced NSCLC, breast, colon, and pancreatic cancer.[119] Another potent MEK1/2 inhibitor that has reached Phase I evaluation is ARRY-142886 (AZD-6244),[120] a member of a group of compounds whose structure has been disclosed only partially but it is known to derive from the anilinobenzimidazole **9.4**.[121]

CI-1040
(PD-184352)

9.4
ARRY-142886 (AZD-6244)

5.3.3. MAPK inhibitors

Activated MEK1 catalyses the phosphorylation of ERK1 and ERK2 on both a Tyr and a Thr residue. These MAP kinases (MAPKs, MKPs) can then phosphorylate a variety of substrates, including transcription factors that control cellular growth. Other similarly activated MAP kinases are JNKs and p38 MAPKs. Although MAP kinases play a role in the regulation of the growth and survival of a range of human tumors, their inhibitors have not reached the clinical evaluation stage as antitumor drugs.[4] Inhibitors of p38 MAPK are promising in arthritic and inflammatory diseases.[122]

6. INHIBITORS OF FARNESYLDIPHOSPHATE SYNTHASE AND GERANYLGERANYLDIPHOSPHATE SYNTHASE

Besides Ras, there are some small GTPases like Rho, Rac, cdc42, and Rab that need to be prenylated by transfer of farnesyl or geranylgeranyl units onto a Cys residue in order to be anchored to cell membranes and to be able to effect protein–protein interactions.

Nitrogen-containing biphosphonates (N-BP) are normally used in therapeutics for the treatment of degenerative bone disease such as osteoporosis. Bisphosphonates belonging to the third generation, such as risedronate, zoledronate, and minodronate, which contain a nitrogen heterocycle, have shown a dual anti-bone resorption and antitumor cell proliferation activity and are undergoing pre-clinical and clinical studies for several cancers including breast, prostate, lung, renal, osteosarcoma, and chondreosarcoma. The antitumor activity of these phosphonates is due to the inhibition of farnesyldiphosphate synthase (FPP) and geranylgeranyl-diphosphate synthase (GGPP) and hence the farnesylation or geranylgeranylation of small GTPases.[84]

Risedronate   Zoledronate   Minodronate

7. ANTICANCER DRUGS ACTING ON APOPTOTIC SIGNALLING PATHWAYS

Apoptosis is normally defined as programmed active cell death. Although at first sight cell death might be viewed as a pathological phenomenon, each second about one million cells in a human body undergo apoptosis. Several genes involved in the apoptosis process have been found to be defective in cancer cells, specially the *BCL2* and caspase-family genes.[123]

Apoptosis is caused by a group of cysteine aspartyl specific proteases called caspases, which cleave their substrates at aspartic acid residues. Caspases are produced as inactive zymogens, which are activated by a hydrolysis reaction at Asp sites. Because both the activation of caspases and the cleavage of their substrates take place at Asp sites, they can act in proteolytic cascade processes.

Most of the caspase-related molecules are not typical drug targets (e.g. cell surface receptors), and for this reason small-molecule drugs are only of limited use and other approaches (monoclonal antibodies, antisense oligonucleotides) are often needed. Many anti-cancer drugs discussed elsewhere in the book, specially those that can induce DNA strand breaks or microtubule damage, are also apoptosis inducers, but this section is dedicated only to those drugs that are aimed at specific targets in the apoptotic pathways,[124–126] which are summarized in Fig. 9.32.

7.1. BCL-2 proteins

BCL-2 is a family of 25 apoptotic and anti-apoptotic proteins. Their main function seems to be the regulation of the release of cytochrome *c* from the mitochondria, which is promoted by pro-apoptotic BCL-2 proteins and inhibited by the anti-apoptotic ones. The ratios of pro-and anti-apoptotic BCL-2 proteins dictate the

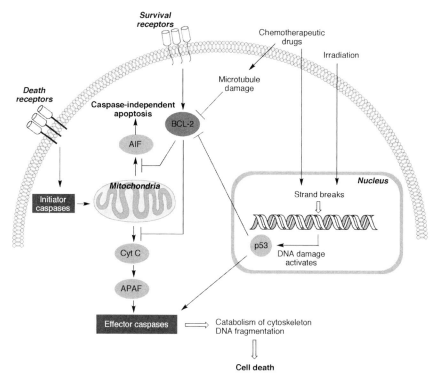

FIGURE 9.32   Drug targets in apoptotic pathways.

ultimate sensitivity or resistance of cells to a number of apoptotic stimuli (hypoxia, radiation, oxidants, Ca^{2+} overload, ceramide, and growth factor/neurotrophin deprivation). BCL-2 proteins are over-expressed in a large number of cancers, including 90–100% of hormone-refractory prostate cancers, 90% of malignant melanomas, 80–90% of estrogen-positive breast cancer, and 50% of non-Hodgkin's lymphoma, among others.

Antisense oligonucleotides that reduce the expression of anti-apoptotic *BCL-2* genes are currently undergoing clinical trials.[127] Thus, oblimersen sodium is an 18-mer oligonucleotide that, in combination with dacarbazine, has been shown to lead to stabilized or improved disease in 57% malignant melanoma patients, while the standard malignant melanoma therapy leads only to 1–20% positive response.[128] Other anti-cancer drugs have been associated with oblimersen for a number of other indications, including chronic lymphocytic leukaemia and acute myelogenous leukaemia. Some small-molecule inhibitors have also been reported that bind to anti-apoptosis BCL-2 proteins,[129] although they have not reached the clinical stage yet. One example are the members of antimycin A family, a group of closely related bis-lactones previously known as inhibitors of mitochondrial electron transfer.[130]

Antimycin A$_1$: R = nC$_4$H$_9$
Antimycin A$_3$: R = nC$_6$H$_{13}$

7.2. p53 proteins

As a transcription factor, the p53 protein does not participate directly in the apoptosis pathway, but it regulates a large number of other genes that lead to apoptosis, and indeed the tumor suppressor gene (*TP53*) is mutated in many cancers. Two *TP53* gene therapy drugs that use an adenovirus as the delivery vehicle are in clinical trials. Thus, INGN201 (Ad-p53) has demonstrated broad-spectrum antitumor activity in many models of human cancer. Combining INGN201 transduction of established tumors with chemotherapy or radiotherapy in these models has resulted in enhanced activity with no apparent increase in toxicity. Clinical development of INGN201 has expanded into multiple Phase II studies, with objective activity demonstrated in head and neck cancer (with 47% positive response), NSCLC (resulting in improved survival rates), and prostate cancer. Other related adenoviruses that have shown promising results in clinical trials are SCH-58500 and ONYX-015, a mutant adenovirus. Although local injection gives good responses, the main problem that these drugs are facing, and that is limiting their more widespread use, is the absence of methods for their systemic delivery.

7.3. Death receptors

A protein known as tumor necrosis factor-related apoptosis-inducing ligand (TRAIL), alternatively called 'APO2L', induces apoptotic cell death via a specific death receptor, DR4 or DR5. Thus, the TRAIL homotrimer induces trimerization of DR4 or DR5 on the surface of cancer cells, resulting in recruitment of an adaptor molecule known as Fas-associated death domain (FADD). FADD activates caspase-8 which subsequently activates caspase-3, a central downstream activator of apoptotic pathways. TRAIL is under clinical trials, and it has also been shown that its combination with conventional anti-cancer drugs may prove to be useful in the treatment of malignancies that express the anti-apoptotic BCL-2 family of proteins.[131]

7.4. Nuclear factor κB

In addition to caspase activation, some proteins containing caspase-associated recruitment domains (CARDs) are involved in controlling the induction of nuclear factor κB (NF-κB). Cancer cells produce higher levels of reactive oxygen species (ROS) because of their high rate of metabolism and inefficient respiration. Furthermore, cancer cells lose their ability to reduce their rate of respiration in the presence of increasing oxidative stress. Chronic activation of NF-κB, which is characteristic of many cancers, is a critical adaptation to these higher levels of oxidative stress, allowing cancer cell survival by preventing activation of the pro-apoptotic kinase JNK by increasing the expression of the JNK-phosphatase MKP1.[132]

A group of synthetic triterpenoids, specially CDDO and CDDO-Me, inhibits NF-κB activity and increases oxidative stress in cancer cells, leading to sustained activation of JNK and triggering caspase-mediated apoptosis. These compounds have shown potent activity in multiple animal models of cancer and in cancer cell samples taken from patients with treatment-resistant cancers, and are in Phase I clinical trials.

NF-κB activity can also be inhibited by interference with its activation processes, which depends on a group of proteins known as IκB kinases (IKK). The pyridyl cyanoguanidine derivative CHS-282 is a potent IKK inhibitor that blocks NF-κB activation.[133] CHS-282 has been evaluated as an anticancer agent in clinical trials, although the results obtained with solid tumors revealed no objective tumor responses.[134]

R = H   CDDO (RTA-401)
R = CH₃   CDDO-Me (RTA-402)

CHS-828

8. INHIBITORS OF HEAT-SHOCK PROTEINS (HSP 90)

Protein folding is catalysed *in vivo* by isomerases and chaperone proteins. Molecular chaperones are ubiquitous proteins that assist folding, assembly, transport, and degradation of proteins within the cell. The first identified chaperones were heat-shock proteins (HSPs), whose names is derived from the elevated levels produced when cells are grown at higher-than-normal temperatures. HSPs stabilize other proteins during their synthesis and assist in protein folding by binding and releasing unfolded or misfolded proteins using an ATP-independent mechanism. Proteins unable to maintain their proper shape are broken down by the proteasome (see Section 1 of Chapter 10) and eliminated, as shown in Fig. 9.33. These events may be favourable if the proteins are previously mutated and hence dangerous for the survival of the cell, but they become a problem if the proteins are necessary for its normal functioning.

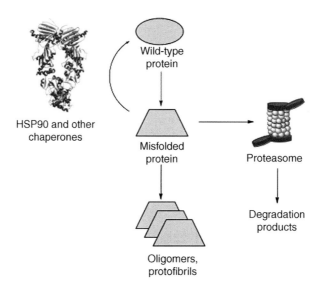

FIGURE 9.33   Function of heat-shock proteins.

HSP 90 is the best known of HSPs and its activity is coupled to an ATPase cycle that is controlled by several cofactors. It has three major domains, namely a highly conserved N-terminal ATPase domain, a middle domain, and a C-terminal dimerization domain. The crystal structure of HSP 90 bound to ATP has shown how this nucleotide is hydrolysed,[135] but the detailed mechanism of protein folding remains unknown.

HSP 90 has emerged as an attractive cancer target because its inhibition blocks a large number of cancer-related signalling pathways since a large number of intra-cellular signalling molecules require association with HSP 90 to achieve their active conformation, correct cellular location, and stability.[136] These include steroid hormone receptors, transcription factors like the tumor suppressor protein p53 and kinases like Src-kinase.

The conformational changes that take place in HSP 90 after binding and hydrolysis of ATP regulate the stabilization and maturation of client proteins, including hypoxia-inducible factor-1 (HIF-1), a relevant anticancer target.[137] This ATP site is known by X-ray crystallography to be very different from that of kinases, allowing the design of inhibitors with high selectivity with regard to other ATP-binding proteins.

The design and study of selective inhibitors of HSP 90 was initially controversial because this protein is critical for the survival of both normal and sick cells. However, HSP does not have much activity under normal conditions. When the cell is under stress by genetic mutations or environmental changes such as heat or infection HSP 90 activity is increased as an emergency response that stabilizes partially unfolded proteins and helps them to achieve their correct shape. This activity also assists the survival of cancer cells despite an abundance of misfolded and unstable proteins, and this is one of the reasons to study HSP 90 as an anticancer target.

The main strategy employed in the design of HSP 90 inhibitors is based in the synthesis of analogues of the natural antitumor geldanamycin, a benzoquinone derivative belonging to the ansamycin class, although some companies working in this field are designing entirely synthetic molecules not related to this compound.

Geldanamycin was originally believed to be a TK inhibitor, but it was later identified as an ATP-competitive inhibitor of HSP 90. It could not be advanced to the clinical stage because it showed unacceptable hepatotoxicity, probably associated with the presence of the electrophilic methoxybenzoquinone moiety. For this reason, displacement of the 17-methoxy group by nucleophiles led to less toxic analogues such as tanespimycin (17-allylaminogeldanamycin, 17-AAG).[138] Another problem associated with geldanamycin is its very low solubility, which was solved with the development of the water-soluble analogue alvespimycin (17-dimethylaminoethylaminogeldanamycin, 17-DMAG).[139] Both analogues were better tolerated than the parent natural product and are under clinical trials. In another approach, the problematic quinone moiety of 17-AAG was reduced to the hydroquinone stage. The resulting compound, IPI-504, can be formulated as a soluble salt that is suitable for intravenous or oral formulations. It has shown encouraging results in Phase I trials in patients with gastrointestinal stromal tumors that were resistant to imatinib, although further clinical development is necessary.

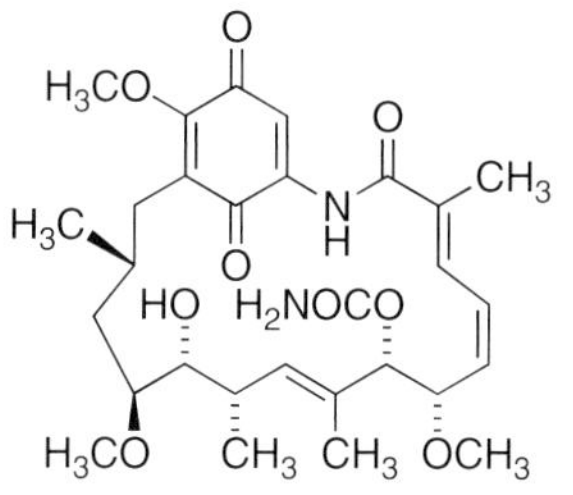

Geldanamycin

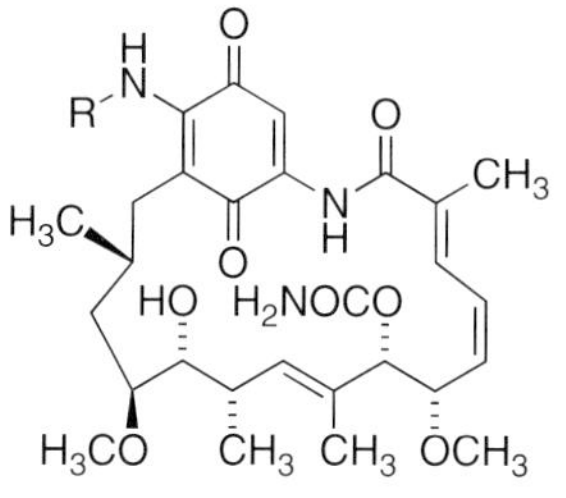

R = CH$_2$CH=CH$_2$ Tanespimycin (17-AAG)
R = (CH$_3$)$_2$NCH$_2$CH$_2$ Alvespimycin (17-DMAG)
(as HCl salt)

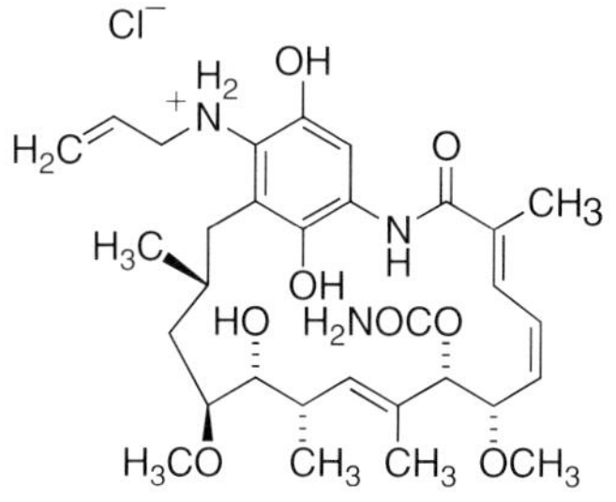

IPI-504

REFERENCES

1. Guillemard, V., and Saragovi, H. U. (2004). *Curr. Cancer Drug Targets* **4**, 313.
2. Dancey, J., and Sausville, E. A. (2003). *Nat. Rev. Drug Discov.* **2**, 296.
3. Collins, I., and Workman, P. (2006). *Curr. Signal Transduct. Ther.* **1**, 13.
4. Kéri, G., Örfi, L., Erös, D., Hegymegi-Barakonyi, B., Szántai-Kis, C., Horváth, Z., Wáczek, F., Marosfalvi, J., Szabadkai, I., Pató, J., Greff, Z., Hafenbradl, D., *et al.* (2006). *Curr. Signal Transduct. Ther.* **1**, 67.
5. Klein, S., and Levitzki, A. (2006). *Curr. Signal Transduct. Ther.* **1**, 1.
6. Tiseo, M., Loprevite, M., and Ardizzoni, A. (2004). *Curr. Med. Chem. Anticancer Agents* **4**, 139.
7. Barker, A. J., Gibson, K. H., Grundy, W., Godfrey, A. A., Barlow, J. J., Healy, M. P., Woodburn, J. R., Ashton, S. E., Curry, B. J., Scarlett, L., Henthorn, L., and Richards, L. (2001). *Bioorg. Med. Chem. Lett.* **11**, 1911.
8. Barker, A. J. (2001). *In* "Medicinal Chemistry into the Millenium," (Campbell, M. M and Blagbrough, I. S, eds.), p. 140. Royal Society of Chemistry, Cambridge.
9. Herbst, R. S., Fukuoka, M., and Baselga, J. (2004). *Nat. Rev. Cancer* **4**, 956.
10. Muhsin, M., Graham, J., and Kirkpatrick, P. (2003). *Nat. Rev. Drug Discov.* **2**, 515.
11. Rosell, R., Ichinose, Y., Taron, M., Sarries, C., Queralt, C., Méndez, P., Sánchez, J. M., Nishiyama, K., Morán, T., Cirauqui, B., Mate, J. L., Besse, B., *et al.* (2005). *Lung Cancer* **40**, 25.
12. Hedge, S., and Schmidt, M. (2005). *Annu. Rep. Med. Chem.* **40**, 443.
13. Dowell, J., Minna, J. D., and Kirkpatrick, P. (2005). *Nat. Rev. Drug Discov.* **4**, 13.
14. Rusnack, D. W., Affleck, K., Cockerill, S. G., Stubberfield, C., Harris, R., Page, M., Smith, K. J., Guntrip, S. B., Carter, M. C., Shaw, R. J., Jowett, A., Stables, J., *et al.* (2001). *Cancer Res.* **61**, 7196.
15. Stamos, J., Sliwkowski, M. X., and Eigenbrot, C. (2002). *J. Biol. Chem.* **277**, 46265.
16. Clark, J., Cools, J., and Gilliland, D. G. (2005). *PloS Med.* **2**, 195.
17. Nyati, M. K., Maheshwari, D., Hanasoge, S., Sreekumar, A., Rynkiewicz, S. D., Chinnaiyan, A. M., Leopold, W. R., Ethier, S. P., and Lawrence, T. S. (2004). *Clin. Cancer Res.* **10**, 691.
18. Tsou, H. R., Mamuya, N., Johnson, B. D., Reich, M. F., Gruber, B. C., Ye, F., Nilakantan, R., Shen, R., Discafani, C., DeBlanc, R., Davis, R., Koehn, F. E., *et al.* (2001). *J. Med. Chem.* **44**, 2719.
19. Sliwkowski, M. X., Lofgren, J. A., Lewis, G. D., Hotaling, T. E., Fendly, B. M., and Fox, J. A. (1999). *Semin. Oncol.* **26**, 60.
20. Scotlandi, K., Manara, M. C., Nicoletti, G., Lollini, P.-L., Lukas, S., Benini, S., Croci, S., Perdichizzi, S., Zambelli, D., Serra, M., García-Echeverría, C., Hofmann, F., *et al.* (2005). *Cancer Res.* **65**, 3868.
21. Mendel, D. B., Laird, A. D., Smolich, B. D., Blake, R. A., Liang, C., Hannah, A. L., Shaheen, R. M., Ellis, L. M., Weitman, S., Shawver, L. K., and Cherrington, J. M. (2000). *Anticancer Drug Des.* **15**, 29.
22. Laird, A. D., Vajkoczy, P., Shawver, L. K., Thurnher, A., Liang, C., Mohammadi, M., Schlessinger, J., Ullrich, A., Hubbard, S. R., Blake, R. A., Fong, T. A., Strawn, L. M., *et al.* (2000). *Cancer Res.* **60**, 4152.
23. Abrams, T. J., Murray, L. J., Pesenti, E., Holway, V. W., Colombo, T., Lee, L. B., Cherrington, J. M., and Pryer, N. K. (2003). *Mol. Cancer Ther.* **2**, 1011.
24. Wood, J. M., Bold, G., Buchdunger, E., Cozens, R., Ferrari, S., Frei, J., Hofmann, F., Mestan, J., Mett, H., O'Reilly, T., Persohn, E., Rosel, J., *et al.* (2000). *Cancer Res.* **60**, 2178.
25. Hecht, R., Trarbach, T., Jaeger, E., Hainsworth, J., Wolff, R., Lloyd, K., Bodoky, G., Borner, M., Laurent, D., and Jacques, C. (2005). *J. Clin. Oncol.* **23**(Suppl., Part I), 3.
26. Manley, P. W., Bold, G., Fendrich, G., Furet, P., Mestan, J., Meyer, T., Meyhack, B., Stark, W., Strauss, A., and Wood, J. (2003). *Cell. Mol. Biol. Lett.* **8**, 532.
27. Hennequin, L. F., Stokes, E. S., Thomas, A. P., Johnstone, C., Ple, P. A., Ogilvie, D. J., Dukes, M., Wedge, S. R., Kendrew, J., and Curwen, J. O. (2002). *J. Med. Chem.* **45**, 1300.
28. Wedge, S. R., Kendrew, J., Hennequin, L. F., Valentine, P. J., Barry, S. T., Brave, S. R., Smith, N. R., James, N. H., Dukes, M., Curwen, J. O., Chester, R., Jackson, J. A., *et al.* (2005). *Cancer Res.* **65**, 4389.
29. Shaheen, P. E., and Bukowski, R. M. (2005). *Expert Opin. Emerg. Drugs* **10**, 773.
30. Rini, B., Campbell, S. C., and Rathmell, W. K. (2006). *Curr. Opin. Oncol.* **18**, 289.
31. Rugo, H. S., Herbst, R. S., Liu, G., Park, J. W., Kies, M. S., Steinfeldt, H. M., Pithavala, Y. K., Reich, S. D., Freddo, J. L., and Wilding, G. (2005). *J. Clin. Oncol.* **23**, 5474.
32. Gingrich, D. E., Reddy, D. R., Iqbal, M. A., Singh, J., Aimone, L. D., Angeles, T. S., Albom, M., Yang, S., Ator, M. A., Meyer, S. L., Robinson, C., Ruggeri, B. A., *et al.* (2003). *J. Med. Chem.* **46**, 5375.
33. Ferrara, N., Hillari, K. J., Gerber, H.-P., and Novotny, W. (2004). *Nat. Rev. Drug Discov.* **3**, 391.

34. Trudel, S., Stewart, A. K., Rom, E., Wei, E., Li, Z. H., Kotzer, S., Chumakov, I., Singer, Y., Chang, H., Liang, S.-B., and Yayon, A. (2006). *Blood* **107,** 4039.
35. Weng, D. E., and Usman, N. (2001). *Curr. Oncol. Rep.* **3,** 141.
36. http://www.clinicaltrials.gov/ct/gui/show/NCT00066768?order=2
37. Kelly, L. M., Yu, J. C., Boulton, C. L., Apatira, M., Li, J., Sullivan, C. M., Williams, I., Amaral, S. M., Curley, D. P., Duclos, N., Neuberg, D., Scarborough, R. M., *et al.* (2002). *Cancer Cell* **1,** 421.
38. http://www.clinicaltrials.gov/ct/show/NCT00297921;jsessionid=162D862FB6AE912B354CFC3BB6F008FF?order=25
39. Smith, B. D., Levis, M., Beran, M., Giles, F., Kantarjian, H., Berg, K., Murphy, K. M., Dauses, T., Allebach, J., and Small, D. (2004). *Blood* **103,** 3669.
40. Monnerat, C., Henriksson, R., Le Chevalier, T., Novello, S., Berthaud, P., Faivre, S., and Raymond, E. (2004). *Ann. Oncol.* **15,** 316.
41. Manley, P. W., Cowan-Jacob, S. W., and Mestan, J. (2005). *Biochim. Biophys. Acta* **1754,** 3.
42. Capdeville, R., Buchdunger, E., Zimmermann, J., and Matter, A. (2002). *Nat. Rev. Drug Discov.* **1,** 493.
43. Zimmermann, J., Buchdunger, E., Mett, H., Meyer, T., and Lydon, N. B. (1997). *Bioorg. Med. Chem. Lett.* **7,** 187.
44. Schindler, T., Bornmann, W., Pellicena, P., Miller, W. T., Clarkson, B., and Kuriyan, J. (2000). *Science* **289,** 1938.
45. Nagar, B., Bornmann, W., Pellicena, P., Schindler, T., Veach, D. R., Miller, W. T., Clarkson, B., and Kuriyan, J. (2002). *Cancer Res.* **62,** 4236.
46. Nowakowski, J., Sridhar, V., Thompson, D. A., Cronin, C. N., Vaughn, D. E., Gangloff, A. R., Sang, B.-C., Zoa, H., Knuth, M. W., Swanson, R. V., Snell, G., Mol, C. D., *et al.* (2003). *Cell. Mol. Biol. Lett.* **8,** 556.
47. Pricl, S., Fermeglia, M., Ferrone, M., and Tamborini, E. (2005). *Mol. Cancer Ther.* **4,** 1167.
48. McLean, S. R., Gana-Weisz, M., Hartzoulakis, B., Frow, R., Whelan, J., Selwood, D., and Boshoff, C. (2005). *Mol. Cancer Ther.* **4,** 2008.
49. Weisberg, E., Manley, P., Mestan, J., Cowan-Jacob, S., Ray, A., and Griffin, J. D. (2006). *Br. J. Cancer* **94,** 1765.
50. Von Bubnoff, N., Manley, P. W., Mestan, J., Sanger, J., Peschel, C., and Duyster, J. (2006). *Blood* **108,** 1328.
51. Gambacorti-Passerini, C., Gasser, M., Ahmed, S., Assouline, S., and Scapozza, L. (2005). *Leukemia* **19,** 1267.
52. Shah, N. P., Tran, C., Lee, F. Y., Chen, P., Norris, D., and Sawyers, C. L. (2004). *Science* **305,** 399.
53. Doggrell, S. A. (2005). *Expert Opin. Investig. Drugs* **14,** 89.
54. Golas, J. M., Arndt, K., Etienne, C., Lucas, J., Nardin, D., Gibbons, J., Frost, P., Ye, F., Boschelli, D. H., and Boschelli, F. (2003). *Cancer Res.* **63,** 375.
55. Martinelli, G., Soverini, S., Rosti, G., Cilloni, D., and Baccarani, M. (2005). *Haematologica* **90,** 534.
56. Summy, J. M., and Gallick, G. E. (2006). *Clin. Cancer Res.* **12,** 1398.
57. Senderowicz, A. M. (2003). *Oncogene* **22,** 6609.
58. Schang, L. M. (2005). *Curr. Drug Targets Infect. Disord.* **5,** 29.
59. Blagosklonny, M. V. (2004). *Cell Cycle* **3,** 1537.
60. Schiller, J. H., Harrington, D., Belani, C. P., Langer, C., Sandler, A., Krook, J., Zhu, J., and Johnson, D. H. (2002). *N. Engl. J. Med.* **346,** 92.
61. Honma, T., Hayashi, K., Aoyama, T., Hashimoto, N. T., Fukasawa, K., Iwama, T., Ikeura, C., Ikuta, M., Suzuki-Takahashi, I., Iwasawa, Y., Hayama, T., Nishimura, S., *et al.* (2001). *J. Med. Chem.* **44,** 4615.
62. Raje, N., Kumar, S., Hideshima, T., Roccaro, A., Ishitsuka, K., Yasui, H., Shiraishi, N., Chauhan, D., Munshi, N. C., Green, S. R., and Anderson, K. C. (2005). *Blood* **106,** 1042.
63. Bach, S., Knockaert, M., Reinhardt, J., Lozach, O., Schmitt, S., Baratte, B., Koken, M., Coburn, S. P., Tang, L., Jiang, T., Liang, D.-C., Galons, H., *et al.* (2005). *J. Biol. Chem.* **280,** 31208.
64. Borman, S. (2003). *Chem. Eng. News* **81,** 29.
65. Kamath, A. V., Chong, S., Chang, M., and Marathe, P. H. (2005). *Cancer Chemother. Pharmacol.* **55,** 110.
66. Fukuoka, K., Usuda, J., Iwamoto, Y., Fukumoto, H., Nakamura, T., Yoneda, T., Narita, N., Saijo, N., and Nishio, K. (2001). *Invest. New Drugs* **19,** 219.

67. Thiry, A., Dogné, J. M., Mesereel, B., and Supuran, C. T. (2006). *Trends Pharmacol. Sci.* **27**, 566.

68. Dittrich, C., Dumez, H., Calvert, H., Hanauske, A., Faber, M., Wanders, J., Yule, M., Ravic, M., and Fumoleau, P. (2003). *Clin. Cancer Res.* **9**, 5195.

69. Tsukahara, K., Watanabe, T., Hata-Sugi, N., Yoshimatsu, K., Okayama, H., and Nagasu, T. (2001). *Mol. Pharmacol.* **60**, 1254.

70. Smyth, J. F., Aamdal, S., Awada, A., Dittrich, C., Caponigro, F., Schöffski, P., Gore, M., Lesimple, T., Djurasinovic, N., Baron, B., Ravic, M., Fumoleau, P., *et al.* (2005). *Ann. Oncol.* **16**, 158.

71. Supuran, C. T. (2003). *Expert Opin. Investig. Drugs* **12**, 283.

72. Fry, M. J. (2001). *Breast Cancer Res.* **3**, 304.

73. Granville, C. A., Memmott, R. M., Gills, J. J., and Dennis, P. A. (2006). *Clin. Cancer Res.* **12**, 679.

74. Machajewski, T., Lin, X., Jefferson, A. B., and Gao, Z. (2005). *Annu. Rep. Med. Chem.* **40**, 263.

75. Luo, Y., Shoemaker, A. R., Liu, X., Woods, K. W., Thomas, S. A., de Jong, R., Han, E. K., Li, T., Stoll, V. S., Powlas, J. A., Oleksijew, A., Mitten, M. J., *et al.* (2005). *Mol. Cancer Ther.* **4**, 977.

76. Posadas, E. M., Gulley, J., Arlen, P. M., Trout, A., Parnes, H. L., Wright, J., Lee, M. J., Chung, E. J., Trepel, J. B., Sparreboom, A., Chen, C., Jones, E., *et al.* (2005). *Cancer Biol. Ther.* **4**, 1133.

77. Morgan-Lappe, S., Woods, K. W., Li, Q., Anderson, M. G., Schurdak, M. E., Luo, Y., Giranda, V. L., Fesik, S. W., and Leverson, J. D. (2006). *Oncogene* **25**, 1340.

78. Graves, P. R., Yu, L. J., Schwarz, J. K., Gales, J., Sausville, E. A., O'Connor, P. M., and Piwnica-Worms, H. (2000). *J. Biol. Chem.* **275**, 5600.

79. Sato, S., Fujita, N., and Tsuruo, T. (2002). *Oncogene* **21**, 1727.

80. Fuse, E., Kuwabara, T., Sparreboom, A., Sausville, E. A., and Figg, W. D. (2005). *J. Clin. Pharmacol.* **45**, 394.

81. Komander, D., Kular, G. S., Bain, J., Elliott, M., Alessi, D. R., and van Aalten, D. M. F. (2003). *Biochem. J.* **375**, 255.

82. Rao, R. D., Buckner, J. C., and Sarkaria, J. N. (2004). *Curr. Drug Targets* **4**, 621.

83. Wullschleger, S., Loewith, R., and Hall, M. N. (2006). *Cell* **124**, 471.

84. Ory, B., Moriceau, G., Redini, F., and Heymann, D. (2007). *Curr. Med. Chem.* **14**, 1381.

85. Vignot, S., Faivre, S., Aguirre, D., and Raymond, E. (2005). *Ann. Oncol.* **16**, 525.

86. Andrews, P. D. (2005). *Oncogene* **24**, 5005.

87. Montembault, E., and Prigent, C. (2005). *Drugs Future* **30**, 4.

88. Fancelli, D., and Moll, J. (2005). *Expert Opin. Ther. Pat.* **15**, 1169.

89. Harrington, E. A., Bebbington, D., Moore, J., Rasmussen, R. K., Ajose-Adeogun, A. O., Nakayama, T., Graham, J. A., Demur, C., Hercend, T., Diu-Hercend, A., Su, M., Golec, J. M. C., *et al.* (2004). *Nat. Med.* **10**, 262.

90. Fancelli, D., Berta, D., Bindi, S., Cameron, A., Cappella, P., Carpinelli, P., Catana, C., Forte, B., Giordano, P., Giorgini, M. L., Mantegani, S., Marsiglio, A., *et al.* (2005). *J. Med. Chem.* **48**, 3080.

91. Jirousek, M. R., and Goekjian, P. G. (2001). *Expert Opin. Investig. Drugs* **10**, 2117.

92. Propper, D., McDonald, A., Thavasu, P., Balkwill, F., Caponigro, F., Yap, A., Champain, K., Csermak, K., Talbot, D., Kaye, S., Harris, A., and Twelves, C. (1998). *Proc. 10th NCI-EORTC Symp. New Drugs Cancer Ther.* **10**, 112.

93. Fine, H. A., Kim, L., and Royce, C. (2005). *J. Clin. Oncol.* **10**, 1504.

94. Force, T., Kuida, K., and Namchuk, M. (2004). *Circulation* **109**, 1196.

95. Utz, I., Spitaler, M., Rybczynska, M., Ludescher, C., Hilbe, W., Regenass, U., Grunicke, H., and Hofmann, J. (1998). *Int. J. Cancer* **77**, 64.

96. Sorbera, L. A., Silvestre, J., Rabasseda, X., and Castaner, J. (2000). *Drugs Future* **10**, 1017.

97. Frank, R. N. (2002). *Am. J. Ophthalmol.* **133**, 693.

98. Madhusudan, S., Protheroe, A., Propper, D., Han, C., Corrie, P., Earl, H., Hancock, B., Vasey, P., Turner, A., Balkwill, F., Hoare, S., and Harris, A. L. (2003). *Br. J. Cancer* **89**, 1418.

99. Cripps, M. C., Figueredo, A. T., Oza, A. M., Taylor, M. J., Fields, A. L., Holmlund, J. T., McIntosh, L. W., Geary, R. S., and Eisenhauer, E. A. (2002). *Clin. Cancer Res.* **8**, 2188.

100. Reuter, C. W. M., Morgan, M. A., and Bergmann, L. (2000). *Blood* **96**, 1655.

101. Adjei, A. A. (2001). *Curr. Pharm. Des.* **7**, 1581.

102. Downward, J. (2003). *Nat. Rev. Cancer* **3**, 11.

103. Morse, M. A. (2001). *Curr. Opin. Mol. Ther.* **3**, 589.

104. Russo, P., Loprevite, M., Cesario, A., and Ardizzoni, A. (2004). *Curr. Med. Chem. Anticancer Agents* **4,** 123.
105. Leonard, D. M. (1997). *J. Med. Chem.* **40,** 2971.
106. Johnston, S. R. D. (2001). *Lancet Oncol.* **2,** 18.
107. Bell, I. M. (2004). *J. Med. Chem.* **47,** 1869.
108. Le, D. T., and Shannon, K. M. (2002). *Curr. Opin. Hematol.* **9,** 308.
109. Caponigro, F., Casale, M., and Bryce, J. (2004). *Expert Opin. Investig. Drugs* **12,** 943.
110. Santucci, R., Mackley, P. A., Sebti, S., and Alsina, M. (2003). *Cancer Control* **10,** 384.
111. Rao, S., Cunningham, D., de Gramont, A., Scheithauer, W., Smakal, M., Humblet, Y., Kourteva, G., Iveson, T., Andre, T., Dostalova, J., Illes, A., Belly, R., *et al.* (2004). *J. Clin. Oncol.* **22,** 3950.
112. Lobell, R. B., Liu, D., Buser, C. A., Davide, J. P., DePuy, E., Hamilton, K., Koblan, K. S., Lee, Y., Mosser, S., Motzel, S. L., Abbruzzese, J. L., Fuchs, C. S., *et al.* (2002). *Mol. Cancer Ther.* **1,** 747.
113. Khuri, F. R., Glisson, B. S., Kim, E. S., Statkevich, P., Thall, P. F., Meyers, M. L., Herbst, R. S., Munden, R. F., Tendler, C., Zhu, Y., Bangert, S., Thompson, E., *et al.* (2004). *Clin. Cancer Res.* **10,** 2968.
114. Reid, T. S., and Beese, L. S. (2004). *Biochemistry* **43,** 6877.
115. Reid, T. S., Long, S. B., and Beese, L. S. (2004). *Biochemistry* **43,** 9000.
116. Honma, T., Yoshizumi, T., Hashimoto, N., Hayashi, K., Kawanishi, N., Fukasawa, K., Takaki, T., Ikeura, C., Ikuta, M., Suzuki-Takahashi, I., Hayama, T., Nishimura, S., *et al.* (2001). *J. Med. Chem.* **44,** 4628.
117. Cripps, M. C., Figueredo, A. T., Oza, A. M., Taylor, M. J., Fields, A. L., Holmlund, J. T., McIntosh, L. W., Geary, R. S., and Eisenhauer, E. A. (2002). *Clin. Cancer Res.* **8,** 2188.
118. Sebolt-Leopold, J. S., Dudley, D. T., Herrera, R., Van Becelaere, K., Wiland, A., Gowan, R. C., Tecle, H., Barrett, S. D., Bridges, A., Przybranowski, S., Leopold, W. R., and Saltiel, A. R. (1999). *Nat. Med.* **5,** 810.
119. Rinehart, J., Adjei, A. A., LoRusso, P. M., Waterhouse, D., Hecht, J. R., Natale, R. B., Hamid, O., Varterasian, M., Asbury, P., Kaldjian, E. P., Gulyas, S., Mitchell, D. Y., *et al.* (2004). *J. Clin. Oncol.* **22,** 4456.
120. Doyle, M. P., Yeh, T. C., Suzy, B., Morrow, M., Lee, P. A., Hughes, A. M., Cartlidge, S., Wallace, E., Lyssikatos, J., Eckhardt, S. G., and Winkler, J. D. (2005). *J. Clin. Oncol.* **23,** 3075.
121. Astra Zeneca AB: WO04004732 & WO04005284 (2004). *Expert Opin. Ther. Pat.* **14,** 1095.
122. Kumar, S., Boehm, J., and Lee, J. C. (2003). *Nat. Rev. Drug Discov.* **2,** 717.
123. Petak, I., Houghton, J. A., and Kopper, L. (2006). *Curr. Signal Transduct. Ther.* **1,** 113.
124. Zhang, J. Y. (2002). *Nat. Rev. Drug Discov.* **1,** 101.
125. Reed, J. C. (2002). *Nat. Rev. Drug Discov.* **1,** 111.
126. Elmore, S. W., Oost, T. K., and Park, C.-M. (2005). *Annu. Rep. Med. Chem.* **40,** 245.
127. Melnikova, I., and Golden, J. (2004). *Nat. Rev. Drug Discov.* **3,** 905.
128. Jansen, B., Wacheck, V., Heere-Ress, E., Schlagbauer-Wadl, H., Hoeller, C., Lucas, T., Hoermann, M., Hollenstein, U., Wolff, K., and Pehamberger, H. (2000). *Lancet* **356**(9243), 1728.
129. Wang, J. L., Liu, D., Zhang, Z.-J., Shan, S., Han, X., Srinivasula, S. M., Croce, C. M., Alnemri, E. S., and Huang, Z. (2000). *Proc. Natl. Acad. Sci. USA* **97,** 7124.
130. Tzung, S. P., Kim, K. M., Basañez, G., Giedt, C. D., Simon, J., Zimmerberg, J., Zhang, K. Y. J., and Hockenbery, D. M. (2001). *Nat. Cell Biol.* **3,** 183.
131. Ballestero, A., Nencioni, A., Boy1, D., Rocco, I., Garuti, A., Mela, G. S., Van Parijs, L., Brossart, P., Wesselborg, S., and Patrone, F. (2004). *Clin. Cancer Res.* **10,** 1463.
132. Kamata, H., Honda, S., Maeda, S., Chang, L., Hirata, H., and Karin, M. (2005). *Cell* **120,** 649.
133. Karin, M., Yamamoto, Y., and Wang, Q. M. (2004). *Nat. Rev. Drug Discov.* **3,** 17.
134. Hovstadius, P., Larsson, R., Jonsson, E., Skov, T., Kissmeyer, A. M., Krasilnikoff, K., Bergh, J., Karlsson, M. O., Lönnebo, A., and Ahlgren, J. (2002). *J. Clin. Cancer Res.* **8,** 2850.
135. Ali, M. M. U., Roe, S. M., Vaughan, C. K., Meyer, P., Panaretou, B., Piper, P. W., Prodromou, C., and Pearl, L. H. (2006). *Nature* **440,** 1013.
136. Chaudhury, S., Welch, T. R., and Blagg, B. S. J. (2006). *Chem. Med. Chem.* **1,** 1331.
137. Giaccia, A., Siim, B. G., and Johnson, R. S. (2003). *Nat. Rev. Drug Discov.* **2,** 1.
138. http://clinicalstudies.info.nih.gov/detail/A_2004-C-0238.html
139. Burger, A. M., Fiebig, H. H., Stinson, S. F., and Sausville, E. A. (2004). *Anticancer Drugs* **15,** 377.

CHAPTER 10

Other Approaches to Targeted Therapy

Contents

1.	Proteasome Inhibitors	307
2.	Antiangiogenic Agents Unrelated to Kinase Signaling	312
	2.1. Inhibitors of proteolytic enzymes of the extracellular matrix: Metalloproteinases	313
	2.2. Inhibitors of other targets related to the extracellular matrix: Heparanase	316
	2.3. Endogenous inhibitors of angiogenesis	318
	2.4. Inhibitors of cellular adhesion molecules	319
	2.5. Miscellaneous antiangiogenic compounds	320
3.	Epigenetic Therapy of Cancer	323
	3.1. Inhibitors of DNA methyltransferases (DNMT)	323
	3.2. Inhibitors of histone deacetylases (HDAC)	330
	3.3. Regulators of histone methylation	337
4.	Inhibitors of Other DNA-Associated Enzymes	337
	4.1. Telomerase inhibitors	337
	4.2. DNA repair system inhibitors	340
5.	Therapy Directed at Other Targets	341
	5.1. Antisense oligonucleotides	341
	5.2. Monoclonal antibodies against cancer cells	343
	5.3. Gene therapy	344
	5.4. Antitumor agents targeted at lysosomes	346
	References	347

1. PROTEASOME INHIBITORS

Protein degradation is essential for the cell to supply fresh amino acids for protein synthesis and also to remove unneeded proteins including excess enzymes and transcription factors that are no longer required or damaged. There are primarily two types of cellular structures that are in charge of protein degradation:

Medicinal Chemistry of Anticancer Drugs
DOI: 10.1016/B978-0-444-52824-7.00010-X

– *Lysosomes*, which exert their proteolytic function on extracellular proteins from endocytosis and phagocytosis mechanisms, and also on transmembrane proteins.
– *Proteasomes*, which act on damaged or unneeded endogenous proteins. These include transcription factors, regulatory proteins, cell cycle cyclins, virus-coded proteins, proteins that are improperly folded because of translation errors, and proteins damaged by cytosol molecules. The average human cell contains 20,000–30,000 proteasomes, which are located in the cytoplasm and nucleus.

The 20S proteasome[1] is a complex of 28 subunits that are organized in four stacked heptameric rings, creating a cylindrical structure. The proteins at the top and bottom rings have sequence similarities and are called α subunits, while the ones in the two inner rings, three of which perform the enzymatic reaction, are called β subunits. To be functional *in vivo*, this 20S proteasome must be capped at both ends by the 19S regulatory complex, leading to the 26S proteasome, a 2.4-MDa structure. This 19S complex contains six ATPases, several other polypeptides, and a "lid." ATP hydrolysis is required for the generation of the 26S proteasome and also to facilitate the unfolding of substrate proteins that must enter into the catalytic inner core. In order to prevent undesirable protein hydrolysis, cells label the proteins to be hydrolyzed by attaching them to a protein called ubiquitin, which binds to the amino group of a lysine unit. The lid of the 19S subunit is essential for the degradation of these ubiquitylated proteins. Proteasomes degrade these proteins to short peptides (about eight amino acids, on the average), and this degradation is followed by hydrolysis of these peptides by cytoplasmic exopeptidases (Fig. 10.1). Recently, the development of fluorescent probes has opened up the possibility of visualizing these protease activities in cells and organisms.[2]

The proteasome is an anticancer target[3] because it controls the levels of several proteins that are essential for the progression of the cell cycle and apoptosis, including cyclins, caspases, BCL-2, the tumor-suppressing factor p53, and nuclear factor-κB (NF-κB). Blocking the proteasome results in the accumulation of various other regulatory proteins, which leads to cell death by a variety of mechanisms. For instance, proteasome inhibition disrupts the regulation of the p53 tumor suppressor, which is mutated in about 50% of human cancers, by the murine double minute 2 (MDM2) protein. This negative regulator exports p53 from the nucleus to the cytoplasm, and, because of its ubiquitin ligase activity, facilitates p53 destruction by the proteasome (Fig. 10.2). For this reason, protease inhibitors may provide a good approach to the treatment of tumors that overexpress the MDM2 factor.

Proteasome inhibitors may also act as anticancer agents by preventing the expression of prosurvival genes. For instance, NF-κB is a survival factor that is inactivated in the cytoplasm through binding to the I-κB inhibitor protein. Phosphorylation of this protein leads to liberation of NF-κB, which translocates to the nucleus and activates the transcription of a number of factors that protect the cell from apoptosis. The phosphorylated I-κB evolves by ubiquitinylation, which is followed by proteasome degradation (Fig. 10.3). Therefore, an approach to the prevention of NF-κB activation consists of inhibiting proteasome activity, thereby stabilizing I-κB. Finally, the failure to degrade cyclins after proteasome

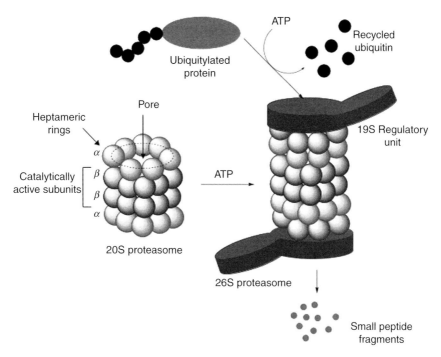

FIGURE 10.1   Structure and function of the proteasome.

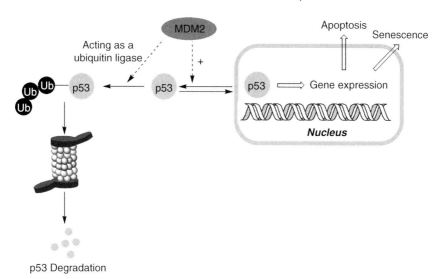

FIGURE 10.2   Negative regulation of p53 by MDM2 and its subsequent degradation by the proteasome.

inhibition prevents completion of the cell cycle and hence the mitotic proliferation of cancer cells.

Proteasome can be classified as an N-terminal nucleophile (Ntn) hydrolase, since the catalytic centers at the β subunits have been identified as N-terminal

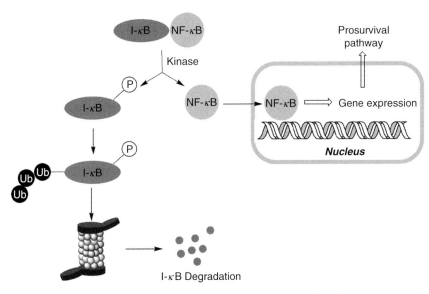

FIGURE 10.3   Proteasome degradation of I-κB stimulates NF-κB-mediated prosurvival pathways in tumor cells.

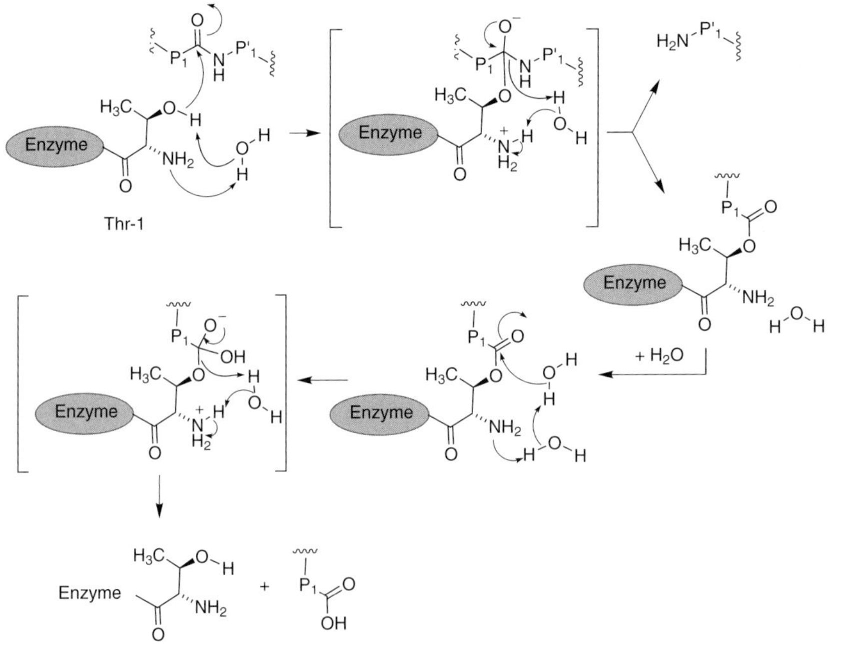

FIGURE 10.4   Mechanism of proteolysis by the proteasome.

threonine residues, acting as nucleophiles through their hydroxyl groups. Considering the general mechanism of action of these enzymes, the mechanism summarized in Fig. 10.4, involving two tetrahedral transition states, has been proposed for the proteolysis mechanism by proteasome.

Most known proteasome inhibitors[4,5] are peptidomimetics containing an electrophilic functional group, and can therefore be classified as site-directed enzyme inhibitors. This group is normally placed at one end of the molecule and reacts with the threonine hydroxyl after its activation. Many of these compounds bear a close relationship with inhibitors of serine proteases (e.g., HIV protease). Some representative examples are given below. Among these compounds, bortezomib was approved in 2003 for the treatment of multiple myeloma, the second most common hematological cancer, and is currently being clinically evaluated for various other malignancies.[6] Bortezomib (PS-341, LDP-341, MLN-341) affects multiple signaling cascades (e.g., NF-κB) within the cell because of proteasome inhibition and induces G2/M phase arrest followed by apoptosis in cancer cells.[7]

MG-132 (peptide aldehyde)

(Peptide α-ketoamide)

NLVS (peptide vinyl sulfone)

Epoxomycin (peptide epoxiketone)

Bortezomib (peptide boronic acid)

Proteasome inhibitors containing aldehyde or ketone functions react reversibly with the threonine hydroxyl to give the corresponding acetals **10.1** and **10.2**. Vinyl sulfones were originally introduced as inhibitors of cysteine proteases,[8] since these Michael acceptors are expected to react with soft nucleophiles like thiols, but it was subsequently found that they also form a covalent adduct **10.3** with the threonine group in the proteasome catalytic site. In the case of epoxyketones, like the natural product epoxomycin, the X-ray crystal structure and spectrometric analysis of a complex between the inhibitor and the yeast *Saccharomyces cerevisiae* 20S proteasome showed the formation of the morpholine derivative **10.5**. The generation of this compound was explained by the formation of hemiacetal **10.4** through reaction of the threonine oxygen with the carbonyl group of the epoxyketone pharmacophore, followed by nucleophilic attack of the amino group onto the more hindered epoxide carbon atom with inversion of configuration.[9]

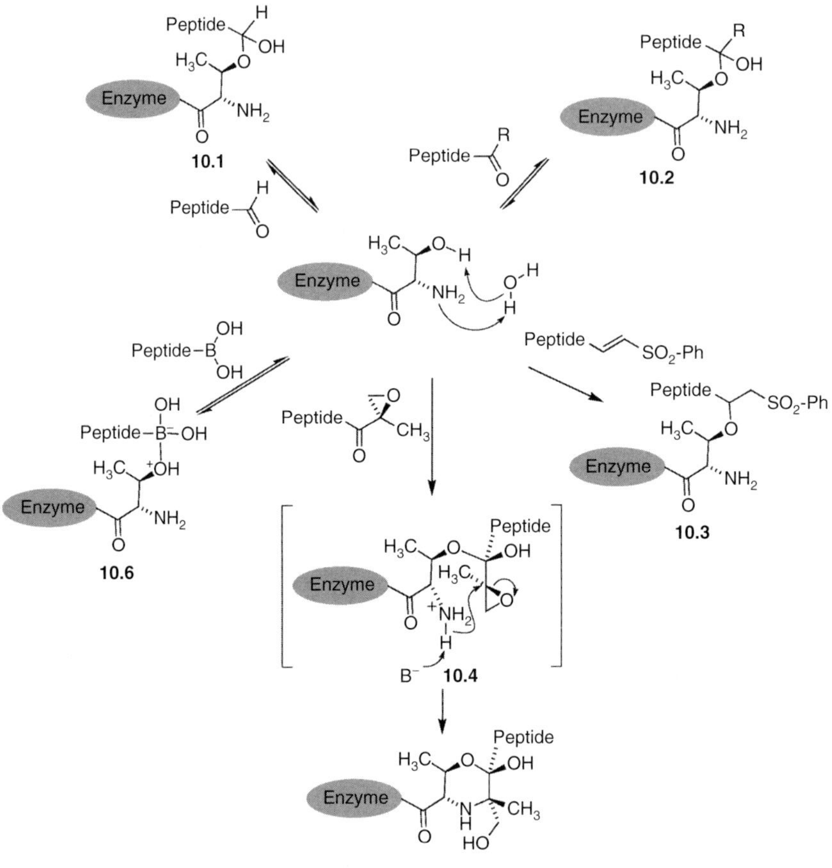

FIGURE 10.5   Several mechanisms for proteasome inhibition.

Finally, peptide boronic acids have extensively been used as serine protease inhibitors. Their interaction with the threonine at the active site can be attributed to the availability of an empty p-orbital on boron, which is well-suited to accept the oxygen lone pair of the N-terminal threonine residues to form stable, reversible tetrahedral intermediates **10.6**.[10] Because of their higher specificity due to their lack of activity on cysteine proteases, a large number of peptide boronic acids and esters were synthesized to target proteasome (Fig. 10. 5).

2. ANTIANGIOGENIC AGENTS UNRELATED TO KINASE SIGNALING

In order for a tumor to grow beyond a size of about 2 mm^3, it needs to develop a network of blood vessels (angiogenesis), a process that is regulated by proangiogenic and antiangiogenic factors. Some proangiogenic factors are involved in signaling pathways and their inhibitors were studied in Section 3.4 of

Chapter 9. Some anticancer drugs targeting preexisting vasculature through tubulin depolymerization were discussed in Section 5 of Chapter 8.

Antiangiogenic drugs[11,12] can be classified into five categories:

- Inhibitors of proangiogenic growth factors, including vascular endothelial cell growth factor (VEGF), fibroblast growth factor (FGF), and platelet-derived growth factor (PDGF). Antitumor drugs targeted at these factors were studied in Section 3.4 of Chapter 9.
- Inhibitors of proteolytic enzymes of the extracellular matrix.
- Inhibitors of other targets related to the extracellular matrix.
- Endogenous inhibitors of angiogenesis.
- Inhibitors of cellular adhesion molecules.
- Miscellaneous antiangiogenic compounds.

2.1. Inhibitors of proteolytic enzymes of the extracellular matrix: Metalloproteinases

In response to angiogenic stimuli, endothelial proteases initiate the breakdown of the surrounding extracellular matrix, which allows the migration of proliferating endothelial cells and their growth to form lumens. Besides their role in cancer treatment,[13] they are also being studied as targets for arthritis and emphysema because of their role in collagen degradation.[14]

Matrix metalloproteinases (MMPs) are zinc-dependent proteolytic endopeptidases. The zinc cation is coordinated by three imidazole side chains from histidine residues, and a water molecule is the fourth ligand. All inhibitors replace this water molecule and coordinate to zinc in a monodentate or bidentate fashion. The general mechanism for peptide hydrolysis by zinc-metalloproteinases is shown in Fig. 10.6, and is based on the enhanced acidity of the water molecule as a consequence of coordination of its oxygen atom with zinc.

2.1.1. First-generation MMP inhibitors: Hydroxamic acid peptidomimetics

The design of the first generation of MMP inhibitors relied on the preparation of peptide and peptide-like compounds that combine backbone features that interact with enzyme subsites and functional groups capable of coordination with zinc. Among these, the hydroxamic acid group is a very potent 1,4-bidentate zinc ligand that binds as an anion with two contacts to the cation and creates a distorted trigonal bipyramidal geometry around the metal.[15] Additionally, it also has a nitrogen atom for binding to the protein backbone. For this reason, peptide-like compounds that contain a hydroxamic acid portion are among the most potent known inhibitors of the MMPs, with potencies in the nanomolar range. Their interaction with the MMP binding domain is shown in Fig. 10.7.

Batimastat (BB-94)[16] and marimastat are hydroxamic acid-based MMP inhibitors with little specificity. Batimastat reached Phase III clinical trials, but it cannot be given orally and it is no longer considered for clinical testing. Marimastat is orally active and it has also undergone several Phase III assays, showing poor performance. Results from clinical trials with this first generation of MMP

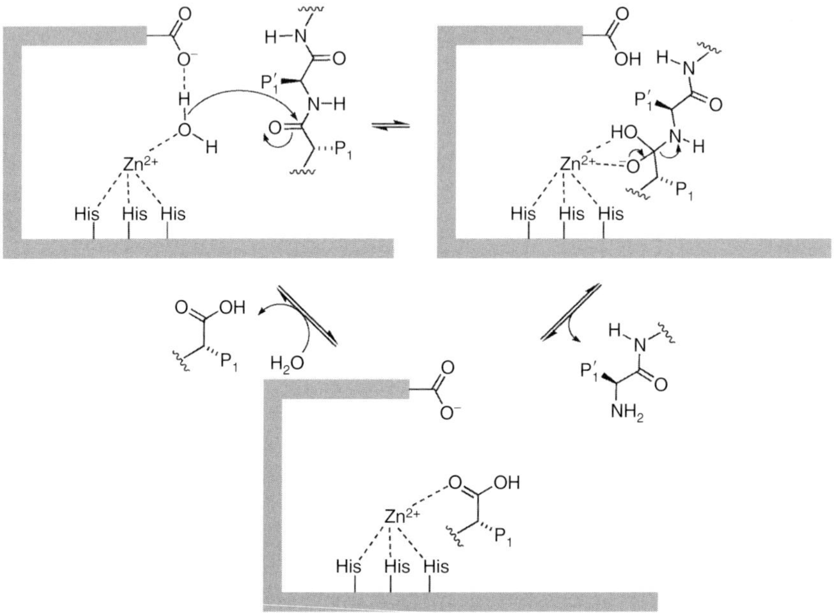

FIGURE 10.6   Catalytic mechanism of matrix metalloproteinases (MMPs).

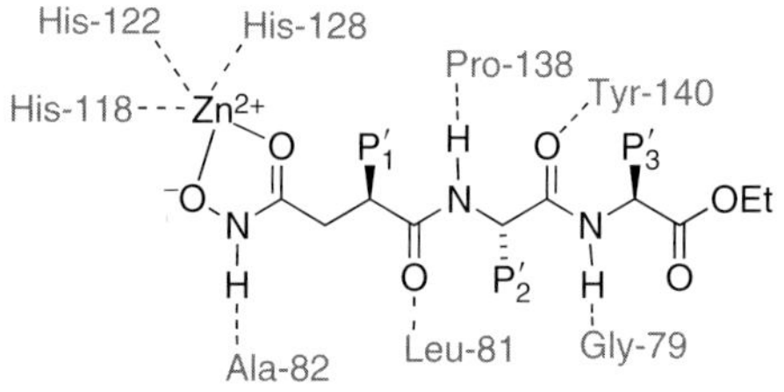

FIGURE 10.7   Interaction of hydroxamic acid peptidomimetics with MMPs.

inhibitors have been disappointing and have led many investigators to conclude that MMPs are not suitable targets for the treatment of human cancer. On the contrary, it has been argued that because MMP inhibition would decrease the rate of tumor progression, the therapeutic benefit obtained from its administration would be minimized for patients undergoing clinical trials, who are normally at late stages of their disease.[17]

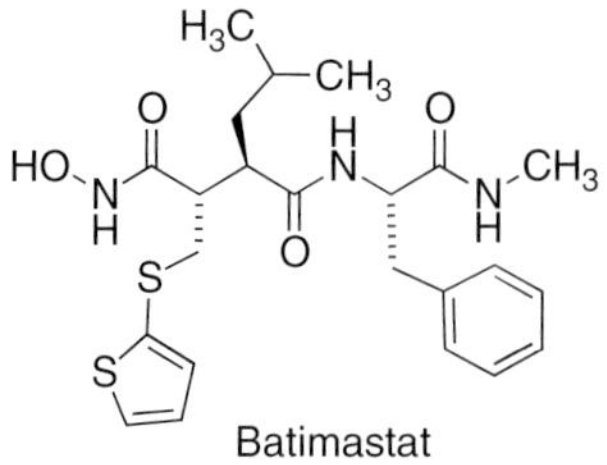

Batimastat

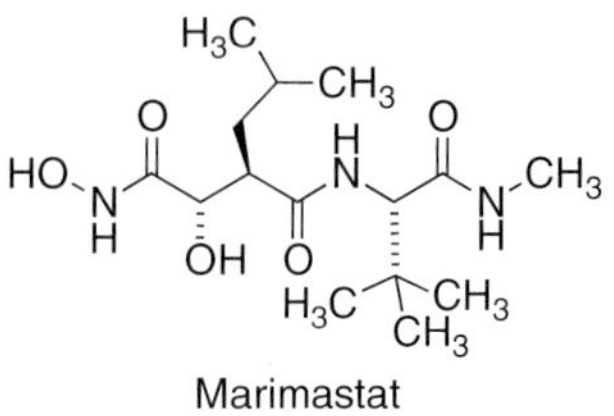

Marimastat

2.1.2. Second-generation MMP inhibitors

These compounds are nonpeptidic and more specific, probably because they have been designed on the basis of structural studies of the MMP active site by NMR and X-ray crystallography. The first subgroup of these inhibitors bear an hydroxamic function and include prinomastat (AG-3340) and MMI-270 (CGS-27023). Phase II clinical studies of prinomastat with early stage cancers are currently in progress, although Phase III trials for advanced prostate and lung cancer were stopped because they did not show beneficial effects.[18] In the case of MMI-270, clinical studies were advanced to Phase II but had to be interrupted because of poor patient tolerance. ABT-518 is a reverse hydroxamate-based inhibitor that has entered early clinical trials for the treatment of solid tumors.

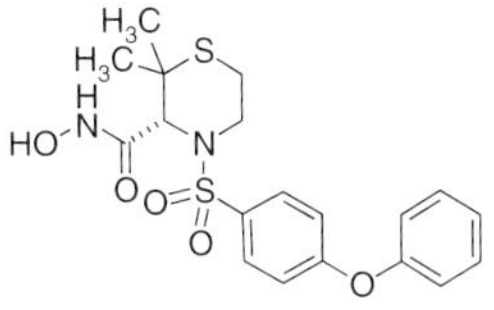

Prinomastat (AG-3340) 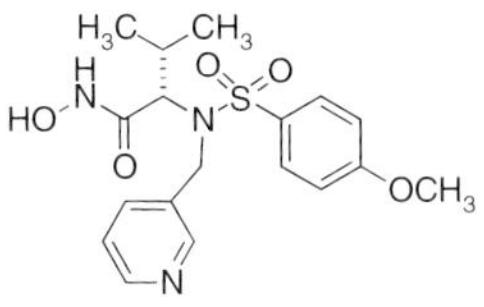   MMI-270 (CGS-27023) 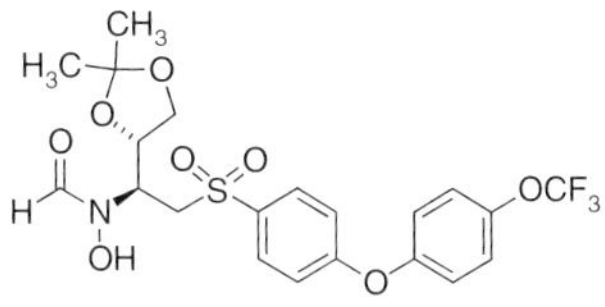   ABT-518

Other functional groups that can interact with the Zn^{2+} cation in MMPs are the carboxy and mercapto moieties. Tanomastat (BAY 12–9566) is a carboxylic acid-based specific inhibitor that failed during Phase III studies for treatment of advanced or small cell lung cancers. Another carboxylic acid-based inhibitor is S-3304, which entered Phase II trials for the treatment of solid tumors. Rebimastat is a thiol-based inhibitor, also in Phase II-III clinical trials. Finally, some tetracyclin derivatives, which are well-known chelating agents, behave as MMP inhibitors. One example is metastat (COL-3), which is under Phase II trials for Kaposi's sarcoma and advanced brain tumors.

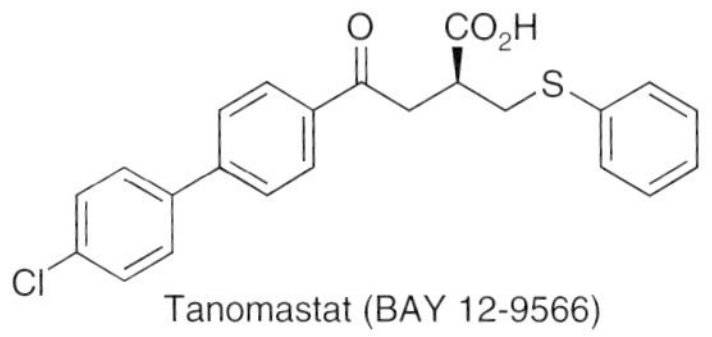

Tanomastat (BAY 12-9566) 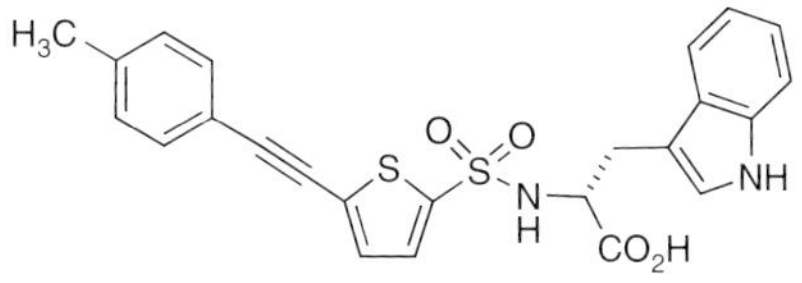   S-3304

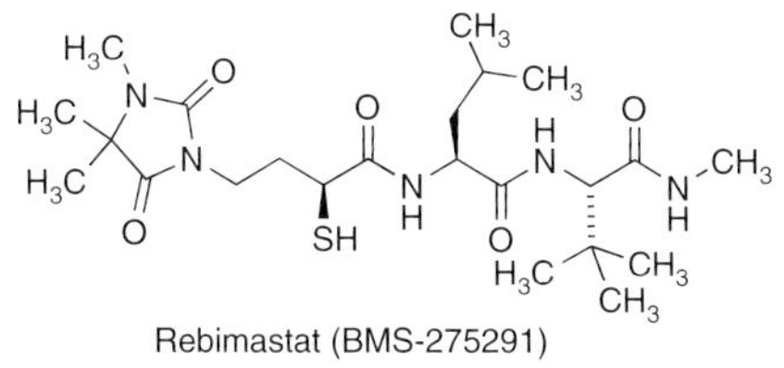

Rebimastat (BMS-275291) 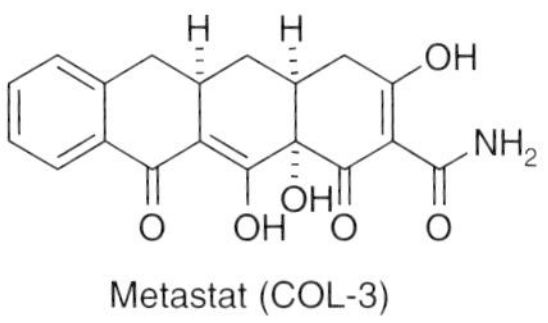   Metastat (COL-3)

We will finally mention neovastat (AE-941), an orally bioavailable standardized extract prepared from shark cartilage that shows significant antiangiogenic and antimetastatic properties *in vivo* by a complex mechanism that includes inhibition of various members of the MMP family. Neovastat is orally bioavailable, shows significant antitumor and antimetastatic properties in animal models, and is currently under evaluation in several clinical studies in patients with lung and renal carcinoma and multiple myeloma.[19]

2.2. Inhibitors of other targets related to the extracellular matrix: Heparanase

Heparan sulfate (HS) is an important component of the heterogeneous mixture of proteins and proteoglycans that make up the extracellular matrix. This is a polysaccharide formed by alternating, repetitive units of D-glucosamine and D-glucuronic acid/L-iduronic acid.

HS is a component of the HS proteoglycans, formed by a protein core covalently bound to HS side chains. These proteoglycans bind to many groups of bioactive molecules, including growth factors, cell adhesion molecules, and cytokines, among many others. These molecules are liberated by heparanase, a β-D-glucuronidase that specifically cleaves HS glycosaminoglycan chains, with profound biological impact. Among other effects, the release of growth factors promotes angiogenesis, tumor growth, invasion, and metastasis. Heparanase is preferentially expressed in many tumor types, and has become an important anticancer target.

Although the substrate specificity of heparanase is not completely understood, recent work suggests that heparanase recognizes sequences as small as a trisaccharide provided they are highly sulfated. The minimum HS recognition sequence[20] is shown in structure **10.7** (Fig. 10.8A) and its catalytic mechanism involves two acidic residues, a proton donor at Glu-225 and a nucleophile at Glu-343 (Fig. 10.8B).[21]

Heparanase inhibitors[22,23] are structurally very heterogeneous, and can be classified into three categories:

– Polysaccharides with O- or N-sulfate groups
– Compounds with C-sulfate groups
– Neutral inhibitors

Additionally, some studies aimed at the production of heparanase antibodies have been reported.

2.2.1. Polysaccharides with O- or N-sulfate groups

Some examples of this class of compounds are the heparins and other sulfated polysaccharides, or synthetic polymers that mimic heparin. These compounds may have a broad range of biological activities, and their main uses are outside the anticancer field. The main goal in this area is the development of compounds

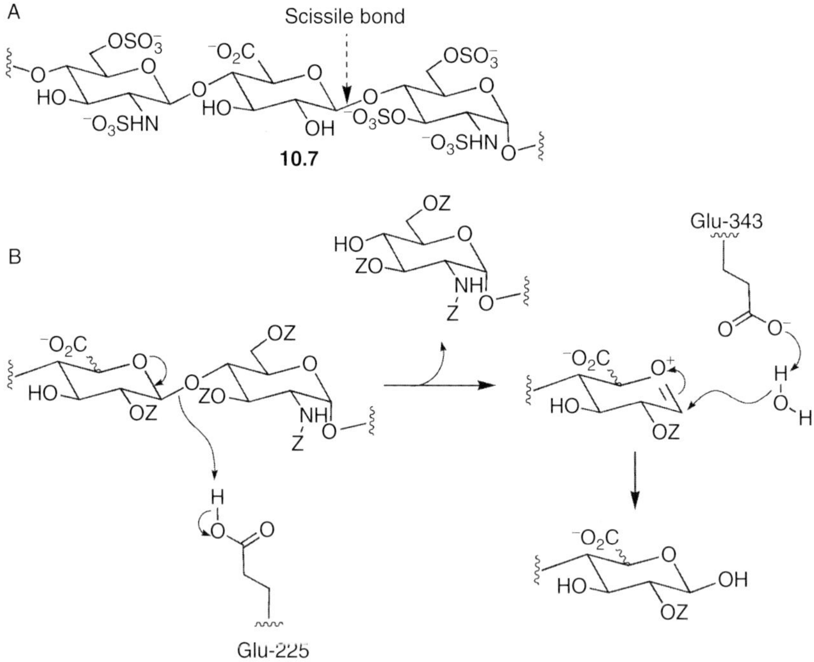

FIGURE 10.8   A. Recognition sequence of heparan sulfate. B. Mechanism of the reaction catalyzed by heparanase.

with reduced molecular sizes, and one of these compounds, the phosphosulfo-mannan PI-88, is in clinical trials in several cancers.[24] PI-88 is a mixture of chemically sulfated oligosaccharides, ranging from di- to hexasaccharides and with the majority (60%) being pentasaccharides. Besides being a heparanase inhibitor, PI-88 also inhibits angiogenesis by antagonizing the interactions of proangiogenic growth factors (e.g., VEGF and bFGF) and their receptors with HS.

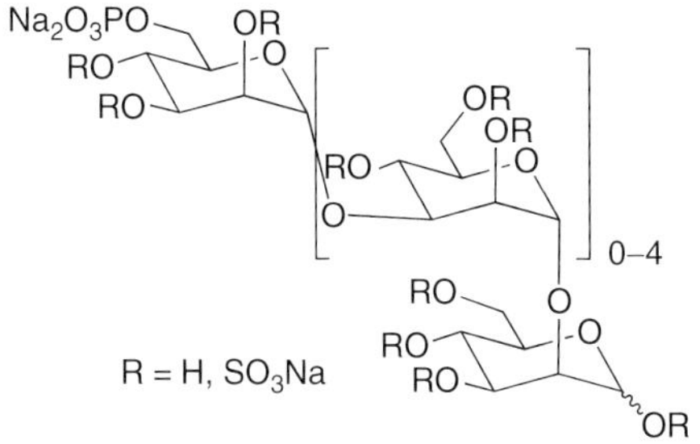

PI-88

2.2.2. Compounds with C-sulfate groups

Suramin, a polysulfonated naphthylurea developed as an antiparasitary agent, is being clinically tested for several tumors. It shows a complex mechanism of action, which includes angiogenesis inhibition (see also Section 3.4.3 of Chapter 9), and it has been shown to be a noncompetitive heparanase inhibitor.[25]

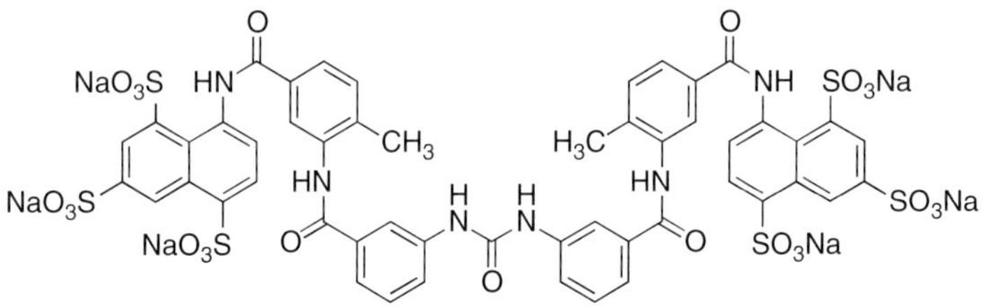

Suramin

2.2.3. Neutral inhibitors

These compounds do not contain sulfate moieties and are structurally very diverse. Among them, some natural and unnatural imino sugars, such as **10.8**, are reversible heparanase inhibitors, acting as putative transition state analogs.[26]

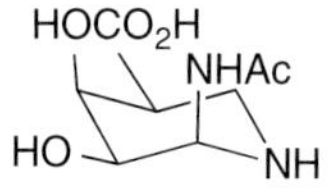

10.8

2.3. Endogenous inhibitors of angiogenesis

Some naturally occurring angiogenesis inhibitors are known, including endostatin, angiostatin, thrombospondin-1 (TSP-1), and platelet-derived factor 4 (PF-4).

Endostatin is a polypeptide of 184 amino acids, corresponding to the globular domain found at the C-terminal of type XVIII collagen, and it is the most studied of the endogenous angiogenesis inhibitors. After promising preclinical trials, where it showed no development of drug resistance over time, it has reached Phase II clinical trials in patients with advanced neuroendocrine tumors,[27] using material prepared by recombinant DNA technology.

Angiostatin is a 57-kDa fragment of plasmin, which is, in turn, a fragment of plasminogen. It is under clinical studies in combination with paclitaxel and carboplatin in patients with non-small cell lung cancer.[28]

Thrombospondins are a family of glycoproteins. One of them (TSP-1) inhibits angiogenesis by interaction with a receptor (CD36) expressed on the surface of endothelial cells. This leads to the expression of FAS ligand (FasL), a transmembrane protein that belongs to the tumor necrosis factor (TNF) family, leading to apoptosis through internalization of its complex with the Fas receptor and final caspase activation. Recent studies have focused on small fragments of TSP-1 that have been shown to be potent inhibitors of angiogenesis. In a related approach, ABT-510 is a thrombospondin-mimetic peptide designed from a heptapeptidic active fragment.[29] It exhibited antiangiogenic and tumor growth inhibition in preclinical models and is undergoing clinical studies.[30]

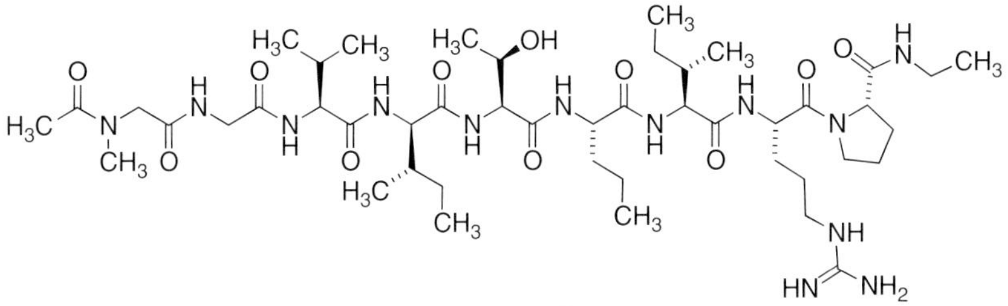

ABT-510

Another possible approach to antiangiogenic therapy related to endogenous inhibitors is based on the observation that certain orally active small molecules seem to raise the plasma levels of endogenous angiogenesis inhibitors by increasing their expression or by alternative means, such as mobilization from matrix or platelets.[31] Some of these molecules are celecoxib, which can increase serum endostatin, doxycycline and rosiglitazone, which can increase expression of TSP-1. The antitumor activity of celecoxib, a well-known anti-inflammatory drug acting by cyclooxygenase-2 inhibition, has been recently recognized, and this compound has reached advanced clinical trials for colon cancer.[32]

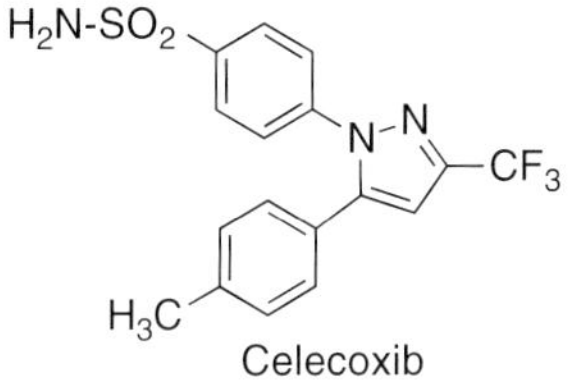

Celecoxib

2.4. Inhibitors of cellular adhesion molecules

Another approach to antiangiogenic therapy is to inhibit the adhesive interactions required by angiogenesis vascular endothelial cells. The migration of endothelial cells is dependent on their adhesion to extracellular matrix proteins through a variety of cell adhesion receptors known as integrins, especially integrin $\alpha v \beta_3$.[33] Integrin binds to an arginine-glycine-aspartic acid (RGD) sequence, which can be found in several extracellular matrix proteins. The antiangiogenic cyclic peptide *cyclo*-(Arg-Gly-Asp-D-Phe-D-NMeVal) (cilengitide, **10.9**) inhibits $\alpha v \beta_3$ and is undergoing clinical trials for brain and solid tumors.

$\alpha v \beta_5$ is another RGD-dependent adhesion receptor that plays a critical role in angiogenesis, and hence selective dual $\alpha v \beta_3 / \alpha v \beta_5$ antagonists, such as SCH-221153, have been proposed as a novel class of angiogenesis and tumor-growth inhibitors.[34]

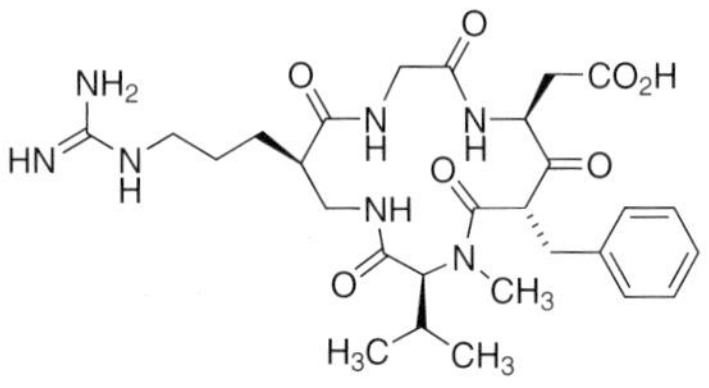

Cilengitide (**10.9**)

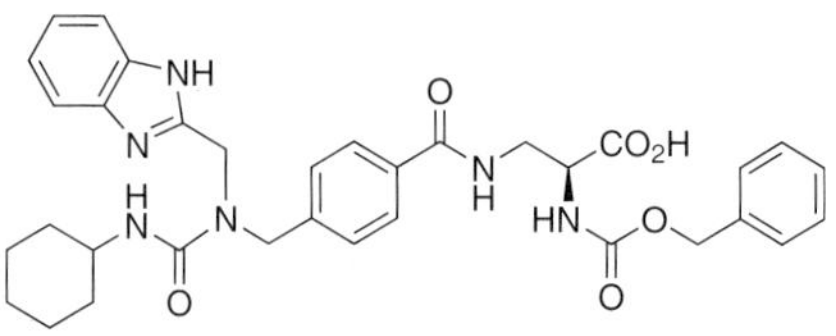

SCH-221153

Vitaxin is a humanized version of LM-609, a monoclonal antibody that functionally blocks the $\alpha v\beta_3$ integrin. This antibody has been shown to target angiogenic blood vessels and cause suppression of tumor growth in various animal models, and is undergoing clinical assays for the treatment of breast carcinoma, melanoma, and Kaposi's sarcoma.[35]

2.5. Miscellaneous antiangiogenic compounds

2.5.1. Squalamine

Squalamine is an antiangiogenic natural cationic steroid that has been isolated from tissues of several species of dogfish shark (*Squalus acanthias*). This compound is currently under clinical studies for several types of cancer, and it has also recently received FDA fast track status for the treatment of "wet" age-related macular degeneration (AMD). It also exhibits potent bactericidal activity against both gram-negative and gram-positive bacteria, is fungicidal, and induces osmotic lysis of protozoa.

Squalamine interrupts and reverses multiple facets of the angiogenic process, including VEGF. It also inhibits integrin expression and reverses cytoskeletal formation, thereby resulting in endothelial cell inactivation and apoptosis.

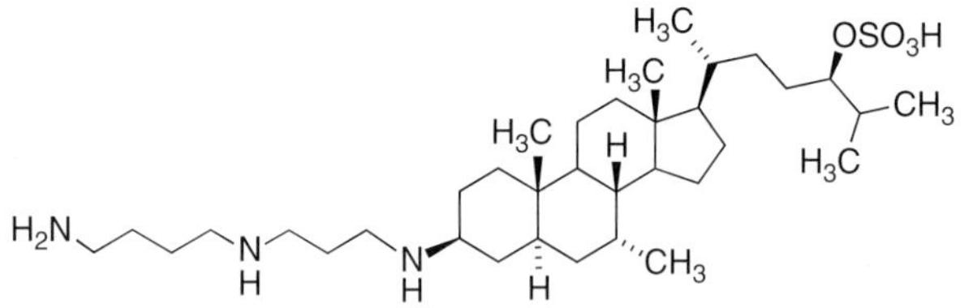

Squalamine

Squalamine specifically inhibits brush-border Na^+/H^+ exchanger isoform NHE3, a sodium-hydrogen exchanger present on cell surfaces that regulates intracellular pH, and is also known to regulate endothelial cell volume and shape.[36]

Cancer cells secrete endothelial cell growth factors that stimulate vascular endothelial cell growth factor receptors (VEGFR), which activates MAP kinase pathways involved in blood vessel growth. Inhibition of the sodium-proton exchanger leads to changes in intracellular pH and subsequent inhibition of MAP kinase activity (Fig. 10.9).[37] Squalamine also interacts with calmodulin and possibly with other signaling pathways.

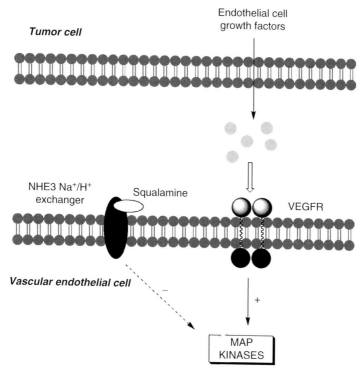

FIGURE 10.9   Inhibition of the NHE3 Na^+/H^+ exchanger by squalamine.

2.5.2. Thalidomide and its analogs

Thalidomide was introduced in the 1950s as a sedative that was prescribed for nausea and insomnia in pregnant women. However, it was found to be the cause of severe birth defects in children whose mothers had taken the drug in their first trimester of pregnancy. In 1965, it was serendipitously discovered that thalidomide was effective at improving the symptoms of patients with erythema nodosum leprosum (ENL), and was approved for this use in 1998. In 1994, thalidomide was found to inhibit angiogenesis through a complex mechanism that includes inhibition of the synthesis by activated monocytes of TNF-α, which seems to have a role in angiogenesis by upregulation of the expression of the endothelial integrin and VEGF, among others. It has been demonstrated that inhibition of angiogenesis by thalidomide requires prior metabolic activation,[38] which has prompted the synthesis and evaluation of a large number of potential metabolites of this lead compound.

Thalidomide is being used, in association with dexamethasone[39] and cytotoxic agents such as cyclophosphamide,[40] for the treatment of multiple myeloma.[41] Its mechanism of antitumor action is complex and, besides the inhibition of angiogenesis, also involves induction of apoptosis and other mechanisms.[42]

Thalidomide has been used as the lead compound in the development of a class of drugs known as immunomodulatory drugs (ImiDs®),[43] which have shown activity in multiple myeloma and other hematological and solid malignancies. The most advanced one is lenalidomide (CC-5013), which has recently been approved by the FDA, in combination with dexamethasone, for the treatment of multiple myeloma patients who have received at least one prior therapy.[44] It has also shown efficacy in the hematological disorders known as the myelodysplastic syndromes (MDS). CC-4047 is another thalidomide analog that is in Phase II trials to determine its potential safety and efficacy as a treatment for multiple myeloma and prostate cancer.[45] The S-isomer of CC-4047 has been reported to be its more potent enantiomer, but it has been shown to undergo rapid racemization in human plasma, a finding that supports the development of the drug in its racemate form.[46]

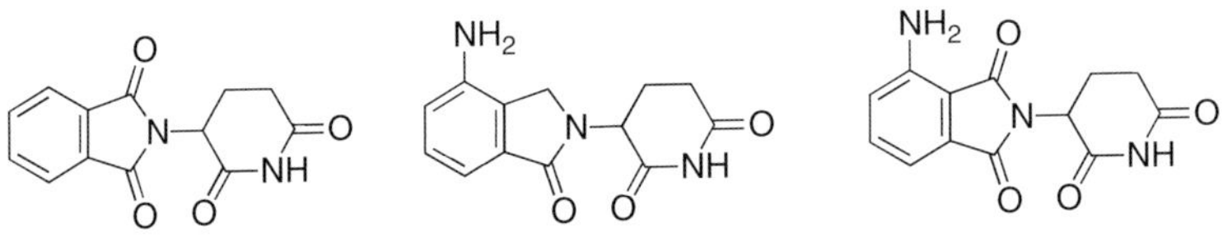

Thalidomide

Lenalidomide
(CC-5013)

CC-4047

2.5.3. TNP-470

Several natural products have shown activity as angiogenesis inhibitors.[47] The best studied, and one of the most potent angiostatic agents, is fumagillin, isolated from *Aspergillus fumigatus* and widely employed as an antifungal in *Nosema apis* infections in honeybees. Fumagillin is an inhibitor of methionine aminopeptidase-2,[48] an enzyme involved in endothelial proliferation. It also inhibits the expression of the ETS1 transcription factor, which regulates the expression of VEGFs.[49] Its toxicity prompted the preparation of analogs, and among them the most advanced one is TNP-470, which is being studied for several lymphomas, acute leukemias, and solid tumors. Because of neurotoxicity problems, conjugates of this compound have been developed in order to prevent its access through the blood–brain barrier.[50]

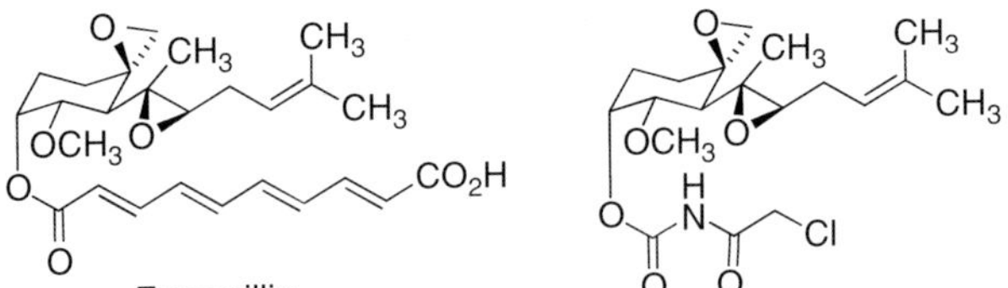

Fumagillin

TNP-470

3. EPIGENETIC THERAPY OF CANCER

The initiation and progression of cancer is controlled by both genetic and epigenetic events. The term "epigenetic" refers to alterations in gene expression that are not associated with changes in DNA sequence. Unlike genetic alterations, epigenetic aberrations are potentially reversible. The best studied epigenetic alterations are DNA methylation and histone tail modifications, and epigenetic gene silencing by these mechanisms has become an attractive anticancer target.[51] The main enzymes involved in establishing epigenetic patterns are the following:

1. DNA methyltransferases (DNMTs)
2. Histone acetylases (HATs)
3. Histone deacetylases (HDACs)
4. Histone methyltransferases (HMTs)

3.1. Inhibitors of DNA methyltransferases (DNMT)

DNMTs are responsible for the methylation of the C-5 position of cytosine, and almost exclusively at CpG dinucleotides. This is an epigenetic mechanism used for long-term silencing of gene expression because structural changes in DNA associated to methylation close to a transcription start site inhibit gene expression either directly, by blocking binding of transcriptional factors, or indirectly, by recruitment of transcription repressors called methyl-binding proteins (MBDs). The methylation pattern is normally maintained throughout life, but in older individuals deviations from this pattern start to appear, and this can lead to genomic instability. One specific goal of epigenetic chemotherapy is to prevent hypermethylation in DNA that could lead to the silencing of genes crucial for normal cell function, usually tumor suppressor genes, and is considered to be one of the early key events in the development of cancer.[52] On the contrary, the use of demethylating agents can potentiate the expression of oncogenes, but it has nevertheless been observed that the overall response to decreased methylation is the abrogation of tumorigenicity (Fig. 10.10). DNA demethylating agents do not cause immediate cell death like most other chemotherapeutic drugs, but they are aimed at the activation genes involved in apoptosis pathways and cell cycle regulation. For this reason, although epigenetic drugs have the advantage of their low toxicity, their effects are transient and the aberrant patterns can be reestablished on removal of the drug.

The DNA methylation reaction uses the S-adenosylmethionine cofactor as a methyl donor, and transforms the cytosine residues **10.10** into their 5-methyl derivatives **10.11**, as shown in Fig. 10.11.

The role of DNMTs in this reaction is twofold. On the one hand, a carboxylic group from the enzyme acts as an acid catalyst by protonation of N-3, and on the other hand, a cysteine residue in the catalytic pocket gives a conjugate addition to the thus activated $C_6=C_5-C_4=N_3$ system to yield the intermediate **10.12**. This compound contains an enamine system that is nucleophilic at the C_5 position, and the enzyme enhances this nucleophilicity by abstraction of the N_3 proton, allowing displacement of the highly electrophilic methyl group attached to the sulfonium unit in S-adenosylmethionine, to give **10.13** and

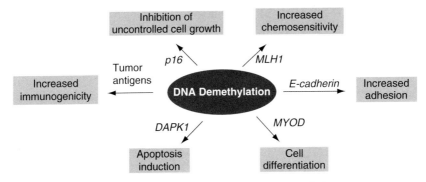

FIGURE 10.10   Events associated to DNA demethylation.

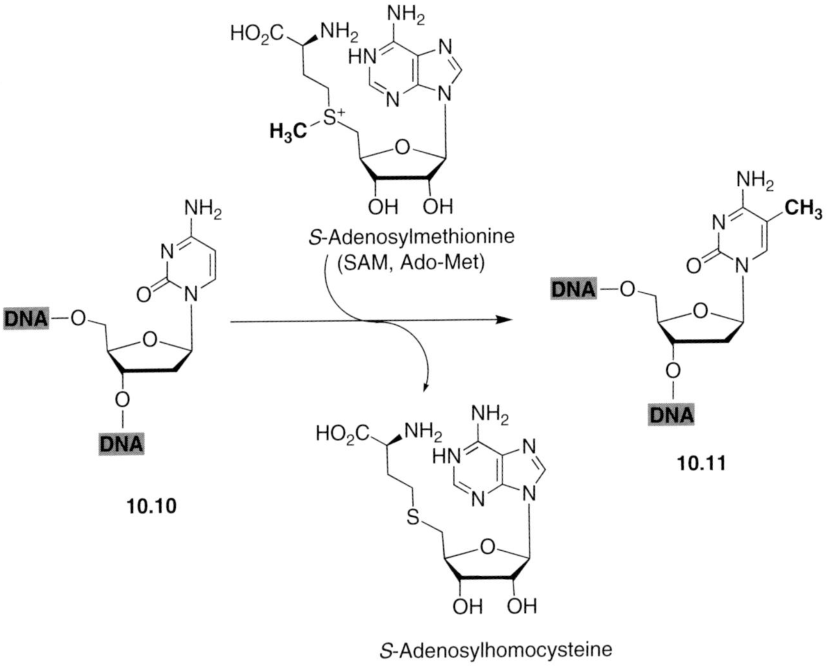

S-Adenosylmethionine
(SAM, Ado-Met)

S-Adenosylhomocysteine

10.10

10.11

FIGURE 10.11   Methylation of cytosine by DNA methyltransferases.

S-adenosylhomocysteine. Finally, the product **10.11** and the free enzyme are released from structure **10.13** by a β-elimination reaction (Fig. 10.12).

3.1.1. Nucleoside inhibitors of DNMT

Some nucleoside analogs that have a modified cytosine ring attached to a ribose or deoxyribose moiety behave as DNMT inhibitors. They are metabolized by kinases and ribonucleotide reductases into deoxynucleotides that can be incorporated into DNA, which allows contact with DNMT and its subsequent inhibition. The most interesting compounds of this class are 5-azacytidine, decitabine, 5-fluoro-2′-deoxycytidine, 5,6-dihydro-5-azacytidine (DHAC), and zebularine.

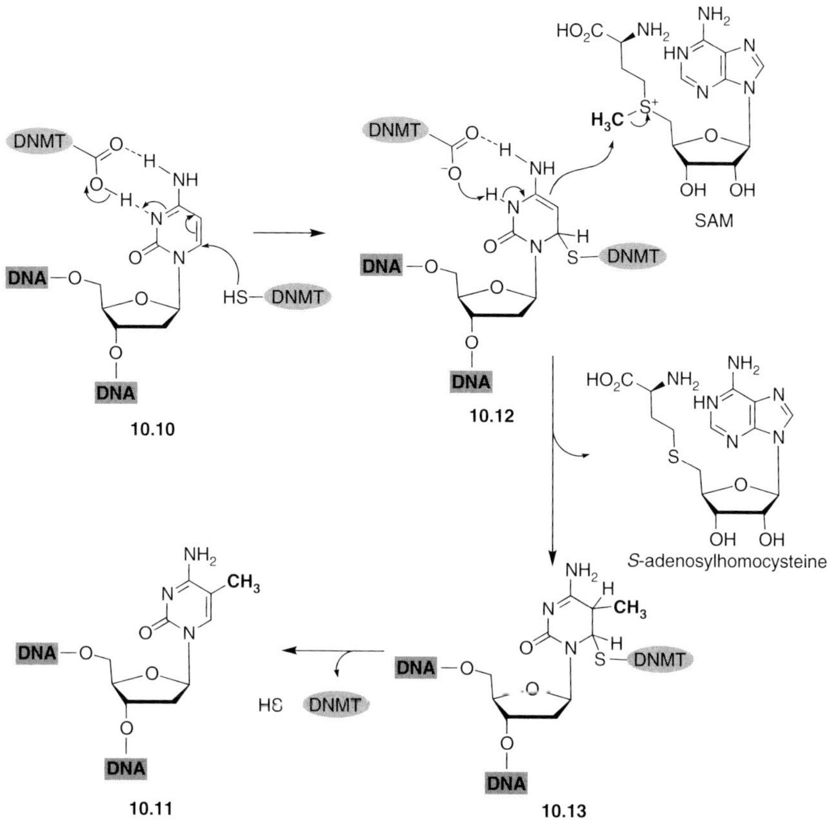
DNMT
DNA
HS—DNMT
10.10
10.12
SAM
S-adenosylhomocysteine
10.11
10.13

FIGURE 10.12 Mechanism of cytosine methylation by DNA methyltransferases.

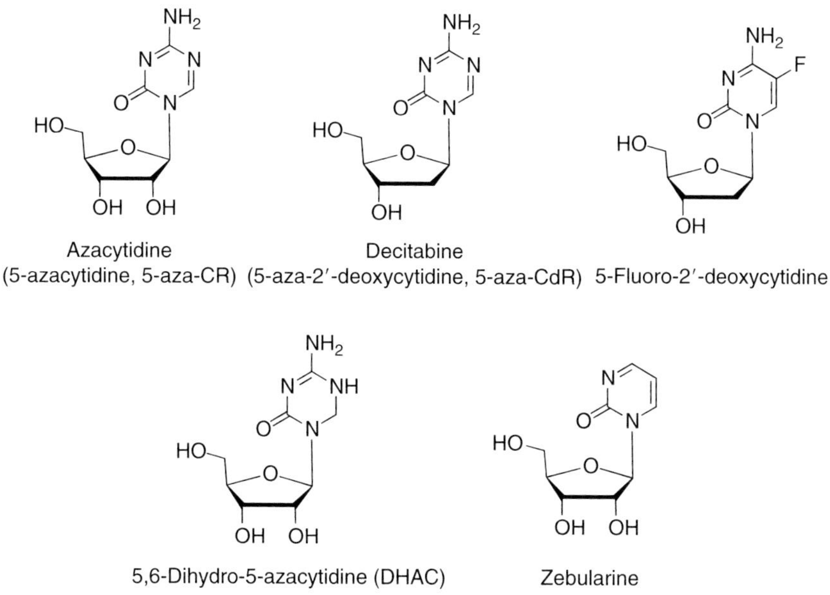
Azacytidine
(5-azacytidine, 5-aza-CR)
Decitabine
(5-aza-2′-deoxycytidine, 5-aza-CdR)
5-Fluoro-2′-deoxycytidine
5,6-Dihydro-5-azacytidine (DHAC)
Zebularine

5-Azacytidine[53] and its 2'-deoxy analog decitabine incorporate into DNA as false nucleotides **10.14**, which are complexed by the DNMT enzyme similar to its natural substrates. Attack of the mercapto group in the active site gives adduct **10.15**, and its methylation at the N-5 position takes place normally to give **10.16**, but the lack of a hydrogen atom at N-5 after methylation prevents the elimination reaction necessary to restore the enzyme, which is thus inactivated (Fig. 10.13).

Although Phase II clinical studies of 5-azacytidine as an antitumor drug took place in 1972, its ability to inhibit DNA methylation was established in 1980. Beginning in 1993, a number of studies proved its efficacy in the treatment of MDS, leading to its approval by FDA for this indication.[54] Because of the poor oral absorption of nucleosides, administration has to be by injection.[55]

Decitabine is also a long-known anticancer drug that was tested in the clinic in the 1970s using the maximum tolerated doses, with myelosuppression as its main side effect. It was not until 2004 that it was shown to have higher efficacy at much lower doses, with a correlation with DNA demethylation being observed.[56] In 2003, decitabine received orphan drug status for treatment of MDS, and it is

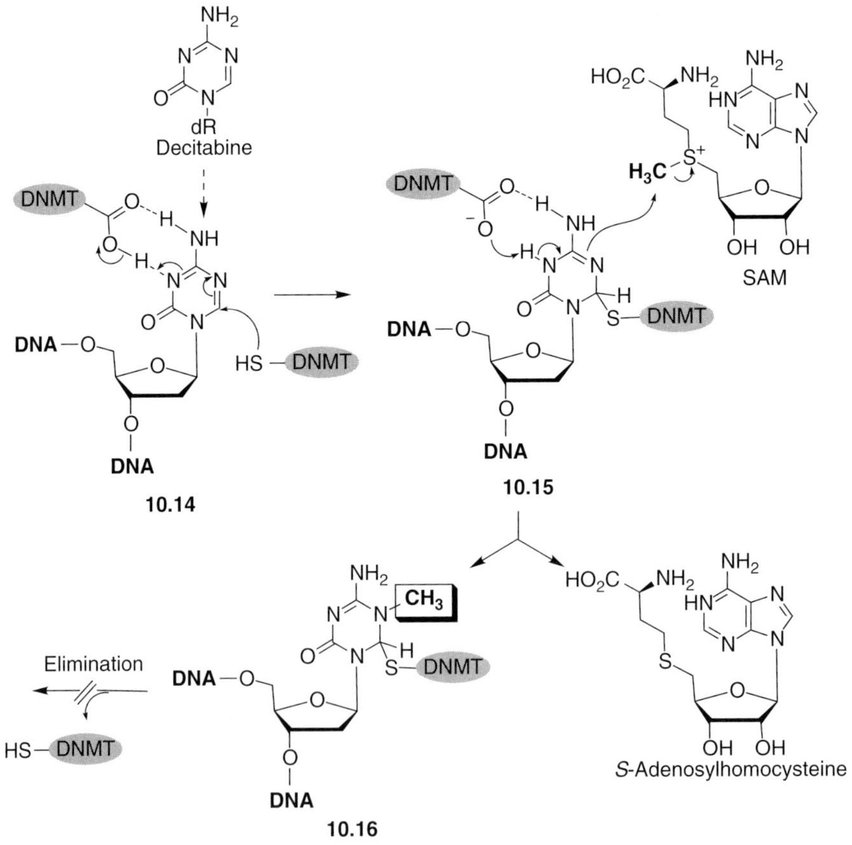

FIGURE 10.13   Mechanism of DNMT inhibition by 5-azacytidine and decitabine.

also being studied in patients with chronic myelogenous leukemia resistant to imatinib.[57]

5-Fluoro-2′-deoxycytidine is another DNA demethylating agent that is currently underogoing Phase I studies in association with tetrahydrouridine.[58] Its mechanism of action involves incorporation into DNA as nucleotide **10.17**, followed by methylation at C-5 mediated by nucleophilic attack of a cysteine residue in the active pocket of DNMT to give intermediate **10.18**, which is methylated by S-adenosylmethionine to **10.19**. The absence of a proton at C-5 prevents the elimination reaction necessary for liberating the free enzyme (Fig. 10.14).

5-Azacytidine, decitabine, and 5-fluoro-2′-deoxycytidine suffer from low *in vitro* and *in vivo* stabilities. The *in vitro* stability can be improved by suppression of the $N_5=C_6$ imine function by either suppression of the double bond or the nitrogen atom, in order to prevent the addition of nucleophiles. Two examples are DHAC and zebularine. Sometimes these compounds are associated with tetrahydrouridine, an inhibitor of cytosine deaminase that behaves as a transition state

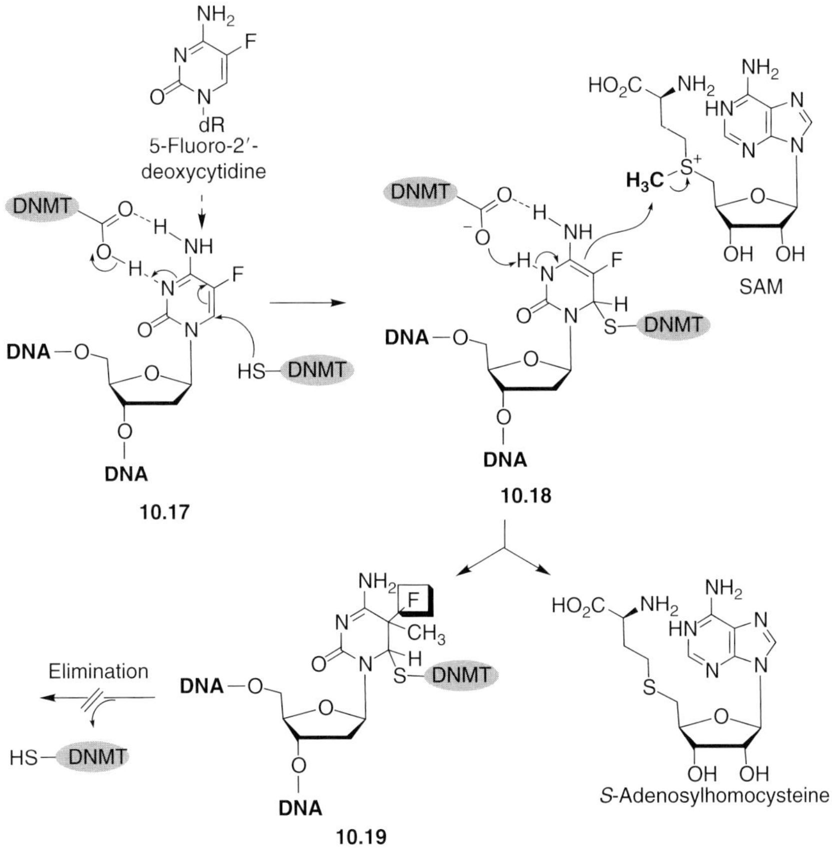

FIGURE 10.14   Mechanism of DNMT inhibition by 5-fluoro-2′-deoxycytidine.

analog. DHAC reached Phase II clinical studies for ovarian cancer and lymphomas, without showing sufficient efficacy, although it is being evaluated for other
indications, such as pleural malignant mesothelioma.[59] Zebularine was originally
developed as a potent cytidine deaminase inhibitor because it lacks an amino
group at position 4 of the pyrimidine ring, and its demethylating activity was not
recognized until 2003.[60] After incorporation into DNA as nucleotide **10.20**, it
forms a stable covalent adduct **10.21** with DNMT (Fig. 10.15), as proved by
X-ray diffraction studies. The formation of **10.21** is not followed by methylation,
for reasons that are not completely clear, but this behavior correlates well with the
low electron density of the C-5 position in **10.21**, according to molecular orbital
calculations.[61]

Zebularine has the remarkable property of showing preference for tumor
cells, since it exhibits greater cell growth inhibition and gene expression in
cancer cell lines compared to normal fibroblasts. It also preferentially depletes
DNMT1 and induces expression of cancer-related antigen genes in cancer cells
relative to normal fibroblasts.[62] Its main drawbacks are its low bioavailability
and the need for high doses, which can be explained by its activity as an
inhibitor of cytidine deaminase. This inhibition is due to analogy between the

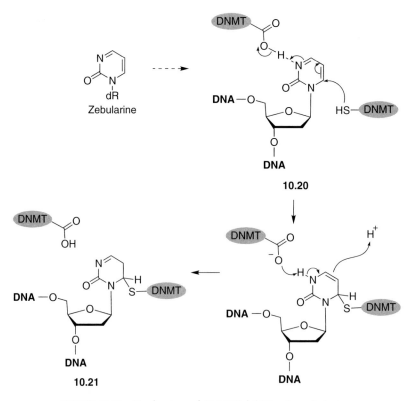

FIGURE 10.15   Mechanism of DNMT inhibition by zebularine.

transition state of the reaction (**10.22**) and zebularine hydrate **10.23**,[63] which is a dehydro analog of the previously mentioned inhibitor tetrahydrouridine (Fig. 10.16). Because of this mechanism for the inhibition of cytidine deaminase, part of the dose of zebularine is sequestered by the enzyme and is not available for DNMT. Additionally, inhibition of cytidine deaminase results in increased levels of deoxycytidine, which competes with zebularine for incorporation into DNA, a necessary step for DNMT inhibition. In spite of the promising preclinical results of zebularine, this drug has not entered clinical trials, and special emphasis is being placed in finding prodrugs that circumvent its bioavailability and metabolic limitations.

3.1.2. Nonnucleoside inhibitors of DNMT

This family of inhibitors has the advantage of binding directly to the catalytic region of the enzyme, without needing to be first incorporated into DNA. Two nonnucleoside natural DNMT inhibitors have undergone preclinical studies, although they have shown lower activity than their nucleoside counterparts. One of them is psammaplin A, isolated from various verongid sponges, which is a dual inhibitor of DNMT and HDAC, the two main epigenetic modifiers of tumor suppressor gene activity. Psammaplin A has also been reported to inhibit topoisomerase II and aminopeptidase N with *in vitro* angiogenesis suppression. However, its physiologic instability has precluded their direct clinical development.[64] Another natural DNMT inhibitor under preclinical study is the polyphenol (−)-epigallocatechin-3-gallate (EGCG), isolated from green tea.[65]

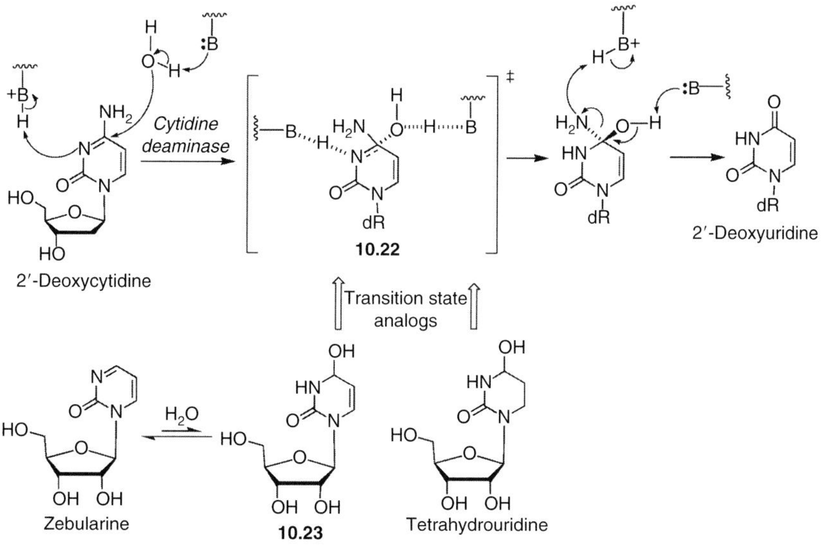

FIGURE 10.16 Inhibition of cytidine deaminase by zebularine hydrate due to its analogy with the transition state.

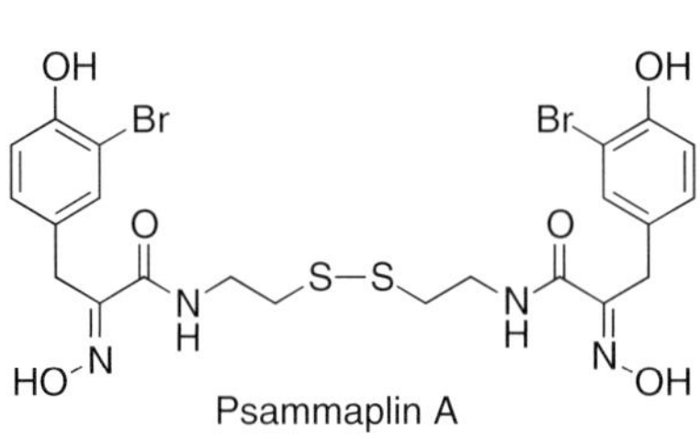

Psammaplin A

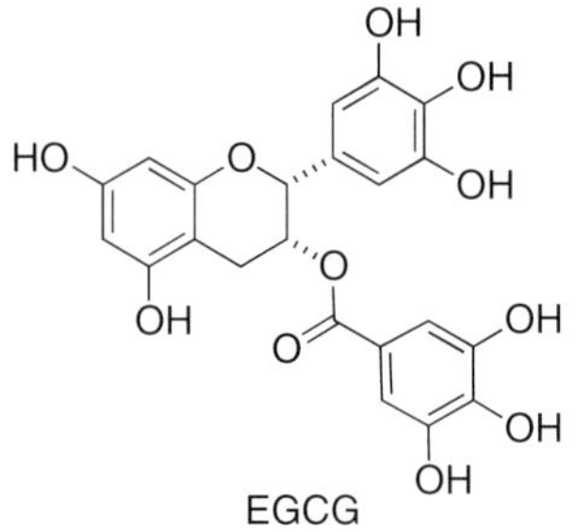

EGCG

Some unnatural DNMT inhibitors under preclinical study are the tryptophan derivative RG-108[66] and the drugs hydralazine and procainamide. MG-98 is an antisense oligonucleotide of human DNMT1, which prevents the translation of the DNMT1 gene into the corresponding mRNA and has reached Phase II clinical studies.[67]

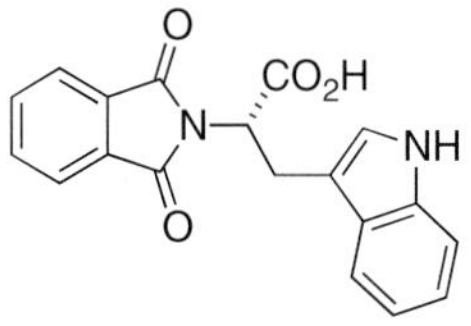

RG-108

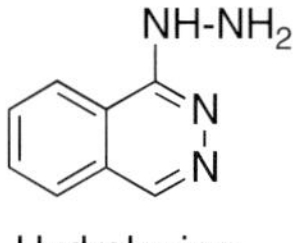

Hydralazine

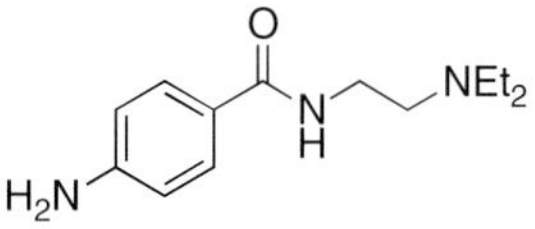

Procainamide

Although X-ray crystallographic structures for human DNMT are not available, the extensive conservation of the catalytic domains of all DNMTs has allowed the use of X-ray structures of bacterial methylases as a basis for ligand design. The model thus derived was validated through the design and evaluation of a new nucleoside analog, namely, N^4-fluoroacetyl-5-azacytidine,[68] and also of nonnucleoside compounds, like RG-108.[66] The binding of the previously mentioned natural inhibitor EGCG to this model[65] is shown in Fig. 10.17.

3.2. Inhibitors of histone deacetylases (HDAC)

Chromatin is the complex of DNA and protein that makes up the chromosome. The human genome corresponds to three billion base pairs of the DNA double helix, two copies of which make up to 2 m of DNA chains that have to be stored within the tiny micron-sized nucleus of each cell. The smallest structural units in chromatin are nucleosomes (10-nm fibers), which are formed by about 200 DNA base pairs wrapped around a core of eight DNA-associated proteins called histones. The N-terminal tails of these proteins protrude out of the nucleosome and are subject to epigenetic transformations that play a regulatory role in gene expression. This control takes place by structural modification of the basic ε-amino groups of lysine units, which are protonated under physiological conditions and interact electrostatically with the negatively charged phosphate

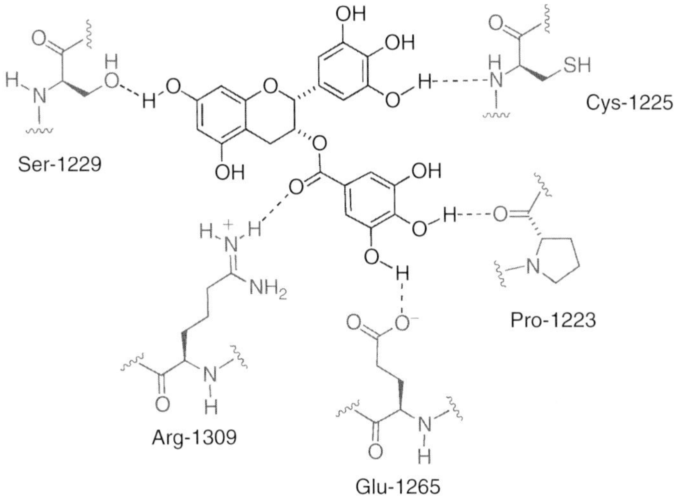

FIGURE 10.17 Interactions between DNMT and its natural inhibitor EGCG.

backbone of DNA. The main posttranscriptional histone transformation is the acetylation of lysine amino groups in these histone tails, which eliminates the positive charge from the lysine ε-amino groups and therefore weakens the above-mentioned electrostatic interactions of histones with DNA. For this reason, acetylation destabilizes the nucleosomes and facilitates the approach and binding of transcription factors to specific sequences in DNA.

The level of histone acetylation is regulated by histone acetyltransferases (HATs) and histone deacetylases (HDACs) that, respectively, add and remove the acetyl groups from lysine. As previously mentioned, loss of lysine acetylation has been identified as the first step in gene silencing, and for this reason there is growing interest in the development of HDAC inhibitors as anticancer agents.[69–73] Almost all known HDAC inhibitors induce the expression of the p21[WAF1/CIP1] gene, which leads to inhibition of the formation of the cyclin D-CDK4 complex, resulting in cell cycle arrest and cell differentiation. On the contrary, HDAC inhibitors also lead to apoptotic and antiangiogenic effects (Fig. 10.18).

The HDAC family of proteins can be divided into zinc-dependent (Class I and II) and zinc-independent, NAD-dependent (Class III) enzymes, with the latter having being only recently implicated in proliferation control. The proposed mechanism for the hydrolysis of the N-acetyllysine residues in a zinc-dependent HDAC belonging to Class I (HDAC1) is based on crystallographic studies of a bacterial deacetylase and is summarized in Fig. 10.19.[74] It involves polarization of the carbonyl oxygen of the acetyl group and activation of a molecule of water by a charge-relay system formed by aspartic and histidine residues (**10.24**), in a process analogous to the one taking place in the activation of the serine hydroxyl in serine proteases or water by glutamic acid in zinc

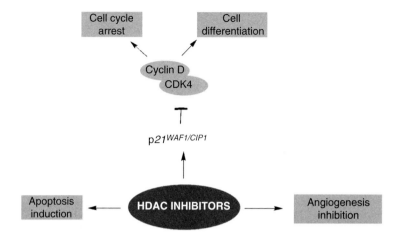

FIGURE 10.18   Biological effects of HDAC inhibitors.

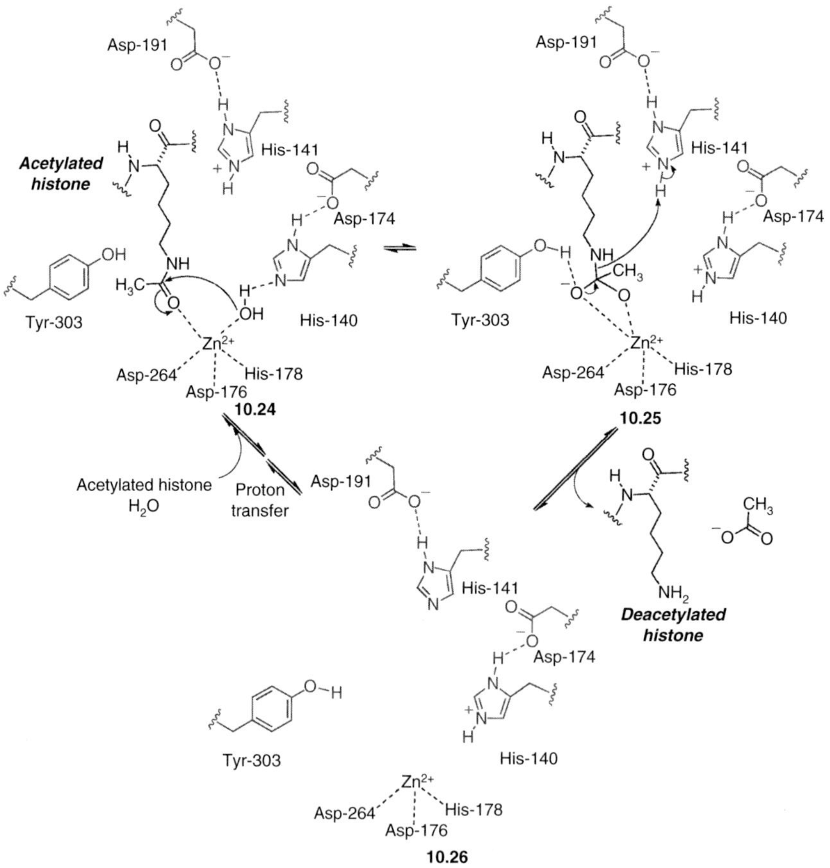

FIGURE 10.19   Proposed mechanism for the reaction catalyzed by Zn^{2+}-dependant HDAC.

proteases. Nucleophilic attack of water onto the carbonyl leads to the formation of a tetrahedral intermediate, stabilized by two zinc–oxygen interactions, similar to zinc proteases, and possibly by a hydrogen bond with the Tyr-303 hydroxyl (**10.25**). In the final step, the tetrahedral intermediate evolves by cleavage of the C–N bond with concomitant protonation from another histidine-aspartic charge-relay system (**10.26**).

HDAC inhibitors can be classified into four main categories, namely, short-chain fatty acids, hydroxamic acids, cyclic tetrapeptides, and benzamides.

3.2.1. Short-chain fatty acids

They normally have low potencies, but have become a useful tool in the study of HDAC inhibitors. Butyric and valproic acids were the first known HDAC inhibitors. Tributyrin is a prodrug of butyric acid with favorable pharmacokinetic and efficacy profiles, which has entered clinical studies for solid tumors.[75] Valproic acid, an anticonvulsant drug, is a dual inhibitor of HDAC1 and HDAC2 and is used for the treatment of acute myelogenous leukemia in elderly patients, in combination with all-*trans* retinoic acid.[76]

Butyric acid

Tributyrin

Valproic acid

3.2.2. Hydroxamic acids

The hydroxamic acid function is a potent zinc chelator, as previously mentioned in the context of matrix metalloproteinase inhibitors (Section 2.1), and some potent inhibitors of HDAC belong to this class of compounds. Trichostatin A (TSA), a natural product isolated from *Streptomyces hygroscopicus*, was first shown to be a potent inducer of cell differentiation and cell cycle arrest, and later reported to have anti-HDAC activity. It is still in preclinical studies.[77] Vorinostat (suberoyla-nilide hydroxamic acid, SAHA) was the first member of this class to enter human clinical trials[78] and has been approved by the FDA for cutaneous T-cell lymphoma (CTCL) for patients who have progressive, persistent, or recurrent disease or following failure of two systemic therapies, making the oral drug the first HDAC inhibitor to reach the market. Pyroxamide, a bioisoster of vorinostat, is also under clinical assays in patients with advanced malignancies.[79] Several hydroxamic derivatives of cinnamic acid, such as PDX-101, LBH-589,[80] and NVP-LAQ-824, are also under clinical evaluation for hematological and solid tumors.

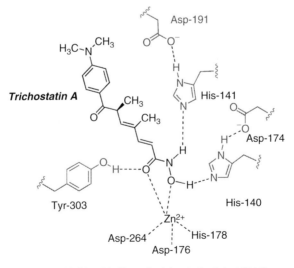

The binding of hydroxamic acid derivatives to the active site of HDACs has been studied mainly for the cases of TSA and SAHA, using a bacterial enzyme. The hydroxamic group coordinates the zinc cation in the active site, using both the hydroxamate and carbonyl oxygens. The hydroxamic acid also establishes hydrogen bonds with both histidines belonging to the charge-relay systems, and also with the Tyr-303 hydroxyl group (Fig. 10.20, where the amino acid residues shown correspond to the human HDAC1 enzyme). The hydroxamic acid hydroxyl group replaces the zinc-bound water molecule of the active structure. Additional van der Waals contacts (not shown) are established between hydrophobic amino acid residues and the lipophilic chain in the inhibitor.[74]

FIGURE 10.20   Binding of trichostatin A to HDAC.

3.2.3. Cyclic tetrapeptides

Some cyclic tetrapeptides are potent inhibitors of HDACs. The best known compound of this group is romidepsin (FK-228, FR901228), a depsipeptide that is currently under clinical studies for the treatment of chronic lymphocytic leukemia and acute myeloid leukemia[81] and T-cell lymphoma. It is a natural product, isolated from *Chromobacterium violaceum*, and it can be considered as a prodrug that is uptaken into the cells and then activated by glutathione. The reduced form (RedFK) has a four-carbon chain between the free sulfhydryl and the cyclic depsipeptide core, and forms a covalent disulfide bond with the only cysteine residue present in the HDAC pocket[82] (Fig. 10.21).

Trapoxins A and B, isolated from the fungus *Helicoma ambiens*, are hydrophobic cyclotetrapeptides that contain, respectively, pipecolinic acid and proline residues, and also two phenylalanines and an unusual amino acid bearing a side chain that contains an epoxide group. These compounds are potent enzyme inactivators that irreversibly inhibit the enzyme, probably by binding covalently through its epoxy group,[83] but are too toxic for clinical use. The α-epoxyketone moiety is not essential for activity, as can be deduced from the structure of apicidin, a fungal metabolite with antiprotozoal activity that also inhibits HDACs through induction of the p21$^{WAF1/CIP1}$ gene[84] and is under preclinical assay. CHAP-31 is a

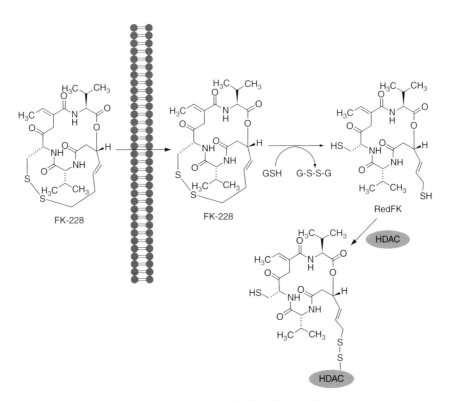

FIGURE 10.21 Inhibition of HDAC by romidepsin.

trapoxin A analog, also under preclinical assay, in which the epoxy group has been replaced with a hydroxamate function,[85] and hence it can be considered as a hydroxamic acid–tetrapeptide hybrid.

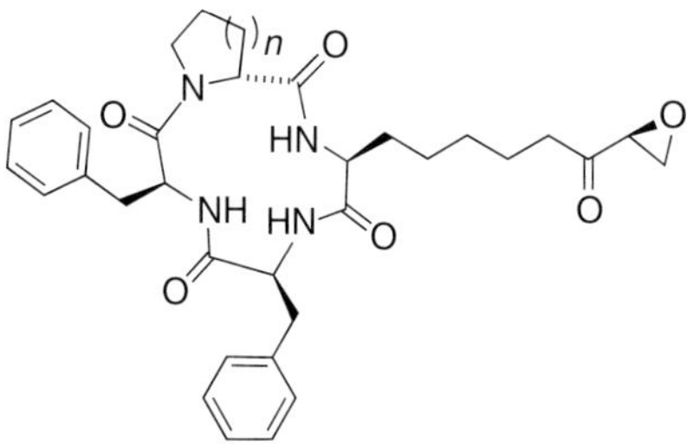

n = 2   Trapoxin A
n = 1   Trapoxin B

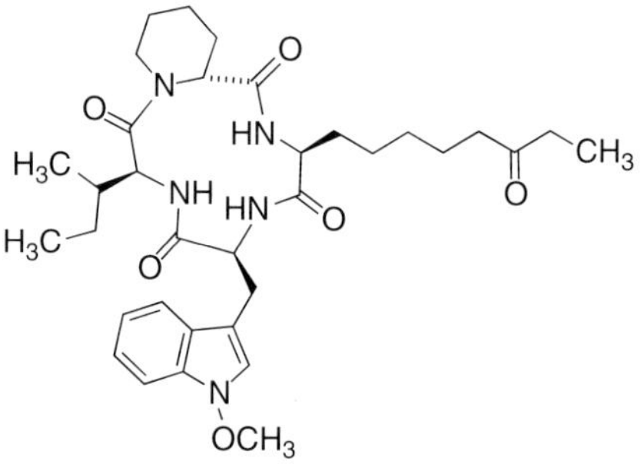

Apicidin

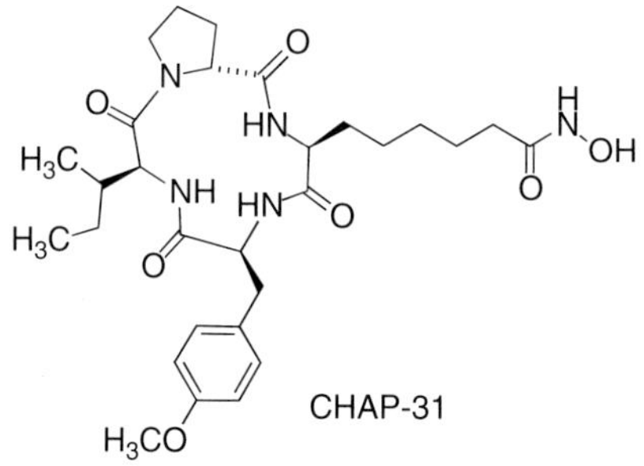

CHAP-31

3.2.4. Benzamides

The synthetic benzamides MS-275,[86] CI-994,[87] and MGCD-0103[88] are being clinically tested in a variety of tumors, alone or in combination with other drugs. The presence of an amino group *ortho* to the benzamide is essential for activity, and therefore it can be assumed to play a key role in the binding to the active site. In the case of MS-275, binding to zinc has been demonstrated.

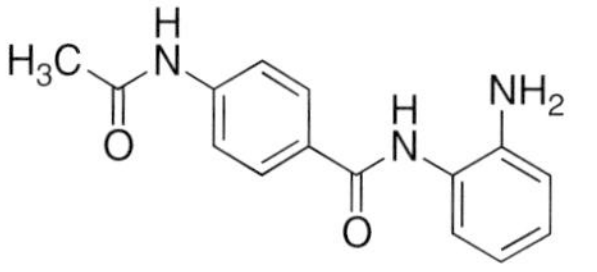

CI-994 (*p-N*-acetyldinaline)

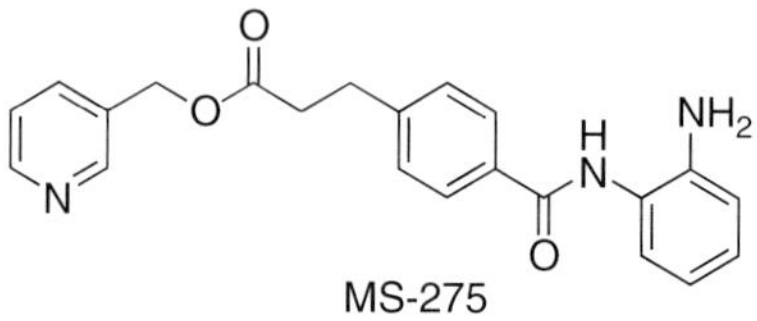

MS-275

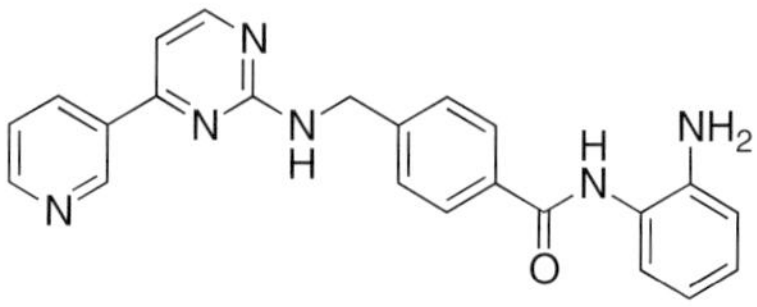

MGCD-0103

3.3. Regulators of histone methylation

Mithramycin A (aureolic acid, plicamycin) is a natural antibiotic that is currently used for the treatment of patients with Paget's disease of the bone as well as with several forms of cancer. It binds to GC-rich regions in DNA and prevents the binding of histone methyltransferase (HMT), an enzyme that adds methyl groups to histones, causing the DNA to coil up and be inaccessible for transcription. Mithramycin A is also a strong activator of the tumor suppressor p53 protein in human hepatoma cells.[89]

Mithramycin A (aureolic acid, plicamycin)

4. INHIBITORS OF OTHER DNA-ASSOCIATED ENZYMES

4.1. Telomerase inhibitors

Eukaryotic chromosomes are linear and have specialized ends called telomeres, which can be defined as regions of highly repetitive DNA at the end of a linear chromosome. The reason for the need for telomeres is that DNA polymerases extend DNA chains in the 5′-3′ direction and require an RNA primer. For this reason, the 3′-5′ chain, which is replicated in the 5′-3′ direction (lead strand), can be replicated to the end, but the complementary chain (lagging strand) has to be replicated discontinuously starting from an RNA primer that is attached to the 5′ end of each segment, resulting in a series of short fragments containing both RNA and DNA, called Okazaki fragments. The RNA fragments from the primer are subsequently degraded and replaced by DNA, leading to the fusion of the successive segments to form a single DNA strand. However, the RNA primer at the end of a complete lagging strand cannot be replaced because the required RNA primer would have no place to bind (Fig. 10.22). Therefore, when removed from the polymerase, the lagging strand of DNA would have an incomplete end, resulting in the loss of the final end and hence of genetic information.

Telomerase is a reverse transcriptase that contains an RNA molecule that generates repeating G-rich sequences (in humans, AGGGTT repeats with an average of 5–15 kb) and adds them to the 3′ end of DNA, allowing the replication of the lagging strand to be completed (Fig. 10.23). Human telomerase is composed of at least two subunits, namely, telomerase RNA (TR or TERC) and telomerase

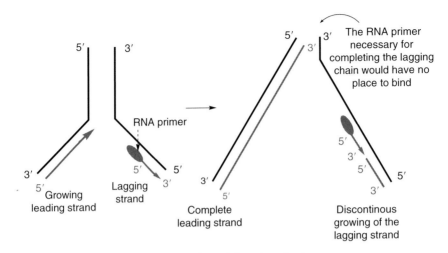

FIGURE 10.22   Biological function of telomerases.

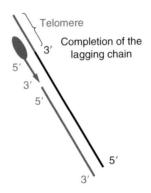

FIGURE 10.23   Addition of telomeres to the 3' end of DNA by telomerase.

reverse transcriptase (TERT), which is a reverse transcriptase with a "mitten" structure that allows it to wrap around the chromosome to add single-stranded telomere repeats. Telomerase inhibition has been considered as a potentially useful anticancer strategy[90–92] because telomerase is present primarily in dividing cells and it is expressed in very low levels, if at all, in most normal cells.

The main approaches that are being pursued for telomerase inhibition are the following:

— Interaction with the telomerase substrate, namely, the telomeric DNA template.
— Inhibition of the catalytic site of reverse transcriptase activity.
— Inhibition of the RNA domain template.

4.1.1. Compounds targeting the telomerase substrate: G-quadruplex ligands

The substrate of telomerase is the single-stranded end of the telomeres, which must be in an unfolded, linear structure in order to fit the telomerase active site. As previously mentioned, telomeric DNA contains G-rich sequences that tend to fold into structures known as G-quadruplex DNA, where guanines are associated

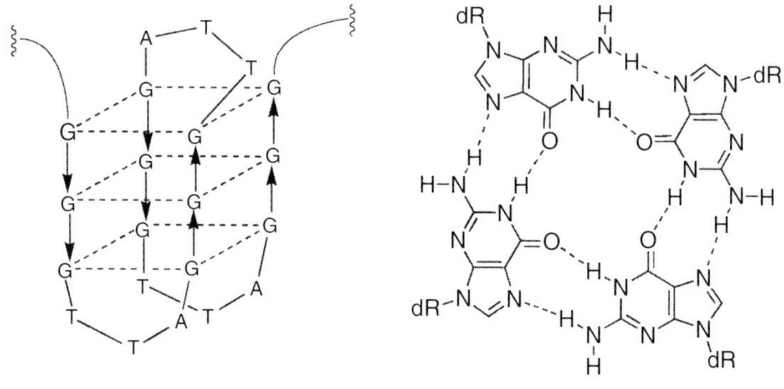

DNA G-quadruplex   Hydrogen bonding in G-quartet

FIGURE 10.24   DNA G-quadruplex in telomeric DNA.

forming three adjacent G-quartets, stabilized through intermolecular hydrogen bonding interactions (Fig. 10.24). G-quadruplex DNA cannot interact with telomerase, and therefore stabilization of the quadruplex structure can be considered as a strategy for telomerase inhibition. However, this approach can lead to undesired toxicity in comparison with the two others mentioned previously because telomerase-negative cells contain telomeres, which have the function of capping the chromosome ends.

Structurally, compounds that interact with the G-quartets are often very similar to intercalating agents, and in fact some of the G-quartet stabilizers, like ethidium bromide, are prototype DNA intercalators. Nevertheless, the quadruplex has structural differences with the DNA double helix, and this provides a basis for selective recognition.[93] Most quadruplex ligands are polyaromatic molecules bearing one or more substituents with positive charges, which seem to interact by stacking on a terminal G-quartet. Some examples are ethidium derivatives, dibenzophenanthrolines, and triazines such as 115405. One exception to this general structure is the natural product telomestatin, isolated from *Streptomyces anulatus*. Most of these compounds have low potencies as telomerase inhibitors.

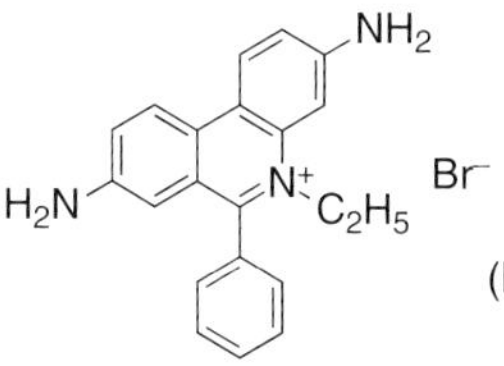

Ethidium bromide

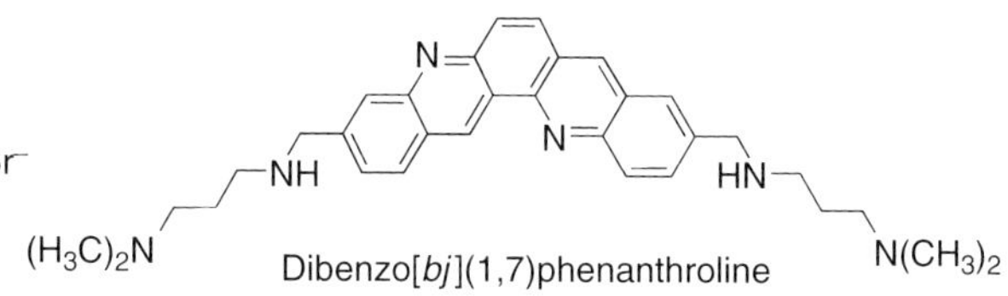

Dibenzo[*bj*](1,7)phenanthroline

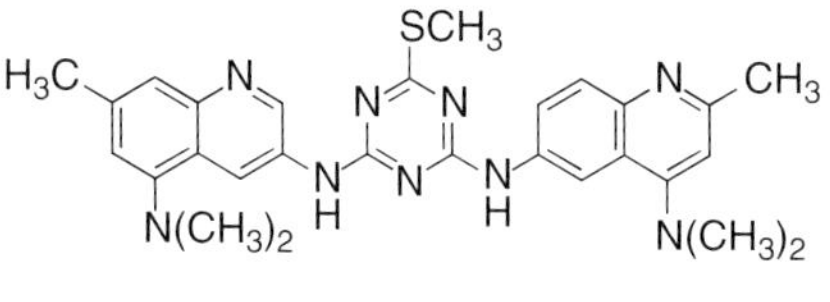

115405

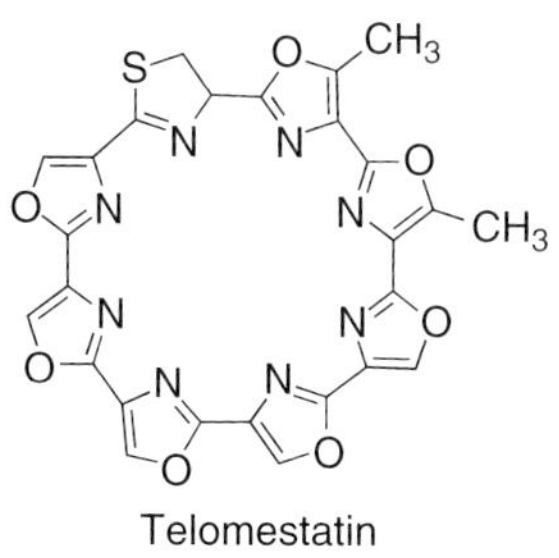

Telomestatin

4.1.2. Compounds targeting the catalytic subunit (hTERT)

Because hTERT acts as a reverse transcriptase, it is not surprising that some nucleo-sides that inhibit HIV-1 reverse transcriptase, like AZT, are also telomerase inhibi-tors, although with poor activity and selectivity. Among the nonnucleoside inhibitors, BIBR-15325 is a mixed-type noncompetitive inhibitor, targeting a bind-ing site distinct from the sites for deoxyribonucleotides and the DNA primer.[94]

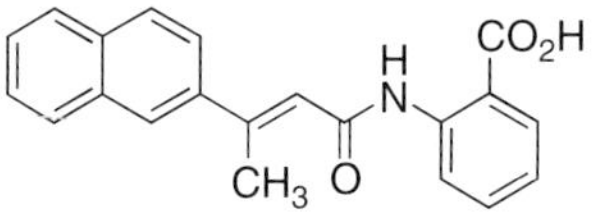

BIBR1532

4.1.3. Compounds targeting the RNA subunit (hTR)

The RNA component of telomerase has also been used as a target, especially using an antisense nucleotide approach. Since hTR is not an mRNA and will not be translated into a protein, an antisense oligomer will not have to compete with the ribosomal machinery and hence its toxicity will be low, provided that a good selectivity can be achieved.

Among the many antisense oligonucleotides targeted at hTR, the most advanced one is GRN-163L, which has entered Phase I clinical trials in patients with chronic lymphocytic leukemia and solid tumors. GRN-163L is a 13-mer oligonucleotide belonging to the N3′-P5′ thiophosphoramidate (NPS) family that is covalently attached to a lipophilic palmitoyl moiety (see Section 5.1 for a more detailed discussion of antisense oligonucleotides). This modification led to enhanced potency.[95]

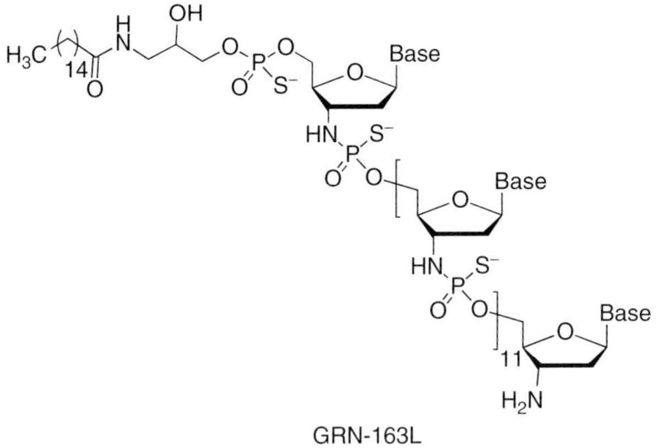

GRN-163L
Base sequence: 5′-Palm-TAGGGTTAGACAA-NH$_2$-3′

4.2. DNA repair system inhibitors

DNA is repeatedly exposed in normal cells to exogenous (e.g., UV light, ionizing radiation) and endogenous toxins (produced as a consequence of natural meta-bolic processes). It is estimated that the average rate of damage is about 10^4 events per cell per day. Therefore, DNA repair systems are vital to preserve the integrity of the genome, but their protective effect can be a disadvantage in cancer cells by reducing the cytotoxicity of antitumor agents, which is a cause of resistance.

Consequently, the different pathways of DNA repair have been studied as potential targets for improving cancer treatments. Some new antitumor drugs are emerging from the study of these targets, particularly those involved in the repair of single-strand damage.[96] Since these compounds are promising as radio- or chemosensitizers, they will be discussed in detail in Chapter 12.

One of these repair mechanisms is the nucleotide excision repair (NER) process, which repairs damage affecting strands of 2–30 bases and recognizes bulky, helix-distorting changes in the DNA such as the formation of thymine dimers, as well as single-strand breaks. The mechanism of action of the previously mentioned marine alkaloid ecteinascidin 743 (ET-743, trabectedin) involves alkylation of guanine-N2 positions in a sequence-specific manner, which leads to its tight binding into the minor groove of DNA (see Section 4 of Chapter 6). This induces a distortion of the helix that would normally trigger the NER process, but ET-743 traps the repair machinery as it attempts to remove the ET-743-DNA adducts and causes the endonuclease components to create lethal single-strand breaks in the DNA rather than repairing it.[97,98] In fact, ET-743 showed decreased activity in NER-deficient cell lines compared to NER-proficient cell lines.[99]

Ecteinascidin-743 (trabectedin)

5. THERAPY DIRECTED AT OTHER TARGETS

5.1. Antisense oligonucleotides

The basic idea of antisense oligonucleotide (ASO)-based therapy is to interrupt the flow of genetic information from a gene to a protein by using synthetic oligonucleotides targeted to specific mRNA sequences, the "sense" sequences, by recognition of Watson–Crick complementary bases. Because ribosomes cannot translate double-stranded RNA, the translation of a given mRNA can be inhibited by a segment of its complementary sequence, the so-called antisense RNA. This results in blocking the translation of the RNA message to generate a specific protein and in the degradation of the mRNA strand by ribonuclease H (Rnase H), as shown in Fig. 10.25. Since overexpression or mutation of specific genes (oncogenes) causes cancer, downregulation of their expression offers the possibility of a selective tumor ablation. To reach this goal, it is necessary for the oligonucleotides not only to have a high and selective affinity toward the target mRNA sequence but also to elude the action of nucleases in cells and body fluids, which rapidly degrade native oligonucleotides, to reach the target cells and to be retained into them.

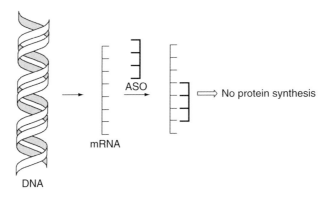

FIGURE 10.25 Mechanism of action of antisense oligonucleotides.

The first-generation antisense nucleotides in clinical use are characterized by having one of the phosphate nonbridging oxygens of the phosphodiester linkages replaced by sulfur (**10.27**). These phosphorothioate (PS) linkages lead to resistance to RNAase H, which slows the degradation of antisense oligonucleotide in the cells. Other common structures are phosphoroamidates (**10.28**) and phosphorothioami-dates (**10.29**). Some structural modifications that increase the affinity of antisense molecules for their specific targets are 2′-methoxylation (**10.30**) and 2′-(2-methoxy) ethoxylation (**10.31**). Peptide nucleic acids (**10.32**) are structures in which the antisense bases are connected to various peptide backbones, a structural feature that improves their half-lives and enhances their hybridization properties.

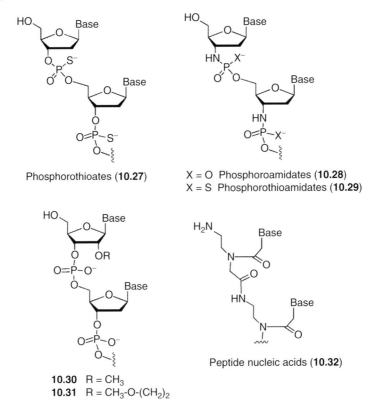

Phosphorothioates (**10.27**)

X = O Phosphoroamidates (**10.28**)
X = S Phosphorothioamidates (**10.29**)

10.30 R = CH₃
10.31 R = CH₃-O-(CH₂)₂

Peptide nucleic acids (**10.32**)

TABLE 10.1   Antisense oligonucleotides in clinical trials as anticancer agents.

Target	Antisense oligonucleotide	Sections
PKC	ISIS-3521 (CGP-64128)	4.4
PKC	ISIS-5132	4.4
Ras	ISIS-2503	5.1
Raf	ISIS-5132	5.3.1
BCL-2	Oblimersen	7.1
RNA subunit of telomerase	GRN-163L	4.1.3

Several antisense oligonucleotides are in clinical trials as anticancer agents[100] and have been previously mentioned in Chapters 9 and 10 (Table 10.1).

5.2. Monoclonal antibodies against cancer cells

Malignant cells present some surface antigens that are not found in normal cells and are therefore excellent targets for the binding of specific antibodies. The development of specific monoclonal antibodies (MoAB) targeted at these antigens is a field of anticancer therapy that is undergoing a very fast growth.[101] The applications of monoclonal antibodies to cancer therapy are summarized in Fig. 10.26. Mechanism (a) will be discussed below, while mechanism (c) was studied in the appropriate sections of Chapter 9 (see also Table 10.2), and mechanisms (b) and (d) will be studied in Chapter 11, together with other strategies of anticancer drug delivery based on the use of prodrugs.

One of the main targets for monoclonal antibodies are cell surface proteins, specially CD (Cluster of Differentiation) proteins, which serve as receptors for antigens, cytokines, or binding molecules on other cells. Several such monoclonal antibodies that have been approved for cancer therapy are discussed below. Most of these drugs normally have toxicities related to myelosuppression.

Rituximab is a chimeric human-murine monoclonal antibody that binds to CD-20, a cell surface protein found almost exclusively on mature B cells. It was the first monoclonal antibody approved for cancer therapy and is employed in refractory B-cell non-Hodgkin lymphoma and other hematological disorders, including, among others, other non-Hodgkin lymphomas, chronic lymphocytic leukemia, and multiple myeloma.

Alemtuzumab is a humanized monoclonal antibody that binds to CD-52, an antigen expressed on B and T lymphocytes. It is approved for patients with B-cell chronic lymphocytic leukemia when other therapy has failed.

Integrin antibodies are also known and are under clinical study. The most important are volociximab (M-200), an anti-$\alpha_5\beta_1$ integrin, which is under clinical evaluation in patients with refractory sloid tumors, specially renal cell carcinoma,[102] and vitaxin, an anti-$\alpha_v\beta_3$ integrin.[103]

Finally, some monoclonal antibodies employed in cancer therapy are directed to the extracellular portions of some receptors associated to signaling pathways, and have been discussed in Chapter 9 (Table 10.2).

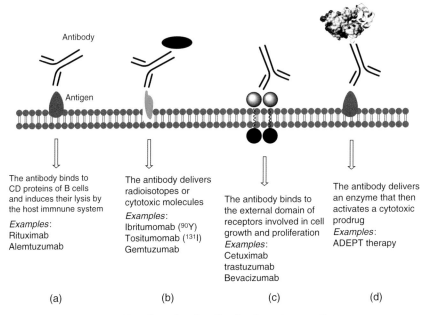

The antibody binds to CD proteins of B cells and induces their lysis by the host immnune system

Examples:
Rituximab
Alemtuzumab

The antibody delivers radioisotopes or cytotoxic molecules

Examples:
Ibritumomab (^{90}Y)
Tositumomab (^{131}I)
Gemtuzumab

The antibody binds to the external domain of receptors involved in cell growth and proliferation
Examples:
Cetuximab
trastuzumab
Bevacizumab

The antibody delivers an enzyme that then activates a cytotoxic prodrug
Examples:
ADEPT therapy

(a)   (b)   (c)   (d)

FIGURE 10.26   The role of antibodies in anticancer therapy.

TABLE 10.2   Anticancer monoclonal antibodies targeting signal receptors.

Target	Monoclonal antibody	Sections
EGFR	Cetuximab	9.3.1
HER-2	Trastuzumab	9.3.2
VEGFR	Bevacizumab	9.3.4.2

5.3. Gene therapy

Gene therapy can be defined as the insertion of a functional gene into the somatic cells of a patient to correct an inborn metabolic error, to repair an acquired genetic abnormality, or to provide a new function to a cell.

The main problem with gene therapy is the lack of efficient and selective vectors to deliver the genes. Viruses, which are the most commonly employed vectors, are not ideal because they trigger an immunological response. Nonviral vectors are safer but less efficient than viruses. The most promising are synthetic cationic liposomes, which have positive charges that interact electrostatically with negative charges in DNA phosphate groups and form complexes that are capable of entering the cells. Some of the positively charged amphiphilic molecules (cationic lipids) used to this purpose, like N-[1-(2,3-dioleyloxy)propyl]-N,N,N-trimethylammonium chloride (DOTMA), dioleoylphosphatidylethanolamine (DOPE) or 5-cholesten-3β-yl N-dimethylaminoethyl carbamate(DC-Chol), are shown below. Unfortunately, because of the low efficiency of DNA delivery by these systems, the amount of liposome currently required is too large to allow clinical use.

DOTMA

DOPE

DC-Chol

Several potential strategies for cancer therapy based on gene therapy are being explored in clinical trials, and are summarized below:[101,104,105]

1. *Replacement of deficient or absent tumor suppressor genes.* These genes are in charge of the control of cell replication, and their decrease or absence is characteristic of many malignancies. The main gene in cancer therapy is *p53*, which is in clinical trials. The gene is transferred using adenoviral vectors by intratumoral injection to patients with accessible cancers like head and neck carcinoma.

2. *Immunomodulatory gene therapy.* This approach is aimed at increasing the immune response of patients against cancer (*vaccine therapy*). This can be achieved by taking cells from the tumor, transducing them *in vitro* with the viral vector containing the cytokine genes, such as those responsible for interleukin 2, TNF, interferon-γ (IFN-γ), and granulocyte-macrophage colony stimulating factor (GM-CSF). The cells are then implanted again in the tumor, where they produce the immunoregulatory cytokine without the toxicity associated with systemic cytokine administration. A large number of Phase I clinical trials have been undertaken to test the efficacy of these cancer vaccines.

3. *Suicide gene therapy.* Viral vectors are used to selectively infect dividing tumor cells. These viruses have been modified to carry a gene for an enzyme that activates an antitumor prodrug, so that after its administration the prodrug is preferentially bioactivated in the tumor cells. One example of this strategy is the transduction of tumor cells with a vector containing the gene for the herpes simplex virus thymidine kinase. Unlike the human thymidine kinase, this viral enzyme is capable of phosphorylating a broad range of nucleosides, such as ganciclovir. This allows the modified tumor cells to activate ganciclovir to its triphosphate, which behaves as a chain terminator when incorporated into DNA because of the absence of the 3'-OH deoxyribose group, blocking the DNA synthesis and killing the cell (Fig. 10.27). This method is in clinical trials for the treatment of glioblastoma multiforme, a malignant brain tumor.

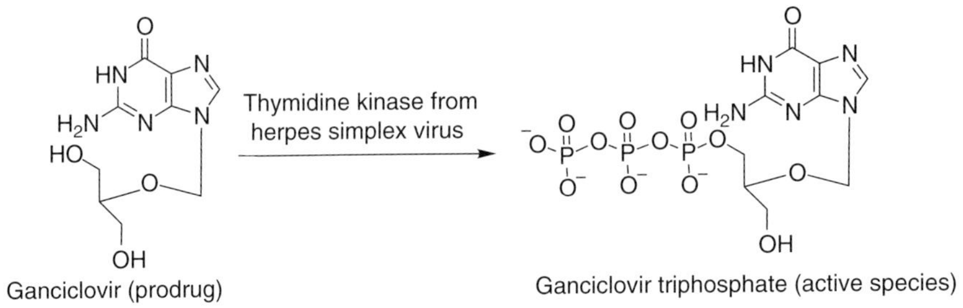

FIGURE 10.27   Bioactivation of ganciclovir.

4. *Chemoprotection*. Before a patient receives chemotherapy, bone marrow cells are withdrawn, transduced *in vitro* with genes responsible for drug resistance, and then given back to the patient. In principle, this should allow higher chemotherapy doses without lethal damage to bone marrow stem cells.

5.4. Antitumor agents targeted at lysosomes

Kahalalide F is a depsipeptide derived from the sea slug *Elysia rufescens*. This compound alters the function of the lysosomal membranes, a mechanism that distinguishes it from all other known antitumor agents. Other mechanisms of action are inhibition of the TGF-α expression, blockade of intracellular signaling pathways downstream of EGF and ErbB2 receptor family, and induction of non-p53-mediated apoptosis. Kahalalide F is currently in Phase II clinical trials in hepatocellular carcinoma, non-small cell lung cancer (NSCLC), and melanoma, and is also being evaluated for the treatment of severe psoriasis. In these studies, kahalalide F has shown limited activity but an excellent tolerability profile that merits further clinical evaluation in combination with other anticancer compounds.

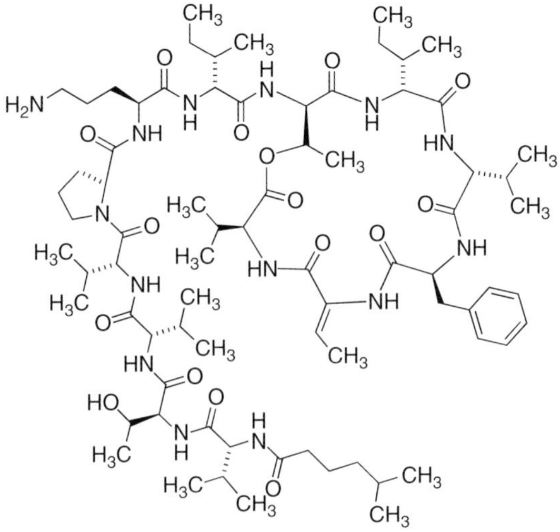

Kahalalide F

REFERENCES

1. Almond, J. B., and Cohen, G. M. (2002). *Leukemia* **26,** 433.
2. Neefjes, J., and Dantuma, M. P. (2004). *Nat. Rev. Drug Discov.* **3,** 58.
3. Adams, J. (2004). *Nat. Rev. Cancer* **4,** 349.
4. Myung, J., Kim, K. B., and Crews, C. M. (2001). *Med. Res. Rev.* **21,** 245.
5. García-Echeverría, C. (2002). *Mini-Rev. Med. Chem.* **2,** 247.
6. Boccadoro, M., Morgan, G., and Cavenagh, J. (2005). *Cancer Cell Int.* **5,** 18.
7. Paramore, A., and Frantz, S. (2003). *Nat. Rev. Drug Discov.* **2,** 611.
8. Palmer, J. T. (1995). *J. Med. Chem.* **38,** 3193.
9. Groll, M., Kim, K. B., Kairies, N., Huber, R., and Crews, C. M. (2000). *J. Am. Chem. Soc.* **122,** 1237.
10. Adams, J., Behnke, M., Chen, S., Cruickshank, A. A., Dick, L. R., Grenier, L., Klunder, J. M., Ma, Y. T., Plamondon, L., and Stein, R. L. (1998). *Bioorg. Med. Chem. Lett.* **8,** 333.
11. Gourley, M., and Williamdon, J. S. (2000). *Curr. Pharm. Des.* **6,** 417.
12. Dhanabal, M., Jeffers, M., and LaRochelle, W. J. (2005). *Curr. Med. Chem. Anticancer Agents* **5,** 115.
13. Rao, B. G. (2005). *Curr. Pharm. Des.* **11,** 295.
14. Borkakoti, N. (2004). *Biochem. Soc. Trans.* **32,** 17.
15. Cross, J. B., Duca, J. S., Kaminski, J. J., and Madison, V. S. (2002). *J. Am. Chem. Soc.* **124,** 1004.
16. Botos, I., Scapozza, L., Zhang, D., Liotta, L. A., and Meyer, E. F. (1996). *Proc. Nat. Acad. Sci. USA* **93,** 2749.
17. Coussens, L. M., Fingleton, B., and Matrisian, L. M. (2002). *Science* **295,** 2387.
18. Bissett, D., O'Byrne, K. J., von Pawel, J., Gatzemeier, U., Price, A., Nicolson, M., Mercier, R., Mazabel, E., Penning, C., Zhang, M. H., Collier, M. A., and Shepherd, F. A. (2005). *J. Clin. Oncol.* **23,** 842.
19. Gingras, D., Boivin, D., Deckers, C., Gendron, S., Barthomeuf, C., and Beliveau, R. (2003). *Anticancer Drugs* **14,** 91.
20. Okada, Y., Yamada, S., Toyoshima, M., Dong, J., Nakajima, M., and Sugahara, K. (2002). *J. Biol. Chem.* **277,** 12188.
21. Hulett, M. D., Hornby, J. R., Ohms, S. J., Zuegg, J., Freeman, C., Gready, J. E., and Parish, C. R. (2000). *Biochemistry* **39,** 15659.
22. Ferro, V., Hammond, E., and Fairweather, J. K. (2004). *Mini-Rev. Med. Chem.* **4,** 693.
23. Miao, H.-Q., Liu, H., Navarro, E., Kussie, P., and Zhu, Z. (2006). *Curr. Med. Chem.* **13,** 2101.
24. Basche, M., Gustafson, D. L., Holden, S. N., O'Bryant, C. L., Gore, L., Witta, S., Schultz, M. K., Morrow, M., Levin, A., Creese, B. R., Kangas, M., Roberts, K., *et al.* (2006). *Clin. Cancer Res.* **12,** 5471.
25. Marchetti, D., Reiland, J., Erwin, B., and Roy, M. (2003). *Int. J. Cancer* **104,** 167.
26. Bols, M., Lillelund, V. H., Jensen, H. H., and Liang, X. (2002). *Chem. Rev.* **102,** 515.
27. Kulke, M. H., Bergsland, E. K., Ryan, D. P., Enzinger, P. C., Lynch, T. J., Zhu, A. X., Meyerhardt, J. A., Heymach, J. V., Fogler, W. E., Sidor, C., Michelini, A., Kinsella, K., Venook, A. P., and Fuchs, C. S. (2006). *J. Clin. Oncol.* **24,** 3555.
28. http://www.clinicaltrials.gov/ct/gui/show/NCT00049790; jsessionid=91EE48B7C2F7D935B96F 12E31D5609E3?order=1
29. Haviv, F., Bradley, M. F., Kalvin, D. M., Schneider, A. J., Davidson, D. J., Majest, S. M., McKay, L. M., Haskell, C. J., Bell, R. L., Nguyen, B., Marsh, K. C., Surber, B. W., *et al.* (2005). *J. Med. Chem.* **48,** 2838.
30. De Vos, F. Y., Hoekstra, R., Eskens, F. A. L. M., De Vries, E. G., VanderGaast, A., Groen, H. J. M., Knight, R., Humerickhouse, R. A., Gietema, J. A., and Verweij, J. (2004). *J. Clin. Oncol.* **22**(14S), 3077.
31. Folkman, J. (2006). *Exp. Cell Res.* **312,** 594.
32. Featherstone, J., and Griffiths, S. (2002). *Nat. Rev. Drug Discov.* **1,** 413.
33. Serini, G., Valdembri, B., and Bussolino, F. (2006). *Exp. Cell Res.* **312,** 651.
34. Kumar, C. C., Malkowski, M., Yin, Z., Tanghetti, E., Yaremko, B., Nechuta, T., Varner, J., Liu, M., Smith, E. M., Neustadt, B., Presta, M., and Armstrong, L. (2001). *Cancer Res.* **61,** 2232.
35. Gutheil, J. C., Campbell, T. N., Pierce, P. R., Watkins, J. D., Huse, W. D., Bodkin, D. J., and Cheresh, D. A. (2000). *Clin. Cancer Res.* **6,** 3056.
36. Akhter, S., Nath, S. K., Tse, C. M., Williams, J., Zasloff, M., and Donowitz, M. (1999). *Am. J. Physiol. Cell Physiol.* **45,** C136.

37. Pietras, R. J., and Weinberg, O. K. (2005). *Evid. Based Complement. Alternat. Med.* **2**, 49.
38. Bauer, K. S., Dixon, S. C., and Figg, W. D. (1998). *Biochem. Pharmacol.* **55**, 1827.
39. Kumar, S., Witzig, T. E., Dispenzieri, A., Lacy, M. Q., Wellik, L. E., Fonseca, R., Lust, J. A., Gertz, M. A., Kyle, R. A., Greipp, P. R., and Rajkumar, S. V. (2004). *Leukemia* **18**, 624.
40. García-Sanz, R., González-Porras, J. R., Hernández, J. M., Polo-Zarzuela, M., Sureda, A., Barrenetxea, C., Palomera, L., López, R., Grande-García, C., Alegre, A., Vargas-Pabón, M., Gutiérrez, O. N., *et al.* (2004). *Leukemia* **18**, 856.
41. Saunders, G. (2005). *J. Oncol. Pharm. Pract.* **11**, 83.
42. Richardson, P., and Anderson, K. (2004). *J. Clin. Oncol.* **22**, 3212.
43. Dredge, K., Dalgleish, A. G., and Marriott, J. B. (2003). *Anticancer Drugs* **14**, 331.
44. Maier, S. K., and Hammond, J. M. (2006). *Ann. Pharmacother.* **40**, 286.
45. Schey, S. A., Fields, P., Bartlett, J. B., Clarke, I. A., Ashan, G., Knight, R. D., Streetly, M., and Dalgleish, A. G. (2004). *J. Clin. Oncol.* **22**, 3269.
46. Teo, S. K., Chen, Y., Muller, G. W., Chen, R. S., Thomas, S. D., Stirling, D. I., and Chandula, R. S. (2003). *Chirality* **15**, 348.
47. Liekens, S., De Clerq, E., and Neyts, J. (2001). *Biochem. Pharmacol.* **61**, 253.
48. Liu, S., Widom, J., Kemp, C. W., Crews, C. M., and Clardy, J. (1998). *Science* **282**, 1324.
49. Wernert, N., Stamjek, A., Kiriakidis, S., Hügel, A., Jha, H. C., Mazitschek, R., and Giannis, A. (1999). *Angew. Chem. Int. Ed.* **38**, 3228.
50. Connell, R. D., and Beebe, J. S. (2001). *Expert Opin. Ther. Patents* **11**, 77.
51. Yoo, C. B., and Jones, P. A. (2006). *Nat. Rev. Drug Discov.* **5**, 37.
52. Yoo, C. B., Cheng, J. C., and Jones, P. A. (2004). *Biochem. Soc. Trans.* **32**, 910.
53. Issa, J.-P., and Kantarjian, H. (2005). *Nat. Rev. Drug Discov.* **4**, S6.
54. Kaminskas, E., Farrell, A. T., Abraham, S., Baird, A., Hsieh, L.-S., Lee, S.-L., Leighton, J. K., Patel, H., Rahman, A., Sridhara, R., Wang, Y.-C., and Pazdur, R. (2005). *Clin. Cancer Res.* **11**, 3604.
55. Kaminskas, E., Farrell, A. T., Wang, Y.-C., Sridhara, R., and Padzur, R. (2005). *Oncologist* **10**, 176.
56. Kuykendall, J. R. (2005). *Ann. Pharmacother.* **39**, 1700.
57. Issa, J.-P. J., Gharibyan, V., Cortes, J., Jelinek, J., Morris, G., Verstovsek, S., Talpaz, M., García-Manero, G., and Kantarjian, H. M. (2005). *J. Clin. Oncol.* **23**, 3948.
58. http://clinicalstudies.info.nih.gov/detail/A_2006-C-0221.html
59. Dhingra, H. M., Murphy, W. K., Winn, R. J., Raber, N. M., and Hong, W. K. (2004). *Invest. New Drugs* **9**, 69.
60. Cheng, J. C., Matsen, C. B., Gonzales, F. A., Ye, W., Greer, S., Marquez, V. E., Jones, P. A., and Selker, E. A. (2003). *J. Natl. Cancer Inst.* **95**, 399.
61. Zhou, L., Cheng, X., Connolly, B. A., Dickman, M. J., Hurd, P. J., and Hornby, D. P. (2002). *J. Mol. Biol.* **321**, 591.
62. Cheng, J. C., Yoo, C. B., Weisenberger, D. J., Chuang, J., Wozniak, C., Liang, G., Márquez, V. E., Greer, S., Orntoft, T. F., Thykjaer, T., and Jones, P. A. (2004). *Cancer Cell* **6**, 151.
63. Jeong, L. S., Buenger, G., McCormack, J. J., Cooney, D. A., Hao, Z., and Márquez, V. E. (1998). *J. Med. Chem.* **41**, 2572.
64. Simmons, T. L., Andrianasolo, E., McPhail, K., Flatt, P., and Gerwick, W. H. (2005). *Mol. Cancer Ther.* **4**, 333.
65. Fang, M. Z., Wang, Y., Ai, N., Hou, Z., Sun, Y., Lu, H., Welsh, W., and Yang, C. S. (2003). *Cancer Res.* **63**, 7563.
66. Brueckner, B., García Boy, R., Siedlecki, P., Musch, T., Kliem, H. C., Zielenkiewicz, P., Suhai, S., Wiessler, M., and Lyko, F. (2005). *Cancer Res.* **65**, 6305.
67. http://clinicaltrials.gov/ct/show/NCT00324220
68. Siedlecki, P., García Boy, R., Comagic, S., Schirrmacher, R., Wiessler, M., Zielenkiewicz, P., Suhai, S., and Lykoc, F. (2003). *Biochem. Biophys. Res. Commun.* **306**, 558.
69. Marks, P. A., Rifkind, R. A., Richon, V. M., Breslow, R., Miller, T., and Kelly, W. K. (2001). *Nat. Rev. Cancer* **1**, 194.
70. Johnstone, R. W. (2002). *Nat. Rev. Drug Discov.* **1**, 287.
71. Monneret, C. (2005). *Eur. J. Med. Chem.* **40**, 1.
72. Moradei, O., Maroun, C. R., Paquin, I., and Vaisburg, A. (2005). *Curr. Med. Chem. Anticancer Agents* **5**, 529–560.

73. Carey, N., and La Thangue, N. B. (2006). *Curr. Opin. Pharmacol.* **6**, 369.

74. Flinnin, M. S., Donigian, J. R., Cohen, A., Richon, V. M., Rifkind, R. A., Marks, P. A., Breslow, R., and Pavletich, N. P. (1999). *Nature* **401**, 188.

75. Khanwani, S. L., Edelman, M. J., and Tait, N. (2001). *Proc. Am. Soc. Clin. Oncol.* **20**, 86a.

76. Raffoux, E., Chaibi, P., Dombret, H., and Degos, L. (2005). *Haematologica* **90**, 986.

77. Vigushin, D. M., Ali, S., Pace, P. E., Mirsaidi, N., Ito, K., Adcock, I., and Coombes, R. C. (2001). *Clin. Cancer Res.* **7**, 971.

78. Duvic, M., Talpur, R., Ni, X., Zhang, C., Hazarika, P., Kelly, C., Chiao, J. H., Reilly, J. F., Ricker, J. L., Richon, V. N., and Frankel, S. (2007). *Blood* **109**, 31.

79. http://www.clinicaltrials.gov/ct/show/NCT00042900; jsessionid=47CCC05C87B745FACD2295 C56507E1A6?order=48

80. Giles, F., Fischer, T., Cortes, J., García-Manero, G., Beck, J., Ravandi, F., Masson, E., Rae, P., Laird, G., Sharma, S., Kantarjian, H., Dugan, M., Albitar, M., and Bhalla, K. (2006). *Clin. Cancer Res.* **12**, 4628.

81. Byrd, J. C., Marcucci, G., Parthun, M. R., Xiao, J. J., Klisovic, R. B., Moran, M., Lin, T. S., Liu, S., Sklenar, A. R., Davis, M. E., Lucas, M. E., Fischer, B., *et al.* (2005). *Blood* **105**, 959.

82. Furamai, R., Matsuyama, A., Kobashi, N., Lee, K.-H., Nishiyama, M., Nakajima, H., Tanaka, A., Komatsu, Y., Nishino, N., Yoshida, M., and Horinouchi, S. (2002). *Cancer Res.* **62**, 4916.

83. Furamai, R., Komatsu, Y., Nishino, N., Khochbin, S., Yoshida, M., and Horinouchi, S. (2001). *Proc. Natl. Acad. Sci. USA* **98**, 87.

84. Kwon, S. H., Ahn, S. H., Kim, Y. K., Bae, G.-U., Yoon, J. W., Hong, S., Lee, H. Y., Lee, Y.-W., Lee, H.-W., and Han, J. W. (2002). *J. Biol. Chem.* **277**, 2073.

85. Komatsu, Y., Tomizaki, K.-Y., Tsukamoto, M., Kato, T., Nishino, N., Sato, S., Yamori, T., Tsuruo, T., Furumai, R., Yoshida, M., Horinouchi, S., and Hayashi, H. (2001). *Cancer Res.* **61**, 4459.

86. http://www.clinicaltrials.gov/ct/show/NCT00101179

87. Undevia, S. D., Kindler, H. L., Janisch, L., Olson, S. C., Schilsky, R. L., Vogelzang, N. J., Kimmel, K. A., Macek, T. A., and Ratain, M. J. (2004). *Ann. Oncol.* **15**, 1705.

88. http://www.clinicaltrials.gov/ct/show/NCT00374296; jsessionid=92563A45C8B57CDD90D1719 43745C815?order=8

89. Koutsodontis, G., and Kardassis, D. (2004). *Oncogene* **23**, 9190.

90. Neidle, S., and Parkinson, G. (2002). *Nat. Rev. Drug Discov.* **1**, 383.

91. Mergny, J.-L., Riou, J.-F., Mailliet, P., Teulade-Fichou, M.-P., and Gilson, E. (2002). *Nucl. Acid Res.* **30**, 839.

92. Cunningham, A. P., Love, W. K., Zhang, R. W., Andrews, L. G., and Tollefsbol, T. O. (2006). *Curr. Med. Chem.* **13**, 2875.

93. Kerwin, S. M. (2000). *Curr. Pharm. Des.* **6**, 441.

94. Ascolo, E., Wenz, C., Lingner, J., Hauel, N., Priepke, H., Kaufmann, I., Garinchesa, P., Rettig, W. J., Damm, K., and Schnapp, A. (2002). *J. Biol. Chem.* **277**, 15566.

95. Herbert, B. S., Gellert, G. C., Hochreiter, A., Pongracz, K., Wright, W. E., Zielinska, D., Chin, A. C., Harley, C. B., Shay, J. W., and Gryaznov, S. M. (2005). *Oncogene* **24**, 5262.

96. Berthet, N., Boturyn, D., and Constant, J.-F. (1999). *Expert Opin. Ther. Patents* **9**, 401.

97. Takebayashi, K., Pourquier, P., Zimonjic, D. B., Nakayama, K., Emmert, S., Ueda, T., Urasaki, Y., Kanzaki, A., Akiyama, S., Popescu, N., Kraemer, K. H., and Pommier, Y. (2001). *Nat. Med.* **7**, 961.

98. Zewail-Foote, M., Ven-Shun, L., Kohn, H., Bearss, D., Guzmán, M., and Hurley, L. H. (2001). *Chem. Biol.* **135**, 1.

99. Damia, G., Silvestri, S., Carrassa, L., Filiberti, L., Faircloth, G. T., Liberi, G., Foiani, M., and D'incalci, M. (2001). *Int. J. Cancer* **92**, 583.

100. Khuri, F. R., and Kurie, J. M. (2000). *Clin. Cancer Res.* **6**, 1607.

101. Segota, E., and Bukowski, R. M. (2004). *Cleve. Clin. J. Med.* **71**, 551.

102. http://clinicaltrials-nccs.nlm.nih.gov/ct/show/NCT00401570; jsessionid=A8186BC084BE2C690 ACBDDE0B44F8330?order=25

103. Posey, J. A., Khazaeli, M. B., DelGrosso, A., Saleh, M. N., Lin, C. Y., Huse, W., and LoBuglio, A. F. (2001). *Cancer Biother. Radiopharm.* **16**, 125.

104. Buchsbaum, D. J., and Curiel, D. T. (2001). *Cancer Biother. Radiopharmacol.* **16**, 275.

105. Bladon, C. M. (2002). *In* ''Pharmaceutical Chemistry: Therapeutic Aspects of Biomacromolecules,'' chapter 5, Wiley, Chichester.

CHAPTER 11

Drug Targeting in Anticancer Chemotherapy

Contents		
	1. Introduction	351
	2. Prodrug-Based Anticancer Drug Targeting: Small-Molecule Prodrugs	352
	2.1. Selective enzyme expression in tumor cells	352
	2.2. Hypoxia-based strategies for tumor-specific prodrug activation	354
	2.3. Gene-directed enzyme prodrug therapy (GDEPT) and virus-directed enzyme prodrug therapy (VDEPT)	363
	2.4. Antibody-directed enzyme prodrug therapy (ADEPT)	364
	3. Polymer-Protein Conjugates	368
	4. Macromolecular Small-Drug Carrier Systems	369
	4.1. N-(2-Hydroxypropyl)methacrylamide polymers	370
	4.2. Poly-(L-glutamic)conjugates	373
	4.3. Neuropeptide Y conjugates	374
	4.4. PEGylated conjugates	375
	4.5. Immunoconjugated drugs	375
	5. Polymer-Directed Enzyme Prodrug Therapy (PDEPT)	377
	6. Folate Receptor-Targeted Chemotherapy and Immunotherapy of Cancer	378
	7. Liposomes and Nanoparticles in Anticancer Drug Targeting	380
	7.1. Liposomes	380
	7.2. Nanoparticle albumin bound technology	383
	References	383

1. INTRODUCTION

Anticancer drugs studied in previous chapters normally have high toxicities, and one of the main purposes of current research in this field is lowering these toxic effects. For this reason, current research efforts to improve the effectiveness of

Medicinal Chemistry of Anticancer Drugs
DOI: 10.1016/B978-0-444-52824-7.00011-1

cancer chemotherapy are focused on the possibility to selectively target and kill the cancer cells while affecting as few healthy cells as possible. This chapter is devoted to the techniques used to achieve this end.

2. PRODRUG-BASED ANTICANCER DRUG TARGETING: SMALL-MOLECULE PRODRUGS

One approach that allows improving the selectivity of cytotoxic compounds in cancer therapy is the use of prodrugs that are selectively activated in tumor tissues.[1] This selective activation may be based on the exploitation of some unique aspects of tumor physiology, such as selective enzyme expression, hypoxia, and low extracellular pH. Other approaches are based on tumor-specific delivery techniques that allow the selective activation of prodrugs by exogenous enzymes, which are delivered into the tumor using monoclonal antibodies [antibody-directed enzyme prodrug therapy (ADEPT)] or generated in tumor cells from DNA constructs that contain the corresponding gene using nonviral [(gene-directed enzyme prodrug therapy (GDEPT)] or viral [virus-directed enzyme prodrug therapy (VDEPT)] vectors.

2.1. Selective enzyme expression in tumor cells

In order to achieve a tumor-specific targeting, the enzyme responsible for prodrug activation should uniquely be present in the tumor cell. Although there is much evidence of pathways involving enzymes that are aberrantly expressed in tumors, these approaches have found varying success because the differences between healthy and tumor tissues are not normally consistent across different species, individuals, or even tumors.

One example, previously discussed in Section 4.3 of Chapter 2, is the selective bioactivation in tumors of capecitabine, a 5-fluorouracil prodrug. This prodrug is rapidly absorbed after oral administration due to its lipophilicity and metabolized by carboxylesterase and cytidine deaminase to 5′-deoxy-5-fluorouridine. The final bioactivation step involves the transformation of the latter intermediate into 5-FU by thymidine phosphorylase (Fig. 11.1), and takes place up to 10 times more efficiently in cancer cells than in normal cells.

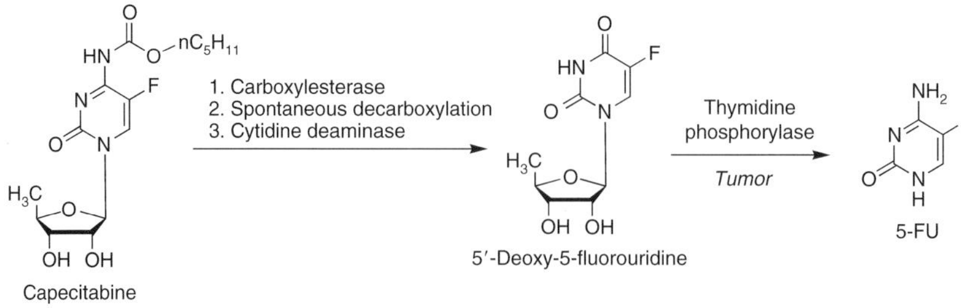

FIGURE 11.1   Selective bioactivation of capecitabine.

Another enzyme that is overexpressed in several tumors, including ovarian, colon, pancreas, and non-small lung cell cancers, is the cytosolic glutathione-S-transferase of the π class (GST-π). The active site of this enzyme contains a tyrosine residue that deprotonates the mercapto group of glutathione in order to increase its nucleophilicity and to allow its reaction with electrophilic toxic metabolites (Fig. 11.2).

The mustard prodrug TLK-286 contains a modified glutathione framework linked to an inactive phosphoramide mustard. The presence of a sulfone group in the linker was designed to enhance the acidity of the α-proton and thus facilitate a β-elimination reaction triggered by the basicity of the deprotonated tyrosine hydroxyl. The negative charge in the liberated phosphoramidate assists the intramolecular nucleophilic displacement reaction that leads to the alkylating aziridinium species (Fig. 11.3). Although the activation of TLK-286 can occur spontaneously, the enzyme facilitates the kinetics of the process. TLK-286 is under Phase III testing for non-small cell lung and ovarian cancers.[2]

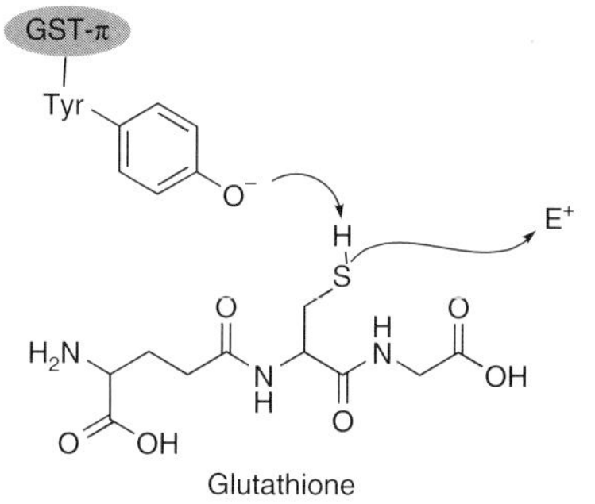

FIGURE 11.2   Activation of glutathion at the active site of GST-π.

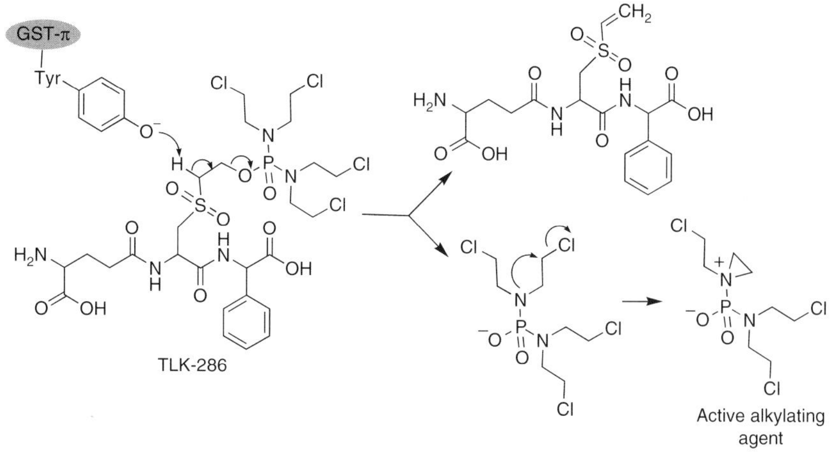

FIGURE 11.3   Selective bioactivation of TLK-286.

2.2. Hypoxia-based strategies for tumor-specific prodrug activation

Hypoxia is a common and unique property of cells in solid tumors, and it is therefore a potential mechanism for tumor-specific prodrug activation.[3] The availability of oxygen electrodes has allowed the accurate measurement of oxygen levels in human tumors, which are highly heterogeneous. Many regions have very low levels, with partial pressures of oxygen around 5 mmHg that corresponds to about 0.7% O_2 in the gas phase or 7 µM in solution. These hypoxic cells are resistant to radiotherapy (see Section 11 of Chapter 4) and can also be considered resistant to most anticancer drugs because of poor diffusion from the distant blood vessels, loss of sensitivity to p53-mediated apoptosis, and upregulation of genes involved in drug resistance. However, the existence of hypoxia and cell necrosis provides an opportunity for tumor-selective therapy, including the development of bioreductive prodrugs[4] specifically activated by hypoxia.

Discrimination between normal (oxygenated) and tumor (hypoxic) tissues can normally be achieved when the prodrug contains a functional group that is susceptible to give an initial reduction (a "trigger"). When oxygen is present, as in the normal tissue, this reduction can be reverted by the transfer of one electron to oxygen, leading to a futile redox cycle that generates superoxide radical-anion (Fig. 11.4A). In the absence of oxygen, the prodrug radical is accumulated and then generates the ultimate cytotoxic species, and hypoxia-selective cytotoxicity is achieved (Fig. 11.4B). Obviously, for this approach to be useful in cancer therapy the above-mentioned radical or its downstream products must have higher cytotoxicity than the superoxide radical-anion arising from redox cycling in oxygenated cells.

The one-electron reduction potential of the functional group acting as a trigger is an important design parameter for hypoxia-selective tumor-activated prodrugs. The main types of triggers are aromatic and aliphatic N-oxides, quinones, aromatic nitro groups, and cobalt complexes, which are discussed below. Other

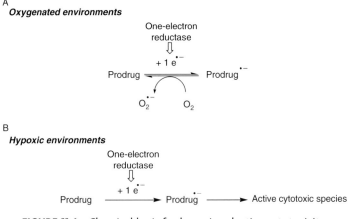

FIGURE 11.4   Chemical basis for hypoxia-selective cytotoxicity.

types of hypoxia-based strategies for tumor-specific prodrug activation will be mentioned in Sections 11.3 (GDEPT therapy) and 11.4 (ADEPT therapy).

One of the enzymes involved in the one-electron reduction reactions needed for hypoxia-selective bioactivation is cytochrome P450 reductase, a flavoprotein that functions as an electron donor for P450. This enzyme is able to reduce aldehydes, quinones, and N-oxides, among other functional groups, directly or via P450s. Some drugs can be reduced by other enzymes, like P450 itself or nitroreductases.

2.2.1. N-oxides

The best-known aromatic N-oxide used as an antitumor drug is tirapazamine (TPZ), which undergoes an enzymatic one-electron reduction to the TPZ radical. In normal cells, this species reacts with oxygen to give back TPZ, together with a superoxide radical. However, in hypoxic environments the TPZ radical undergoes two different types of fragmentation reactions (see Section 9 of Chapter 4), leading to hydroxyl and benzotriazinyl (BTZ) radicals, which cause DNA strand cleavage and topoisomerase II poisoning (Fig. 11.5). One advantage of TPZ is its potentiation of the efficacy under hypoxic conditions of radiotherapy and some chemotherapeutic drugs, including cisplatin.

Aliphatic N-oxides can be considered as good prodrugs of intercalating agents bearing side chains with basic tertiary amino groups. The rationale for the use of these compounds as prodrugs is that they have a greatly decreased affinity for DNA because the negatively charged N-oxide oxygen atoms prevent their interaction with the anionic phosphate groups in DNA.[5] The best-known aliphatic N-oxide hypoxia-activated prodrug is the anthraquinone AQ4N, which is under clinical trials.[6] Its reduction followed by protonation furnishes the active species

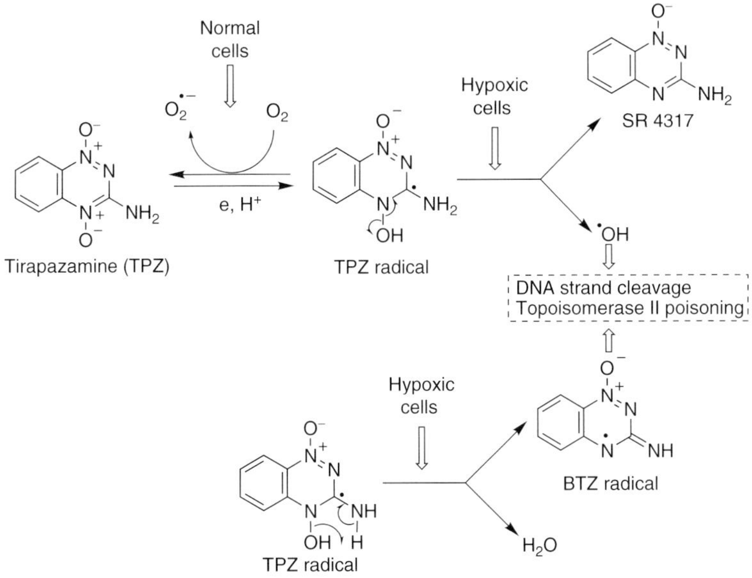

FIGURE 11.5   Reactions of the tirapazamine radical relevant to its anticancer activity.

AQ4, which shows a tight binding to DNA by intercalation and subsequent interference with the topoisomerase II function (Fig. 11.6). AQ4 is unusual among hypoxia-activated prodrugs in being activated by two-electron reduction. In humans, this reaction is effected mainly by the CYP3A members of the cytochrome P450 family, which are overexpressed in some tumors,[7] and is inhibited by oxygen due to competition for the reduced heme group in the enzyme active site rather than from redox cycling.[8]

2.2.2. Quinones

Quinone derivatives were among the first compounds studied as hypoxia-selective tumor-activated prodrugs. Quinones can undergo reduction by cytochrome P450 reductase, leading to captodative-stabilized semiquinone radical anions (see Section 2 of Chapter 4), that can be back-oxidized by molecular oxygen in normal, well-oxygenated cells. On the other hand, quinones are also good substrates for two-electron reductases, particularly DT-diaphorase (Fig. 11.7).

The first examples of reductively activated quinones were compounds having a good leaving group at the α position of a side chain placed at the quinone C-2 carbon.

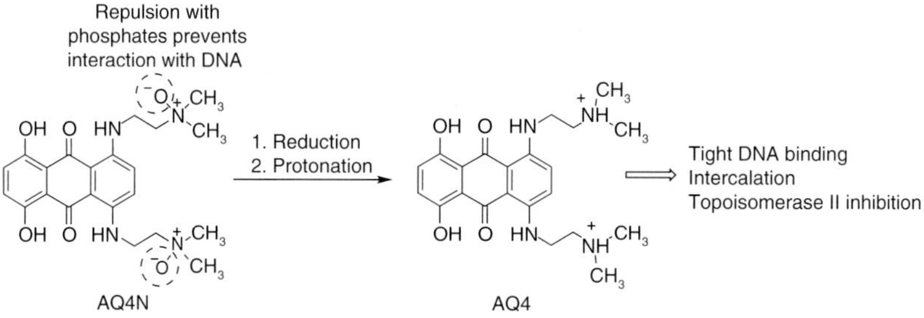

FIGURE 11.6 Hypoxia-activation of the anthraquinone prodrug AQ4N.

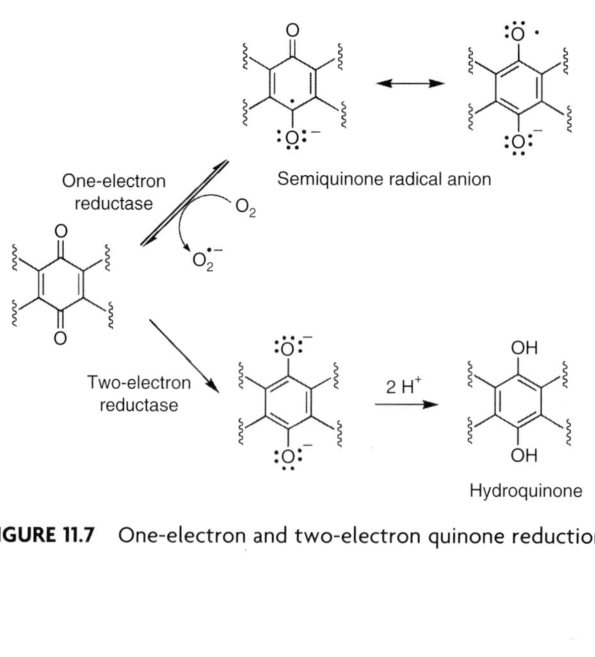

FIGURE 11.7 One-electron and two-electron quinone reduction.

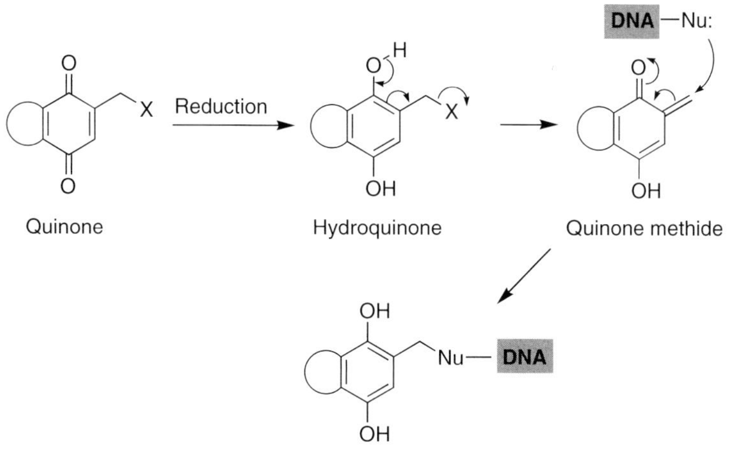

FIGURE 11.8   Reductive generation of electrophilic quinone methides from quinones.

After reduction, these compounds generate highly reactive quinone methides that behave as DNA alkylators (Fig. 11.8).

Two simple examples of antitumor compounds designed using this strategy are quinones **11.1**[9] and **11.2**,[10] though they show only a marginal hypoxic selectivity. The natural products mitomycin C and porfiromycin are also activated by bioreductive mechanisms (see Section 3 of Chapter 6).

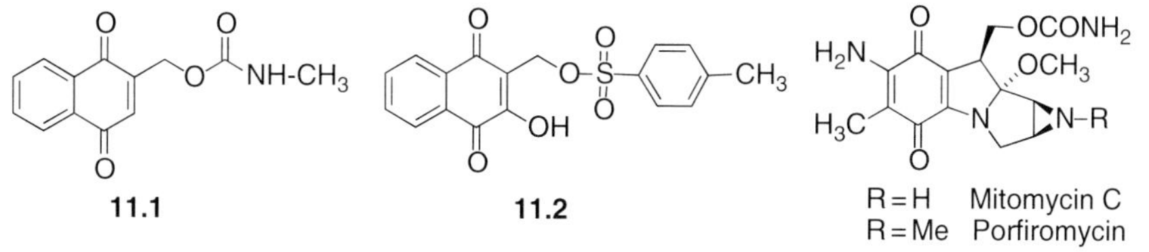

11.1   **11.2**   R = H   Mitomycin C
                                                  R = Me   Porfiromycin

The second structural type of bioreductively activated quinones is aziridinyl-quinones, represented by the benzoquinone derivative diaziquone and by indo-lequinone EO-9 (see also Section 3 of Chapter 5). These quinones are bioactivated by two-electron reductases, particularly DT-diaphorase (Fig. 11.9), an enzyme that is overexpressed in many tumors, but their clinical results have not been particularly successful.

A final application of quinones in bioreductive activation processes is their use as triggers for the release of alkylating species, especially nitrogen mustards. One example is compound **11.3**, which liberates a molecule of melphalan upon lacto-nization of its reduced hydroquinone form (see also Section 2.4 of Chapter 5). In the case of **11.4**, reduction to hydroquinone is followed by C–N bond cleavage to release the aliphatic mustard **11.5**. This reaction is not possible before the reduc-tion step because of the electron-withdrawing effect of the quinone moiety on the indole nitrogen (Fig. 11.10).

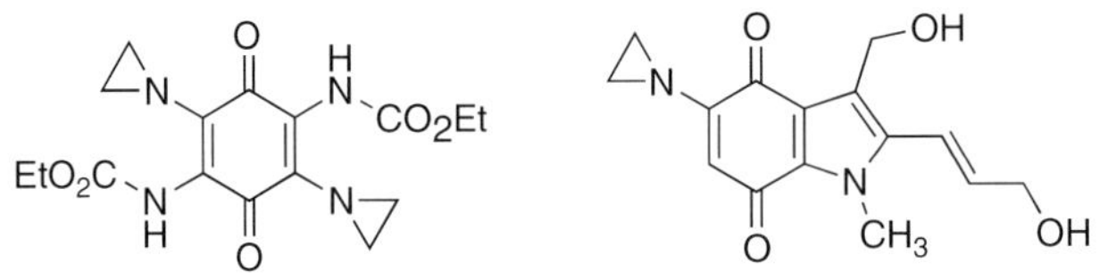

Diaziquone (AZQ)   EO-9

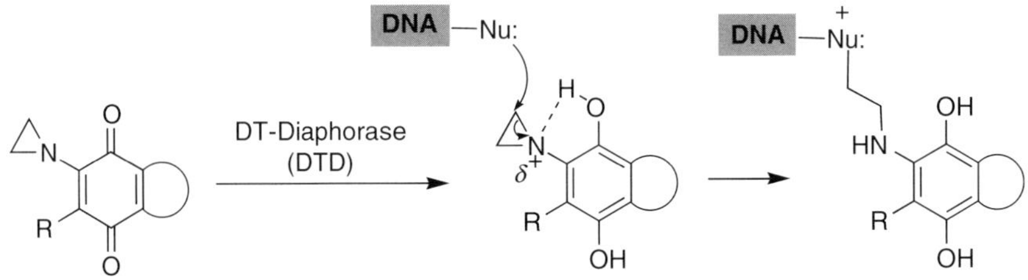

FIGURE 11.9   Reductive bioactivation of aziridinylquinones.

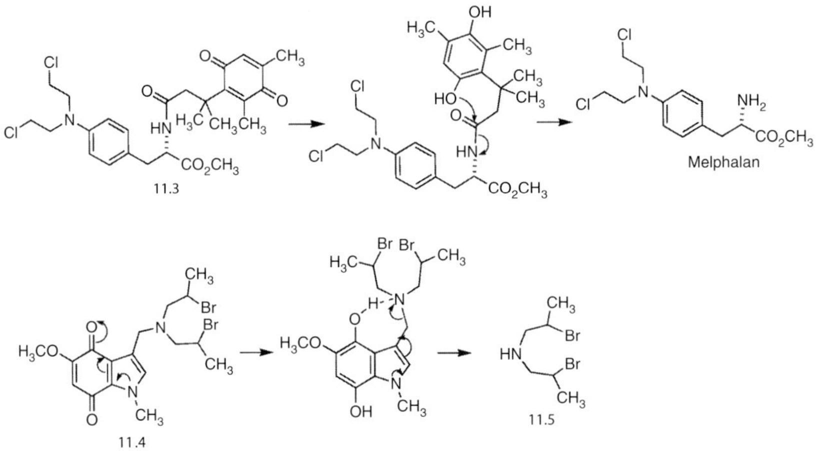

FIGURE 11.10   Release of alkylating species through reductive bioactivation of quinones.

2.2.3. Aromatic nitro derivatives

Nitroaromatic compounds are reduced by several nitroreductases, which are flavoprotein enzymes that catalyze the stepwise addition of up to six electrons, though the major metabolite is normally the hydroxylamine formed by addition of four electrons. In nitroaromatic compounds with suitable reduction potentials (around −330 to −450 mV), the first radical anion formed by one-electron addition can be scavenged efficiently by molecular oxygen, and consequently its formation is restricted to hypoxic cells. Compounds with reduction potentials outside this range are less useful, either because they are too easily reduced and therefore show less selectivity for hypoxic tissues (reduction potentials higher than $-330\,\mathrm{mV}$) or because they are too difficult to activate (reduction potentials below $-450\,\mathrm{mV}$).

The main nitroaromatic compounds used in cancer chemotherapy are nitroimidazoles. These compounds were introduced as radiosensitizers (see Section 11 of Chapter 4), but it was later shown that they were able to induce cell death in hypoxic environments in the absence of radiation. This cytotoxic activity is mainly due to the nitro radical anion **11.6** and hydroxylamine (**11.8**) metabolites. Thus, **11.6** or its protonated derivative **11.7** can oxidize DNA chains (see also Section 11 of Chapter 4), while the *O*-acetyl derivative of hydroxylamine **11.8** may give covalent DNA adducts (Fig. 11.11).[11]

Although the observation of cytotoxic activity in the absence of radiation normally requires concentrations of the nitro derivative that are too high to be found in clinical situations, the presence of two alkylating moieties can lead to improved activity. For instance, RSU-1069 behaves as a DNA monoalkylator in normal tissues and as a bisalkylator under hypoxic environments, where it is 50–100 times more cytotoxic (Fig. 11.12). Unfortunately, clinical studies of this compound showed a high-intestinal toxicity that prevented its further development.

Nitracrine is another nitro derivative with selective cytotoxicity in hypoxic cell cultures, and it has been shown that besides its DNA intercalating properties it is able to alkylate DNA following reduction by thiols or enzymes, though the nature of the electrophilic metabolites generated in the bioreductive process is still debated. Unfortunately, the hypoxia selectivity has not been observed in solid tumors, probably because the high-reduction potential (–303 mV) and the tight DNA binding of this compound slows its diffusion into hypoxic areas.

Since the alkylating reactivity of aromatic mustards is greatly determined by the electron density in the mustard nitrogen, enzymatic reduction of a nitro group on the aromatic ring to a hydroxylamine derivative can result in a higher potency

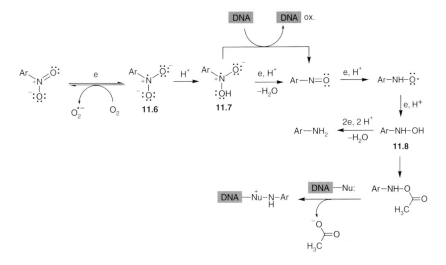

FIGURE 11.11 Reductive bioactivation of cytotoxic nitroaromatic compounds.

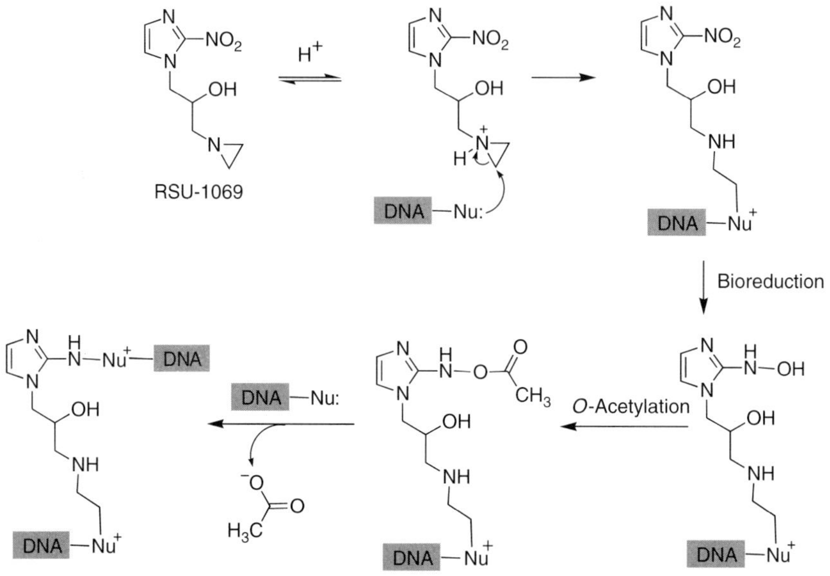

FIGURE 11.12   Enhanced cytotoxicity of RSU-1069 in hypoxic environments.

of these compounds as DNA alkylating agents (see Section 2.4 of Chapter 5). The simplest such prodrug is the nitrophenyl mustard (**11.9**), but it shows only a modest hypoxic selectivity because, due to its low-reduction potential of about −515 mV, only a small amount of the drug is likely to be reduced. Accordingly, its 2,4-dinitro analogue (SN-23862), in which the electron-attracting properties of the second nitro group induce a higher-reduction potential, has a higher-hypoxic selectivity. Overall, this strategy is not very useful, because the presence of two or more electron-deficient groups onto the benzene ring of a nitrophenyl mustard to ensure a high enough reduction potential results in a low cytotoxicity even after reductive activation of part of these groups. This is also true for analogues based on heteroaromatic mustards such as **11.10**.

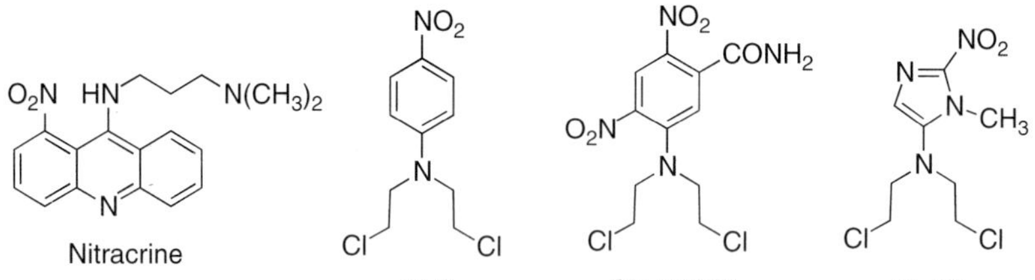

Further problems associated with the presence of several nitro groups attached to the benzene ring of a nitrogen mustard are due to metabolic side reactions that contribute to its deactivation. For instance, the reductive metabolism of SN-23862

involves the predominant reduction of the nitro group *ortho* to the mustard moiety, which affords a mixture of hydroxylamino (**11.11**) and amino (**11.12**) reduction products. These metabolites undergo a fast intramolecular cyclization to tetrahydroquinoxaline derivatives **11.13**[12] where most antitumor activity has been lost (Fig. 11.13).

Another mechanism studied involves the generation of an active fragment after a bioreductive process. For instance, reduction of nitrobenzyl carbamates such as **11.14** to its hydroxylamino metabolite generates an electrophilic quinoneimine methide **11.15** together with amine R–NH₂, though the reduction potential is too low and for this reason this bioreduction is inefficient (Fig. 11.14).

The same problem related to a too low value for the reduction potential has been shown in the bioreductive activation of the fluorouracil prodrug **11.16**, which has been designed to generate the active drug by a "through-space" cyclization-extrusion process in the reduced metabolite **11.17** (Fig. 11.15).

2.2.4. Cobalt complexes

As already mentioned in Section 2.4 of Chapter 5, another strategy to design hypoxic-selective nitrogen mustards has been the complexation of both nitrogen atoms from bidentate mustards with transition metals such as cobalt. Complexes in the low-spin Co (III) oxidation state, such as SN-24771, are very stable and have appropriate reduction potential values to be reduced by cellular reductases. This reduction is competitively inhibited by oxygen, but under hypoxia the unstable high-spin Co (II) species resulting from reduction rapidly releases its ligands to

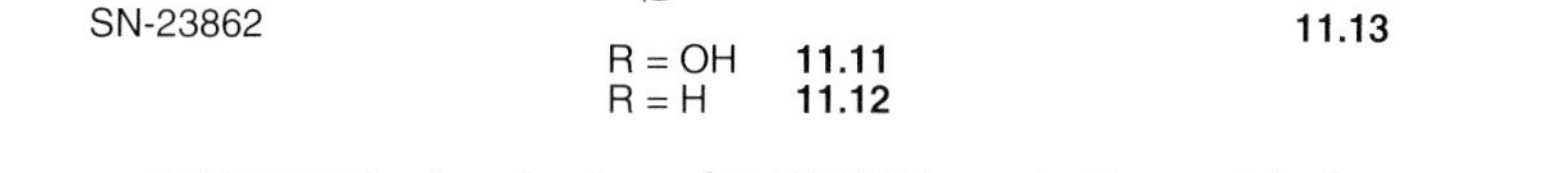

FIGURE 11.13 Inactivation of SN-23862 by reductive metabolism.

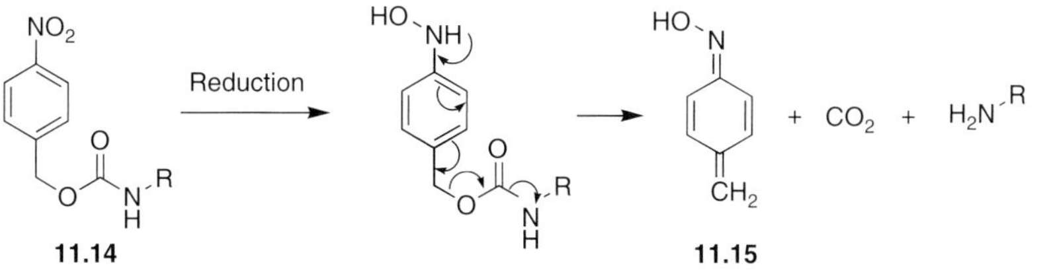

FIGURE 11.14 Reductive bioactivation of nitrobenzyl carbamates.

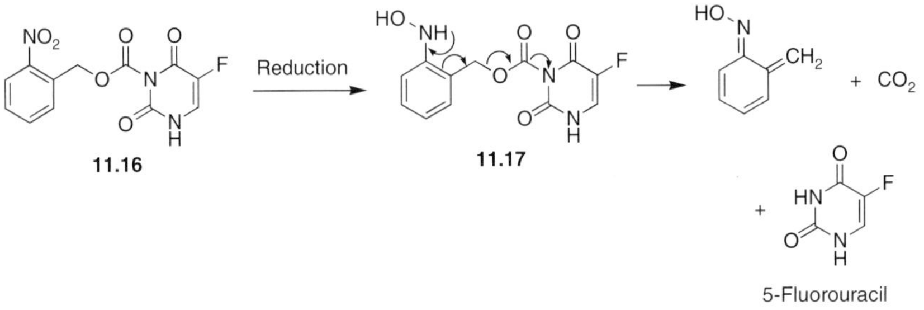

FIGURE 11.15   Reductive bioactivation of a 5-fluorouracil prodrug.

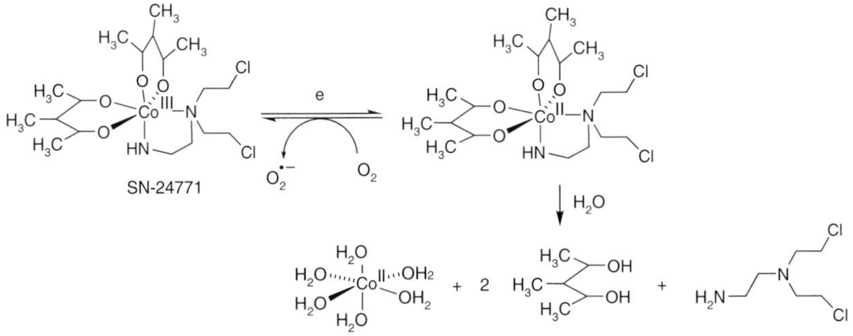

FIGURE 11.16   Hypoxia-selective activation of a Co(III)-complexed nitrogen mustard.

coordinate with water molecules forming stable hexa-aquo Co (II) species (Fig. 11.16).[13] The limited activity showed *in vivo* by this compound discouraged its further development.

2.2.5. Prodrugs activated by therapeutic radiation

Since severely hypoxic tissues are necrotic and therefore they lack the enzymes and cofactors required for the reductive activation of cytotoxic prodrugs, it may be useful to employ ionizing radiation for this purpose. This methodology has the advantage that radiotherapy focuses the radiation field on the tumor.

Irradiation of water in cells during radiotherapy generates hydrated electrons that can be used to activate antitumor prodrugs because they are much more powerful reducing agents than enzymes. However, their very low yield, coupled with competition with other endogenous electron acceptors, makes necessary the design of prodrugs that liberate very potent cytotoxic species.

Some examples of prodrugs that can be activated by ionizing radiation under hypoxia are heterocyclic nitroarylmethyl quaternary ammonium salts,[14] 1-(2'-oxopropyl)-5-fluorouracil (OFU001),[15] and some Co (III) complexes, but they have not demonstrated sufficiently high activity.

2.3. Gene-directed enzyme prodrug therapy (GDEPT) and virus-directed enzyme prodrug therapy (VDEPT)

In these approaches, "suicide" genes encoding prodrug activating enzymes are targeted to tumor cells, which are followed by prodrug administration.[16] In GDEPT, nonviral vectors, such as cationic lipids, peptides, or naked DNA, are used for gene targeting. In VDEPT, gene targeting is accomplished using viral vectors, especially retroviruses and adenoviruses. In both cases, the vector needs to be taken up by the target cells, the encoded enzyme must be expressed (transduction) and the prodrug must enter the target cells and be activated intracellularly. Finally, because it is not possible to target genes to every cell, the locally activated drug must also be able to kill nonexpressing cells, a phenomenon known as "bystander effect" (Fig. 11.17).

Some reductases from anaerobic bacteria are more efficient than human enzymes for the hypoxia-selective reductive activation of certain prodrugs. In these cases, it is possible to administer the prodrug associated to a viral vector that transports the gene responsible for the production of the required microbial enzyme. One example that has entered clinical trials[17] is the association of the

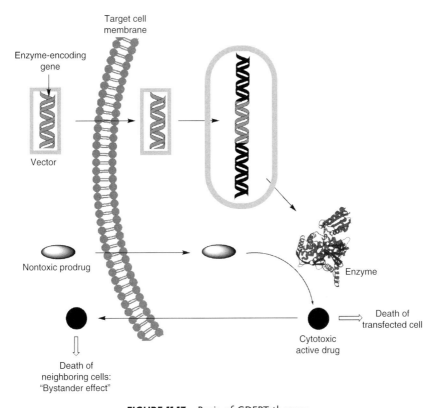

FIGURE 11.17 Basis of GDEPT therapy.

aziridine derivative CB-1954, related to the previously mentioned SN-23862, with a non-replicating adenoviral vector that expresses the *nfsB* gene, corresponding to the *Escherichia coli* nitroreductase (NTR). This enzyme is a two-electron reductase that reduces either of the two nitro groups in CB-1954. The key metabolite seems to be the 2-hydroxylamino compound **11.18**. A subsequent acetylation by acetylcoenzyme A affords **11.19**, a potent DNA cross-linking agent[18] (Fig. 11.18).

VDEPT approaches have also been used in the case of *N*-oxide bioreductive prodrugs by transfecting tumor cells with a mammalian expression vector, mainly adenovirus, containing the genes encoding for the enzymes necessary for their activation, namely CYP3A4 in the case of AQ4N[19] and cytochrome 450 reductase (P450R) in the case of tirapazamine.[20] VDEPT therapy must not be confused with the use of the so-called oncolytic viruses as anticancer "drugs."[21]

GDEPT methodologies are not restricted to hypoxia-selective prodrug activation. For instance, a GDEPT has been developed from cyclophosphamide and the CYP2B1 gene for the treatment of brain tumors. Cyclophosphamide is not active in the brain for two reasons, namely because it requires oxidative metabolism, which takes place mainly in the liver to yield its cytotoxic metabolites (see Section 2.4 of Chapter 5), and also because these metabolites are poorly transported across the blood–brain barrier and P450 activity in brain is low.

2.4. Antibody-directed enzyme prodrug therapy (ADEPT)

Another approach to achieve high local concentration of antitumor drugs is the so-called "antibody-directed enzyme prodrug therapy", in which antigens expressed on tumor cells are used to target enzymes to the tumor site by means of suitable monoclonal antibodies. The direct use of antibodies as antitumor agents has been discussed in Section 5.2 of Chapter 10.

In ADEPT therapy, an immunoconjugate of the proposed activating enzyme and an antibody specifically directed at a tumor antigen are administered. After allowing some time for the non-bound enzyme to be eliminated from the general circulation, a prodrug that is activated by the enzyme is administered. This activation takes place at the cell surface, and the active species is then

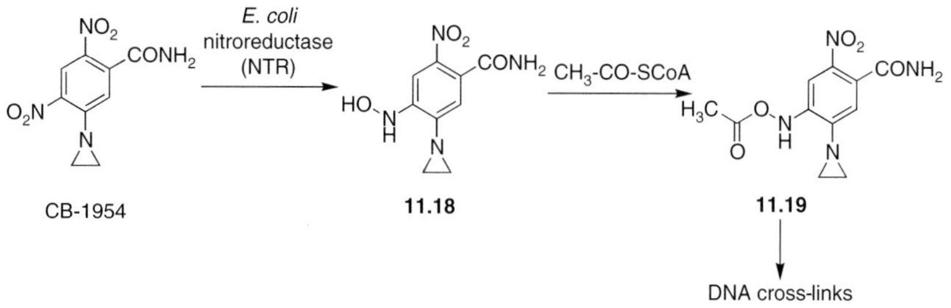

FIGURE 11.18 Bioactivation of the prodrug CB-1954.

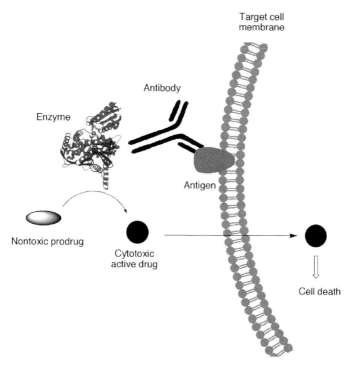

FIGURE 11.19   Basis of ADEPT therapy.

uptaken into the tumor cells (Fig. 11.19). One advantage of this approach is the possibility of using nonhuman enzymes, which may be more active for prodrug activation. Its main drawbacks are the scarcity of tumor-selective antigens, the possibility of immune reactions if nonhuman proteins are employed and the need for the active species to cross the cell membrane, since activation occurs extracellularly.

ADEPT strategies appear to be promising to target glucuronidated prodrugs to tumor cells because glucuronidated prodrugs are very poorly taken up by cells and hence are suitable for extracellular activation. β-Glucuronidase is widely used as an activating enzyme in ADEPT. One technique that has proved to have general value for this purpose is the use of β-glucuronyl self-immolative carbamate prodrugs, which is exemplified in Fig. 11.20 for the case of the anthracycline prodrug DOX-GA3 which showed improved antitumor activity in mice compared with DOX-GA3 administration alone.[22] Prodrug activation can be assumed to take place by glucuronide hydrolysis to phenol **11.20**, followed by spontaneous loss of the *p*-hydroxybenzyl group through a 1,6-elimination reaction[23] and final decarboxylation of the carbamic acid **11.21** thus generated.

In a related approach, an *Escherichia coli* nitroreductase can be used to activate prodrugs containing a *p*-nitrobenzylcarbamate substituent. One example is the mitomycin C prodrug **11.22**, whose mechanism of bioactivation involves again a 1,6-elimination process (Fig. 11.21).[24]

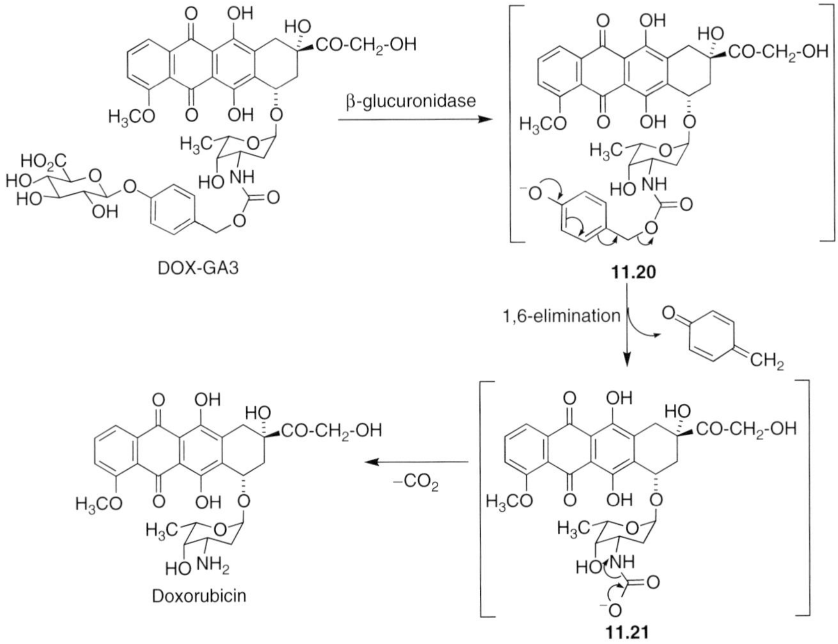

FIGURE 11.20   Bioactivation of DOX-GA3 in ADEPT therapy.

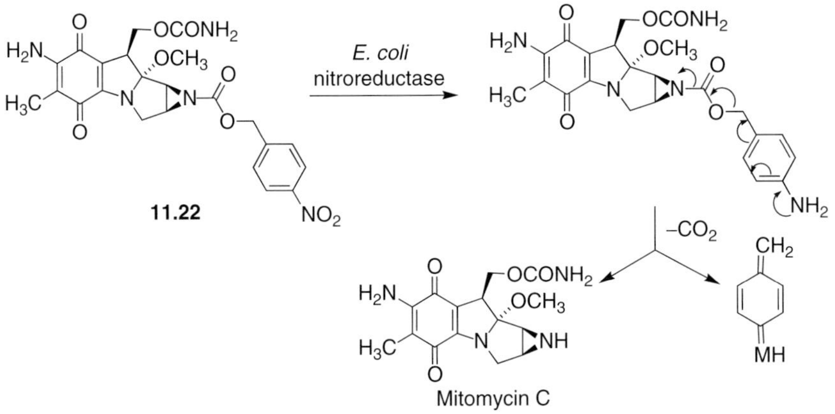

FIGURE 11.21   Bioactivation of a mitomycin C prodrug in ADEPT therapy.

Phosphatases have also been used as activating enzymes in ADEPT approaches. For instance, etopophos is activated to etoposide by a monoclonal antibody-alkaline phosphatase immunoconjugate (Fig. 11.22).

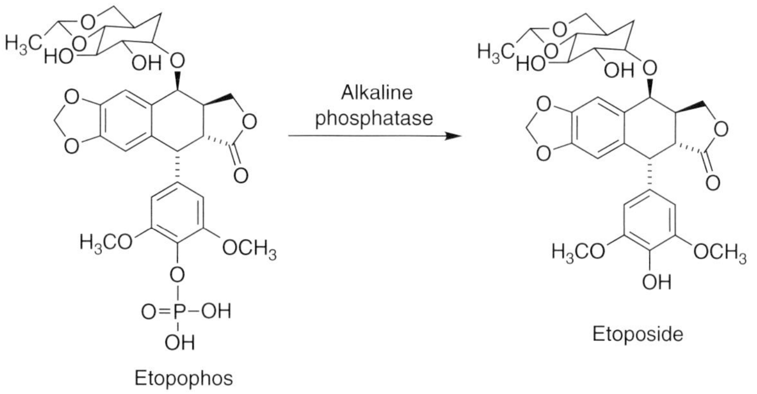

FIGURE 11.22 Bioactivation of etopophos in ADEPT therapy.

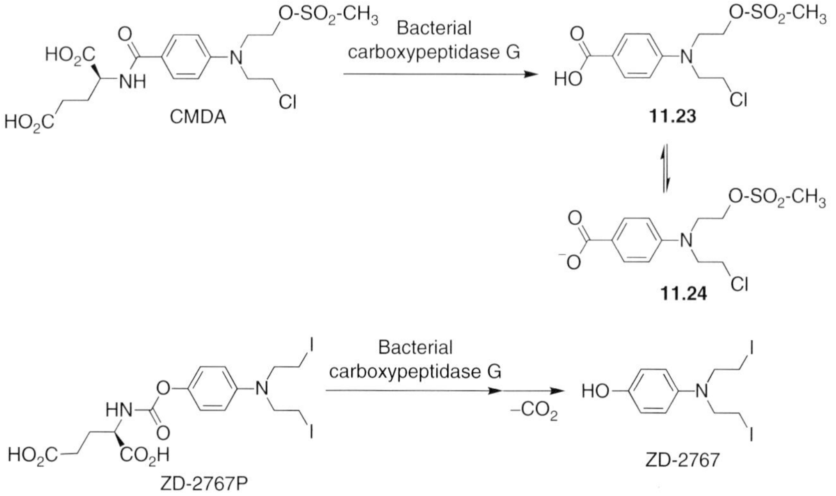

FIGURE 11.23 ADEPT approaches to chemotherapy with nitrogen mustards.

The first example of a locally activated prodrug using and ADEPT approach that reached clinical trials was the mustard prodrug CMDA in combination with bacterial carboxypeptidase G and cyclosporin to counteract the immune response to the conjugate.[25] The activity of **11.23** is probably associated with its ionized form **11.24**, where the electron density of the nitrogen atom is increased. It is also relevant to note that **11.23** shows a higher activity than its bischloroethyl analogue (compound **5.13**, Section 2.3 of Chapter 5), which can be ascribed to the higher ability of the mesylate unit to act as a leaving group. A related carbamate prodrug is ZD-2767P, which releases the corresponding iodo nitrogen mustard and has also undergone Phase I clinical trials[26] (Fig. 11.23).

3. POLYMER-PROTEIN CONJUGATES

The term "polymer therapeutics" has been coined to describe water-soluble devices that use polymers as carriers and that are designed for parenteral administration. They include polymer-drug or polymer-protein conjugates and polymeric micelles to which a drug is covalently attached. Therapeutic polymers may be considered as one of the first nanodrugs, which can be defined as nanometer-scale complexes that contain at least two components, one of them being a bioactive agent (see also Section 11.7).

Besides being water-soluble, the polymer has to be nontoxic, non-immunogenic, and suitable for repeated administration, and it has to be chosen taking into account that its physico-chemical properties govern biodistribution, elimination, and metabolism of the conjugate. The most widely tested polymers in clinical assays are polyethylene glycol (PEG), N-(2-hydroxypropylmethacrylamide) (HPMA), and polyglutamic acid (PGA). Because PEG and HPMA copolymers are not biodegradable, their use has to be limited to masses below 40 kDa to ensure eventual renal elimination, while this limitation does not affect PGA copolymers.

Several polymer-protein conjugates containing a therapeutic protein, mostly PEGylated enzymes or cytoquines, have entered into routine clinical use in oncology.[27] Polyethylene glycol is a unique polyether diol, usually manufactured by the aqueous anionic polymerization of ethylene oxide. If this polymerization is initiated with anhydrous methanol or other alcohol derivatives it results in monoalkyl capped polyethylene glycols such as methoxy PEG (mPEG).

PEG   mPEG

These polymers are amphiphilic and dissolve well both in organic solvents and in water, and their conjugation to proteins is accomplished mainly by the reaction of an available amino group or other reactive sites such as histidine or cysteine residues.

PEGylation of proteins enhances their stability, reduces their immunogenicity, and prolongs their plasma half-life and consequently the patient requires less frequent dosing.[28] On the negative side, the PEGylation process can lead to reduction or even complete loss of the bioactivity of the therapeutic protein associated with the alteration of the overall protein charge and to the reduction of its substrate- or receptor-binding affinity.

The first antitumor PEGylated protein approved for clinical use was PEG-L-asparaginase (pegaspargase).[29] It is used to treat acute lymphoblastic leukemia, a disease that requires L-asparagine (see Section 9 of Chapter 2). Pegaspargase has advantages as compared with the native enzyme because of its reduced immunogenicity and its much longer plasma half-life. Other PEG-enzyme conjugates that have entered clinical trials are PEG-recombinant arginine deiminase (ADI-PEG20) and PEGylated-glutaminase (PEG-PGA). The first copolymer depletes arginine, and it is being developed for hepatocellular carcinoma as a single agent or in combination with 5-FU.[30] The second is being clinically evaluated in combination with the previously mentioned glutamine antimetabolite DON (see Section 6.3 of Chapter 2), based on the idea that this drug should be more effective when glutamine levels are depleted.[31]

Among PEG-cytokine conjugates, the granulocyte colony-stimulating factor (GCSF), used to prevent chemotherapy-induced neutropenia, is used in its PEGylated form (PEG-GCSF, pegfilgrastim), which has a longer half-life and fewer allergic reactions than the free protein.[32]

4. MACROMOLECULAR SMALL-DRUG CARRIER SYSTEMS

In macromolecular drug carrier systems, an active drug is covalently attached to a macromolecule. These conjugates may target solid tumor tissues passively by a mechanism known as "enhanced permeability and retention" (EPR) effect, which is based on the increased permeability of vascular endothelium in tumors due to its poor organization (Fig. 11.24). This phenomenon allows that relatively large particles loaded with an antitumor drug can extravasate and accumulate inside the interstitial space, where the drug can be released as a result of normal carrier degradation.[33]

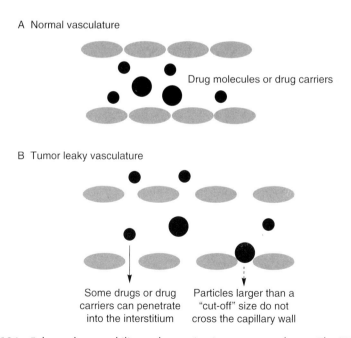

A Normal vasculature

Drug molecules or drug carriers

B Tumor leaky vasculature

Some drugs or drug carriers can penetrate into the interstitium

Particles larger than a "cut-off" size do not cross the capillary wall

FIGURE 11.24   Enhanced permeability and retention in tumor vasculature: The EPR effect.

More specific targeting may be achieved by using as a part of the macromolecular component an antibody directed to a tumor antigen or a peptide whose receptors are overexpressed in tumor cells. The conjugate approach has been particularly studied in the case of the anthracyclines.[34] These conjugates do not cross cell membranes, and they need to access the intracellular space by receptor-mediated endocytosis, adsorptive endocytosis, or fluid-phase endocytosis. In these processes, the cell membrane invaginates the particle and then forms an intracellular vesicle (endosome) that eventually fuses with lysosomes. The macromolecular transporter is hydrolyzed and the active drug is released as a consequence of lowered pH values both at the endosomes and at the lysosomes, and also to the presence of hydrolytic enzymes in the latter vesicles (Fig. 11.25). Furthermore, some extracellular drug release may also be produced because of the more acidic tumor environment (often 0.5–1 pH units lower than normal tissues) and to the overexpression in tumors of some extracellular proteases, such as matrix metalloproteinases and plasmin.

4.1. N-(2-Hydroxypropyl)methacrylamide polymers

Several of these polymer-drug conjugates have entered clinical trials for anticancer therapy.[35] They are copolymers of N-(2-HPMA and a Gly-Phe-Leu-Gly linker designed to facilitate intralysosomal liberation of the drug by cysteine proteases.

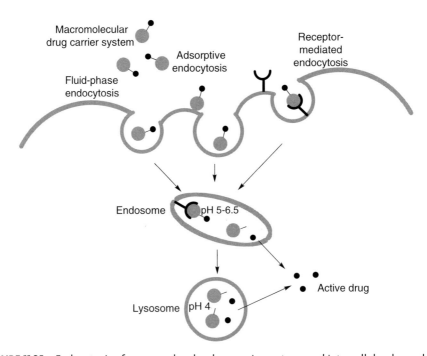

FIGURE 11.25 Endocytosis of macromolecular drug carrier systems and intracellular drug release.

The HPMA polymer has not shown evidence of toxicity or immunogenicity in man, which represents a great advantage over previously studied natural polymers that led to immunogenic reactions. On the other hand, HPMA has the disadvantage of not being biodegradable and for this reason the molecular mass of administered copolymers has to be lower than 40 kDa in order to ensure its direct renal elimination. The best-known compound among this group of agents is the doxorubicin conjugate PK-1 (FCE-28068),[36] which has a greatly reduced toxicity compared with free doxorubicin and was active in chemotherapy-refractory patients. Other HPMA conjugates that have entered clinical studies are the paclitaxel conjugate PNU-166945[37] and the camptothecin derivative **11.25**.[38]

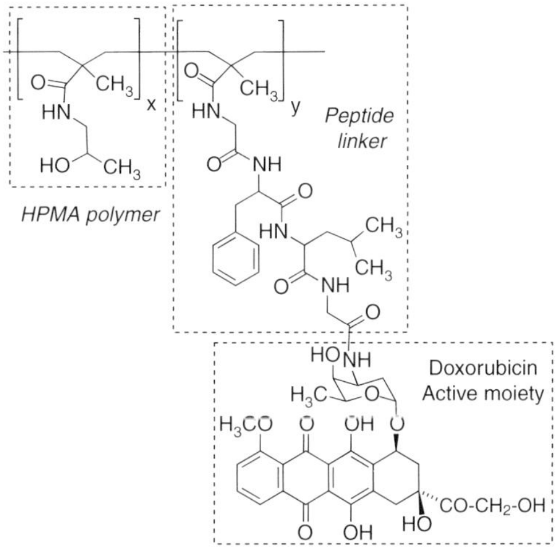

PK-1 (FCE-28068)

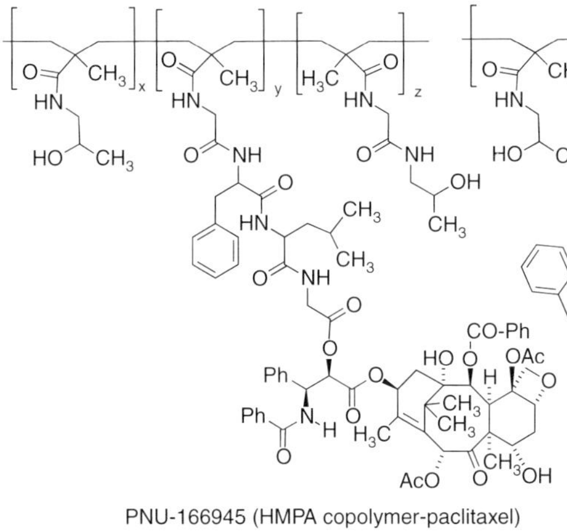

PNU-166945 (HMPA copolymer-paclitaxel)

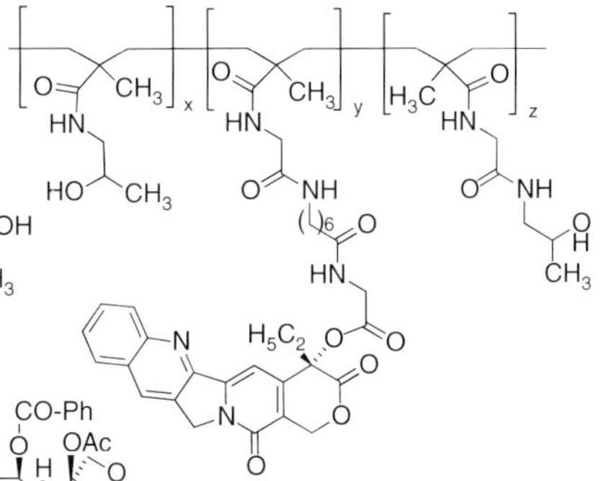

HMPA copolymer-camptothecin (**11.25**)

Cisplatin is one of the main anticancer agents currently in use, but it shows severe side effects, the most prominent being nephrotoxicity, neurotoxicity, nausea, and vomiting. Also, intrinsic or acquired tumor resistance is a major problem.

Such limitations, coupled with a narrow therapeutic index and poor solubility, have been the driving force behind a sustained research effort into the discovery of novel platinum agents or novel formulations and delivery methods of existing platinum agents. Two HPMA copolymer-platinate agents known as AP-5280[39,40] and AP-5346[41] are under clinical development.

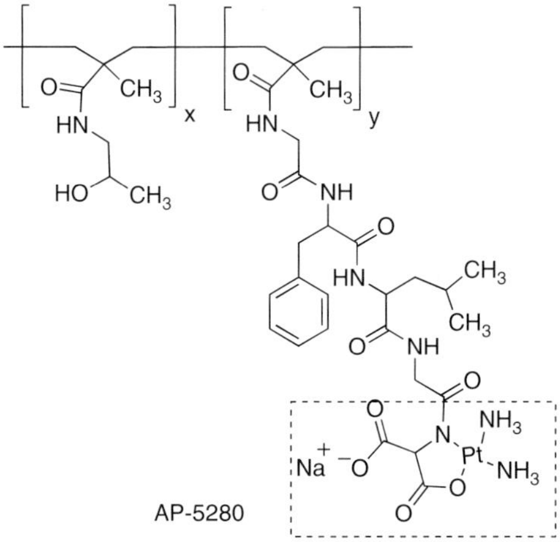

AP-5280

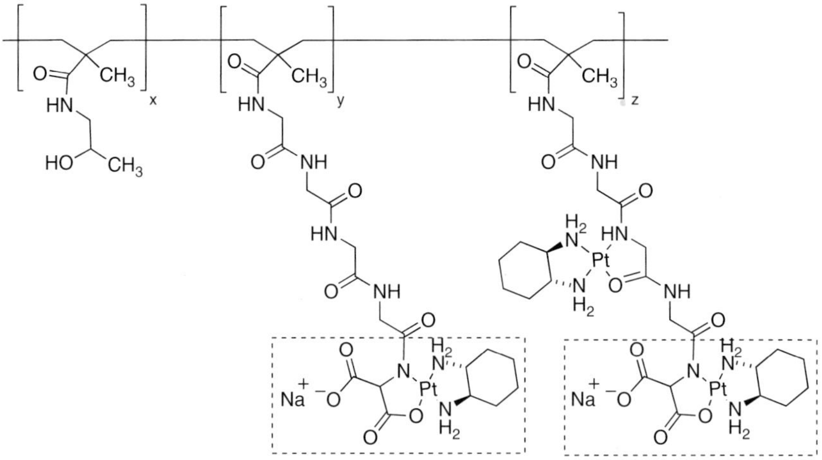

AP-5346

In a more sophisticated approach, an HPMA conjugate known as PK-2 (FCE-28069) was designed for tumor targeting using receptor-mediated endocytosis. This copolymer contains the HPMA polymer, a Gly-Phe-Leu-Gly peptide linker, doxorubicin and also galactosamine units that are targeted at the asialoglycoprotein receptor. Since this receptor is present in hepatocytes, the prodrug is expected to be useful in hepatocarcinomas.[42] Other ligands different to galactosamine are being explored for targeting.

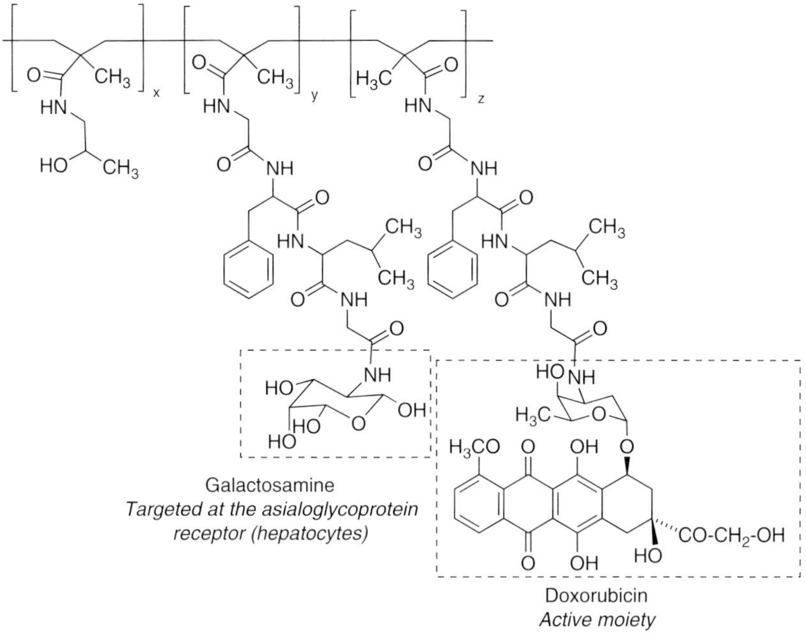

Galactosamine
*Targeted at the asialoglycoprotein
receptor (hepatocytes)*

Doxorubicin
Active moiety

PK-2 (FCE-28069)

4.2. Poly-(L-glutamic)conjugates

Another types of polymers designed for passive targeting through the EPR effect that are under clinical trials are the conjugates of poly-(L-glutamic) acid (PGA). These polymers have the advantage over others (HPMA, PEG) of being biodegradable and therefore not subject to the previously mentioned 40 kDa limit in molecular mass. The main PGA conjugates under study are those with paclitaxel (paclitaxel polyglumex, CT-2103)[43] and camptothecin (CT-2106). CT-2103 is the most advanced anticancer drug conjugate in clinical trials and has shown activity against several cancers. Phase III studies have shown promising activity against non-small lung cell cancer.[44]

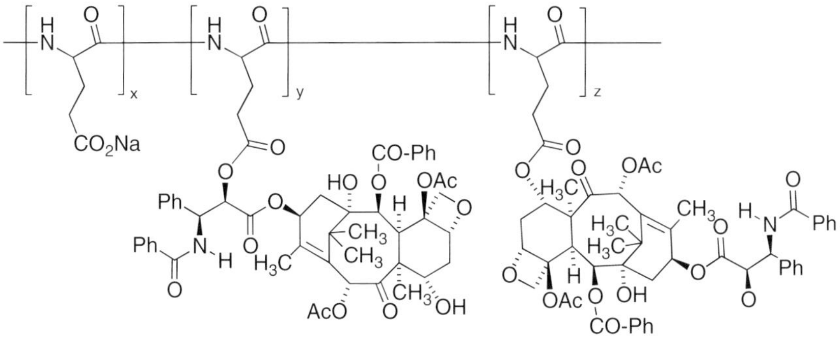

CT-2103

CT-2106

4.3. Neuropeptide Y conjugates

These cell-surface-selective polypeptide-prodrug conjugates have been directed to neuroblastomas. Receptors of neuropeptide Y(NPY), a 36-amino acid peptide of the pancreatic polypeptide family, are often overexpressed in these tumors. For this reason, conjugates of daunorubicin or doxorubicin with this neuropeptide bind to these cells and, after being internalized, they release the free drug. A Cys residue at the position 15 of NPY was used for attaching maleimide anthracycline derivatives without significant loss of binding to the receptor.[45]

4.4. PEGylated conjugates

Although some low-molecular weight anticancer PEG-drug conjugates have been studied, commercial products have thus far not been reported. However, higher-molecular weight PEG-drug conjugates, particularly those with a mass of 40,000, have led to a clinical candidate studied for several solid tumors indications.[46] This is PEG-camptothecin (CPT), an ester-based prodrug that includes an alanine spacer linked to the hydroxy group of the drug. Cleavage of the amide bond between PEG and the amino acid by exo-peptidases in the tumor results in an amino acid-CPT ester conjugate, which would still have its bioavailability enhanced by lactone stabilization. The ester bond would subsequently be cleaved to release CPT. Clinical studies have shown that the maximal concentration of free camptothecin was proportional to the administered dose of PEG-CPT, but these values were much lower than those observed for similar doses of CPT in the form of sodium camptothecinate.[47]

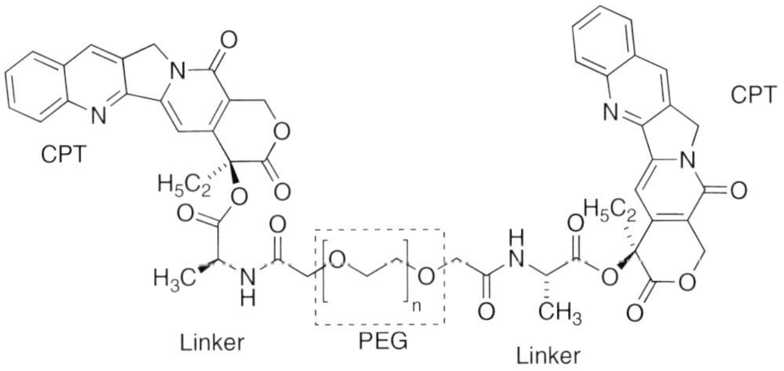

4.5. Immunoconjugated drugs

Selective monoclonal antibodies (mAbs) may be linked to anticancer agents to reduce the exposure of sensitive organs and tissues to drugs while enhancing the exposure of the tumor and metastatic foci. Additionally, although most antibodies normally remain bound to the cell surface, some of them may be endocytosed which permits to increase the potency of a drug when the antibody is internalized after binding to the corresponding tumor antigen. Here also peptide linkers allow for selective release of the drug in the lysosomal or endosome environments where occur proteolysis.

In vitro studies have been carried out with immunoconjugates of several antitumor drugs such as camptothecin[48] and a Co (II) complex of tallysomycin S_{10b}, a bleomycin analogue.[49] The structure of the latter complex is shown below. After complexation with Cu (II), which involves the nitrogen atoms marked with asterisks in the structure shown below, only two amino groups, marked with arrows, are available for acylation. A carbamate with p-aminobenzyl alcohol was used as the spacer between the dipeptide linker and the drug to ensure that the scissile bond is not sterically encumbered, and a maleimide group was employed as a handle for conjugation to the antibody (BR-96) via a cysteine residue. This conjugate enhanced the activity of the free drug by up to 825-fold.

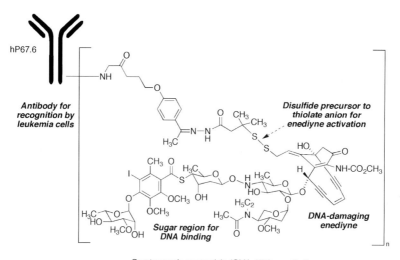

Gemtuzumab ozogamicin is a conjugate of a humanized mAb known as hP67.6. This antibody binds specifically to CD-33, a sialic acid-dependent adhesion protein found on the surface of normal and leukemic myeloid cells, including acute myeloid leukemia blasts, but not on normal bone marrow hematopoietic stem cells. In gemtuzumab ozogamicin, hP67.6 is coupled to a prodrug form of the natural product calicheamicin, which belongs to the enediyne class. After binding, the internalized conjugate breaks down allowing calicheamicin to interact with the minor groove of DNA (see Section 8 of Chapter 4). As the antigen is not expressed on normal hematopoietic cells, this conjugate is highly selective for leukemia cells. Gemtuzumab ozogamicin was the first approved antibody-chemotherapeutic agent complex, and is indicated for patients with CD-33-positive acute myeloid leukemia that have relapsed after initial treatment and are considered ineligible for more aggressive cytotoxic chemotherapy, such as the elderly.[50]

Monoclonal antibodies can also be employed to target radioactive nuclides to specific tumor cells.[51] Thus, ibritumomab tiuxetan consists of two parts, namely, the murine anti-CD-20 ibritumomab, that targets mature B cells, and the EDTA analogue tiuxetan, that provides a chelation site for yttrium-90 or indium-111. This was the first radioconjugate targeted agent approved for cancer treatment, and is indicated for refractory B-cell non-Hodgkin's lymphoma. Tositumomab is also a radioconjugate consisting of an anti-CD-20 antibody and radioactive iodine-131, and is approved for follicular non-Hodgkin lymphoma.[52] Similarly, the combination of the antibody tositumomab and its radioactive derivative [^{131}I]-tositumomab is the basis of an antineoplastic radioimmunotherapeutic monoclonal antibody-based regimen that is indicated for the treatment of patients with CD-20 antigen-expressing non-Hodgkin's lymphoma. Tositumomab itself is a murine IgG2a monoclonal antibody directed against the CD-20 antigen, which is found on the surface of normal and malignant B lymphocytes.

5. POLYMER-DIRECTED ENZYME PRODRUG THERAPY (PDEPT)

Polymer-directed enzyme prodrug therapy is a two-step antitumor approach that uses a combination of a polymeric prodrug and a polymer-enzyme conjugate to generate selective cytotoxicity. Thus, in a preliminary study of this approach, administration of the previously mentioned doxorubicin conjugate PK-1 was followed by the administration of a conjugate of the proteolytic enzyme cathepsin B, present in all mammalian cell lysosomes. This conjugate also used the copolymer of HPMA and the Gly-Phe-Leu-Gly tetrapeptide linker and the antitumor activity of this combination in mice showed advantages compared with PK-1 alone.[53]

The PDEPT strategy has been claimed to have advantages over ADEPT and GDEPT because the polymer-enzyme conjugates have reduced immunogenicity and the polymeric prodrug has a relatively short residence time in plasma which allows subsequent administration of polymer-enzyme without prodrug activation in the circulation.

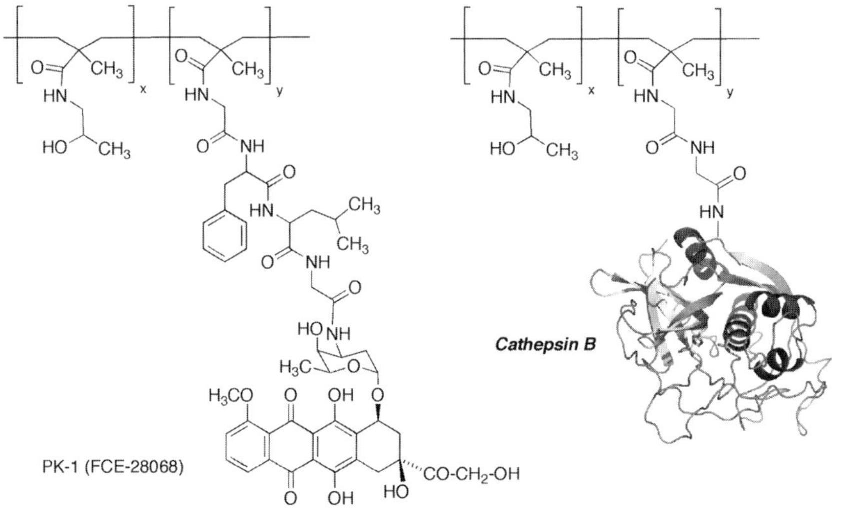

Cathepsin B

PK-1 (FCE-28068)

6. FOLATE RECEPTOR-TARGETED CHEMOTHERAPY AND IMMUNOTHERAPY OF CANCER

Folic acid has become a useful ligand for targeted cancer therapies because it binds to a tumor-associated antigen known as the folate receptor (FR). The human FR (FRα) is a glycophosphatidylinositol-anchored membrane glycoprotein that binds physiological folates and mediates their intracellular transport via receptor-mediated endocytosis. It is upregulated in many tumors and appears to increase as the cancer progresses. It is possible to link folic acid to drugs specifically for FR-positive tumor cells, in which these folate-drug conjugates are internalized after binding, with subsequent drug delivery.

Initial folate-targeting studies were conducted with radiolabeled and fluorescent proteins covalently attached to folic acid, but subsequently this technique has been extended to conjugates of radiopharmaceutical agents, magnetic resonance imaging (MRI) contrast agents, low-molecular weight chemotheraputic agents, antisense oligonucleotides and ribozymes, proteins, liposomes with entrapped drugs, drug-loaded nanoparticles, and plasmids.[54]

A typical structure for a folate-drug conjugate contains pteroic acid, a linker to avoid the lower affinity of the conjugate for the FR that occurs when the drug is positioned too close to the pteroic acid core, a cleavable bond which is very often a disulfide moiety and, finally, the drug. The linker usually is a peptide that contains a glutamic acid residue attached to the pteroate portion, thus giving rise to a folic acid moiety. It may also be a polymer or a carbohydrate.

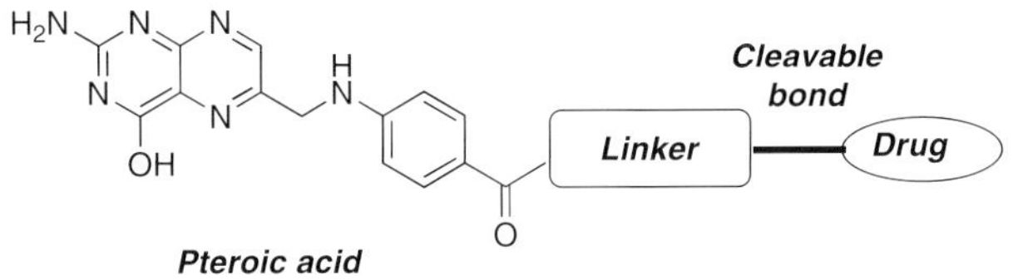

Pteroic acid

Many folate-drug conjugates have been preclinically studied. The structure of one of these drugs, namely the EC-16-mitomycin C conjugate, is given. Among those that have reached clinical trials we will mention EC-145, which is a folate-targeted conjugate of a *Vinca* alkaloid in clinical stage development as a treatment for patients with refractory or metastatic folate-receptor positive cancers. Another example is EC-0225, which contains both a vinca alkaloid and a mitomycin C attached to a single folate molecule.

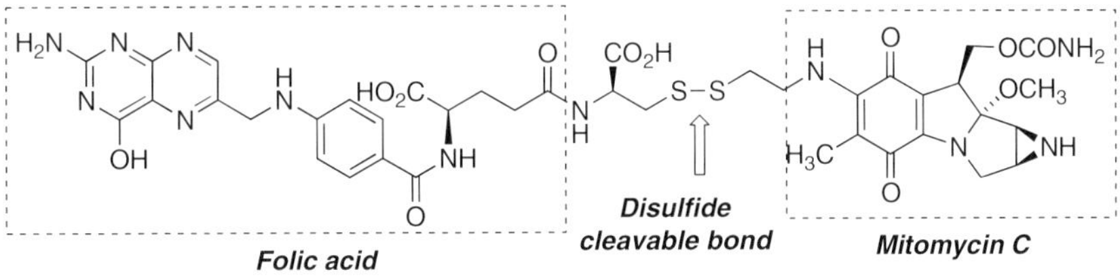

EC16-mitomycin

In a new approach to cancer immunotherapy[55] that aims at rendering the tumors more immunogenic, we will mention EC-17, a folate-targeted hapten (a highly antigenic molecule) studied as a potential treatment of metastatic renal and ovarian cancer. The general strategy of this multistep process can be summarized as follows (Fig. 11.26):

1. The surface of FR-positive tumor cells is saturated with a folate-hapten conjugate (in this case EC-17) against which the cancer-bearing host has a preexisting or induced immunity.
2. When these tumor cells are saturated with millions of folate receptor-targeted haptens, they attract anti-hapten antibodies to the tumor cell surface.
3. The antibody-coated tumor cells are recognized by immune cells containing surface proteins known as Fc receptors, such as natural killer cells, macrophages, neutrophils and mast cells, and stimulation of Fc receptor mounts an antitumor response against the anti-hapten antibody opsonized tumor cells that leads to their destruction.

Finally, we will mention EC-20, a folate-targeted radiopharmaceutical imaging agent used to identify folate-receptor positive cancers. It allows to identify tumors that overexpress this receptor without the need for a tissue biopsy and hence to select the patients that will be most likely to respond to folate-targeted therapy.

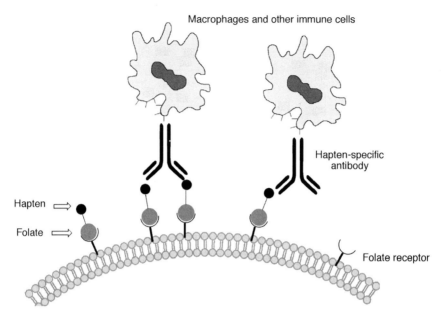

Macrophages and other immune cells

Hapten-specific
antibody

Hapten ⇨

Folate ⇨

Folate receptor

FIGURE 11.26   Cancer immunotherapy with a folate-targeted hapten.

7. LIPOSOMES AND NANOPARTICLES IN ANTICANCER DRUG TARGETING

A critical advantage in treating cancer with non–solution-based therapies is the previously mentioned leaky vasculature inherently present in cancerous tissues due to the rapid vascularization. However, the injected nanoparticles will usually be taken up by the liver, spleen, and other parts of the reticuloendothelial system (RES), depending on their surface characteristics and size. To obtain particles with longer circulation times, and hence greater ability to target to a given tumor, they should be 100 nm or less in diameter and have a hydrophilic surface in order to reduce clearance by macrophages. Additionally, coating of hydrophilic polymers can originate a cloud of chains at their surface that will repel plasma proteins.[56]

Cancer-related nanotechnological devices include liposomes for the therapy of different cancers,[57] nanosized magnetic resonance imaging (MRI) contrast agents for neuro-oncological interventions[58] and novel nanoparticle-based methods for the high-specificity detection of DNA and proteins.[59]

7.1. Liposomes

Since the observation that phospholipids form closed bilayered structures in aqueous systems, liposomes have become quite common pharmaceutical carriers.[60] In general, drugs can be loaded into any of the three areas of a liposome: the internal aqueous compartment (A), where hydrophilic drugs such as doxorubicin are usually carried; the lipid bilayer (B), where lipid soluble drugs are usually carried, and the interface between the lipid bilayer and the aqueous compartment (C), as is shown in Fig. 11.27. The drug-loaded liposomes enter the tumor tissues through the previously mentioned EPR effect. They can then be adsorbed or fused with the cell membrane and release their contents into the cytoplasm or use the endocytosis process. Classical liposomes are thus designed to concentrate in the tumor mass and provide a more targeted delivery of drugs, but soon after their injection they may be attacked by proteins and then broken down by the monocyte–phagocyte system, with premature release of the drug.

More recently, liposomes coated with a protective polymer have been developed to avoid the interaction with opsonizing proteins. The most common polymer is PEG, which provides a water-soluble coating. PEGylation has permitted the development of "stealth" liposomes that can evade the immune system. Current research on this topic is focused on attaching PEG to the liposomes in such a way that it can be removed in order to facilitate cell uptake under local pathologic conditions, specially the decreased pH commonly found in tumors. This can be achieved by linking the polymer to the phosphatidylethanolamine molecules that make up the liposome through an N-glutaryl spacer (Fig. 11.28).

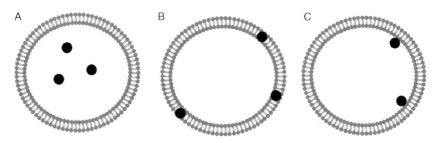

FIGURE 11.27   Possible locations of drugs in a liposome.

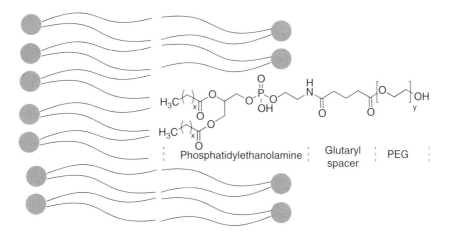

FIGURE 11.28   An example of a PEGylated bilayered phospholipid.

Daunorubicin and doxorubicin are two of the drugs most commonly formulated as liposomes, and PEGylated liposomal doxorubicin (doxil) is employed against Kaposi's sarcoma and other solid tumors with mild myelosuppression, minimal hair loss, and a low risk of cardiotoxicity.[61] In these liposomes, doxorubicin is transported in the hydrophilic internal aqueous compartment (Fig. 11.29).

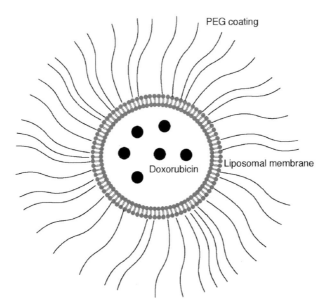

FIGURE 11.29   A doxorubicin-carrying PEGylated liposome (doxil).

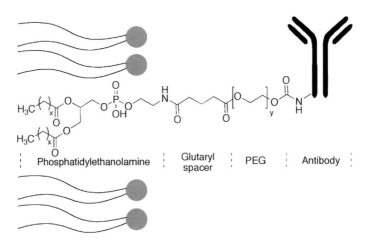

FIGURE 11.30   Antibody-containing immunoliposomens.

DaunoXome is another liposome formulation that is used for first-line chemotherapy in advanced AIDS-related Kaposi's sarcoma. This formulation contains a solution of daunorubicin encapsulated within liposomes composed of a lipid bilayer of L-α-distearoylphosphatidylcholine (DSPC) and cholesterol.[62]

Antibody-targeted immunoliposomes may have the antibody covalently coupled, either to the reactive phospholipids in the membrane or to the PEG hydroxy groups (Fig. 11.30). Alternatively, they may be hydrophobically anchored into the liposomal membrane after modifying the antibody by the attachment of a lipophilic moiety.

7.2. Nanoparticle albumin bound technology

Besides angiogenesis, tumors have adapted other mechanisms to meet their increased need for nutrients. One of them is the gp60 pathway, by which nutrients are preferentially transported across the endothelial barrier when attached to albumin. They also secrete a specialized protein called SPARC (Secreted Protein Acidic and Rich in Cysteine) into the tumor's interstitium. The SPARC protein acts as a highly charged receptor to specifically attract and bind albumin and albumin-bound nutrients to concentrate them within the tumor's interstitium avoiding their diffusion outside the tumor cell. On the basis of these mechanisms, it has been developed a nanoparticle albumin-bound technology to transport and deliver drugs into tumors, instead of nutrients. Obviously, these drugs have to be previously bound to albumin. Nanoparticles that incorporate an albumin-bound taxane (Abraxane) are used for the treatment of metastatic breast cancer.[63,64]

REFERENCES

1. Rooseboom, M., Commandeur, J. N. M., and Vermeulen, N. P. E. (2004). *Pharmacol. Rev.* **56**, 53.
2. Tew, K. D. (2005). *Expert Opin. Investig. Drugs* **14**, 1047.
3. Brown, J. M., and Wilson, W. R. (2004). *Nat. Rev. Cancer* **4**, 437.
4. Naylor, M. A., and Thomson, P. (2001). *Mini-Rev. Med. Chem.* **1**, 17.
5. Patterson, L. H. (1993). *Cancer Metastasis Rev.* **12**, 119.
6. http://www.clinicaltrials.gov/ct/show/NCT00394628.
7. Patterson, L. H. (2002). *Drug Metab. Rev.* **34**, 581.
8. Patterson, L. H., and Murray, G. I. (2002). *Curr. Pharm. Des.* **8**, 1335.
9. Antonini, I., Lin, T. S., Cosby, L. A., Dai, Y. R., and Sartorelli, A. C. (1982). *J. Med. Chem.* **25**, 730.
10. Hatzigrigoriou, E., Papadopoulou, M. V., Shields, D., and Bloomer, W. D. (1993). *Oncol. Res.* **5**, 29.
11. De Oliveira, R. B., and Alves, R. J. (2002). *Quim. Nova* **25**, 976.
12. Palmer, B. D., van Zijl, P., Denny, W. A., and Wilson, W. R. (1995). *J. Med. Chem.* **38**, 1229.
13. Ware, D. C., Palmer, B. D., Wilson, W. R., and Denny, W. A. (1993). *J. Med. Chem.* **36**, 1839.
14. Kriste, A. G., Tercel, M., Anderson, R. F., Ferry, D. M., and Wilson, W. R. (2002). *Radiat. Res.* **158**, 753.
15. Shibamoto, Y., Ling, Z., Hatta, H., Mori, M., and Nishimoto, S.-I. (2000). *Jpn. J. Cancer Res.* **91**, 433.
16. Aghi, M., Hochberg, F., and Breakfield, X. O. (2000). *J. Gene Med.* **2**, 148.
17. Chung-Faye, G., Palmer, D., Anderson, D., Clark, J., Downes, M., Baddeley, J., Hussain, S., Murray, P. I., Searle, P., Seymour, L., Harris, P. A., Ferry, D., *et al.* (2001). *Clin. Cancer Res.* **7**, 2662.
18. Knox, R. J., Friedlos, F., Jaman, M., and Roberts, J. J. (1988). *Biochem. Pharmacol.* **37**, 4661.
19. McCarthy, H. O., Yakkundi, A., McErlane, V., Hughes, C. M., Keilty, G., Murray, M., Patterson, L. H., Hirst, D. G., McKeown, S. R., and Robson, T. (2003). *Cancer Gene Ther.* **10**, 40.

20. Cowen, R. L., Williams, K. J., Chinje, E. C., Jaffar, M., Sheppard, F. C. D., Telfer, B. A., Wind, N. S., and Stratford, I. J. (2004). *Cancer Res.* **64,** 1396.
21. Russell, S. J., and Peng, K. W. (2007). *Trends Pharmacol. Sci.* **28,** 326.
22. Houba1, P. H. J., Boven, E., van der Meulen-Muileman, I. H., Leenders, L. G. G., Scheeren, J. W., Pinedo, H. M., and Haisma, H. J. (2001). *Int. J. Cancer* **91,** 550.
23. Springer, C. J., and Nicolescu-Duvaz, I. (2000). *J. Clin. Invest.* **105,** 1161.
24. Mauger, A. B., Burke, P. J., Somani, H. F., Friedlos, F., and Knox, R. J. (1994). *J. Med. Chem.* **37,** 3452.
25. Basgshawe, K. D., and Begent, R. H. J. (1996). *Adv. Drug Deliv. Rev.* **22,** 365.
26. Francis, R. J., Sharma, S. K., Springer, C., Green, A. J., Hope-Stone, L. D., Sena, L., Martin, J., Adamson, K. L., Robbins, A., Gumbrell, L., O'Malley, D., Tsiompanou, E., *et al.* (2002). *Br. J. Cancer* **87,** 600.
27. Vicent, M. J., and Duncan, R. (2006). *Trends Biotechnol.* **24,** 39.
28. Delgado, C., Francis, G. E., and Fischer, D. (1992). *Crit. Rev. Ther. Drug Carrier Syst.* **9,** 249.
29. Graham, M. L. (2003). *Adv. Drug Deliv. Rev.* **55,** 1293.
30. Delman, K. A., Brown, T. D., Thomas, M., Ensor, C. M., Holtsberg, F. W., Bomalaski, J. S., Clark, M. A., and Curley, S. A. (2005). *Proc. Am. Soc. Clin. Oncol.* Abstract 4139.
31. Unger, C., Müller, C., Jäger, E., Bausch, M., Roberts, J., Al-Batran, S., and Sethuraman, N. (2005). *Proc. Am. Soc. Clin. Oncol.* Abstract 3130.
32. Campos, L. T., Folbe, M., Meza, L., Charu, V., Dansey, R., and Xie, F. (2005). *Proc. Am. Soc. Clin. Oncol.* Abstract 8115.
33. Jain, R. K. (1987). *Cancer Metastasis Rev.* **6,** 559.
34. Kratz, F., Warnecke, A., Schmid, B., Chung, D.-E., and Gitzel, M. (2006). *Curr. Med. Chem.* **13,** 477.
35. Vicent, M. J., and Duncan, R. (2006). *Trends Biotechnol.* **24,** 39.
36. Vasey, P. A., Twelves, C., Kaye, S. B., Wilson, P., Morrison, R., Duncan, R., Thomson, A. H., Hilditch, T. E., Murray, T., Burtles, S., and Cassidy, J. (1999). *Clin. Cancer Res.* **5,** 83.
37. Meerum Terwogt, J. M., Bokkel Huinink, W. W., Schellens, J. H. M., Schot, M., Mandjes, I. A. M., Zurlo, M. G., Rocchetti, M., Rosing, H., Koopman, F. J., and Beijnen, J. H. (2001). *Anticancer Drugs* **12,** 315.
38. Caiolfa, V. R., Zamal, M., Fiorini, A., Frigerio, E., D'Argy, R., Ghigleri, A., Farao, M., Angelucci, F., and Suarato, A. (2000). *J. Controlled Release* **65,** 105.
39. Gianasi, E., Wasil, M., Evagorou, E. G., Keddle, A., Wislon, G., and Duncan, R. (1999). *Eur. J. Cancer* **3,** 994.
40. Rademaker-Lakhai, J. M., Terret, C., Howell, S. B., Baud, C. M., de Boer, R. F., Pluim, D., Beijnen, J. H., Schellens, J. H. M., and Droz, J.-P. (2004). *Clin. Cancer Res.* **10,** 3386.
41. Sood, P., Thurmond, K. B., Jacob, J. E., Waller, L. K., Silva, G. O., Stewart, D. R., and Nowotnik, D. P. (2006). *Bioconjugate Chem.* **17,** 1270.
42. Seymour, L. W., Ferry, D. R., Anderson, D., Hesslewood, S., Julyan, P. J., Poyner, R., Doran, J., Young, A. M., Burtles, S., and Kerr, D. J. (2002). *J. Clin. Oncol.* **20,** 1668.
43. Shaffer, S. A., Baker Lee, C., Kumar, A., and Singer, J. W. (2002). *Eur. J. Cancer* **38,** S129.
44. Singer, J. W., Shaffer, S., Baker, B., Bernareggi, A., Stromatt, S., Nienstedt, D., and Besman, M. (2005). *Anticancer Drugs* **16,** 243.
45. Langer, M., Kratz, F., Rothen-Rutishauser, B., Wunderli-Allenspach, H., and Beck-Sickinger, A. G. (2001). *J. Med. Chem.* **44,** 1341.
46. Greenwald, R. B., Conover, C. D., and Choe, Y. H. (2003). *Crit. Rev. Ther. Drug Carrier Syst.* **55,** 217.
47. Ochoa, L., Tolcher, A. W., Rizzo, J., Schwartz, G. H., Patnaik, A., Hammond, L., McCreery, H., Denis, L., Hidalgo, M., Kwiatek, J., Mcguire, J., and Rowinsky, E. K. (2000). *J. Clin. Oncol.* **19,** 198a.
48. Walker, M. A., Dubowchik, G. M., Hofstead, S. J., Trail, P. A., and Firestone, R. A. (2002). *Biorg. Med. Chem. Lett.* **12,** 217.
49. Walker, M. A., King, H. D., Dalterio, R. A., Trail, P. A., Firestone, R. A., and Dubowchik, G. M. (2004). *Bioorg. Med. Chem. Lett.* **14,** 4323.
50. Larson, R. A., Sievers, E. L., Stadtmauer, E. A., Löwenberg, B., Estey, E. H., Dombret, H., Theobald, M., Voliotis, D., Bennett, J. M., Richie, M., Leopold, L. H., Berger, M. S., *et al.* (2005). *Cancer* **104,** 1442.
51. Milenic, D. E., Brady, E. D., and Brechwiel, M. W. (2004). *Nat. Rev. Drug Discov.* **3,** 488.
52. Hedge, S., and Carter, J. (2004). *Annu. Rep. Med. Chem.* **39,** 337.

53. Satchi, R., and Duncan, R. (2001). *Brit. J. Cancer* **85,** 1070.
54. Leamon, C. P., and Reddy, J. A. (2004). *Adv. Drug Deliv. Rev.* **56,** 1127.
55. Lu, Y., Sega, E., Leamon, C. P., and Low, P. S. (2004). *Adv. Drug Deliv. Rev.* **56,** 1161.
56. Brannon-Peppas, L., and Blanchette, J. O. (2004). *Adv. Drug Deliv. Rev.* **56,** 1649.
57. Park, J. W. (2002). *Breast Cancer Res.* **4,** 95.
58. Kircher, M. F., Mahmood, U., King, R. S., Weissleder, R., and Josephson, L. (2003). *Cancer Res.* **63,** 8122.
59. Ferrari, M. (2005). *Nat. Rev. Cancer* **5,** 161.
60. Torchilin, V. P. (2005). *Nat. Rev. Drug Discov.* **4,** 145.
61. O'Shaughnessy, J. A. (2003). *Clin. Breast Cancer* **4,** 318.
62. Forssen, E. A. (1997). *Adv. Drug Deliv. Rev.* **24,** 133.
63. Brigger, I., Dubernet, C., and Couvreur, P. (2002). *Adv. Drug Deliv. Rev.* **54,** 631.
64. Moghimi, S. M., Hunter, A. C., and Murray, J. C. (2005). *FASEB J.* **19,** 311.

CHAPTER **12**

Drugs That Modulate Resistance to Antitumor Agents

Contents

1. ATP-Binding Cassette Efflux Pumps in Anticancer
   Drug Resistance   388
   1.1. General features of ABC efflux pumps   388
   1.2. P-glycoprotein   390
2. Glutathione and Glutathione-*S*-Transferase in Anticancer
   Drug Resistance   397
   2.1. Inhibitors of glutathione biosynthesis   398
   2.2. Inhibitors of glutathione-*S*-transferase   399
3. Chemosensitizers Targeting DNA-Repair Systems   401
   3.1. Inhibitors of O^6-alkylguanine-DNA alkyltransferase   403
   3.2. Potential antitumor adjuvants targeting the BER process   404
   3.3. Inhibitors of enzymes involved in double-strand DNA break
        repair pathways   411
4. Antitumor Drug Resistance Related to Extracellular pH:
   Tumor-Associated Carbonic Anhydrase as an Anticancer Target   412
   References   414

Most drugs that are able to cure or prolong life of patients in several types of cancer become ineffective some time after their first application, because cancer cells elude chemotherapy through a myriad ways. This problem will continue to be present even if personalized cancer treatments become possible in the future.[1]

For instance, when an essential protein is therapeutically inactivated, the selective pressure thus created makes tumor cells evolve mechanisms of resistance in a manner similar to the bacterial resistance after exposure to anti-microbial agents. These mechanisms include the following:

1. Production of a drug-resistant variant of the targeted protein.
2. Substitution of its cellular function by upregulating alternate pathways.
3. Enhanced expression and function of transporters involved in drug efflux.

Medicinal Chemistry of Anticancer Drugs
DOI: 10.1016/B978-0-444-52824-7.00012-3

The existence of chemotherapy-sensitive and -resistant tumor cells was known very soon, but the interpretation of this phenomenon had to wait until 1973, when it was demonstrated that a major factor in resistance of cancer cells was a reduced drug accumulation due to overexpression of drug efflux transporters. It was also shown that after the development of a resistance mechanism to a single drug, cells could display cross-resistance to other structural and mechanistically unrelated drugs, a phenomenon known as multidrug resistance (MDR),[2] which is one of the main obstacles in the chemotherapy of cancer. Its inhibition, by combination of chemosensitizers with antitumor compounds, continues to be an active field of research because the availability of safe and potent reversal agents would be very beneficial for clinical use.

Additionally, resistance to cancer chemotherapy is also associated with a failure of the apoptotic pathways, because cells induce a network of upstream factors that transmit pro- and anti-apoptotic signals in response to damaged DNA. For instance, p53 and Bcl-2 are upstream factors that appear to be involved in cisplatin resistance.

1. ATP-BINDING CASSETTE EFFLUX PUMPS IN ANTICANCER DRUG RESISTANCE

The MDR phenotype is mostly associated with the overexpression of P-glycoprotein (P-gp, P-170) and multidrug resistance-associated protein 1 (MRP1). Both proteins are members of the superfamily of membrane transport carriers known as ATP-binding cassette (ABC) proteins, which hydrolyse ATP as an energy source to drive the outwardly directed transport of substrates against a concentration gradient and therefore reduce their intracellular concentration.[3] To date, most studied compounds that reverse this event (MDR modulators, resistance modifiers, chemosensitizers) are P-gp inhibitors. Three generations of these inhibitors have been developed but, although they have enhanced the understanding of the mechanisms involved in chemotherapy resistance, their success in clinical applications has been limited so far since no drug acting through this mechanism has reached the market.

1.1. General features of ABC efflux pumps

ABC transporters are 'pump' proteins found in the membranes of bacteria and human cells. They are present in organs related to digestion and excretion as a protective mechanism that eliminates toxic chemicals, and have a great importance in drug absorption through biological membranes like those found in the intestinal wall. These transporters are the biggest single cause for failure of anticancer chemotherapy, and the genes responsible for their synthesis are activated by environmental stress (e.g., by foreign chemicals or heat). They act by removing the anticancer drugs from the cell (Fig. 12.1A), and much effort has been placed in

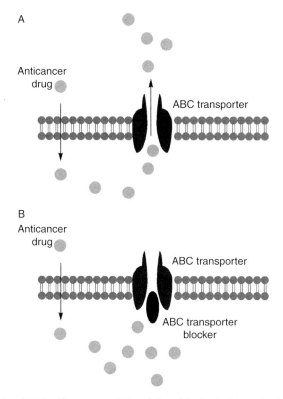

FIGURE 12.1   Effects of ABC efflux pumps (A) and their blockade (B) on the intracellular concentrations of anticancer drugs.

the development of compounds that behave as blockers of the transport protein and hence can restore the sensitivity of the cell to the anticancer drug (Fig. 12.1B).

P-gp, a member of the ABCB transporter subfamily, is a membrane-associated 170-kDa glycoprotein that effluxes ~50% of all anticancer agents used clinically today without chemically modifying them. It is overexpressed in many intrinsically resistant tumors and in others that acquire resistance during chemotherapy treatment. When the *mdr* gene, which encodes P-gp, is transfected into drug-sensitive cells they became resistant to these agents.[4]

Another functionally related member of the ABC transporter subfamily is MRP1, which confers resistance to the vinca alkaloids, anthracyclines, epidophyllotoxins, and glucuronide-, glutathione-, and sulfate conjugates of drugs. Other members of this subfamily that transport the same drugs are MRP2 and MRP3, while MRP4 and MRP5 transport nucleotide and nucleoside analogs. Another ABC transporter is the breast cancer resistance protein (BCRP), a member of the ABCG transporter subfamily that partially overlaps the substrate specificity of P-gp and MRPs, conferring resistance to mitoxantrone, methotrexate, topotecan, and SN-38.[5]

The ABC transporters are asymmetrically distributed when they are present in the same cell. For example, in intestinal epithelium cells, P-gp, MRP2, and BCRP are located at the brush borders while MRP1 and MRP3 are located at the basolateral surface.

The ABC transporters are also differently expressed in normal conditions. Thus, P-gp is expressed in several organs such as intestine, lung, kidney, liver, adrenal gland, certain hematological cells, blood–brain barrier, and placenta, which suggests that it is important in limiting the oral absorption of xenobiotics and may help to limit access to the central nervous system through the blood–brain barrier. Several of these roles have been confirmed in knockout mice lacking one or both of the two murine genes for P-gp, *mdr 1a*, and *mdr1b*. MRP1 is expressed in all tissues, although knockout mice lacking both alleles of *mrp1* gene are viable, while MRP2 and MRP3 have very limited expression. BCRP is expressed in breast ducts and lobules, the intestine epithelium, and the liver canalicular membrane.

Most MDR modulators act by binding to P-gp and MRP, inhibiting their drug-effluxing activity. Some others act by indirect mechanisms, including inhibition of the expression of the *mdr1* gene.[6] General structure–activity studies of this therapeutic group are hampered by the very heterogeneous chemical structure of compounds that have showed this activity, although some conclusions regarding the location of binding domains of P-gp and the structural requirements for MDR reversal have been drawn.

These membrane-bound proteins are very difficult to study by nuclear magnetic resonance (NMR) or X-ray diffraction techniques, and currently there is no detailed information on the structures of these proteins and their substrate or inhibitor binding sites, so far preventing *de novo* design approaches.

1.2. P-glycoprotein

Expulsion of drugs from the cell by P-gp is explained by the traditional 'hydrophobic vacuum cleaner' model, although overexpression of the *mdr1* gene triggers other mechanisms that can partially explain resistance.[7] P-gp contains two transmembrane domains that form a single barrel with a central pore that is open to the extracellular surface and spans much of the membrane depth. After ATP binding, a major conformational change is induced and the central pore is opened along its length, allowing access of hydrophobic substrates from the membrane and their ejection to the outside. Chemosensitizers are P-gp modulators that are able to reverse this activity through a direct binding to the transporter. The existence of at least three P-gp modulator binding sites has been established, although probably not all of them are capable of drug transport.[8] Other mechanisms to reverse this resistance involve perturbation of the membrane environment and interference with drug sequestration by cellular organelles (Fig. 12.2).

The extensive list of traditional P-gp substrates includes the anthracyclines (doxorubicin, daunorubicin), *Vinca* alkaloids (vinblastine, vincristine), colchicine, epipodophyllotoxins (etoposide, teniposide), and paclitaxel, among others. Besides these compounds, some of the new antitumor drugs, such as the antileukaemia drug imatinib, the marine natural product ecteinascidin 743, and the

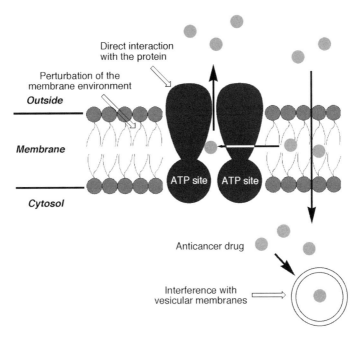

FIGURE 12.2   Modes of action of P-gp modulators.

calicheamicin conjugate gemtuzumab ozogamicin, have been shown to be excreted by this mechanism.

Because MDR is a very complex process for which there is no precise molecular-level description, great difficulty is found in establishing structure–activity relationships. A complicating factor is the above-mentioned existence of several binding sites in P-gp. These sites are located near to another binding ligands according to the distribution of their hydrophobic and polar elements rather than their chemical motifs.[9] In this regard, a difficulty found in SAR studies is the use of inhibitory concentration (IC_{50}) values without considering whether modulators acted by the same mechanism and binding mode. A better alternative for determining the biological activity of chemosensitizers appears to be the measurement of the inhibition of P-gp ATPase activity.[10]

1.2.1. P-gp inhibitors

P-gp inhibitors are non-cytotoxic agents that, when used in combination with drugs pumped by P-gp, restore the sensitivity to these therapeutic agents maintaining their intracellular concentration.[11,12] The pharmacological approach to circumvention of MDR began with the report by Tsuruo that the calcium channel blocker verapamil and the phenothiazine derivative trifluperazine potentiate the activity of vincristine.[13]

Since that time, the identification of lead compounds in this area has been based mainly on serendipity. The first generation of P-gp inhibitors included compounds that were developed for other therapeutic purposes but showed their resistance modulation effect when administered in combination with some anticancer treatments. Consequently, they showed undesirable side effects at concentrations necessary to inhibit P-gp clinically. Among them, we find the previously mentioned calcium channel blocker verapamil or the immunosuppressive agent cyclosporin A. Verapamil, vinblastine, and digoxin appear to have superimposable binding sites in spite of their structural differences, which is explained by the fact that different drugs can occupy different receptor points in different binding modes.[14]

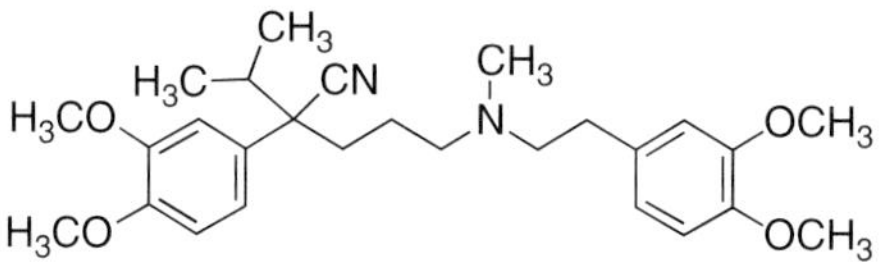

Verapamil

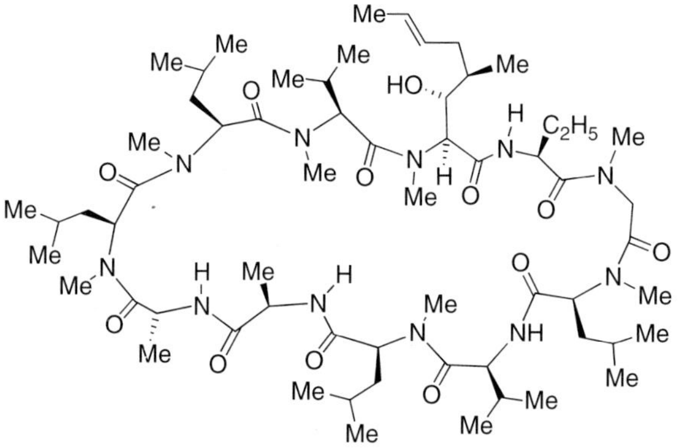

Cyclosporin A

The second generation of chemosensitizers includes analogs of the above-mentioned compounds that were designed to reduce their toxicity. Among them, the (R)-isomer of verapamil, named dexverapamil, lacks its cardiac effects while retaining the ability to inhibit P-gp. Similarly, PSC-833 (valspodar) is a structural analogue of cyclosporin A that lacks its immunosuppressive effects. However, in spite of their improved activity, both compounds are non-selective. For instance, PSC-833 inhibits P-gp and MRP2, as well as other proteins of the ABC superfamily. The clinical value of these agents is also uncertain because, as it will be mentioned later, their substrate specificity for P-gp is similar to the one they show for cytochrome P450, which explains why PSC-833 is involved in pharmacokinetic interactions with most anticancer drugs, requiring dose adjustment and leading to a high interpatient variability.[15] It is worth mentioning that it has been suggested that valspodar and cyclosporin may have an anticancer effect independently of their action on MDR.[16]

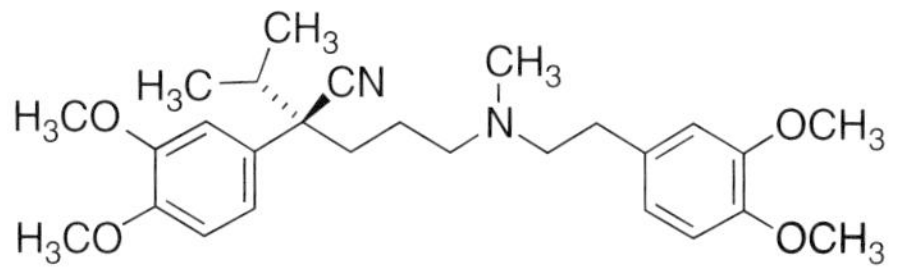

Dexverapamil

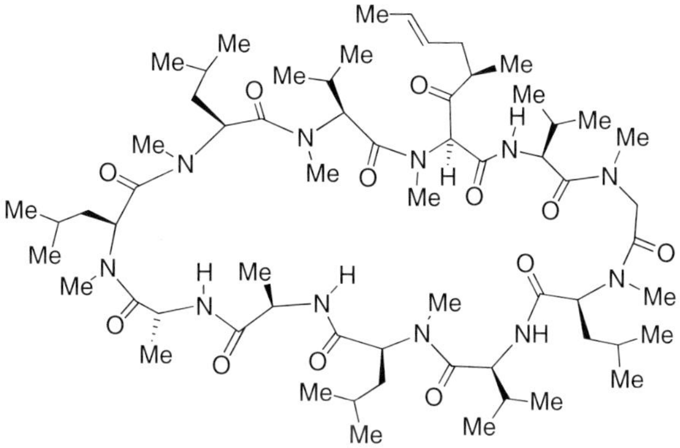

PSC-833 (Valspodar)

The third generation of chemosensitizers attempted the development of compounds more specific and more potent as P-gp inhibitors than the earlier studied agents. Such inhibitors would have fewer undesirable effects than compounds that inhibit two or more transporters with overlapping functions. Among the P-gp inhibitors of the third generation that have been evaluated clinically, VX-710 (biricodar) and MS-209 (dofequidar) inhibit P-gp and MRP1, elacridar (GF120918) inhibits P-gp and BCRP, while LY-335979 (zosuquidar), XR9576 (tariquidar), and ONT-093 (OC-144–093) are selective inhibitors of P-gp. Biricodar is a simplified analogue of tacrolimus, an immunosuppressive macrolactone which has an activity similar to cyclosporin. It has shown an optimal pharmacological profile in combination with paclitaxel,[17] and a Phase II study has demonstrated its good safety and tolerability.[18] Dofequidar, in combination with etoposide or adriamycin, resulted in marked inhibition of methastases in refractory small-cell lung cancer patients,[19] and other clinical study showed that it increases the antitumor efficiency of docetaxel.[20] The related compound MS-073 has been used to study the brain distribution of several neurokinin-1 antagonists, proving that some of them are effectively transported by P-gp across the blood–brain barrier.[21] Zosuquidar (LY-335979) is one of the most potent P-gp inhibitors described to date.[22] It has fewer pharmacokinetic interactions than other MDR modulators because of its low affinity for P450 cytochromes, and it entered advanced clinical studies on acute myeloid leukaemia patients.[23] Pharmacokinetic studies with ONT-093 (OC-144–093) showed that this compound does not interact significantly with the metabolism of paclitaxel because it is not a cytochrome P4503A (CYP3A) substrate,[24] and that it is selective towards P-gp being a good clinical candidate as a MDR modulator.

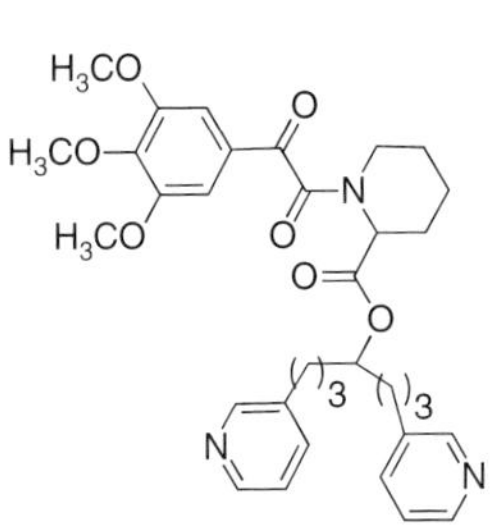

VX-710 (biricodar)

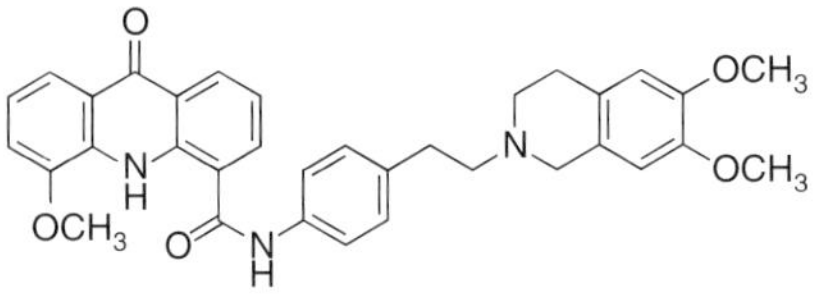

Elacridar
GF120918

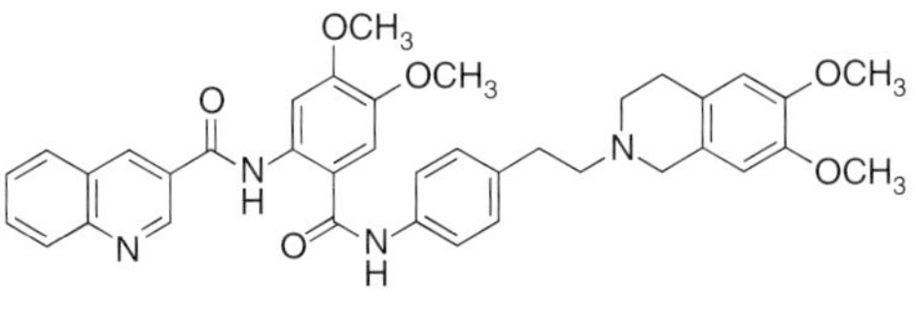

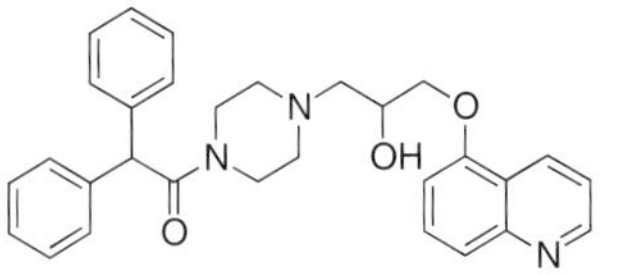

MS-209 (dofequidar)

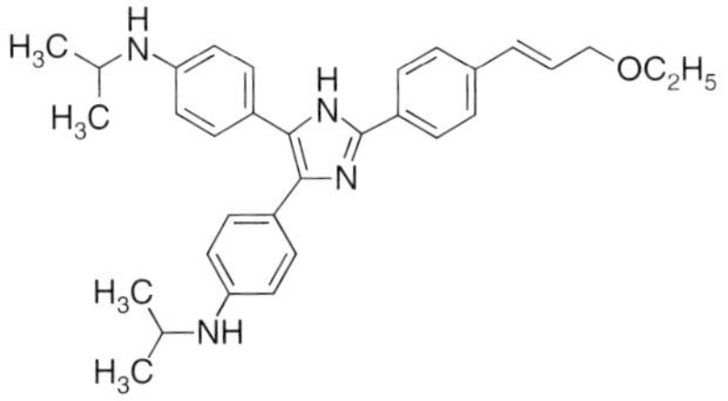

XR9576 (tariquidar)

LY-335979 (zosuquidar)

ONT-093
OC-144-093

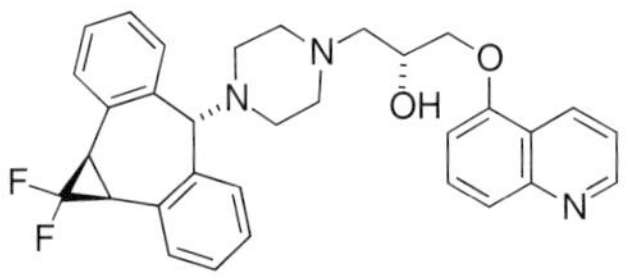

Laniquidar is a potent orally active MDR inhibitor that is undergoing Phase II clinical trials in metastatic breast cancer in combination with taxols.[25] The triazineaminopiperidine derivative S-9788, which inhibits P-gp specifically with regard to MRPs, showed cardiac toxicity in Phase I clinical trials, but this drawback can be circumvented if this compound is combined with verapamil or PSC-833.[26] Other P-pg inhibitors that are in advanced clinical trials as MDR modulators[2,29] are SN-22995, ethacrynic acid, and irofulven.

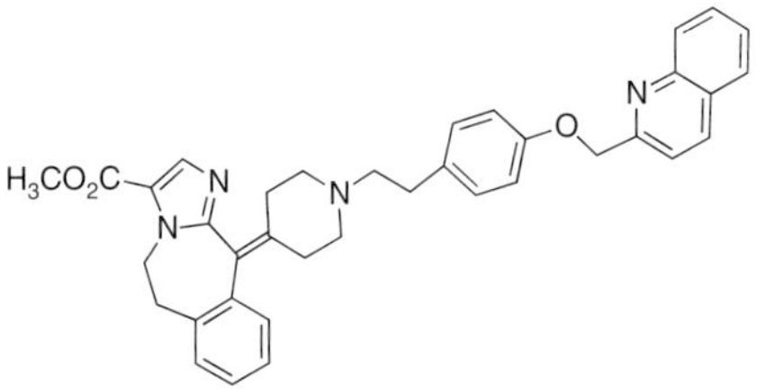

Laniquidar (R-101933)

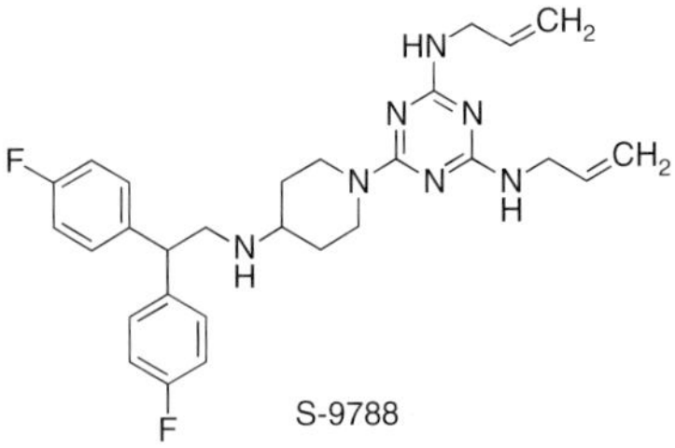

S-9788

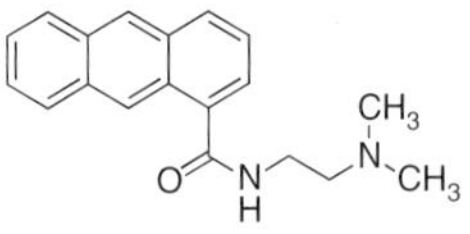

SN-22995

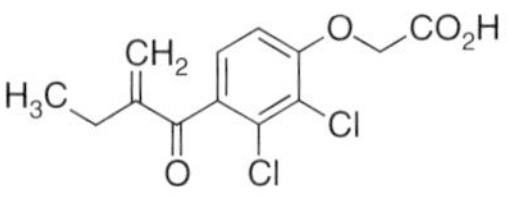

Ethacrynic acid

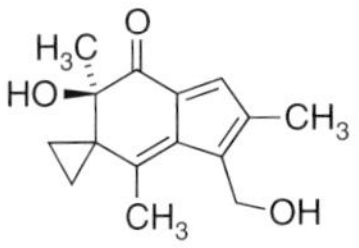

Irofulven

An ideal resistance modulator through inhibition of P-gp would have to inhibit it selectively, that is without affecting other membrane transporters or inhibiting CYP3A4. As we have previously mentioned, the most obvious reason for enhanced toxicity in the presence of an efflux blocker is the increased plasma concentration of the parent oncolytic because the substrate specificity of P-gp is similar to that of cytochrome P450 enzyme CYP3A4, which is important in the metabolism of many antitumor drugs. Consequently, inhibitors of both proteins will result in drug–drug interactions and a significant reduction in the clearance of the co-administered anticancer drugs. In order to try to circumvent this toxicity, clinical studies with MDR modulators have been conducted with reduced doses of chemotherapy, as compared to those routinely used in clinical practice, and these doses may be too low for some patients or still too high for others. The most promising compound that seems to overcome this serious problem is zosuquidar, which has a P-gp/CYP3A4 affinity ratio of around 60.[27]

The current situation is that, although the existence of multiple and heterogeneous resistance mechanisms and the own toxicity of modulators due to alterations in the pharmacokinetics of the associated cytotoxic agents have arisen serious doubts about the clinical relevance of P-gp inhibition in cancer chemotherapy, it is expected that the use of optimized modulators will lead to a significant improvement in cancer chemotherapy, specially in hematological malignancies.[28]

The first attempts to identify a pharmacophore for P-gp[29] inhibition used a software package to analyze a set of structurally diverse ligands, which led to the identification of a number of pharmacophoric substructures (Fig. 12.3).[30] However, this conclusion was not particularly helpful in the design of new ligands as these fragments can be found in almost all bioactive molecules.

A subsequent study of more than 100 P-gp substrates led to the proposal of a well-defined set of structural elements for P-gp recognition, which is mainly based on the formation of hydrogen bonds.[31] Two different types of recognition elements were identified:

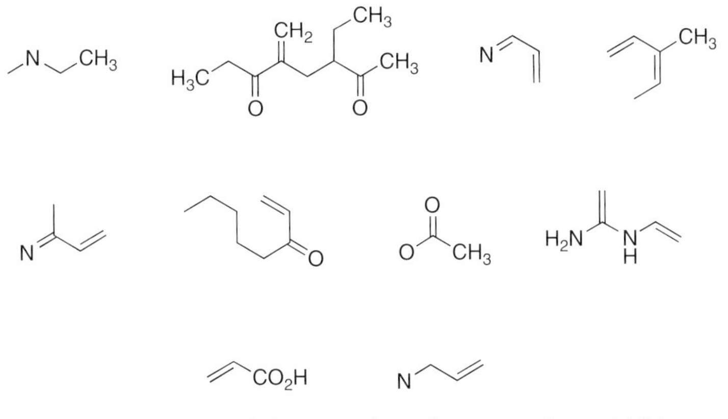

FIGURE 12.3   Proposed pharmacophoric fragments of P-gp inhibitors.

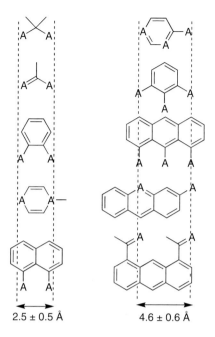

A = Hydrogen bonding acceptor group
(electron donor group)

FIGURE 12.4   Proposed structural elements for P-gp recognition.

1. Type I units, which contain two hydrogen bond acceptor (electron donor) groups with a separation of 2.5 ± 0.5 Å.
2. Type II units, which contain either three electron donor groups with a separation of 4.6 ± 0.6 Å between the outer units, or two electron donor groups with the same spatial separation (Fig. 12.4).[32 33]

All molecules containing at least one Type I or Type II unit are predicted to be P-gp substrates, and the number and strength of these hydrogen bonds is related to the affinity to the protein. Further rationale for this theory comes from the fact that the transmembrane sequences of P-gp involved in substrate interaction contain a high number of amino acids with hydrogen bond donor sites such as the OH groups of Ser, Thr and Tyr, the NH_2 group of Gln, the indolic NH group of Trp, and the SH group of Cys.

Another computer-aided substructural search coupled to a QSAR study of 609 compounds showed several pharmacophores, the most important of which was the fragment C–C–X–C–C, where X = N, O, nitrogen being preferentially tertiary. The most significant physicochemical property was found to be lipophilicity as measured by the $(\log P)^2$ parameter, while hydrophilic fragments such as carboxylic acids, phenols, anilines, and quaternary ammonium compounds are deactivating.[34] These findings correlate well with an independent study concluding that an effective P-gp modulator candidate should have a log P higher than 2.92, a molecular axis with at least 18 atoms, a high energy value for the Highest Occupied Molecular Orbital (HOMO), and at least one tertiary, basic nitrogen atom.[35] The role of lipids in MDR cells and the changes induced in the properties of membrane lipids by MDR modulators has been reviewed,[36] and, in this context, it has been proposed that MDR reversers should be designed to be lipophilic (log $P \approx$ 4) monobasic drugs with a near neutral pK_a (7–8) in order to maximize favourable drug–membrane interactions.[37] In addition, electrostatic interactions between the modulator and the membrane phospholipids also play an important role.

1.2.2. Structural manipulation of anticancer drugs aimed at circumventing P-gp

An alternative to the use of P-gp inhibitors is to introduce structural modifications in its substrates in order to increase passive diffusion, since the efflux pump cannot maintain a gradient and its pumping efficiency is poor when passive diffusion is sufficiently fast. This can be achieved by eliminating groups that solvate in water, decreasing their hydrogen bonding capacity by promoting intramolecular hydrogen bonds, and introducing lipophilic substituents such as halogen atoms, although there are still few published examples of this approach.[38]

1.2.3. Indirect inhibitors of MDR

The P-gp expression and function is influenced by several enzymes that, as cyclooxygenase 2 (COX-2)[39] or glucosylceramide synthase,[40] can be indirect targets in MDR inhibition. Certain compounds, such as the anticancer drug ecteinascidin-743, can prevent *mdr1* gene expression,[41] which can also be achieved by RNA interference through small RNA (siRNA) constructs.[42] However, inhibition of the biosynthesis of the transport proteins by use of antisense oligonucleotides related to MRP or P-gp mRNAs seems to be of low clinical relevance in spite of previous good *in vitro* results.[43]

Because of the ATPase activity of P-gp, intracellular ATP concentration is important for P-gp function, and inhibitors of the ATPase activity of P-gp, like vanadate ion, have been proposed as adjuvants in the chemotherapy of solid tumors.[44]

Finally, besides MDR inhibition, a number of alternative approaches can be used to kill cells expressing the MDR phenotype. One of these approaches is based on optimization of drug delivery by use of nanoparticles or liposomes[45] combined with hyperthermia.[46] Another obvious alternative to circumvent P-gp resistance is the design of new anticancer agents that are not substrates of this transporter, but this aim would require that neither of the other ABC transporters be involved in chemoresistance.

2. GLUTATHIONE AND GLUTATHIONE-S-TRANSFERASE IN ANTICANCER DRUG RESISTANCE

Glutathione (GSH) is a ubiquitous cysteine-containing tripeptide that is the predominant cellular thiol. GSH is a radical scavenger through its transformation to the disulphide derivative, but it is also a nucleophile that reacts with electrophiles to form deactivated conjugates readily excreted by a glutathione synthase (GS)-conjugated export pump, in a reaction that may occur spontaneously or with the help of the enzyme glutathione-S-transferase (GST).[47] In addition, GSH may directly or indirectly participate in DNA repair because it modulates the expression of transcription factors that potentially affect DNA repair and apoptosis, such as c-fos and c-jun,[48] and may protect tumor cells against apoptotic cell death through the preservation of protein mercapto groups in a reduced state because of its antioxidant properties.[49] Owing to its reactivity and high intracellular concentrations, glutathione (GSH) has been implicated in resistance of several chemotherapeutic agents, such as platinum-containing compounds,[50] alkylating agents,[51] and anthracyclines,[52] and research efforts have been directed to find compounds that modulate its activity.

2.1. Inhibitors of glutathione biosynthesis

Glutathione is synthesized in two steps from amino acid precursors: the first step, where glutamic acid and cysteine are joined, is catalyzed by γ-glutamylcysteine synthetase (γ-GCS), while addition of glycine takes place at the second step by the catalysis of GS (Fig. 12.5).

Since γ-GCS is the enzyme involved in the rate-limiting step of the GSH synthesis, depletion of intracellular GSH levels has been pursued by using inhibitors of this enzyme. Among these inhibitors, diazenes and ethacrynic acid have been preclinically evaluated, while L-buthionine-(S,R)-sulfoximine (L-BSO) has been further studied.[53]

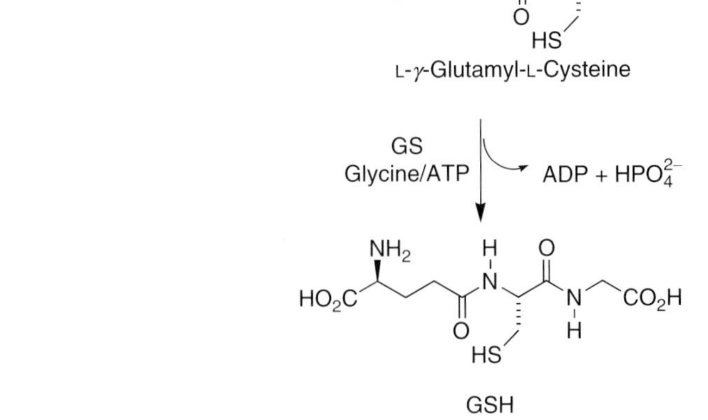

FIGURE 12.5 Biosynthesis of glutathione and its inhibition by L-BSO.

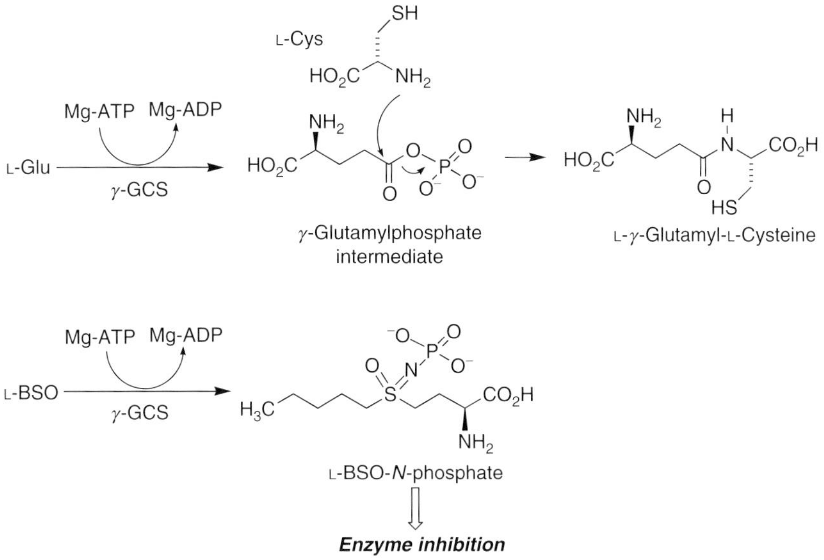

FIGURE 12.6   Inhibition of γ-GCS by L-BSO.

It is known that L-glutamate is phosphorylated by MgATP to form the enzyme-bound intermediate γ-glutamylphosphate, which subsequently reacts with the amino group of cysteine. Similarly, L-BSO is phosphorylated on the sulfoximine nitrogen. This phosphorylated product is tightly, although not covalently, bound to the active site of the enzyme γ-GCS, which remains inhibited until this product and MgADP are dissociated. The geometry of the sulfoximine group resembles the tetrahedral adduct formed in the attack of the cysteine amino group to the mixed anhydride γ-glutamylphosphate and it is considered as a transition state analogue (Fig. 12.6). The L-buthionine-(S)-sulfoximine causes essentially irreversible inhibition, while the L-buthionine-(R)-sulfoximine is a reversible inhibitor that binds competitively with respect to L-glutamate.[54]

L-BSO has proven its efficacy as an enhancer of the antitumor activity of the alkylating agent melphalan in Phase I and II clinical trials, while other clinical trials have shown that administration of L-BSO depletes intracellular GSH levels in circulating white blood cells as much as 60–80%. However, the extent to which this depletion enhances tumor cell sensitivity without augmenting toxicity to normal cells remains to be determined.[55]

The second strategy that has not been still tested clinically involves the use of a hammerhead ribozyme against γ-GCS mRNA (a ribozyme to cleave the γ-GCS mRNA), to downregulate specifically the enzyme levels.[56]

2.2. Inhibitors of glutathione-S-transferase

Glutathione-S-transferases are a family of Phase II metabolic enzymes that catalyze the conjugation of glutathione to a large variety of endogenous and exogenous electrophilic compounds. GSTs have been implicated in the resistance

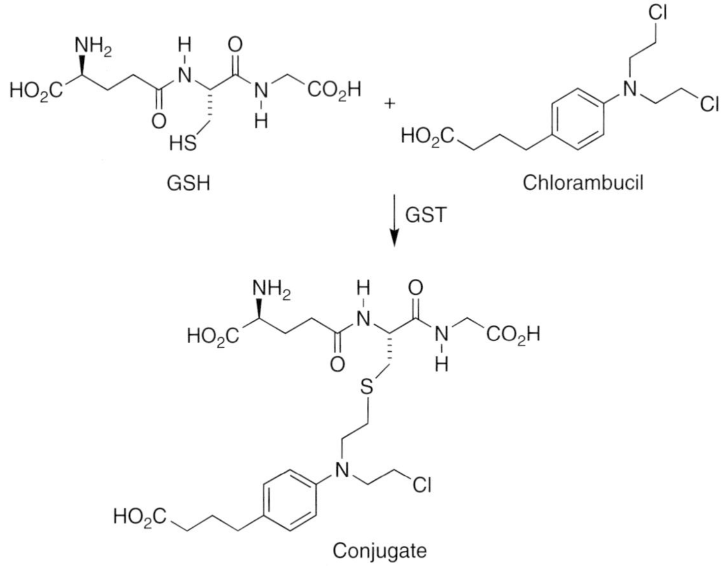

FIGURE 12.7   Mechanism of GST-mediated resistance to chlorambucyl.

towards electrophilic antitumor agents, specially alkylating agents such as some nitrogen mustards and nitrosoureas, because they catalyze their conjugation with glutathione (Fig. 12.7).

Besides direct detoxification, the π and μ classes of cytosolic GSTs have a regulatory role in cancer as inhibitors of the MAP-kinase pathway via protein–protein interactions. More specifically, GSTπ is an inhibitor of c-Jun N-terminal kinase 1 (JNK1), which is involved in stress response, apoptosis, and cellular proliferation. The GSTπ enzyme is particularly important in resistance, and many efforts have been addressed at the development of specific inhibitors of this isoform. The human GSTπ is a homodimer with 209 residues per monomer. The glutathione binding site (G site) is located in a cleft located between the N-terminal and C-terminal ends, but most residues that interact with glutathione belong to the N-terminal domain. The binding site for hydrophobic electrophiles (H site) is adjacent to the G site.

The diuretic drug ethacrynic acid is a GST inhibitor that was clinically evaluated as a resistance modulator, but it lacked specificity for the GST isoforms and its usefulness was limited by its diuretic activity. In addition to being an inhibitor of GST, ethacrynic acid is a substrate, thereby leading to glutathione depletion. Ethacrynic acid forms a conjugate with glutathione via Michael addition to its α,β-unsaturated ketone moiety, both spontaneously and by GST catalysis. The Michael adduct also acts as an inhibitor of human GSTπ, which is more potent than the parent compound[57] (Fig. 12.8).

Another interesting compound is TLK-199, which is a prodrug of TLK-117, a glutathione peptidomimetic analogue that specifically inhibits GSTπ (Fig. 12.9). TLK-199 has entered clinical trials as a modulator of drug resistance mediated by this enzyme.[58]

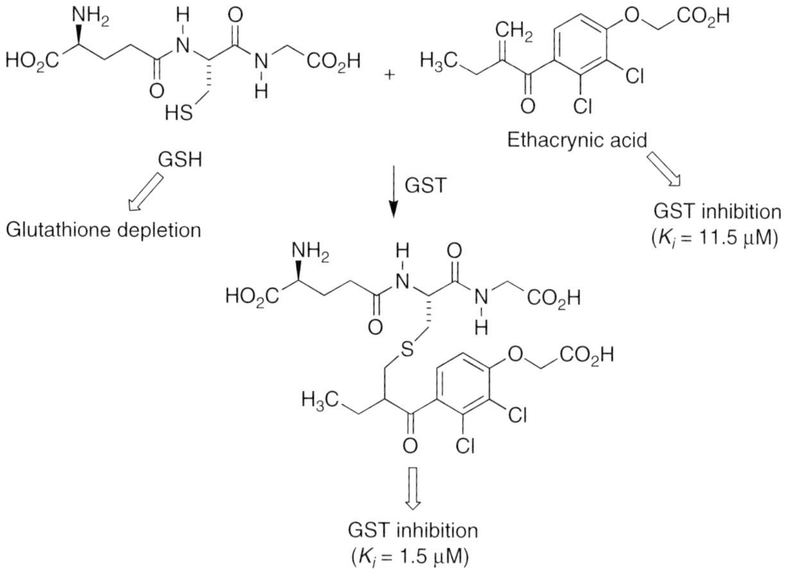

FIGURE 12.8   Mechanism of GST inhibition by ethacrynic acid.

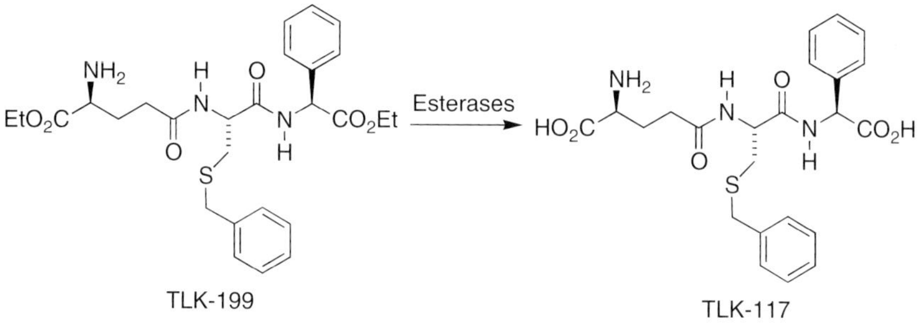

FIGURE 12.9   Bioactivation of the GST inhibitor prodrug TLK-199.

3. CHEMOSENSITIZERS TARGETING DNA-REPAIR SYSTEMS

The DNA-repair machinery of cells is activated triggering distinct repair pathways in response to different types of DNA damage. However, certain DNA-repair inhibitors capable of modulating DNA repair have the potential to act as anti-carcinogenic compounds by promoting cell death, rather than repair of potentially carcinogenic DNA damage mediated by error-prone DNA-repair processes.[59] The discovery of changes in the DNA-repair pathways produced in various chemoresistant and radioresistant phenotypes, and their understanding, has identified the disruption of this process as a novel strategy to overcome intrinsic and/or acquired resistance, especially to ionizing radiation and DNA-damaging agents.

Several compounds that specifically target distinct factors in various DNA-repair pathways have been investigated for these purposes, and some of them have entered clinical trials.[60,61,62] Unfortunately, the enhanced therapeutic efficacy of antitumor drugs when they are administered with these chemosensitizers may be linked to undesirable effects derived from inhibition of DNA repair in normal tissues. Furthermore, these agents may improve the risk of secondary malignancies, because of the potential mutagenesis and carcinogenesis that may take place after inhibition of DNA repair.

Six damage-type-specific DNA-repair pathways are known, but only four of them have led to new targets against which adjuvant cancer therapeutics are under investigation at preclinical or clinical stages (Fig. 12.10):

1. Direct repair (DR) pathway, which restricts the therapeutic response of tumors to chloroethylating or methylating agents through the repair factor O^6-alkylguanine-DNA alkyltransferase (AGT) (see also Section 6 of Chapter 5).[63]
2. Base-excision repair (BER) pathway, which reduces tumor sensitivity to alkylating or oxidative agents by repairing oxidized–reduced, alkylated, or deaminated bases through multiple factors that include DNA glycosylases, apurinic-apyrimidinic endonuclease 1 (APE1), DNA polimerase β (DNA Polβ), poly(ADP-ribose) (PAR), and poly(ADP-ribose) polymerase-1 (PARP-1). DNA glycosylases remove the damaged base generating an apurinic-apyrimidic (AP) site, APE1 cleaves the phosphodiester bonds at the 5′ end of the AP site, and Polβ is recruited to fill this gap with assistance from PAR-synthesized PARP-1.

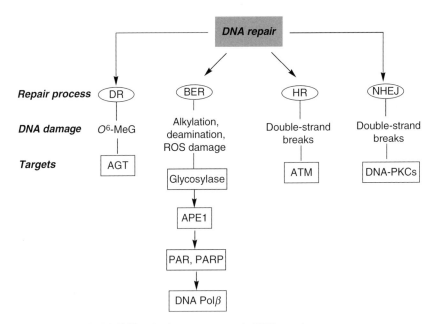

FIGURE 12.10   Anticancer targets in DNA repair processes.

3. and 4. Homology recombination (HR) and non-homologous end-joining (NHEJ) pathways repair double-strand breaks (DSBs) produced after use of ionizing radiation or administration of drugs that generate reactive oxygen species (ROS), alkylating agents, and topoisomerase inhibitors.

3.1. Inhibitors of O^6-alkylguanine-DNA alkyltransferase

As mentioned in Chapter 5, DNA damage by several types of alkylating agents, such as nitrosoureas and temozolomide, is initiated by alkylation of the guanine O-6 atom. This damage is repaired by alkylguanine transferase (AGT), which covalently transfers its active group to a cysteine-45 residue in its active site before mispairing of bases or covalent cross-links can occur (Fig. 12.11). This reaction is stoichiometric in terms of AGT, which is deactivated and cannot therefore be considered as a true enzyme and has instead been defined as a sacrificial or suicide enzyme. AGT is an interesting anticancer target for combination therapy, since its inhibition potentiates the antitumor effect of those alkylating agents for which O-6 alkylation is the determinant of cancer cell death,[64] specially carmustune and temozolamide.[65] It must be remembered, however, that alkylating agents also react at other DNA positions, specially guanine N-7 and adenine N-3, and this damage is repaired by the BER system.

The main type of AGT inhibitors are O^6-alkylguanine derivatives,[66] which act as pseudosubstrates and inactivate AGT by transferring their O^6-alkyl group to the active site Cys-45 residue (Fig. 12.12). The main inhibitors are O^6-benzylguanine and lomeguatrib, which are being clinically evaluated in combination with temozolomide[67] or 1, 3-bis(2-chloroethyl)nitrosourea (BCNU). Triple combinations including a topoisomerase I inhibitor, such as irinotecan, are also under clinical evaluation.[68]

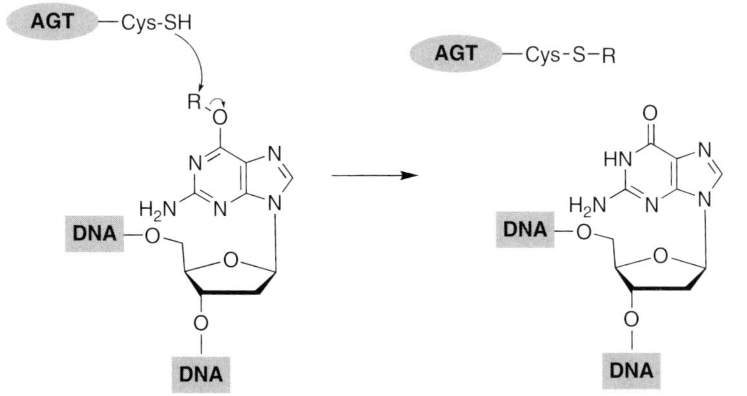

FIGURE 12.11   Repair of O^6-alkylguanine residues by alkylguanine transferase (AGT).

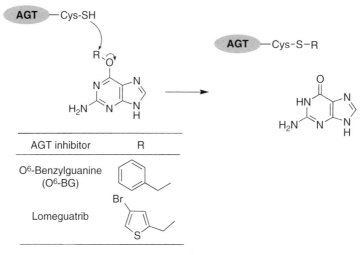

FIGURE 12.12   AGT inactivation by O^6-benzylguanine and lomeguatrib.

Platinum anticancer drugs, which are not influenced by the AGT proteins because their primary mode of action involves interaction with the guanine N-7, can reduce O^6-methylguanine DNA methyltransferase (MGMT) expression by downregulation of the corresponding mRNA. For this reason, clinical assays have been carried out to study the combination of cisplatinum with nitrosoureas (such as nimustine) and temozolomide.[69]

3.2. Potential antitumor adjuvants targeting the BER process

The major pathway for the repair of a DNA damaged at a base is the 'short-patch' BER mechanism. This mechanism is crucial for restoring DNA damage generated by ROS, alkylation, and deamination, and involves the following steps:

1. Removal of the incorrect or damaged base by a DNA glycosylase. This generates an apurinic or apyrimidinic (AP) site.
2. Cleavage of the AP site by an AP endonuclease-3'-phosphodiesterase (APE-1). This leads to the formation of a single-strand break.
3. Replacement of the damaged base and DNA religation.

A summary of the BER pathway is given in Fig. 12.13. Most compounds targeting enzymes in this pathway are under preclinical studies.

3.2.1. Inhibitors of DNA glycosylases

DNA glycosylases monitor the presence of aberrant bases in order to remove them. All of these glycosylases flip the damaged nucleotide out of the double helix and place it into the active site of the enzyme, where bases are bound through π-stacking interactions. Monofunctional glycosylases hydrolyze the N-glycosidic bond that links these bases to the DNA backbone and normally are involved in

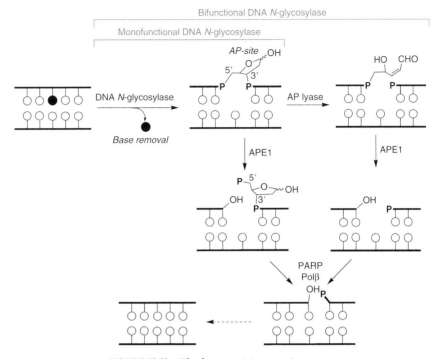

FIGURE 12.13   The base-excision repair process.

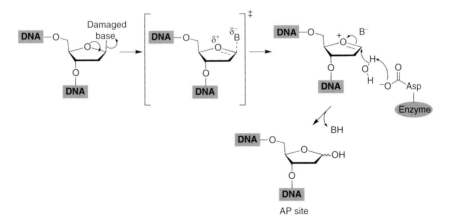

FIGURE 12.14   Mechanism of the reaction catalyzed by DNA glycosilases.

the repair of deaminated or alkylated bases. The hydrolysis is carried out by a hydroxide anion generated by deprotonation of a molecule of water by a Asn or Asp residue (Fig. 12.14).[70]

Bifunctional glycosylases normally remove bases that have suffered oxidative damage. The catalytic cycle of these enzymes involves an initial S_N1-like attack at the C-1' position by Lys or Pro residues that removes the aberrant base. In the second step, and because of their purinic/apyrimidinic (AP) lyase activity, they catalyze a subsequent β-elimination reaction of the 3'-phosphodiester bond on the protonated Schiff base intermediate and subsequent hydrolysis. As shown in Fig. 12.15, this mechanism results in strand scission.

Three classes of DNA glycosylase inhibitors are known,[71,72] all of which are oligonucleotides obtained using solid phase DNA synthetic methodology[73]:

1. Abasic site analogues that are reduced and chemically more stable (e.g., compound **12.1**). These compounds bind to glycosylases because these enzymes are end product-inhibited.
2. Oligonucleotides that contain pyrrolidine moieties that mimic the positive charge at the transition state (e.g., **12.2**).
3. Nucleotides with stabilized glycosidic bonds, which cannot be processed by the DNA glycosylases (e.g., **12.3**)

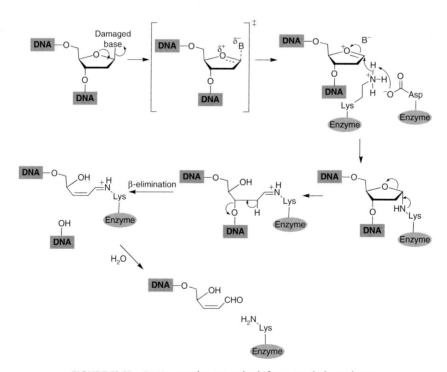

FIGURE 12.15 DNA strand scission by bifunctional glycosilases.

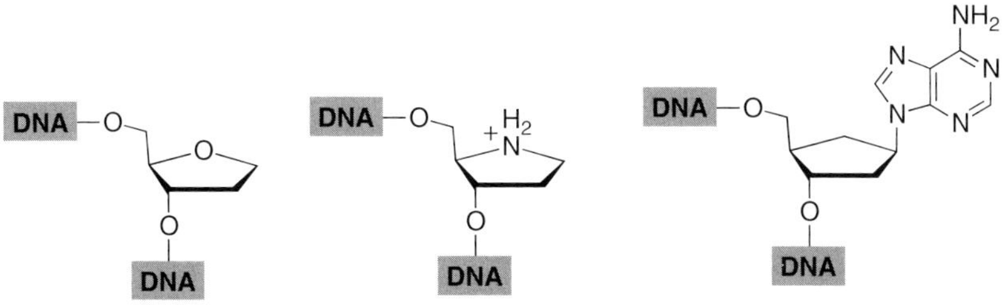

12.1   12.2   12.3

Although inhibition of DNA glycosylase activity can in principle be used to potentiate the activity of base-damaging anticancer drugs or radiation therapy, there are still no useful drugs based on this concept.

3.2.2. Inhibitors of APE-1 and compounds targeting the AP site at DNA

APE-1 cleaves the phosphodiester bonds at the 5' end of the AP sites (Fig. 12.16). Increased APE-1 expression is correlated with resistance to chemotherapy and radiotherapy, making it an attractive anticancer target.

One example of a selective APE-1 inhibitor that was identified through a high-throughput screening assay of a chemical library of 5,000 compounds was 7-nitroindole-2-carboxylic acid (CRT-0044876). This compound potentiates the cytotoxicity of several DNA base-targeting drugs and molecular modelling studies showed that it binds to the APE-1 active site.[74] Another specific APE-1 inhibitor that has been shown in preclinical studies to sensitize cancer cells to DNA alkylating agents, such as temozolomide, is the anti-parasitic drug lucanthone.[75]

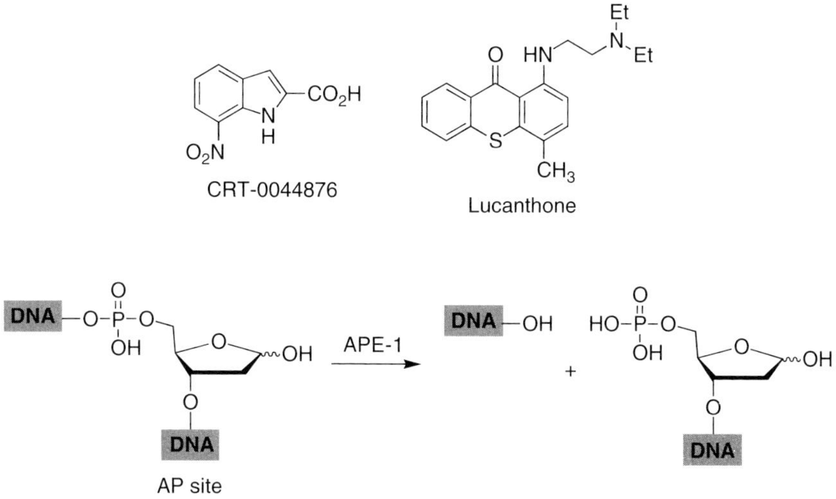

CRT-0044876

Lucanthone

AP site

FIGURE 12.16 Reaction catalyzed by APE-1 and some inhibitors of this enzyme.

An indirect strategy to achieve inhibition of the APE-1 function is to chemically modify AP sites, making them unsuitable for APE-1 binding. Thus, methoxyamine potentiates the antitumor efficacy of alkylating agents such as temozolomide and carmustine in colon cancer and malignant glyoma xenogratfs[76] and is being tested in Phase I clinical assays in humans. Furthermore, it has been found that pretreatment with 5-iodouridine-deoxyribose (IUdR) and methoxyamine enhances the effects of ionizing radiation by causing a prolonged G1 cell cycle arrest and by promoting stress-induced premature senescence.[77]

The mechanism of action of methoxyamine involves its condensation with the tautomeric open-ring form of deoxyribose produced by DNA glycosylases, in a reaction that is faster than APE-1 binding and thus blocks the BER pathway (Fig. 12.17).

Methoxyamine is mutagenic in itself because it converts cytosine bases into their N^4-methoxycytosine analogues. Because of the electron-withdrawing effect of the methoxy group, the methoxycytosine derivative can exist as enamino or imino tautomeric forms (Fig. 12.18A). While the enamino structure pairs with guanine forming three hydrogen bonds, the same as unsubstituted cytosine, the imino tautomer is able to pair with adenine (Fig. 12.18B).[78]

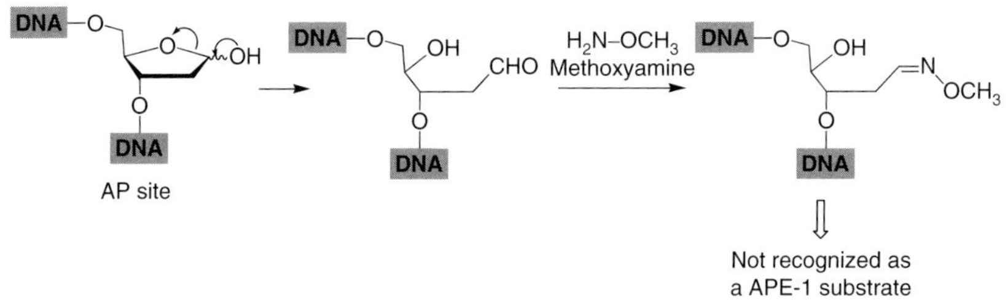

FIGURE 12.17 Inhibition of APE-1 following blockade of the AP sites by methoxyamine.

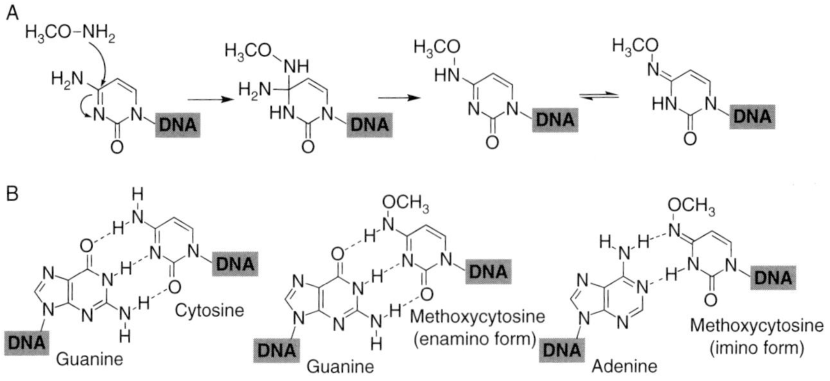

FIGURE 12.18 Chemical basis for the mutagenic activity of methoxyamine.

3.2.3. Inhibitors of poly(ADP-ribose) polymerase (PARP)

The last step of the BER pathway is a complex process that involves binding of DNA to PARP-1, which functions as a sensor of the strand breaks generated by APE-1. When PARP-1 binds to the nicked site, it becomes poly(ADP-ribosylated), and after some intermediate steps it recruits DNA β-polymerase (Polβ).

PARP-1 is a ubiquitous zinc-finger DNA-binding enzyme that is activated by binding to DNA breaks and then catalyzes the synthesis of the branched polymer PAR using NAD^+ as the building block. PARP-1 activity is enhanced in many tumors and its inhibition is associated with increased sensitivity to antitumor agents that cause DNA strand breaks, including alkylating agents, topoisomerase I inhibitors, and ionizing radiation. For these reasons, PARP-1 seems to be pivotal in DNA-repair processes and has become a target for anticancer therapy.[79,80]

PARP-1 catalyzes the reaction of acceptor proteins, including PARP itself, histones, or p53, with a NAD^+ molecule with displacement of nicotinamide to yield precursor **12.4**, which then undergoes linear or branched polymerization to PAR, as shown in Fig. 12.19. Because of their negative charge due to the ionized

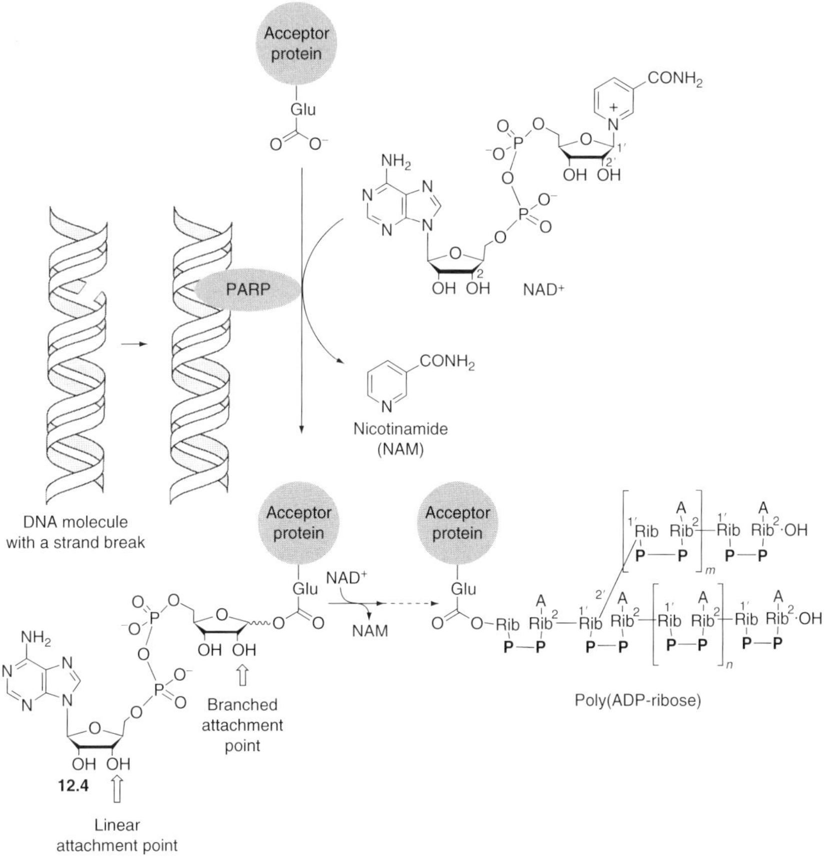

FIGURE 12.19   Poly-ADP-ribosylation of nuclear proteins.

phosphate groups, the presence of these polymers helps to open up the damaged DNA to allow access to other enzymes involved in the repair process such as DNA polymerases and DNA ligases.[81] In this way, poly-ADP-ribosylation of nuclear proteins by PARP-1 converts DNA damage into intracellular signals that activate DNA repair by either the base-excision pathway or cell death.

The first generation of PARP inhibitors was designed on the basis of their NAD^+ binding site. Nicotinamide, the second product of the PARP-catalyzed reaction, is itself a weak PARP inhibitor and the first inhibitors (e.g., 3-aminobenzamide) were designed around its structure, but they suffered from low activity and specificity. A subsequent screening of 170 compounds allowed to identify several heterocyclic systems that were used as leads for subsequent optimization, and it also allowed to establish some structural features that are required for potent PARP inhibitory activity. These include an electron-rich aromatic or heteroaromatic system with a non-cleavable bond at the position corresponding to C-3 of the benzamides, restricted rotation around the Ar–CO bond so that the carbonyl group is *anti* with respect to the C_1–C_2 bond of the aromatic ring, and finally one amide group for hydrogen bonding.[82] These SAR conclusions were rationalized by the subsequent resolution of the crystal structure of the PARP catalytic domain complexed by some inhibitors, which showed that the carbonyl oxygen forms two hydrogen bonds, with Ser-904 and Gly-863, and the amide nitrogen is a hydrogen bond donor to Gly-863 (Fig. 12.20).

The knowledge gained from these studies led to the preparation of several fused tricyclic indoles and benzimidazoles containing lactam bonds. Some of these compounds, including AG-014699[83] and INO-1001,[84] are in clinical trials for several types of cancer in combination with temozolomide.

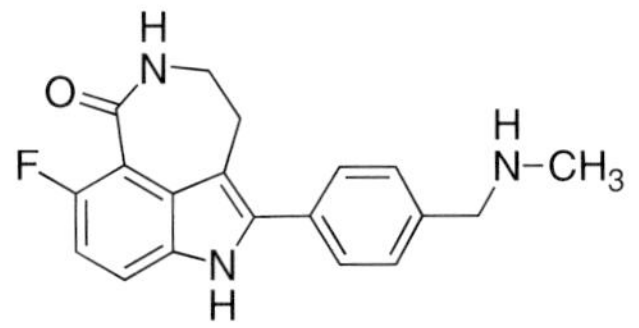

AG-014699

PARP is believed to be one of the last effectors in the cascade of cell and tissue damage caused by ischemia and reperfusion injury. In situations of excessive

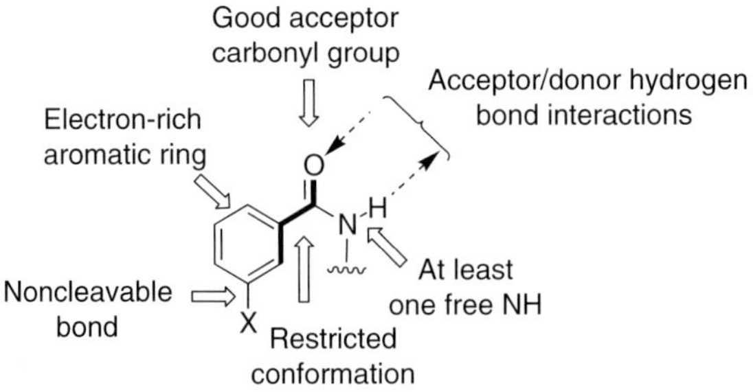

FIGURE 12.20 SAR conclusions for PARP inhibitors.

DNA damage (such as acute exposure to a large pathological insult), overactivation of PARP results in cell-based energetic failure leading to cellular necrosis, tissue injury, and organ damage or failure. For this reason, some PARP inhibitors are being assayed for pathologies associated with damage caused by ROS, and INO-1001 has received orphan drug status from the Food and Drug Administration (FDA) to prevent post-surgical complications of aortic aneurysm repair.

3.3. Inhibitors of enzymes involved in double-strand DNA break repair pathways

Double strand breaks generated by ionizing radiation and ROS, or indirectly by DNA-damaging anticancer drugs such as alkylating agents and topoisomerase inhibitors, are repaired by either the HR or the NHEJ pathways. The enzymes involved in these pathways are members of the phosphatidylinositol 3-kinase (PI3K) superfamily and have become anticancer targets because their inhibition confers radio- or chemosensitization to tumor cells.[85] These enzymes can be considered as molecular sensor of DSBs, and the most relevant targets in this area[86] are

Ataxia telangiectasia mutated (ATM) kinase, which is involved in the HR pathway and plays a critical role in the maintenance of genome integrity by triggering DNA damage sensors through phosphorylation of downstream targets such as p53.[87]
DNA-dependant protein kinase (DNA-PK), which is involved in the NHEJ pathway.

The search for drugs that inhibit these pathways started from two non-selective PI-3 kinase inhibitors, namely wortmannin and LY-294002, that inhibit ATP binding within the catalytic site of the kinases. As shown in Fig. 12.21, the mechanism of inhibition by wortmannin relies on its reactivity as a Michael acceptor and involves the irreversible alkylation of a lysine unit that resides in the active site and is critical for the phosphate transfer (Lys-802 in the case of DNA-PK). Wortmannin is an effective radiosensitizer of a variety of normal and cancer cells, but its further development was hampered by its poor water solubility and its toxicity.

LY-294002 is another non-selective, competitive inhibitor of PI-3 kinases. Although this compound significantly sensitizers ATM-proficient cells to ionizing radiation and DBS-inducing chemotherapeutics, such as etoposide, doxorubicin, and camptothecin, its relatively low stability, fast metabolic degradation, and *in vivo* toxicity have prevented its clinical evaluation in humans. However, LY-294002 has been used as a lead compound in the development of further inhibitors. Thus, the ATM-selective inhibitor KU-55933 was discovered by screening a combinatorial library based around LY-294002,[88] while the structurally related NU7026 demonstrated 70-fold more selectivity for DNA-PK compared to other PI-3 kinases and more than fivefold more selectivity with regard to ATM.

LY-294002   KU-55933   NU7026

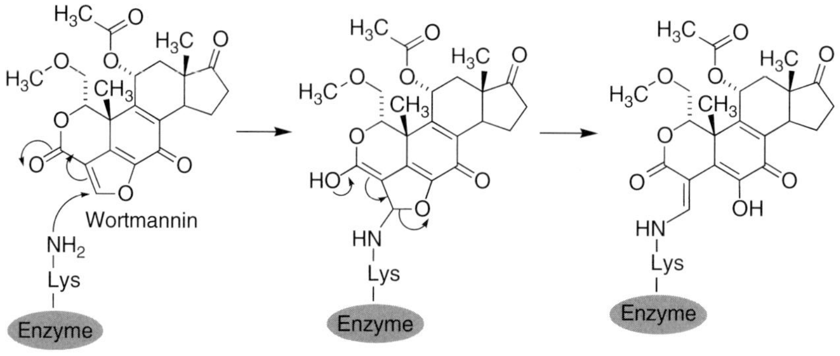

FIGURE 12.21   Kynase inactivation by wortmannin.

The topoisomerase II inhibitor salvicine, which is under Phase II clinical trials, simultaneously damages DNA and disrupts DNA repair by inhibiting DNA-PK activity, being extremely effective against tumor cells. The mechanism of suppression of DNA-PK activity by salvicine involves the generation of ROS, which is probably associated with its *ortho*-quinone structure.[89]

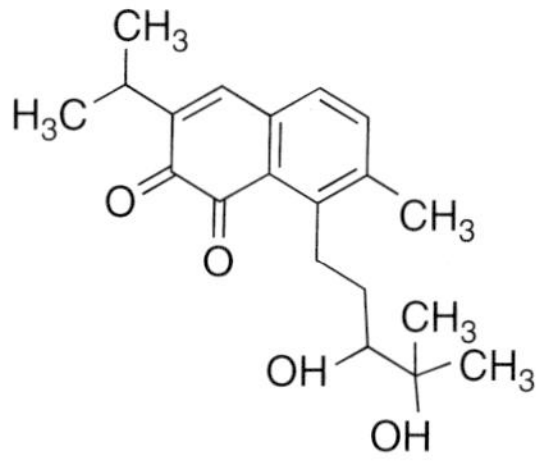

Salvicine

4. ANTITUMOR DRUG RESISTANCE RELATED TO EXTRACELLULAR PH: TUMOR-ASSOCIATED CARBONIC ANHYDRASE AS AN ANTICANCER TARGET

Tumor cells decrease their extracellular pH by two mechanisms, namely production of lactic acid as a consequence of a higher glycolysis rate, and CO_2 hydration catalyzed by the tumor-associated carbonic anhydrase IX (CA IX) isoform, specially in hypoxic conditions. Thus, most hypoxic tumors are acidic (pH $\approx$ 6), in contrast to normal tissues (pH $\approx$ 7.4).

Drugs that are weakly ionized (e.g., mitoxantrone, paclitaxel, and topotecan) enter cells by passive diffusion in their non-ionized form, and variations in extracellular pH alter this ionization-dependant diffusion. Acidic extracellular pH values hamper the uptake of basic drugs into the tumor cells, because the predominant ionized form is not diffused through cell membranes. Indeed, enhancement of the extracellular pH by chronic ingestion of a sodium bicarbonate solution has been found to improve the cytotoxicity of these drugs.

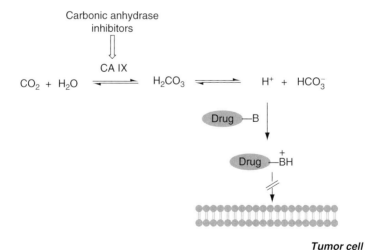

Mitoxantrone

Topotecan

The isoform IX of CA IX is highly overexpressed in many types of cancer and is induced by hypoxia because its expression is regulated by the hypoxia-inducible factor 1 (HIF-1) transcription factor (see Section 4.2.1 of Chapter 9). High levels of CA IX correlate with chemoresistance to weakly basic anticancer drugs because, due to the existence of a CA IX extracellular catalytic domain, this enzyme contributes to acidification of the tumor environment by catalyzing the hydration of carbon dioxide to bicarbonate and protons (Fig. 12.22). Other effects of lowered extracellular pH include extracellular matrix breakdown, migration, invasion, and induction of cell growth factors and protease activation. CA IX inhibitors produce other effects, including inhibition of the expression of aquaporin, a water channel protein that might be implicated in vascular permeability in tumors.

The involvement of CA IX in alterations of the pH balance in tumor tissues explains the antitumor effects found for many CA IX inhibitors.[90] The most advanced one is the sulfonamide indisulam (E-7070), which has a complex

Carbonic anhydrase
inhibitors

CA IX

$$CO_2 + H_2O \rightleftharpoons H_2CO_3 \rightleftharpoons H^+ + HCO_3^-$$

Drug—B

Drug—BH$^+$

Tumor cell

FIGURE 12.22   Acidification of tumor environments by tumor-associated carbonic anhydrase IX.

mechanism of antitumor action and is under clinical development for the treatment of solid tumors (see Section 4.1 of Chapter 9).[91]

Indisulam (E-7070)

REFERENCES

1. Kerr, D., and Middleton, M. (2006). *Curr. Opin. Pharmacol.* **6,** 321.
2. Gottesman, M. M., Fojo, T., and Bates, S. E. (2002). *Nat. Rev. Cancer* **2,** 48.
3. Flügge, U. I., and van Meer, G. (2006). *FEBS Lett.* **580,** 997.
4. Gottesman, M. M., and Ling, V. (2006). *FEBS Lett.* **580,** 998.
5. Dantzig, A. H., Alwis, D. P., and Burgess, M. (2003). *Adv. Drug Deliv. Rev.* **55,** 133.
6. Modok, S., Mellor, H. R., and Callaghan, R. (2006). *Curr. Opin. Pharmacol.* **6,** 350.
7. Larsen, A. K., Escargueil, A. E., and Skladanowski, A. (2000). *Pharmacol. Ther.* **85,** 217.
8. Schmid, D., Ecker, G., Kopp, S., Hitzler, M., and Chiba, P. (1999). *Biochem. Pharmacol.* **58,** 1447.
9. Garrigues, A., Loiseau, N., Delaforge, M., Ferté, J., Garrigos, M., André, F., and Orlowski, S. (2002). *Mol. Pharmacol.* **62,** 1288.
10. Wiese, M., and Pajeva, I. K. (2001). *Curr. Med. Chem.* **8,** 685.
11. Avendaño, C., and Menéndez, J. C. (2002). *Curr. Med. Chem.* **9,** 159.
12. Avendaño, C., and Menéndez, J. C. (2004). *Med. Res. Rev. Online* **1,** 419.
13. Tsuruo, T., Iida, H., Tsukagoshi, S., and Sakurai, Y. (1981). *Cancer Res.* **41,** 1967.
14. Ekins, S., Kim, R. B., Leake, B. F., Dantzig, A. H., Schuet, E. G., Lan, L. B., Yasuda, K., Shephard, R. L., Winter, M. A., Schuet, J. D., Wikel, J. H., and Wrighton, S.A (2002). *Mol. Pharmacol.* **61,** 974.
15. Bates, S., Kang, M., Meadows, B., Bakke, S., Choyke, P., Merino, M., Goldspiel, B., Chico, I., Smith, T., Chen, C., Robay, R., Bergan, R., *et al.* (2001). *Cancer* **92,** 1577.
16. Kreis, W., Budman, D. R., and Calabro, A. (2001). *Cancer Chemother. Pharmacol.* **47,** 78.
17. Yanagisawa, T., Newman, A., Coley, H., Renshaw, J., Pinkerton, C. R., and Pritchard Jones, K. (1999). *Br. J. Cancer* **80,** 1190.
18. Toppmeyer, D., Seidman, A. D., Pollak, M., Russell, C., Tkaczuk, K., Verma, S., Overmoyer, B., Garg, V., Ette, E., Harding, M. W., and Demetri, G. D. (2002). *Clin. Cancer Res.* **8,** 670.
19. Nokihara, H., Yano, S., Nishioka, Y., Hanibuchi, M., Higasida, T., Tsuruo, T., and Sone, S. (2001). *Jpn. J. Cancer Res.* **92,** 785.
20. Naito, M., Matsuba, Y., Sato, S., Hirata, H., and Tsuruo, T. (2002). *Clin. Cancer Res.* **8,** 582.
21. Smith, B. J., Doran, A. C., McLean, S., Tingley, F. D., III, O' Neill, B. T., and Kajiji, S. M. (2001). *J. Pharmacol. Exp. Ther.* **298,** 1252.
22. Sorbera, L. A., Castaner, J., Silvestre, J. S., and Bayes, M. (2003). *Drugs Future* **28,** 125.
23. http://www.clinicaltrials.gov/ct/show/NCT00046930.
24. Guns, E. S., Denyssevych, T., Dixon, R., Bally, M. B., and Mayer, L. (2002). *Eur. J. Drug Metab. Pharmacokinet.* **27,** 119.
25. http://www.clinicaltrials.gov/ct/gui/show/NCT00028873.
26. Moins, N., Cayre, A., Chevillard, S., Maublant, J., Verrelle, P., and Finat-Duclos, F. (2000). *Anticancer Res.* **20,** 2617.
27. Dantzig, A. H., Alwis, D. P., and Burgess, M. (2003). *Adv. Drug Deliv. Rev.* **55,** 133.
28. Sonneveld, P. (2000). *J. Intern. Med.* **247,** 521.
29. Pleban, K., and Ecker, G. F. (2005). *Mini-Rev. Med. Chem.* **5,** 153.

30. Klopman, G., Srivastava, S., Kolossvary, I., Epand, R. F., Ahmed, N., and Epand, R. M. (1992). *Cancer Res.* **52,** 4121.
31. Seelig, A. (1998). *Eur. J. Biochem.* **251,** 252.
32. Seelig, A., and Gatlik-Landwojtowicz, E. (2005). *Mini-Rev. Med. Chem.* **5,** 135.
33. Seelig, A., Landwojtowicz, E., Fischer, H., and Blatter, X.-L. (2003).   Towards P-glycoprotein structure-activity relationships. *In* ''Drug Bioavailability,'' (H. van de Waterbeemd, H. Lennernäs, and P. Artursson, eds.). Wiley-VCH, Weinheim chapter 20.
34. Klopman, G., Shi, L. M., and Ramu, A. (1997). *Mol. Pharmacol.* **52,** 323.
35. Wang, R. B., Kuo, C. L., Lien, L. L., and Lien, E. J. (2003). *J. Clin. Pharm. Ther.* **28,** 203.
36. Hendrich, A. B., and Michalak, K. (2003). *Curr. Drug Targets* **4,** 23.
37. Castaing, M., Loiseau, A., and Dani, M. (2001). *J. Pharm. Pharmacol.* **53,** 1021.
38. Raub, T. J. (2005). *Mol. Pharmaceutics* **3,** 3.
39. Patel, V. A., Dunn, M. J., and Sorojin, A. (2002). *J. Biol. Chem.* **277,** 38915.
40. Plo, I., Lehne, G., Beckstrom, K. J., Maestre, N., Bettaieb, A., Laurent, G., and Lutier, D. (2002). *Mol. Pharmacol.* **62,** 304.
41. Jin, S., Gorfajn, B., Faircloth, G., and Scoto, K. W. (2000). *Proc. Natl. Acad. Sci. USA* **97,** 6775.
42. Wu, H., Hait, W. N., and Yang, J. M. (2003). *Cancer Res.* **63,** 1515.
43. Dassow, H., Lassner, D., Remke, H., and Preiss, R. (2000). *Int. J. Clin. Pharmacol. Ther.* **38,** 209.
44. Capella, L. S., Alcantara, J. S. M., Moura-Neto, V., Lopes, A. G., and Capella, M. A. M. (2000). *Tumor Biol.* **21,** 54.
45. Brigger, I., Dubernet, C., and Couvreur, P. (2002). *Adv. Drug Deliv. Rev.* **54,** 631.
46. Gaber, M. H. (2002). *J. Biochem. Mol. Biol. Biophys.* **6,** 309.
47. Wang, W., and Ballatori, N. (1998). *Pharmacol. Rev.* **50,** 335.
48. Zejia, Y., Faustino, P. J., Andrews, P. A., Monastra, R., Rasmussen, A. A., Ellison, C. D., and Cullen, K. J. (2000). *Cancer Chemother. Pharmacol.* **46,** 255.
49. Voehringer, D. (1999). *Free Radical Biol. Med.* **27,** 945.
50. Yao, K. S., Godwing, A. K., Johnson, S. W., Ozols, R. F., O'Dwyer, P. J., and Hamilton, T. C. (1995). *Cancer Res.* **55,** 4367.
51. Sipos, E. P., Witham, T. F., Ratan, R., Burger, P. C., Baraban, J., Li, K. W., Piantadosi, S., and Brem, H. (2001). *Neurosurgery* **48,** 392.
52. Lai, G. M., Moscow, J. A., Álvarez, M. G., Fojo, A. T., and Bates, S. E. (1991). *Int. J. Cancer* **49,** 688.
53. Chen, X., Carystinos, G. D., and Batist, G. (1982). *Chem. Biol. Interact.* **111,** 263.
54. Griffith, O. W. (1982). *J. Biol. Chem.* **257,** 13704.
55. Fojo, T., and Bates, S. (2003). *Oncogene* **22,** 7512.
56. Nagata, J., Kijima, H., Hatanaka, H., Asai, S., Miyachi, H., Takagi, A., Miwa, T., Mine, T., Yamazaki, H., Nakamura, M., Kondo, T., Scanlon, K. J., *et al.* (2001). *Biochem. Biophys. Res. Commun.* **286,** 406.
57. Oakley, A. J., Lo Bello, M., Mazzetti, A. P., Federici, G., and Parker, M. W. (1997). *FEBS Lett.* **419,** 32.
58. Townsend, D. M., and Tew, K. D. (2003). *Oncogene* **22,** 7369.
59. Bentle, M. S., Bey, E. A., Dong, Y., Reinicke, K. E., and Boothman, D. A. (2006). *J. Mol. Histol.* **37,** 1567.
60. Madhusudan, S., and Hickson, I. D. (2005). *Trends Mol. Med.* **11,** 503.
61. Ding, J., Miao, Z.-H., Meng, L.-H., and Geng, M-Y. (2006). *Trends Pharmacol. Sci.* **27,** 338.
62. Curtin, N. (2007). *Expert Opin. Ther. Targets* **11,** 783.
63. Gerson, S. L. (2002). *J. Clin. Oncol.* **20,** 2388.
64. Sabharwal, A., and Middleton, M. R. (2006). *Curr. Opin. Pharmacol.* **6,** 355.
65. Bobola, M. S., Silber, J. R., Ellenbogen, R. G., Geyer, J. R., Blank, A., and Goff, R. D. (2005). *Clin. Cancer Res.* **11,** 2747.
66. Gerson, G. L. (2004). *Nat. Rev. Cancer* **4,** 296.
67. Ranson, M., Middleton, M. R., Bridgewater, J., Lee, S. M., Dawson, M., Jowle, D., Halbert, G., Waller, S., McGrath, H., Gumbrell, L., McElhinney, R. S., Donnelly, D., *et al.* (2006). *Clin. Cancer Res.* **12,** 1577.
68. Friedman, H. S., Keir, S., Pegg, A. E., Houghton, P. J., Colvin, O. M., Moschel, R. C., Bigner, D. D., and Dolan, M. E. (2002). *Mol. Cancer Ther.* **1,** 943.

69. Silvani, A., Eoli, M., Salmaggi, A., Lamperti, E., Maccagnano, E., Broggi, G., and Boiardi, A. (2004). *J. Neurooncol.* **66,** 203.

70. Dinner, A. R., Blackburn, G. M., and Karplus, M. (2001). *Nature* **413,** 752.

71. Ide, H., and Kotera, M. (2004). *Biol. Pharm. Bull.* **27,** 480.

72. Schärer, O. D., and Jiricny, J. (2001). *BioEssays* **23,** 270.

73. Deng, L., Schärer, O. D., and Verdine, G. L. (1997). *J. Am. Chem. Soc.* **119,** 7865.

74. Madhusudan, S., Smart, F., Shrimpton, P., Parsons, J. L., Gardiner, L., Houlbrook, S., Talbot, D. C., Hammonds, T., Freemont, P. A., Sternberg, M. J. E., Dianov, G. L., and Hickson, I. D. (2005). *Nucleic Acid Res.* **33,** 4711.

75. Luo, M., and Kelley, M. R. (2004). *Anticancer Res.* **24,** 2127.

76. Liu, L., and Gerson, S. L. (2004). *Curr. Opin. Investig. Drugs* **5,** 623.

77. Yan, T., Seo, Y., Schupp, J. E., Zeng, X., Desai, A. B., and Kinsella, T. J. (2006). *Mol Cancer Ther.* **5,** 893.

78. Gdaniec, Z., Ban, B., Sowers, L. C., and Fazakerley, G. V. (1996). *Eur. J. Biochem.* **242,** 271.

79. Curtin, N. J. (2005). *Expert Rev. Mol. Med.* **7,** 1.

80. Haince, J.-F., Rouleau, M., Hendzel, M. J., Masson, J.-Y., and Poirier, G. G. (2005). *Trends Mol. Med.* **11,** 456.

81. Plummer, E. R. (2006). *Curr. Opin. Pharmacol.* **6,** 364.

82. Banasik, M., Komura, H., Shimoyama, M., and Ueda, K. (1992). *J. Biol. Chem.* **267,** 1569.

83. Plummer, R., Lorigan, P., Evans, J., Steven, N., Middleton, M., Wilson, R., Snow, K., Dewji, R., and Calvert, H. (2006). *J. Clin. Oncol.* **24,** 8013.

84. Wang, C., Bedikian, A., Kim, K., Papadopoulos, N., Hwu, W., and Hwu, P. (2006). *J. Clin. Oncol.* **24,** 12015.

85. Lord, C. J., Garrett, M. D., and Ashworth, A. (2006). *Clin. Cancer Res.* **12,** 4463.

86. Collis, S. J., DeWeese, T. L., Jeggo, P. A., and Parker, A. R. (2005). *Oncogene* **24,** 949.

87. Bakkenist, C. J., and Kastan, M. B. (2004). *Cell* **118,** 9.

88. Hickson, I., Zhao, Y., Richardson, C. J., Green, S. J., Martin, N. M. B., Orr, A. I., Reaper, P. M., Jackson, S. P., Curtin, N. J., and Smith, G. C. M. (2004). *Cancer Res.* **64,** 9152.

89. Lu, H. R., Zhu, H., Huang, M., Chen, Y., Cai, Y.-J., Miao, Z. H., Zhang, J. S., and Ding, J. (2005). *Mol. Pharmacol.* **68,** 983.

90. Thiry, A., Dogné, J.-M., Mesereel, B., and Supuran, C. T. (2006). *Trends Pharmacol. Sci.* **27,** 566.

91. Oratz, R., Blum, J., Rowland, K., Cunningham, C., Jacobs, S., Arseneau, J., Richards, D., Renshaw, F. G., Holmes, F., and O'Shaughnessy, J. (2005). *J. Clin. Oncol.* **23,** 685.

CHAPTER 13

Cancer Chemoprevention

Contents

1. Introduction   417
2. Ligands for Nuclear Receptors in Cancer Chemoprevention   418
3. Anti-Inflammatory Agents and Antioxidants in Cancer
   Chemoprevention   421
   3.1. COX-2 inhibitors and other anti-inflammatory agents   422
   3.2. Antioxidants   422
4. Chromatin Modifiers in Cancer Chemoprevention   425
5. Miscellaneous Agents for Chemoprevention   426
6. Cancer Vaccines   428
   References   428

1. INTRODUCTION

Cancer may be prevented in some cases through lifestyle modification like an adequate diet and physical activity. The aim of chemotherapy is to kill cancer cells in the hope of preventing further cancer progression, while chemoprevention is the attempt to use natural or synthetic chemical agents to avoid cancer. In contrast to the successful chemoprevention of cardiovascular diseases by using antihypertensive agents or statins, chemoprevention of cancer is a highly controversial topic. To achieve a significant positive change in the mortality currently produced from the common forms of cancer, despite immense advances in the understanding of carcinogenesis and in bringing potent new drugs to the clinic, a much greater emphasis would be necessary toward cancer prevention before the complex series of genetic and epigenetic events that result in metastasis have occurred.

A distinction can be made between blocking agents, which are inhibitors of tumor initiation, and suppressing agents, which inhibit tumor promotion/progression.[1] Tumor suppressor genes and proto-oncogenes encode proteins involved in cell cycle control, signal transduction, and transcriptional regulation.

Medicinal Chemistry of Anticancer Drugs
DOI: 10.1016/B978-0-444-52824-7.00013-5

They affect three different carcinogenic stages: initiation (in which carcinogens are binding to DNA), promotion (in which epigenetic mechanisms lead to prema-lignancy), and progression to cancer. With rare exceptions, the first stage is initiated decades before promotion and progression stages. This knowledge supports strategies to prevent *de novo* malignancies in healthy population, especially in individuals with high-risk features such as women who have a *BRCA1* or a *BRCA2* mutation, who are likely to develop breast cancer, or patients with familial adenomatous polyposis, who are almost certain to develop colon cancer. Consequently, its success depends on a correct determination and analysis of biomarkers. In secondary prevention, the progression of a premalignant lesion such as a colon adenoma into cancer is focused, while tertiary prevention attempts that patients cured of an initial cancer or premalignant lesion develop a second primary tumor and is directed to reverse, suppress, or prevent carcinogenic progression to invasive cancer. Metastatic tumors are the leading cause of mortality in several cancers and, even if total cure of advanced malignancy cannot be achieved because an absolute prevention is not possible, extension of the latency period of carcinogenesis so that the patients can have a higher quality of life is highly desirable.

Many new drugs that prevent cancer in experimental animals are now available for further studies and some drugs have been approved for prevention of some types of cancer.[2] Head and neck squamous cell cancers have been one of the most studied in chemoprevention because of their high prevalence and morbidity.[3] Skin cancer prevention, focused on nutritional supplements such as β-carotene or selenium, had a limited success and systemic retinoids have given mixed results. Clinical results in chemoprevention in lung cancer, the leading cause of cancer death in the world, and in bladder cancer have been so far rather discouraging. Regarding prostate cancer prevention, although hormonal therapy with the 5α-reductase inhibitor finasteride was promising, it has sexual side effects, and the malignancies developed after its administration are very aggressive.

The most promising targets for cancer chemoprevention so far discovered are ligands for nuclear receptors, anti-inflammatory agents, chromatin modifiers, and processes leading to the generation of free radicals.

2. LIGANDS FOR NUCLEAR RECEPTORS IN CANCER CHEMOPREVENTION

The nuclear receptors superfamily are transcription factors that regulate cell differentiation and proliferation in specific organs that are important for carcinogenesis. They may be directly activated after the binding of specific ligands, but this binding may also trigger transcription in other cellular contexts because of the selective recruitment of other proteins, such as transcriptional coactivators and corepressors, that interact with transcription factors themselves. Nuclear receptors are ideal targets for chemoprevention, being the most studied the estrogen receptors ERα and ERβ; the androgen receptor; the retinoic receptors RARα, β, and γ; the retinoid X receptors RXRα, β, and γ; the vitamin D receptor (VDR); and the peroxisome proliferative receptor-γ (PPARγ).[4]

In the estrogen receptors context, we have previously explained why tamoxifen is not an estrogen antagonist but a selective estrogen receptor modulator (SERM) that may be antiestrogenic in some organs, such as breast, and proestrogenic in others, such as uterus or bone (see Section 3.1 of Chapter 3). Since estrogens enhance the growth of almost all breast cancer cells during early stages of carcinogenesis, the chronic administration of antiestrogens is useful in breast cancer prevention. In this regard, the FDA approval of tamoxifen for breast cancer prevention[5] was a landmark in chemoprevention research. The associated risk of endometrial cancer and thromboembolic events, which precludes its use in certain populations, lead to clinical trials with other SERMs such as raloxifene.[6] Good clinical results have also been obtained with arzoxifene.[7] Besides their utility in breast cancer, chemopreventive use of SERMs may be extended to other cancers such as prostate and colon in which ERα and ERβ play a carcinogenic role.

Tamoxifen

R = H   Raloxifene
R = CH$_3$ Arzoxifene

Vitamin A and its analogs, collectively known as retinoids, have profound effects in cell growth and differentiation, and the loss of retinoid function is linked to carcinogenesis in some cancers (see Section 9 of Chapter 3). In the context of the retinoic receptors RARα, β, and γ, and the retinoid X receptors RXRα, β, and γ, several retinoids have shown promising activity as antitumor and cancer chemopreventive agents by inhibiting carcinogenesis at the initiation, promotion, and progression stages.[8] The development of a malignant phenotype frequently includes a block in the normal differentiation process and numerous compounds, such as retinoids or vitamin D$_3$ analogs, have been studied with this approach in mind.

Besides the success of retinoids in the therapy of acute promyelocytic leukemia (APL), some of them are also of interest in the prevention of several other cancers (oral cavity, head and neck, breast, skin, and liver). In fact, the RAR receptor ligand 13-*cis*-retinoic acid (isotretinoin) is one of the standard treatments for the prevention of oral cancer.[9]

13-*Cis*-retinoic acid
(isotretinoin)

Several atypical retinoids have also been assayed for cancer chemoprevention. Fenretinide, an amide of tretinoin that acts as a ligand of RARβ and γ, has entered clinical trials showing a beneficial effect in the prevention of premenopausal breast cancer in combination with tamoxifen.[10] Polyprenoic acid, also called acyclic retinoid, has shown RAR, RXR, and PPAR activities and is useful in the prevention of hepatocellular carcinoma.[11] Finally, adapalene prevents cancer in patients with cervical intraepithelial neoplasia.

4-hydroxyphenylretinamide (fenretinide)

Acyclic retinoid
(polyprenoic acid)

Adapalene

The ligands of RXRs are known as rexinoids. Some of them, such as the rigid analog of cis-retinoic acid LG100268, are another very promising group of compounds in cancer chemoprevention. Rexinoids may modulate the activity of other transcription factors because their receptors form heterodimers with other nuclear receptors, such as RARs, VDR, and PPARγ.[12] Preclinical studies have shown that these compounds appear to maintain the cancer prevention potential of retinoids with less toxicity. When combined with a SERM, they can also effectively kill breast cancer cells.[13] Bexarotene, a rexinoid approved as an oral antineoplastic agent indicated by for cutaneous T cell lymphoma, has entered clinical trials for primary prevention of breast cancer after encouraging preclinical results.[14]

LG100268

Bexarotene

The VDR is another transcription factor that exerts a direct control of gene expression and interacts with regulatory pathways such as SMAD3, which is a component of the signal-transduction pathway that regulates the cytokine transforming growth factor-β (TGF-β) that helps to prevent carcinogenesis. Vitamin D intake diminishes the risk of colon cancer, protecting the colon from the carcinogenic effects of bile acids.[15] However, ingestion of large amounts of this vitamin results in hypercalcemia. Synthetic analogs of vitamin D named deltanoids, such as Ro24-5531, (which is a hexafluoro-1α,25-dihydroxyvitamin D_3 derivative), have shown potent differentiative and antiproliferative activities with less propensity to cause hypercalcemia.[16]

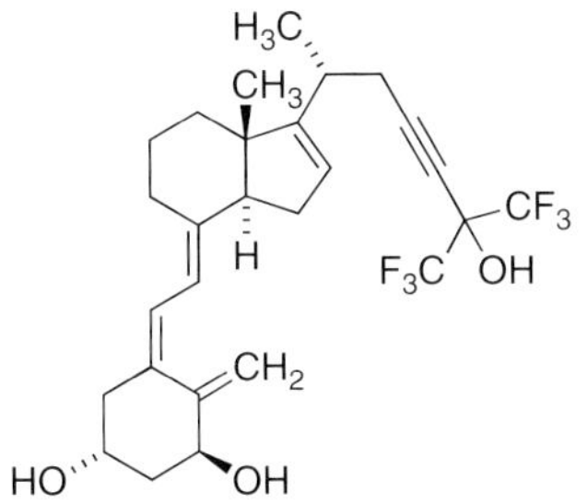

Ro24-5531

Selective PPARγ modulators (SPARMs) are also important in cancer chemoprevention. Among them, GW7845, a high affinity ligand for PPARγ, inhibits mammary carcinogenesis in animal models.[17] Clinical trials are in progress to study its preventive activity against breast, colon, and prostate cancer.

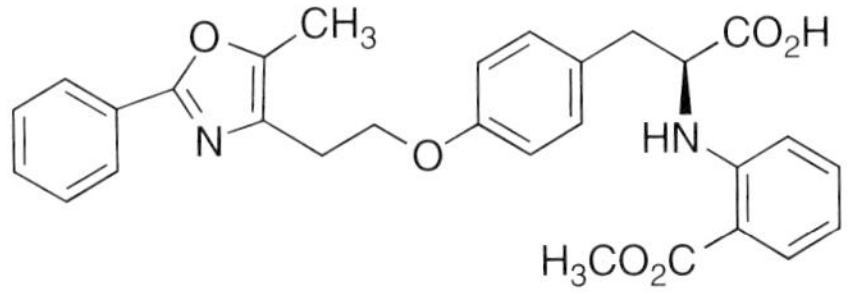

GW7845

3. ANTI-INFLAMMATORY AGENTS AND ANTIOXIDANTS IN CANCER CHEMOPREVENTION

Free radicals are generated by normal physiological processes, including aerobic metabolism and inflammatory responses to eliminate invading pathogenic microorganisms. A chronic cell injury initiates an inflammatory response and the activation of cytoquines or receptor molecules to recruit mast cells and leukocytes to the damaged place. This "respiratory burst" leads to an increased uptake of oxygen, and the subsequent release of free radicals from leucocytes: reactive oxygen species (ROS) as hydroxyl and superoxide radicals, and nitrogen oxide reactive species (RNOS) as nitric oxide, peroxynitrite, and nitrous anhydride.

ROS can activate lipid peroxidation and the arachidonic acid cascade, with the production of cell-proliferation-stimulating eicosanoids. They can also damage DNA modifying its structure and function, as well as that of cancer-related proteins, while other DNA-damaging agents, such as malondialdehyde (MDA), are byproducts of the arachidonic acid cascade (see Section 2 of Chapter 4).[18] Other effects of radicals include mutations in cancer-related genes, posttranslational modification of cancer-related proteins, and activation of signal-transduction pathways resulting in the transcriptional induction of proto-oncogenes (like c-FOS, c-JUN, and c-MYC) and hence an increase in cancer risk. In summary, chronic inflammation deregulates cellular homeostasis and can drive carcinogenesis. It has been estimated that chronic inflammations contribute to about one-fourth of cancers.

3.1. COX-2 inhibitors and other anti-inflammatory agents

Inhibition of prostaglandin formation from arachidonic acid has been found useful in cancer chemoprevention. The main target enzyme in this respect is cyclooxygenase-2 (COX-2), which is not detected in most normal tissues but is induced by inflammatory and mitogenic stimuli; COX-2 is overexpressed in many premalignant and malignant tissues. COX-2 inhibitors inhibit colon carcinogenesis in animal models[19] and reduce the number of colorectal polyps in humans. More specifically, the selective COX-2 antagonist celecoxib received FDA approval for the treatment of patients with familial adenomatous polyposis.[20]

The chemopreventive effects of COX-2 inhibitors seem to be mediated by their effects on stromal cells of the intestine, especially angiogenesis suppression.[21] Clinical trials examining the use of celecoxib, with or without eflornithine, in the prevention of colorectal cancer in patients with familial adenomatous polyposis are in progress.[22] Eflornithine is a suicide inhibitor of ornithine decarboxylase, an enzyme that regulates cell division by catalyzing the first step in polyamine biosynthesis.

Other compounds, such as the natural product curcumin, are blockers of activation or transcription activity of the transcriptional factor nuclear factor-κB (NF-κB) (see Section 6.4 of Chapter 9), and have both anti-inflammatory and anticarcinogenic activity. Clinical trials of these compounds as chemopreventive agents were planned. However, suppression of NF-κB activity can increase susceptibility to infections.[23]

Celecoxib   Eflornithine   Curcumin

3.2. Antioxidants

Several compounds with radical scavenging properties are being studied for cancer chemoprevention. However, it must be noted that, although many patients being treated for cancer use antioxidants in the hope of reducing the toxicity of chemotherapy and radiotherapy, mechanistic considerations suggest that antioxidants might reduce the effects of conventional cytotoxic therapies and a limited number of clinical studies have not found any benefit in these associations.[24] The main antioxidants that are claimed to behave as chemoprotective agents are found in foodstuffs, especially of a vegetal origin, and are ascorbic acid, ergothioneine, green tea polyphenols, and lycopene.

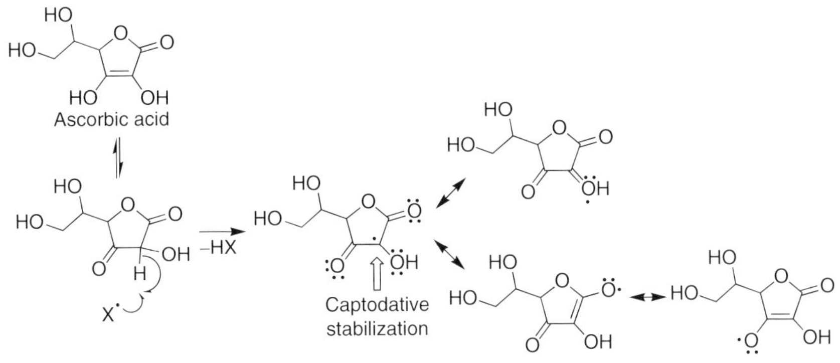

FIGURE 13.1   Ascorbic acid as an antioxidant.

3.2.1. Ascorbic acid

Ascorbic acid (vitamin C) is the main hydrophilic radical scavenger present in the human body. Its antioxidant properties are related to its ability to generate a stabilized radical at its C-3 position because of the operation of the captodative effect (Fig. 13.1). This allows ascorbic acid to react with harmful, more reactive species, particularly the hydroxyl radical, and prevent their interaction with biomolecules. Ascorbic acid has been recommended for many years to prevent the appearance of gastrointestinal cancers, although a recent statistical study including more than 170,000 patients in risk of this type of cancer showed no evidence of benefit.[25] Interestingly, a similar study had previously shown that β-carotene consumption actually increases the risk of lung cancer.[26]

3.2.2. Ergothioneine

Ergothioneine is a component of white button mushrooms that is considered as an antioxidant with cancer chemopreventive properties. Its antioxidant properties appear to be related to at least four molecular activities:

1. The ability to scavenge free radicals,[27] which can be proposed to arise from the easy one-electron oxidation of its mercapto group to a disulfide (Fig. 13.2).
2. Chelating properties toward divalent metallic cations (see Section 1 of Chapter 4), which is due to its α-amino acid moiety.

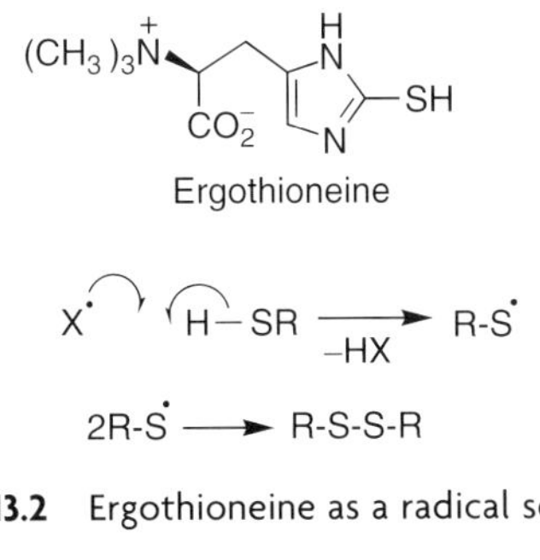

Ergothioneine

FIGURE 13.2   Ergothioneine as a radical scavenger.

3. Activation of antioxidant enzymes such as glutathione peroxidase (Se-GPx) and Mn superoxide dismutase (SOD) and inhibition of superoxide-generating enzymes such as NADPH-cytochrome c reductase.
4. Its ability to affect the oxidation of various hemoproteins such as hemoglobin and myoglobin.

3.2.3. Green tea polyphenols

Green tea polyphenols (e.g., epicatechin gallate and epigallocatechin gallate) are potent radical scavengers that are being extensively studied as chemopreventive agents. In this case, the stabilization of the phenolic radical is due to extensive delocalization of the unpaired electron around the aromatic ring and into the p-acyl substituent, and also to the steric hindrance provided by the neighboring hydroxyl groups (Fig. 13.3). A Phase II clinical assay studied the modulation by these substances of the urinary excretion of 8-hydroxydeoxyguanosine (8-OHdG), an oxidative DNA damage biomarker. The results obtained suggest that chemoprevention with green tea polyphenols is effective in diminishing oxidative DNA damage.[28]

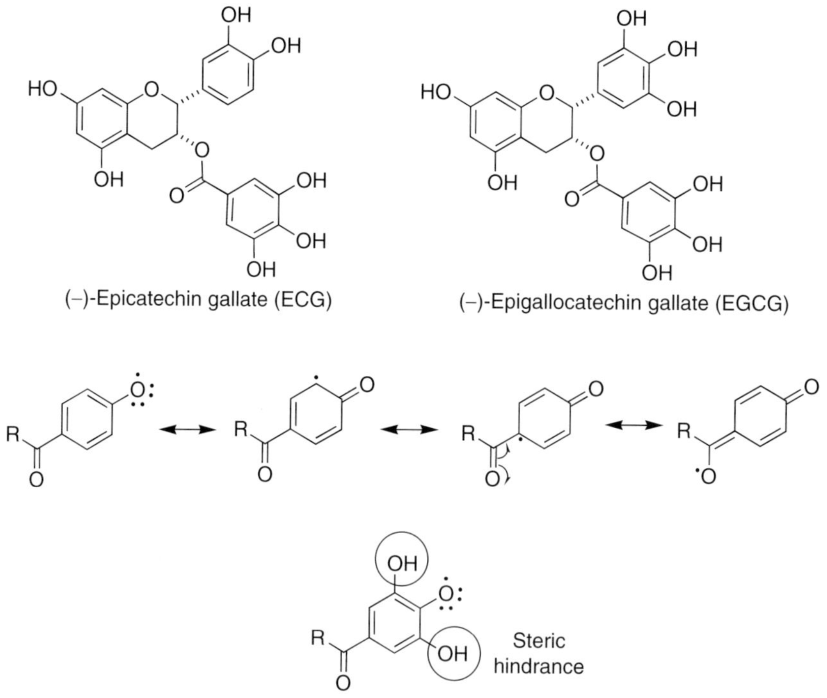

(−)-Epicatechin gallate (ECG)   (−)-Epigallocatechin gallate (EGCG)

FIGURE 13.3   Green tea polyphenols as radical scavengers.

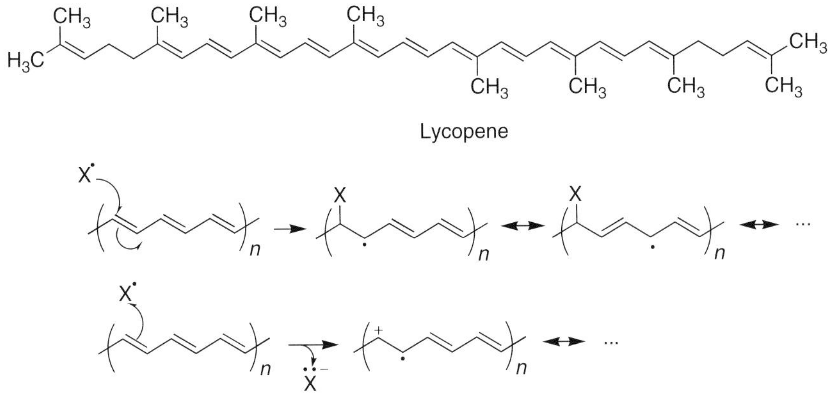

FIGURE 13.4   Lycopene as a radical scavenger.

3.2.4. Lycopene

Lycopene is an open-chain carotenoid found in several fruits, especially in tomatoes, which is accumulated in high concentrations in several tissues. It reacts with hydroxyl radicals giving a stabilized, highly delocalized species (Fig. 13.4). Chemoprevention with lycopene has shown definite results in prostate cancer.[29]

4. CHROMATIN MODIFIERS IN CANCER CHEMOPREVENTION

Chromatin is the complex of DNA and protein that makes up the chromosome. The human genome corresponds to 3 billion base pairs of the DNA double helix, two copies of which make up 2 m of DNA chains that have to be stored within the tiny micron-sized nucleus of each cell. These 2 m are composed of 46 shorter DNA pieces, each of which, if not condensed, would form a swollen coil of roughly 100 μm diameter. Chromatin is a suitable compact structure that allows for certain proteins to access specific portions of the DNA. In chromatin, DNA is folded in a hierarchical fashion. On the first level, named the nucleosome or the "10-nm fiber," about 200 bp DNA are associated with a globular octameric aggregate formed by two molecules of the four histone proteins H2A, H2B, H3, and H4. Under physiological conditions, this structure folds into a chromatin fiber that has a diameter of 30 nm. Other higher-order foldings vary with the cell cycle. Thus, before cell division, the DNA chain and its copy are folded into a chromosome prepared to be distributed into the two daughter cells.

Chromatin structure may be modified by increasing the acetylation of histones through histone deacetylase (HDAC) inhibition (see Section 3.2 of Chapter 10), or by demethylation of cytosine residues in DNA through inhibition of DNA methyltransferases (DNMTs) (see Section 3.1.1 of Chapter 10). Both types of agents are interactive and increase the ability of transcription factors to stimulate gene expression and have been successfully tested as cancer chemopreventors in experimental animals. Trichostatin A, an antifungal antibiotic and an HDAC inhibitor, as well as 5-aza-2'-deoxycytidine, a DNA demethylating agent, enhance the ability of all-*trans* retinoic acid to differentiate human leukemia cells[30] or to suppress breast cancer cells proliferation,[31] but their high toxicity have limited their use. The development of new less toxic drugs, such as the HDAC inhibitor vorinostat (SAHA),[32] indicates that the toxicity associated to chromatin modifiers may be diminished, thus opening the way to possible chemopreventive agents.

Trichostatin A (TSA)

Vorinostat
(suberoylanilide hydroxamic acid, SAHA)

5-Aza-2'-deoxycytidine

5. MISCELLANEOUS AGENTS FOR CHEMOPREVENTION

1,2-Dithiol-3-thiones, reported constituents of cruciferous vegetables, are five-membered cyclic sulfur-containing compounds with antioxidant, chemotherapeutic, and chemoprotective activities. In this context, oltipraz, which was originally developed as an antischistosomal agent, was found to protect against chemically induced carcinogens in the lung, stomach, colon, and urinary bladder in animals.[33] Its utility as a cancer chemopreventive agent is thought to depend on the induction of enzymes involved in Phase II xenobiotic detoxification.[34] Polycyclic aromatic hydrocarbons, *N*-nitrosamines, and other compounds produce electrophilic carcinogenic metabolites. Thus, the fungal toxic secondary metabolite aflatoxin B1 (AFB1) may contaminate food and by epoxydation of a furane double bond by a P450 cytochrome (Fig. 13.5) give carcinogenic compounds that are inactivated by glutathione addition catalyzed by glutathione *S* (GSH)-transferase (see Section 2.1 of Chapter 11). Oltipraz stimulates this enzyme[35] and can be effective in patients with histories of *Schistosoma haematobium* bladder infections that are at increased risk for developing bladder cancer (Fig. 13.6).[36]

Sulforophane is another component of cruciferous vegetables (e.g., broccoli) that has been proposed as a chemoprotector. This compound bears an unusual isothiocyanate function and is generated from its precursor glucoraphanin by the myrosinase enzyme on damage to the plant (e.g., from chewing), as shown in Fig. 13.7. Similarly to the previously mentioned oltipraz, sulforophane is an inducer of Phase II metabolizing enzymes and is being clinically studied as a chemopreventive agent in several cancers.[37]

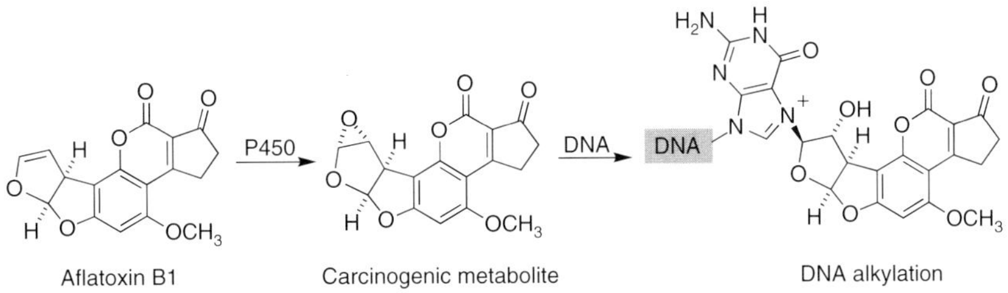

FIGURE 13.5   Carcinogenesis by aflatoxin B₁.

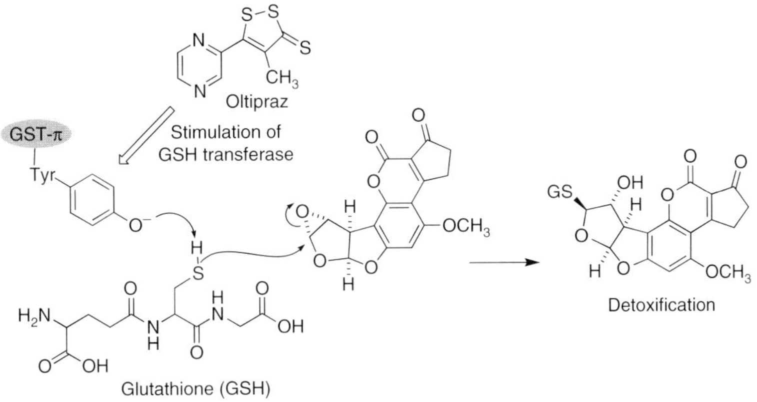

FIGURE 13.6   Aflatoxin B₁ detoxification stimulated by oltipraz.

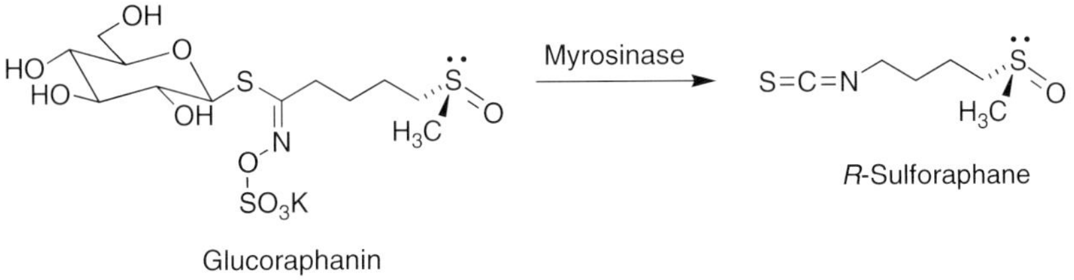

FIGURE 13.7   Bioactivation of glucoraphanin.

Resveratrol is a phytoalexin that is found in many plants, especially in the skin of red grapes, and is therefore present in red wine. It induces quinone reductase, which is a Phase II enzyme that metabolizes carcinogens. Some clinical trials are in progress regarding the use of resveratrol in cancer chemoprevention.[38]

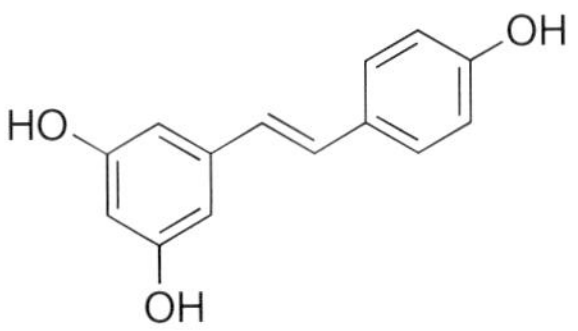

Resveratrol

6. CANCER VACCINES

During the past two decades tremendous research efforts have been focused to the development of cancer vaccines, which are intended either to treat existing cancers (therapeutic vaccines) or to prevent the development of cancer (prophylactic vaccines). Some of these cancer vaccines have reached Phase III clinical trials,[39] and the strategies developed to stimulate the immuno response to cancer include:

1. Use of cancer cell antigens that are rarely present on normal cells. These antigens may be isolated from the same patient suffering the disease (personalized vaccines) or from another patient. The prime candidates as vaccination antigens have been antiapoptotic molecules such as IAP (inhibitor of apoptosis protein) and BCL-2 (see Section 6 of Chapter 9) because these proteins enhance the survival of cancer cells and facilitate their escape from cytotoxic therapies.[40]
2. Enhancement of the immunogenicity of the tumor-associated antigen by altering its structure in order to make it more clearly foreign.
3. Administration of antigen-presenting cells (APCs), such as the specialized white blood cells known as dendritic cells that have previously been stimulated with the patient's own cancer antigens. Once injected, these vaccines activate the immune system's T cells, which are expected to attack tumor cells that express that antigen.
4. Idiotype vaccines. Antibodies produced by certain cancer cells, called idiotype antibodies, are unique to each patient and can be used to trigger an immune response in a manner similar to antigen vaccines.

REFERENCES

1. Tsao, A. N., Kim, E. S., and Hong, W. K. (2004). *CA Cancer J. Clin.* **54**, 150.
2. Sporn, M. B., and Suh, N. (2002). *Nat. Rev. Cancer* **2**, 537.
3. Hong, W. K., Lippman, S. M., Hittleman, W. N., and Lotan, R. (1995). *Clin. Cancer Res.* **1**, 677.
4. Sporn, M. B., and Suh, N. (2000). *Carcinogenesis* **21**, 525.
5. Fisher, B., Costantino, J. P., Wickerham, D. L., Redmond, C. K., Kavanah, M., Cronin, W. M., Vogel, V., Robidoux, A., Dimitrov, N., Atkins, J., Daly, M., Wieand, S., *et al.* (1998). *J. Natl. Cancer Inst.* **90**, 1371.
6. Cauley, J. A., Norton, L., Lippman, M. E., Eckert, S., Krueger, K. A., Purdie, D. W., Farrerons, J., Karasik, A., Mellstrom, D., Ng, K. W., Stepan, J. J., Powles, T. J., *et al.* (2001). *Breast Cancer Res. Treat.* **65**, 125.
7. Suh, N., Glasebrook, A. L., Palkowitz, A. D., Bryant, H. U., Burris, L. L., Starling, J. J., Pearce, H. L., Williams, C., Peer, C., Wang, Y., and Sporn, M. B. (2001). *Cancer Res.* **61**, 8412.
8. Okuno, M., Kojima, S., Matsushima-Nishigaki, R., Tsurumi, H., Muto, Y., Friedman, S. L., and Moriwaki, H. (2004). *Curr. Cancer Drug Targets* **4**, 285.
9. Lee, J. J., Hong, W. K., Hittelman, W. N., Mao, L., Lotan, R., Shin, D. M., Benner, S. E., Xu, X.-C., Lee, J. S., Papadimitrakopoulou, V. M., Geyer, C., Pérez, C., *et al.* (2000). *Clin. Cancer Res.* **6**, 1702.
10. Decensi, A., and Costa, A. (2000). *Eur. J. Cancer* **36**, 694.
11. Muto, Y., Moriwaki, H., and Saito, A. (1999). *N. Engl. J. Med.* **340**, 1046.
12. Chawla, A., Repa, J. J., Evans, R. M., and Mangelsdorf, D. J. (2001). *Science* **294**, 1866.

13. Hede, K. (2004). *J. Nat. Cancer Inst.* **96,** 1807.
14. Arun, B., Mohsin, S., Miller, A., Isaacs, C., Saxton, K., Hilsenbeck, S., Lamph, W., Johnson, K., Brown, P., and Elledge, R. (2005). *J. Clin. Oncol.* **23**(16S), 1002.
15. Makishima, M., Makishima, M., Lu, T. T., Xie, W., Whitfield, G. K., Domoto, H., Evans, R. M., Haussler, M. R., and Mangelsdorf, D. J. (2002). *Science* **296,** 1313.
16. Guyton, K. Z., Kensler, T. W., and Posner, G. H. (2001). *Annu. Rev. Toxicol.* **41,** 421.
17. Suh, N., Wang, Y., Williams, C. R., Risingsong, R., Gilmer, T., Willson, T. M., and Sporn, M. B. (1999). *Cancer Res.* **59,** 5671.
18. Hussain, S. P., Hofseth, L. J., and Harris, C. C. (2003). *Nat. Rev. Cancer* **3,** 276.
19. Reddy, B. S., Hirose, Y., Lubet, R., Steele, V., Kelloff, G., Paulson, S., Seibert, K., and Rao, C. V. (2000). *Cancer Res.* **60,** 293.
20. Steinbach, G., Lynch, P. M., Phillips, R. K. S., Wallace, M. H., Hawk, E., Gordon, G. B., Wakabayashi, N., Saunders, B., Shen, Y., Fujimura, T., Su, L.-K., Levin, B., *et al.* (2000). *N. Engl. J. Med.* **342,** 1946.
21. Gupta, R. A., and Dubois, R. N. (2001). *Nat. Rev. Cancer* **1,** 11.
22. http://clinicaltrials.gov/ct/show/NCT00033371;jsessionid=14A1950A717BDE8B1E1404757F3BBC82?order=6
23. Bharti, A. C., and Aggarwal, B. B. (2002). *Biochem. Parmacol.* **64,** 883.
24. D'Andrea, G. M. (2005). *Cancer J. Clin.* **55,** 319.
25. Bjelakovic, G., Nikolova, D., Simonetti, R. G., and Gluud, C. (2004). *Lancet* **364,** 1219.
26. Forman, D., and Altman, D. (2004). *Lancet* **364,** 1193.
27. Franzoni, F., Colognato, R., Galetta, F., Laurenza, I., Barsotti, M., Di Stefano, R., Bocchetti, R., Regoli, F., Carpi, A., Balbarini, A., Migliore, L., and Santoro, G. (2006). *Biomed. Pharmacother.* **60,** 453.
28. Luo, H., Tang, L., Tang, M., Billam, M., Huang, T., Yu, J., Wei, Z., Liang, Y., Wang, K., Zhang, Z.-Q., Zhang, L., Sun, S., *et al.* (2006). *Carcinogenesis* **27,** 262.
29. Mohanty, N. K., Saxena, S., Singh, U. P., Goyal, N. K., and Arora, R. P. (2005). *Urol. Oncol.* **23,** 383.
30. Ferrara, F. F., Fazi, F., Bianchini, A., Padula, F., Gelmetti, V., Minucci, S., Mancini, M., Pelicci, P. G., Lo Coco, F., and Nervi, C. (2001). *Cancer Res.* **61,** 2.
31. Widschwendter, M., Berger, J., Hermann, M., Müller, H. M., Amberger, A., Zeschnigk, M., Widschwendter, A., Abendstein, B., Zeimet, A. G., Daxenbichler, G., and Marth, C. (2000). *J. Natl. Cancer Inst.* **92,** 826.
32. Marks, P. A., Rifkind, R. A., Richon, V. M., Breslow, R., Miller, T., and Kelly, W. K. (2001). *Nat. Rev. Cancer* **1,** 194.
33. Kensler, T. W., Groopman, J. D., Sutter, T. R., Curphey, T. J., and Roebuck, B. D. (1999). *Chem. Res. Toxicol.* **12,** 113.
34. Auyeung, D. J., Kessler, F. K., and Ritter, J. K. (2003). *Mol. Phamacol.* **63,** 119.
35. Kensler, T. W., Egner, P. A., Dolan, P. M., Groopman, J. D., and Roebuck, B. D. (1987). *Cancer Res.* **47,** 4271.
36. Glintborg, B., Weimann, A., Kensler, T. W., and Poulsen, H. E. (2006). *Free Radic. Biol. Med.* **41,** 1010.
37. Cornblatt, B. S., Ye, L., Dinkova-Kostova, A. T., Erb, M., Fahey, J. W., Singh, N. K., Chen, M.-S. A., Stierer, T., Garrett-Meyer, E., Argani, P., Davidson, N. E., Talalay, P., *et al.* (2007). *Carcinogenesis* **28** doi:10.1093/carcin/bgm049.
38. http://clinicaltrials.gov/ct/show/NCT00098969;jsessionid=9628876D173ADEF448DE62395C60762D?order=8
39. http://www.cancer.gov/cancertopics/factsheet/cancervaccine
40. Andersen, M. H., Becker, J. C., and Straten, P. (2005). *Nat. Rev. Drug Discov.* **4,** 399.

A

A-443654, 279
AAG113–161, 38
AAL-993, 267
Abarelix, 84
ABC transporters, 388
Abelson kinase (see BCR-ABL kinase)
Abiraterone acetate, 77
ABJ879, 241
ABT-510, 318
ABT-518, 315
ABT-751, 236
ABX-EGF, 264
Aclarubicin (aclacinomycin A), 110, 212, 215, 219
Aconitase, 105
Acridines, as intercalating agents, 206
Actinomycin D (dactinomycin), 114–115, 204
"Activated" bleomycin, 118
Acute promyelocytic leukemia (APL), 87
Acyclic retinoid, 420
Adapalene, 89, 420
Adaphostin, 274
Adenosine deaminase inhibitors, 42
ADEPT, 352, 355, 364–367, 377
Adiol, 74
ADI-PEG, 20 (see PEG-recombinant arginine
     deiminase)
Adozelesin, 194
ADR-925, 106
Adrenocortical cancer, 85
Adriamycin, (see doxorubicin)
AEW-541, 265
Aflatoxin B1, 426
AG-014699, 409
AG-2037, 38
AGT inhibitors, 279, 403
AKT, 279–280
   inhibitors, 279
Alemtuzumab, 343
Alimta, (see pemetrexed)
Alitretinoin, 87
Allopurinol, 42
Altratamine, (see hexamethylmelamine)
Alvespimycin, 301
Alvocidib (flavopiridol), 253, 276
Ametantrone, 112

Aminoglutethimide, 72
5-aminolevulinic acid (ALA), 133
Aminopterin (AM), 33
   deaza analogues, 36
Amonafide, 205
Amsacrine (mAMSA), 213
Anamycin, 112
Anaplastic astrocytoma, 166
Anastrazole, 72
1,4-Androstadiene-3,17-dione, 70
Angiogenesis, 265, 269, 279, 312, 316
   endogenous inhibitors, 318–319
Angiostatin, 318
Angiozyme, 269
Anthracyclines, 102, 178, 200, 206, 214–216, 219,
     365, 370, 373, 389, 398
   cardiac toxicity, 104–105
   effects on iron regulation, 105–107
   formaldehyde DNA adducts, 108–110
Anthramycin, 196
Antiandrogens, 76, 80
Antiangiogenic agents, 312, 318–322, 328, 332
Antibody-directed enzyme prodrug
     therapy (see ADEPT)
Antiestrogens, 58
   non-steroidal, 58–62
   steroidal, 62–65
Antifolate drugs, 28, 31–41
Anti-inflammatory agents, in cancer
     chemoprevention, 421–425
Antimetabolite enzymes, 50
Antimetabolites, definition, 10
Antimycin A, 298
Antioxidants, in cancer chemoprevention,
     421–422, 425
Antisense oligonucleotide, 257, 285, 288, 295, 297,
     298, 319, 340–343
AP-23573, 281
AP-5280, 372
AP-5346, 372
APE-l inhibitors, 407
Apicidin, 335
APO2L (see TRAIL)
Apoptosis, 10, 23, 33, 103, 213, 232, 265, 279, 296,
     299, 308–311, 318, 320, 322–324, 332, 346, 355,
     398, 400, 428
AQ4N, 355

Ara-C (see cytarabine)
   non-steroidal, 72–73
   steroidal, 68–72
Aromatase inhibitors, 65
   nonsteroidal, 72–73
   steroidal, 68–72
Aromatase mechanism of action, 66–68
ARRY-142886 (AZD-6244), 295
Arzoxifene, 419
AS-1404, 246
Ascorbic Acid, 423
L-Asparaginase, 50
Aspartate transcarbamoylase, 11
Asulacrine, 214
ATM kinase, 411
ATP analogues (ATP mimics), 253, 258, 262–263,
   267–283, 295, 301
ATP-binding cassette efflux pumps, 388
   inhibitors, 388–397
Aureolic acid, 337
Auristatin PE, 234
Aurora kinase inhibitors, 283–284
AVE8062A, 245
Axitinib (AG-013736), 268
5-Azacytidine, 325
Azacitidine, 48
Azaserine, 39
Azathioprine (imuran), 42
AZD-0530, 274
AZD-1152, 283
AZD-2171, 268
AZD-3409, 291
Azinomycins, 158
Aziridine alkaloids, 182–189
Aziridines (ethyleneimines), 154–158
Aziridinylquinones, 155–157, 357
AZQ (see diaziquone)

B

BAPP, 117
Batimastat (BB-94), 313
BAY43–9006, 295
BBR 3464, 172
BC-2626, 277
BCL-2 proteins, 296–298
BCNU (carmustine), 161, 403
BCR-ABL kinase, 271
   dual inhibitors of BCR-ABL and Src,
      274–275
   inhibitors, 271–275
Bendamustin, 145–146
Benzotriazinyl radical, 127–128
BER repair pathway, 402–404, 408–409
Bergmann reaction, 123–125

Bevacizumab, 269
Bexarotene, 89, 420
BIBR-1532, 340
Bicalutamide, 76
Bifurcated (three-centred) hydrogen
   bonds, 180
Bioreductive activation, 126, 131, 155, 183,
   354–364
Bioxalomycins, 190
Biricodar (VX-710), 393
Bis(dioxopiperazines), 219–220
Bizelesin, 194
Blenoxane, 116
Bleomycins (BLMs), 116–121, 178
BMS-184476, 239
BMS-188797, 239
BMS-214662, 291
BMS-239091, 277
BMS-247550, 241
BMS-275183, 239
BMS-310705, 241
BMS-387032, 277
BOF-AZ (see emitefur)
Bortezomib, 311
Brostallicin (PNU-166196), 181
Bryostatin 1, 284
Buserelin, 81–82
Busulfan, 159
BZQ, 155

C

2C4, 264
Calicheamicins, 122–124
Camptothecins (CPTs), 221–223
   HMPA copolymer, 371
   PEG conjugate, 375
Cancer vaccines, 428
Canertinib (CI-1003), 263
Capecitabine, 25–26, 352
Captodative effect, 103
Carbamoylaspartate, 11
Carbonic anhydrase as anticancer target,
   412–413
Carboplatin, 171–172
Carboquone, 155
Carboxypeptidase G, 367
Carmustine (see BCNU)
Carzinophilin, 158
Caspases, 296–297, 299
CB-1954, 364
CB-300638, 31
CC-1065, 193
CC-5013 (see lenalidomide)
CC-4047, 322

CDDO, 299
CDDO-Me, 299
CDKs, 255, 275–276
    inhibitors, 275–278
Celecoxib, 319, 422
Cemadotin, 234
CDHP, 28
CEP-5214, 269
CEP-701, 270
CEP-7055, 269
Cetrorelix, 83–84
Cetuximab (IMC-C225), 264
CGP 64128A, 285
CGP-41251, 284
CHAP-31, 335
Chaperones, 300
Chartreusin, 116, 206
Chimeric proteins, 264
Chlorambucil, 145–147
Chlorozotocin, 161
Chromatin, 330
        modifiers in cancer chemoprevention,
        425–426
Chronic myeloid leukaemia (CML), 271
CHS-282, 299
CI-1040, 295
CI-994, 336
Cisplatin (CDDP), 169–172
    resistence to, 388–404
Cladribine, 49
Clofarabine, 49–50
Clomiphene, 58
CMDA, 367
CNDAC, 48
Cobalt complexes, 361
Coformycin (CF), 42, 45
Colchicines, 231, 236–237, 245, 390
Combretastatins, 236–237, 245
Coumate, 74
COX-2 inhibitors, 422
CPT (see camptothecin)
CPT-11 (see irinotecan)
Criegee rearrangement, 99
CRT-0044876, 407
Cryptophycins, 233–235
CT-2103, 373
CT-2106, 373–374
CT-53518, 270
Curcumin, 422
CYC-202 (see roscovitine)
CYC-682 (CS-682), 49
Cyclin-dependent kinases (see CDKs)
Cyclophosphamide, 149–150, 159, 321
Cyclopropylindole alkylating agents, 193
Cyclosporin A, 392

Cyproterone, 76
Cytarabine (Ara-C), 47
Cytochrome P450 reductase, 355

D

DACA (XR5000), 214
Dacarbazine (DTIC), 165
Dactinomycin (see actinomycin D)
Dasatinib (BMS-354825), 274
DAUF, 108
Daunorubicin (daunomycin), 102, 107, 390
DaunoXome, 383
Death receptors, 298–299
Decitabine, 325
Deltanoids, 420
14α-Demethylase inhibitors, 77
Deoxyepothilone B, 241
Detirelix, 83
Dexamethasone, 321
Dexaminoglutethimide, 72
Dexrazoxane (ICRF-159), 106
Dexverapamil, 392
dFdC (see gemcitabine)
DHFR (see dihydrofolate reductase)
Diaziquone (AZQ), 155, 357
Dibenzophenanthrolines, 339
Didox, 14
Diflomotecan, 221
Dihydrofolate reductase (DHFR), 19–22, 28
    inhibitors, 32–38
Dihydroorotate dehydrogenase, 11
5,6-Dihydro-5-azacytidine (DHAC), 325–326
Dihydropyrimidine dehydrogenase
    (DPD), 27
5,6-Dimethylxanthenone acetic acid, 246
Discodermolide, 244
Distal activation, 152
Distamycin A, 178–182, 194
Ditercalinium, 207
DMXAA, 246
DNA biosynthesis, summary, 10
DNA crosslinking, 140–141
    by aziridines, 155–156
    by epoxides, 158–159
    by methanesulfonates, 159–160
    by mitomycin C, 183–185
    by mitosenes, 186–187
    by nitrogen mustards, 144–146
    by nitrosoureas, 163–164
DNA glycosylase, 402
        inhibitors, 404–408
DNA intercalation, 200–201
DNA methyltransferases (DNMTs), 323
        inhibitors, 323–330

DNA microarrays, 6
DNA oxopropenylation, 98
DNA-PK, 402, 411–412
DNA-repair pathways, 340, 402
    chemosensitizers acting on, 401–412
    in double-strand DNA breaks, 411
    inhibitors, 340
DNA repair system inhibitors, 340
DNA strand cleavage (scission),
    by oxidative stress, 98–99, 112, 118–121,
        127–128
    following DNA alkylation, 144–145
    mediated by topoisomerases, 203, 209–213, 218,
        221, 223–225
DNA topoisomerases (see topoisomerases)
Docetaxel, 238
Dofequidar, 393
Dolastatin 10, 233
DON (6-diazo-5-oxo-L-norleucine), 39, 369
DOXF, 108
DOX-GA3, 365, Doxifluridine, 24
Doxil (see PEGylated liposomal doxorubicin)
Doxorubicin (adriamycin), 102–103, 107,
        372–373, 390
    HPMA polymer conjugates, 371–373, 377–378
    liposome formulations, 380–383
    neuropeptide conjugate, 374
    prodrug in ADEPT strategy, 365–366
Droloxifene, 59
DT-diaphorase (DTD), 155
Duocarmycins, 194
Dutasteride, 79
Dynemicin A, 122, 125

                                    E

E2-3,4-Q, 57
E7389 (ER0865), 5–6, 233
EC-16-mitomycin C conjugate, 379
EC-20, 379
Echinomycin, 207
Ecteinascidin 743 (ET-743, trabectedin),
        191–182, 341, 390
Edatrexate, 36
Edotecarin, 224
Eflornithine, 422
EGFR (HER-1), 254–255
    inhibitors, 258–264
EKB-569, 263
EKI-785, 263
Electroradiochemotherapy, 127
Eleutherobin, 243
Elinafide, 207
Ellipticine, 201
Elomotecan, 221

Elsamicin A, 116, 206
EMD-72000, 264
Emitefur, 26
Endostatin, 318
Enedyine(s), 122–123, 125, 178
Enhanced permeability and retention (EPR)
        effect, 6, 369
Eniluracil (5-ethynyluracil), 28
Enzastaurin (LY-317615), 284
EO4, 186
EO9, 155, 186, 357
Epicatechin gallate, 424
Epidermal growth factor, (see EGFR)
Epigallocatechin-3-gallate (EGCG), 329, 424
Epigenetic therapy of cancer, 323–337
Epirubicin (EPI), 108
Epothilones A and B, 243 D, 243
Epoxides as DNA alkylating agents, 158–159
ER-086526, 233
ErbB2, 261
Erbstatin, 259
Ergothioneine, 423
Erlotinib (OSI-774), 253, 261
Esperamicins, 122–124
Estradiol, 54, 61–66, 73–74
Estradiol-2,3-quinone (E2-2,3-Q), 56, 58
Estradiol-3,4-quinone (E2-3,4-Q), 56
Estramustine, 147–148
Estramustine binding protein (EMBP), 148
Estramustine phosphate, 245
Estrogen receptor (ER), 55–56, 61–64
Estrogens involvement in carcinogenesis, 54–58
Estrone, 54
ET-743 (see ecteinascidin 743)
Etanidazole, 131
Ethacrynic acid, 394, 398–401
Ethidium bromide, 339
Ethyleneimines (see aziridines)
Etopophos, 216, 366–367
Etoposide, 216, 366, 390
Everolimus (RAD-001), 281
Exatecan, 221
Exemestane, 70–71

                                    F

Fadrozole, 72
FapyAde, 100
FapyGua, 100–101
Farnesyldiphosphate synthase inhibitors, 296
Farnesyl pyrophosphate (FPP), 290
Farnesyl transferase (FTase), 287–288
        inhibitors, 289–294
Fazarabine, 47
Fenretinide, 89, 419

Fenton reaction, 94, 97
Figianolide B (*see* laulimalide)
Finasteride, 78
Finrazole, 73
Flavopiridol (alvocidib), 253, 276
Floxuridine (5-FUdR), 21
FLT-3 inhibitors, 270
Fludarabine, 49
Flutamide, 76
5-Fluoro-2'-deoxycytidine, 325
5-Fluoro-2-pyrimidinone (5-FP), 27
5-Fluorouracil (5-FU), 11, 21–24
    modulation, 27–29
    prodrugs, 24–27, 369
Folate-based TS inhibitors, 29
Folate receptor (FR), 378
Folate receptor-targeted chemotherapy, 378
Folate-targeted radiopharmaceutical, 379
Folinic acids, 32, 35
Folylpolyglutamate synthetase
    (FPGS), 30–31
Formaldehyde generation in oxidative
    stress, 102
Formestane, 69–70
Formyltransferase, 41
Forodesine (*see* immucillin H)
FR-69979, 158, 184
FR-900482, 158, 184
FTase (*see* farnesyltransferase)
FTI-276, 291
FTI-277, 291
Ftorafur (tegafur), 24
Fulvestrant, 62–64
Fumagillin, 322

G

Galactosamine, 372–373
Ganciclovir, 345
Ganirelix, 84
GARFT inhibitors, 37–39
GCSF, 369
Gefitinib (ZD-1839), 261, 262
Gefitinib (ZO-1839), 259
Geldanamycin, 301
Gemcitabine (dFdC), 16, 47
Gemtuzumab ozogamicin, 123, 376, 391
Gene-directed enzyme prodrug therapy,
    (GDEPT), 363–364, 377
Gene therapy, 298, 344
Geranylgeranyl-diphosphate synthase (GGPP)
    inhibitors, 296
Gestagens as antitumor agents, 85
GF120918, 393
Gimatecan, 221

Gimestat, 28–29
Glioblastoma multiforme, 345
Glucocorticoids as antitumor agents, 85
Glucuronidated prodrugs, 365
Glutathione, 129
    biosynthesis inhibition, 398
Glutathione-S-transferase (GST)
    in anti-cancer drug resistance, 181, 397
    of π class (GST-π), 353
Glyceraldehyde-3-phosphate dehydrogenase
    (GAPDH), 190
Glycinamide rebonucleotide formyltransferase
    (see GARFT)
GnRH (LHRH) agonists, 81
GnRH (LHRH) antagonists, 82
GnRH hormone, 81
Gonadotropin-releasing hormone
    (GnRH, LHRH), 79
Goserelin, 82
G-quadruplex ligands, 338
Granulocyte colony-stimulating factor
    (see GCSF)
Green tea polyphenols, 424
GRN-163L, 340
GTPase activating proteins (GAPs), 287
Guaneran (see thiamiprine)
GW7845, 421
GW-786034, 268

H

Haber-Weiss reaction, 94
Halichondrin B, 5–6, 233
"Hard" electrophiles, 140
HATs, 331
HDAC, inhibitors, 323
    inhibitors, 330–336
Heat-shock proteins (see HSPs)
Hemiasterlin, 234
Heparan sulfate (HS), 316
Heparanase inhibitors, 316
Hepsulfam, 159
HER-1 (see EFGR)
HER-2, 258, 261, 263
    inhibitors, 264
Herpes simplex virus thymidine kinase, 345
Hexamethylmelamine
    (HMM, altretamine), 167
Histone acetylation, 331
Histone deacetylases (see HDAC)
Histone methylation, 337
Histones, 330
HKI-272, 263
HMPA copolymer-camptothecin, 371
HMPA copolymer-paclitaxel, 371

Hoechst 33258 (*see* pibenzimol)
Homocamptothecins, 221
HR22C16 (*see* monastroline)
HSPs (heat-shock proteins), 297, 300
    inhibitors, 300–301
HTI-284, 234
Hydralazine, 329
Hydroxamic acid, 313
Hydroxyl radical, 94–96, 100–105, 116, 118,
    127–129, 421, 424–425
17α-Hydroxylase inhibitors, 77
4-Hydroxyestradiol (4-OHE2), 56
Hydroxyurea, 13
Hypoxia-based strategies for tumor-specific
    prodrug activation, 354–362
Hypoxia-inducible factor 1 (HIF-1), 207
Hypoxic-selective nitrogen mustards, 361

I

Ibritumomab tiuxetan, 377
ICI-182780, 62
ICRF-154, 220
ICRF-159 (*see* dexrazoxane)
ICRF-193, 220
Idarubicin (IDA), 108
Idoxifene, 59
Ifosfamide, 149
IGFR-1 inhibitors, 265
Imatinib (STI-571), 253, 271, 390
Immucillin H (forodesine), 18, 20, 49–50
Immunoconjugated drugs, 375–377
Immunomodulatory drugs, 322
Immunomodulatory gene therapy, 345
Improsulfan, 159
Indisulam (E-7070), 277, 413–414
Indolocarbazoles, 223
INGN201 (Ad-p53), 298
INO-1001, 409
Insulin-like growth factors (*see* IGFR-1)
Integrins, 319
Intercalating agents, 201-206
    bifunctional (bisintercalators), 206–209
Intercalation (see DNA intercalation)
Intoplicine, 203
IPI-504, 301
Iproplatin, 171
Irinotecan (CPT-11), 221, 403
Irofulven, 394
IRP-1, 106
ISIS-2503, 288
ISIS 3521, 285
ISIS 5132, 285, 295
Isotretinoin, 87
Ispinesib (SB-715992), 247

IST-622, 206
Itaconic acid, 259
Ixabepilone, 241
IκB kinases (IKK), 299

J

J-107088, 224
JNK kinase, 295, 299

K

Kahalalide F, 346
Karenitecin, 221
Ketoconazole, 77
Kinase inhibitors summary, 255–258
Kinases and cancer, 252–254
Kinesin inhibitors, 246–247
KOS-862, 241
KU-55933, 411
KW-2149, 187
KW-2170, 214
KW-2189, 194

L

L-739750, 291
L-744832, 291
L-778123, 291
Lamellarins, 224–225
Laniquidar, 394
Lapatinib (GW-2016), 261, 264
Laulimalide (figianolide B), 244
LBH-589, 333
L-buthionine-(*S*,*R*)-sulfoximine (L-BSO), 398–399
Leinamycin, 173
Lenalidomide (CC-5013), 322
Letrozole, 72
Leucovorin (LV), 28–29, 35, 38
Leuprolide, 81–82
Leuprorelin, 82
LG100268, 420
LHRH (*see* GnRH)
Liblomycin, 117
Liposomes, 378, 380–383
    stealth, 381
Lomeguatrib, 403
Lometrexol, 37
Lomustine (CCNU), 161
Lonafarnib (SCH-66336), 291–292
Lucanthone, 407
Lurtotecan, 221
LV (see leucvorin)
LY-231514 (*see* pemetrexed)
LY-294002, 411

LY-309887, 38
LY-333531, 284
LY-335979 (see zosuquidar)
LY-355703, 235
Lycopene, 425
Lysosomes, 308

M

Malondialdehyde generation, 96–98
MAPK, 255, 258, 284, 287
    inhibitors, 296
Marimastat, 313
Matrix metalloproteinases (see MMPs)
Maytansine 1, 235
MCX-210, 264
MDX-447, 264
MDR, 388–391
    indirect inhibitors, 397
    inhibitors (modulators), 391–397
Mechlorethamine, 142
Medroxyprogesterone acetate, 85
Me-DZQ, 156
Megestrol acetate, 85
MEK, 255, 287, 289, 295
    inhibitors, 295
Melphalan, 147, 153, 357
Membrane folate receptor (see MFR)
Membrane phospholipid peroxidation, 95–97
Menogaril (TUT-7), 110
Merbarone, 219
6-Mercaptopurine (MP), 37, 41–44
Mesna, 149
Metastat (COL-3), 315
Methanesulfonates, 159–160
Methotrexate (MTX), 28–29, 33
Methoxsalen, 135
Methoxyamine, 408
2-Methoxyestradiol, 236
8-Methoxypsoralen, 135
Methylhydrazines, 166
Metronidazole, 130
MFR (α-FR), 31, 38–139
MG-98, 329
MGCD-0103, 336
Microtubules, 229–230
    bundling, 238
Minodronate, 296
Misonidazole, 130
Mithramycin A, 337
Mitobronitol, 158
Mitomycins, 158, 182–189
Mitomycin C, 182–185
    prodrug, 357, 365–366, 379
Mitonafide, 205

Mitosenes, 186–187
Mitotane, 85–86
Mitotic kinesin inhibitors (see kinesin inhibitors)
Mitoxantrone, 112, 215
MLN-518, 270
MMI270 (CGS 27023A), 315
MMPs, 313
    inhibitors, 313–316
Monastrol, 246–247
Monastroline (HR22C16), 246–247
Monoclonal antibodies, 259, 263–264, 269–297,
    320, 343–344, 352, 364, 366, 375, 377
8-MOP, 135
MRP1, 388–390, 393
MS-209 (see dofequidar)
MS-275, 336
mTOR, 279–282
    inhibitors, 281, 282
MTX (see methotrexate)
Multidrug resistance (see MDR)
Multidrug resistance-associated protein 1
    (see MRP1)
Multiple sclerosis, 112
Mustine, 142
Myers reaction, 123

N

N-(2-Hydroxypropyl)methacrylamide
    polymers, 370
N-acetylcystein, 149
Nanodrugs, 368
Nanoparticles, 378, 380, 383
Nanotechnology in cancer therapy, 6, 380
Nanovectors, 6
Naphthalimides, 205
Napthyridinomycin, 189–190
Natural products in cancer therapy, 5–6
NB-506, 223
Nedaplatin, 171
Nelarabine, 49–50
Nemorubicin (MMRA), 111
Neocarzinostatin, 122, 124
Neovastat (AE-941), 315
NER, 192, 207, 341
Netropsin, 178
Neuropeptide Y conjugates, 374
NFκB, 299, 308–311
    inhibitors, 299
Nicotinamide, 164
Nilotinib (AMN-107), 271, 273
Nilutamide, 76
Nimorazole, 131
Nimustine (ACNU), 161
Nitracrine, 359–360

Nitroaromatic compounds, 358–361
Nitrogen mustards, 141–153, 357, 361
    Co (III) complexes, 151
    prodrugs, 147–153, 353, 357, 359–361, 367
    SAR, 144
Nitroimidazoles, 130, 359
Nitrosoureas, 140, 160, 164
Nitro radical anions, 130–131
N-methyl-9-hydroxyellipticinium (NMHE), 202
Nogalamycin, 110, 215
Nolatrexed (thymitaq, AG-337), 30
Non-intercalating topoisomerase II
    poisons, 216–218
Nonnucleoside inhibitors of DNMT, 328
Nonsteroidal aromatase inhibitors, 72
Norethisterone acetate, 85 N-oxides, 355
N-phosphonoacetyl-L-aspartate (see PALA),
NSC-639829, 245
NSC-655649 (BMY-27557–14, XL-119), 223
NSC-703147, 241
NU7026, 411
Nuclear factor κB (see NFκB)
Nucleoside diphosphate reductase (NDPR),
    (see RNR)
Nucleotide excision repair (see NER)
NVP-LAQ-824, 333

O

O^6-alkylguanine derivatives, 403
    association with DNA alkyltransferase
        inhibitors, 403
Oblimersen sodium, 298
OFU001, 362
Oltipraz, 426–427
ON-012380, 274
ONT-093 (OC-144–093), 393
ONYX-015, 298
Ornidazole, 131
Orotate phosphoribosyl transferase, 11
Orotidylate decarboxylase, 11
Ortataxel, 239
Orzel, 28
Oxaliplatin, 171
Oxidation of DNA bases in oxidative stress,
    100–102
Oxidative stress by hydroxyl radicals, 95–98
Oxonic acid, 29
"Oxygen effect", 129

P

p53 proteins, 277, 283, 298, 300, 308-309, 337,
    345–346, 354, 388, 409, 411
    activation by TS inhibitors, 23–24

Paclitaxel (taxol), 237–238, 390
    analogues, 239–240
    HMPA copolymer, 371
    polyglumex conjugate, 373
    SAR, 239–240
PALA, 11
Panitumumab, 264
PARP, 402, 405
    inhibitors, 409–410
Patupilone, 241
PDGF, 259–265
    inhibitors, 270
PD-115934, 214
PDEPT, 377–378
PDK1, 279–280
    inhibitors, 280
PDT (see photodynamic therapy)
PDX, 36
PDX-101, 333
PEG (polyethyleneglycol), 368
Pegaspargase (see PEG-L-asparaginase)
Pegfilgrastim (see PEG-GCSF)
PEG-camptothecin, 375
PEG-cytokine conjugates, 369
PEG-drug conjugates, 375
PEG-GCSF, 369
PEG-L-asparaginase, 368
PEG-recombinant arginine deiminase
    (ADI-PEG20), 368
PEGylated liposomal doxorubicin (doxil),
    382
PEGylated-glutaminase (PEG-PGA), 368
PEGylation of proteins, 368
Pemetrexed (alimta, LY-231514), 30, 38
Penclomedine, 128
Pentostatin (dCF), 42, 45
Peptidomimetics, 83, 290–291, 311, 313, 400
Perifosine, 279
Peroxisome proliferator activating receptors
    (see PPAR)
P-gp, (P-glycoprotein), 388, 390, 391
    inhibitors, 391–397
PHA-739358, 283
Pharmacogenetics, 2
Phosphatases in ADEPT, 366
Phosphatidylinositol-3-kinase (see PI3K)
Phosphoramidases, 149
Phosphoramide mustard, 149
Phosphoribosylformylglycinamidine synthetase
    inhibitors, 39
Phosphoribosylpyrophosphate amidotransferase
    (see PRPP amidotransferase)
Phosphoroamidates, 342
Phosphorothioamidates, 342
Phosphorothioates, 342

Photodynamic therapy (PDT), 132–135
Photophrin, 133–134
Photosensitivity, 165
Photosensitizers, 132
Phthalascidin, 193
PI3K–AKT–mTOR pathway, 279
PI3K superfamily, 279, 411
PI-88, 317
Pibenzimol, 182
Pimonidazole, 131
Pipobroman, 173
Piposulfan, 159
Pirarubicin, 110
Piritrexim, 36
Pixantrone, 114, 215
PK-1 (FCE-28068), 371, 377
PK-2 (FCE-28069), 372
PKC-412, 270, 284
PKC, 284–285
    modulators, 284–286
Platelet-derived growth factor (see PDGF)
Platinum complexes, 169–173
Plicamycin, 337
Plomestane, 68
PM00104/50, 193
PNP, 18
PNU-159548, 111
PNU-166945, 37
Podophyllotoxin, 216, 237
Poly(ADP-ribose)polymerase (see PARP)
Poly-(L-glutamic) conjugates, 373
Polycythemia vera, 173
Polyelectrolyte effect, 201
Polyethylene glycol (see PEG)
Polymer-directed enzyme prodrug therapy
    (see PDEPT)
Polymer therapeutics, 368
Polyprenoic acid, 89, 420
Porfiromycin, 131, 182, 357
Porphyrin, 133, 134
PPAR, 87, 89
    selective modulators (SPPARMs), 421
Prednisone, 85
Prinomastat (AG3400), 315
PRO-001, 269
Procainamide, 329
Procarbazine, 166, 168
Prodrug-based anticancer drug targeting,
    352–367
Prodrugs activated by therapeutic radiation,
    362
Proteasome, 297, 308
    inhibitors, 307–312
Protein kinases in cancer, 252–254
Protoporphirin IX, 133

PRPP amidotransferase, 36
    inhibitors, 36–37
Psammaplin A, 328
PSC-833 (valspodar), 392
Psoralens, 135
PTA, 42
PTK 787, 267
Purine biosynthesis inhibitors, 36
Purine nucleoside phosphorylase (see PNP)
Purine nucleosides, 49–50
Pyrimidine nucleosides, 47–49
Pyroxamide, 333
Pyrrolo[1,4]benzodiazepines, 196

R

Radical scavengers, 423–424
    as inhibitors of RNR, 13
Radiochemotherapy, 127
Radioconjugate targeted agent, 377
Radiosensitizers, 129–130
Radiotherapy, 129
Raf proteins, 295
    inhibitors, 295
Raloxifene, 60–61, 419
Raltitrexed (TOM), 30–31
Rapamycin (sirolimus), 281
Ras proteins, 286
    inhibitors, 287–295
RARE (see retinoic acid response elements)
Reactive oxygen species (see ROS)
Rebeccamycin, 223
Rebimastat, 315
Reduced folate carrier, 28, 30–31, 35, 38–39
5α-Reductase inhibitors, 77
Reductively activated alkylating agents
    (see bioreductive alkylation)
Reductively activated quinones (see bioreductive
    activation)
REPSA, 181
Resveratrol, 427
Retinoic acid response elements, 87
Retinoids, 86–87
    in cancer chemoprevention, 419–420
Rexinoids, 86
RFC (see reduced folate carrier)
RG-108, 330
RH1^{32}, 156
RH3, 264
Ribonucleotide reductase (see RNR)
Ribozymes, 269
Risedronate, 296
Rituximab, 343
Ro24-5531, 420
Romidepsin (FK-228, FR901228), 335

RNR, 11
   catalytic cycle, 12–13
   inhibitors, 13–18, 46
ROS, 93, 95, 299
   as signaling molecules, 102
Roscovitine (seleciclib), 253
Rosiglitazone, 319
RSU-1069, 131, 359
Rubitecan, 221
Ruboxistaurin, 284

S

S-1 formulation, 41
S-16020, 203
S-3304, 315
S-9788, 394
Saframycin A, 189
Saframycin S, 189
SAHA (suberoylanilide hydroxamic acid)
   (see vorinostat)
Salvicine, 217, 412
SARMs (see selective androgen receptor
   modulators)
SERMs (see selective estrogen receptor
   modulators)
Sarcodictyins, 243
Satraplatin (JM 216), 171
SCH-221153, 319
SCH-226374, 291
SCH-58500, 298
SELDI-TOF mass spectrometry, 6
Seleciclib (see roscovitine)
Selective androgen receptor modulators, 76
Selective estrogen receptor modulators,
   58, 419
Semaxanib (SU-5416), 253, 266
Semustine, 161
Serine hydroxymethyl transferase
   (SHMT), 19
Serine-threonine kinase inhibitors, 275–286
Sibiromycin, 196
Sickle cell anemia, 13
Sirolimus (see rapamycin)
SKI-2053R, 171
SKI-606, 274
SMANCS, 122–123
SN-24771, 151, 153
SN-22995, 394
SN-23862, 360
SN-24771, 361
SN-38, 221
Soblidotin, 234
Sobuzoxane (MST-16), 218
''Soft'' electrophiles, 140

Sorafenib, 253, 294
SPARC protein, 383
Spermine, 108
SPIKET-P, 235
Spongistatin 1, 235
SPPARMs (see PPAR)
Squalamine, 320
Src kinase, 274
   inhibitors, 274–275
Staurosporine, 223, 253, 269
Stealth liposomes, 381
Steroid hormone receptors, 54–56
Streptozotocin (streptozocin), 161
STX-64, 74
Styrene maleic acid neocarzinostatin copolymers
   (see SMANCS)
SU-6668, 266
Sulfatase inhibitors, 73–75
Sulforophane, 426
Sunitinib (SU-11248), 266
Superoxide dismutase (SOD), 94
Superoxide radical, 94, 127
Suramin, 270, 317
Synthadotin, 234

T

Tafluposide, 217
Talaporphin, 133–134
Tallimustine, 181
Tallysomycin S10b (TLM S10b), 117,
   375–376
Tamoxifen, 58, 60, 64, 419
Tandutinib, 270
Tanespimycin, 301
Tanomastat (BAY 12–9566), 315
Tariquidar, 393
TAS-103, 204–205
Taxane site, 237
Taxanes, 237–240
Taxol (see paclitaxel)
TDDP, 172
Telomerase, 337–338
   inhibitors, 337–340
Telomestatin, 339
Temozolomide, 166, 403
Teniposide, 216, 390
Tensirolimus (CCI-779), 281
Testolactone, 70–71
Testosterone, 75
Tetrahydroisoquinoline alkaloids, 189–193
Tetrahydrouridine, 326–327
Tetraplatin, 171
Tezacitabine (FMdC), 15
Thalidomide, 321–322

Thiamiprine (guaneran), 42
Thioguanine (TG), 41
Thioinosinic acid, 41
Thiopurines, 41
Thiopurine methyltransferase (TPMT), 42, 44
Thiosemicarbazones, 13
Thiotepa, 154
Thrombospondins, 318
Thymidine phosphorylase (TP), 24
Thymidylate cycle, 19–20
Thymidylate synthase (TS), 18, 20
    inhibitors, 21–31
Tipifarnib (R-115777), 291
Tirapazamine (TPZ), 126, 131, 355
TLK-117, 400
TLK-199, 400
TLK-286, 353
TNP-470, 322
TOM (see raltitrexed)
Tomaymycin, 196
TOP-53, 217
Topoisomerases, 209–213
    cleavable complex, 209
    inhibitors, 212
    poisons, 212
Topoisomerase I, 204, 209
    inhibitors, 219–225
    mechanism, 209
Topoisomerase II, 204, 209
    catalytic inhibitors, 218–220
    mechanism, 211
    poisons, 128, 213–218
Topotecan, 221
Toremifene, 59
Tositumomab, 377
TPMT (see thiopurine methyltransferase)
    TPZ (see tirapazmine)
Trabectedin, 191
TRAIL, 298
Transition state analogs, 11, 18, 20, 43, 45, 318, 326–327, 330
Trapoxins A and B, 335
Trastuzumab, 264
Treosulfan, 158–159
Tretinoin, 87
Triapine, 13
1,3,5-Triazines, 167–339
Triazenes, 165
Triaziquone, 155
Tributyrin, 333
Trichostatin A (TSA), 333, 425
Triethylenemelamine (TEM), 154
Triethylenephosphoramide (TEPA), 154
Trilostane, 65

Trimelamol, 167, 169
Trimetrexate, 36
Trimidox, 14
Triptorelin, 82
Troglitazone, 89
TS (see thymidylate synthase)
TSP-1, 318
Tubulin, 229–232
Tumor-associated carbonic anhydrase IX (CA IX), 412
Tumorigenic events, 1
Tumor necrosis factor-related apoptosis-induced ligand (see TRAIL)
Tumor suppressor gene (TP53), 298
Tyrosine kinases (TKs), 252, 254–274, 289
    inhibitors, 254–275
Tyrosine mimics, 274
TUT-7 (see menogaril)
Tyrphostin (AG-213), 258
TZT-1027, 234, 246

U

U-80224, 194
UCN-01, 223, 280, 284
UFT formulation, 27
Uracyl mustard, 147
Uridylic acid biosynthesis, 10–11
Uvadex, 135

V

Vaccine therapy, 345
Valproic acid, 333
Valrubicin, 110
Vandetanib, 267
Vatalanib, 267
VDEPT, 363
VEGF(R), 265–266
    inhibitors, 266–269, 313–317, 320–322, 344
Verapamil, 392
Vinblastine, 231, 390
Vinca alkaloids, 231
Vinca site (domain), 232
    ligands, 231–235
Vincristine, 231, 390
Vindesine, 231
Vinflunine, 231
Vinorelbine, 231
Virus-directed enzyme prodrug therapy (see VDEPT)
Vitamin A, 86, 419
Vitaxin, 320, 343
Volociximab (M-200), 343
Vorinostat (SAHA, suberoylanilide hydroxamic acid), 333, 426

Vorozole, 72
VX-680, 283
VX-710 (*see* biricodar), 393

W

Wortmannin, 411
WV15, 186

X

XR9576 (*see* tariquidar)

Z

ZD-0473, 171

ZD-2171, 268
ZD-2767P, 367
ZD6126, 245
ZD6474, 267
ZD-9331, 30
Zebularine, 324, 327
Zinc-finger protein transcription
    factor, 170–171
Zinostatin (see neocarzinostatin)
ZK-222584, 267
ZK-epothilone, 241
Zoledronate, 296
Zorubicin, 110
Zosuquidar (LY-335979), 393